Classification of Nursing Diagnoses

Proceedings of the Thirteenth Conference

Classification of Nursing Diagnoses

Proceedings of the Thirteenth Conference

North American Nursing Diagnosis Association

Celebrating the 25th Anniversary of NANDA

Edited by

Marilyn J. Rantz, PhD, RN, FAAN
Associate Professor, Sinclair School of Nursing
University Professor, University Hospitals & Clinics
University of Missouri-Columbia
Columbia, Missouri

Priscilla LeMone, DSN, RN, FAAN
Associate Professor, Sinclair School of Nursing
University of Missouri-Columbia
Columbia, Missouri

Cinahl Information Systems

Production: Myrna Esposo, John Shoreen, Ginny Chaskey
Book/Cover Design: Ernest R. Razo, BFA
Printer and Bindery: Advance Business Graphics

ISBN 0-910478-62-7

Any procedure or practice described in this book should be applied by the health care practitioner under appropriate supervision in accordance with professional standards of care used with regard to the unique circumstances that apply in each practice situation. Care has been taken to confirm the accuracy of information presented and to describe generally accepted practices. However, the authors, editors, and publisher cannot accept any responsibility for errors or omissions or for any consequences from application of the information in this book and make no warranty, express or implied, with respect to the contents of this book.

Every effort has been made to ensure drug selections and dosages are in accordance with current recommendations and practice. Because of ongoing research, changes in government regulations, and the constant flow of information on drug therapy, reactions and interactions, the reader is cautioned to check the package insert for each drug for the indications, dosages, warnings, and precautions, particularly if the drug is new or infrequently used.

Preface

The Thirteenth Conference on the Classification of Nursing Diagnoses, held April 22-26, 1998 in St. Louis, Missouri, centered around the theme "Nursing Diagnosis: Gateway to the Future of Nursing Language – Visiting Our Past, Envisioning Our Future." This conference presented exciting information about new developments in the development of nursing language and clinical uses of nursing diagnoses. It also celebrated NANDA's first 25 years, and recommitted the membership to the development and refinement of nursing diagnosis and its use in clinical practice, education and research in the next 25 years.

The objectives of the conference were to:
1. Discuss the evolution and future of the nursing diagnosis movement.
2. Develop a comprehensive framework for the use and study of nursing diagnosis in clinical, educational, and research settings.
3. Analyze the uses of nursing diagnosis in professional nursing practice, including advanced practice.
4. Collaborate in the development of NANDA's classification of nursing diagnosis and other classification systems.
5. Address national and international issues and trends related to the use and development of nursing diagnosis.

The conference planning committee, under the guidance of the NANDA Board of Directors, designed and implemented the program to include "Pearls" of conferences through the years; preconference work groups and educational sessions; invited presentations highlighting collaboration with NIC, NOC, and NDEC; international information; clinical specialty perspectives; refereed paper and poster presentations, recognitions and honors, and a wonderful dinner. Members of the Conference Committee members were Mary Ann Lavin (Chair), Georgia Whitley, Vici Cole Schonlau, Ros Alfaro-LeFevre, Carol Matz, and Anne Perry.

This written report of the proceedings of the thirteenth conference is organized in sections as follows:

Section 1: Preconference Presentation
Section 2: Pearls
Section 3: General Session Presentations
Section 4: Paper Presentations
Section 5: Poster Abstracts
Section 6: Workgroup Reports
Section 7 Business of the Organization
Appendix

We wish to thank the many individuals who made this published proceedings a reality.

Marilyn Rantz
Priscilla LeMone

Contributors

Invited and Paper Presentations

Ana Cristina Freitas Vilhena Abrao, MNSC
Univers. Fed. de S. Paulo
Sao Paulo - SP - Brazil

Betty Ackley, MSN, RN, EdS
Jackson Community College
Jackson, MI

Joan M. Agretelis
Doctoral candidate, Boston College
Somerville, MA

Mercedes Ugalde Apalategui, RN, CNS
University of Barcelona
Spain

Jean M. Arnold, EdD, RNC
Rutgers College of Nursing
The State University of New Jersey
Newark, NJ

Alba Lucia Botura Leite de Barros, RN, PhD
Universidade Federal de Sao Paulo
Brazil

Jean Krajicek Bartek, PhD, ARNP, CARN
University of Nebraska
Omaha, NE

Beverly J. Bartlett, PhD, RN
Gannon University
Erie, PA

Suzanne C. Beyea, RN, CS, PhD
Co-Director Perioperative Nursing Research
Association of Operating Room Nurses

Margaret E. Briody, MSN, RN
University of Rochester
Rochester, NY

Gloria M. Bulechek, PhD, RN, FAAN
University of Iowa
Iowa City, IA

Judith H. Carlson, MSN, RN, CS, GNP
St. Louis University
St. Louis, MO

Judy Carlson-Catalano, MSN, RN
Radford University
Radford, VA

Rose Mary Carroll-Johnson, MN, RN
Valencia, CA

Roberta Cavendish, PhD, RN, CPN
The College of Staten Island
Staten Island, NY

Susan K. Chase, EdD, RNCS, FNP
Boston College
Chestnut Hill, MA

Amanda Coakley, RNC, PhD(c)
Massachusetts General Hospital
Brookline, MA

Amy Coenen, PhD, RN, CS
Marquette University
Milwaukee, WI

Marga Simon Coler, EdD, RN, CS, CTN, FAAN
Federal University of Paraiba, Brazil
University of Connecticut, USA

Katherine Collopy
Doctoral Candidate, Boston College
Durham, NH

Martha Craft-Rosenberg, PhD, RN, FAAN
University of Iowa
Iowa City, IA

Jessie Daniels, MA, RN
University of Minnesota
Minneapolis, MN

Gail C. Davis, RN, EdD
Texas Woman's University
Denton, TX

Connie Delaney, PhD, RN, FAAN
University of Iowa
Iowa City, IA

Janice Denehy, PhD, RN
University of Iowa
Iowa City, IA

Mary DeWys, RN, BSN
Grand Rapids, MI

Cynthia M. Dougherty, RN, PhD, ARNP
VA Puget Sound Medical Center
Seattle, WA

Joyce M. Dungan, RN, MSN, EdD
ECHO Health Center
Evansville, IN

Takako Egawa, PhD, RN
Osaka University
Japan

Nancy Fairchild, MS, CAES, RN
Boston College
Chestnut Hill, MA

Maria de Oliveira Ferreira Filha, MS, Enf.
Federal University of Paraiba
Brazil

Jane M. Flanagan, RNC, MSN
Massachusetts General Hospital
Brookline, MA

Susan A. Ford, RN, MSN, CCRN
Glen Oaks Medical Center
Glendale Heights, IL

K. Fujisaki
Japan

Telma Ribeiro Garcia, RN, DNS
Universidade Federal da Paraiba
Brazil

Donna Jean Gardner, MSN, CNS
Commander United States Navy
Portsmouth Naval Medical Center, VA

Kristine M. Gebbie, DrPH, RN, FAAN
Columbia University School of Nursing
New York, NY

Marjory Gordon, PhD, RN, FAAN
Boston College
Chestnut Hill, MA

Don Gorman, RN, DipNEd, BEd, MEd, EdD, FANZCMHN, FRCNA
La Trobe University
Australia

Cyd Q. Grafft, MSN, ARNP
Special Education Nurse
Cedar Falls, IA

Maria Gaby Rivero de Gutierrez, DNSC
Univers. Fed. de S. Paulo
Sao Paulo - SP - Brazil

Jane Hokanson Hawks, DNSc, RN, C
Midland Lutheran College
Fremont, NE

Kathryn Van Dyke Hayes, DNSc, RN, C
Holy Family College
Philadelphia, PA

Elizabeth F. Hiltunen, MS, RN, CS
Harvard School of Public Health
Boston, MA

Mildred Hogstel, RN, C, PhD
Texas Christian University
Fort Worth, TX

Lois M. Hoskins, PhD, RN, FAAN
Catholic University of America
Washington, DC

Marion Johnson, PhD, RN
University of Iowa
Iowa City, IA

Dorothy A. Jones, EdD, RNC, FAAN
NANDA President-Elect
Boston College
Chestnut Hill, MA

Aileen R. Killen, RN, PhD, CNOR
Datmouth Hitchcock Medical Center
Hanover, NH

Barbara Krainovich-Miller, EdD, RN, CS
Teachers College, Columbia University
New York, NY

Barbara Kraynyak-Luise, EdD, RN
The College of Staten Island
Staten Island, NY

Yasuko Kume, MSN, RN
Osaka University
Japan

Gail Ladwig, RN, MSN, CHTP
Jackson Community College
Jackson, MI

Mary Ann Lavin, ScD, RN, CS, FAAN
St. Louis University School of Nursing
St. Louis, MO

Priscilla LeMone, RN, DSN, FAAN
University of Missouri-Columbia
Columbia, MO

Jean D'Meza Leuner, PhD, RN
Medical University of South Carolina
Charleston, SC

Rona F. Levin, PhD, RN
Felician College
Lodi, NJ

Marlene G. Lindeman, MSN, RN, CS
University of Nebraska Medical Center
Omaha, NE

Maria Helena Baena de Moraes Lopes
Brazil

Margaret Lunney, PhD, RN, CS
The College of Staten Island
Staten Island, NY

Kim Lutzen, RN, PhD
Karolinska Institute
Sweden

Eiko Masutani, MSEd, RN
Osaka University
Japan

Mitsuko Matsuki, PhD, RN
Fukui University
Japan

Joanne McCloskey, PhD, RN, FAAN
University of Iowa
Iowa City, IA

Ann McCourt
Ormond Beach, FL

Cynthia Medich, PhD, RN
Simmons College
Boston, MA

Geralyn Meyer, MSN(R), RN, CS
St. Louis University
St. Louis, MO

Jeanne Lilane Marlene Michel, RN, BS
Universidade Federal de Sao Paulo
Brazil

Winnifred C. Mills, RN, MEd
Western Consulting Associates
Vancouver, British Columbia, Canada

Sue Moorhead, PhD, RN
University of Iowa
Iowa City, IA

T. Nakaki
Japan

Maria Miriam Lima da Nobrega, RN, MS
Universidade Federal da Pariba
Brazil

Chie Ogasawara, PhD, RN
Osaka University
Japan

Yuko Ohno, PhD, RN
Osaka University
Japan

Jean A. O'Neil, EdD, RN, C
Boston College
Chestnut Hill, MA

Nico Oud, RN, Dip. N. Adm., MNSc
Broens & Oud
The Netherlands

Gulten Ozalting, PhD, RN
Marmara University
Turkey

Margaret Padnos, RN, BA, BSN

Laurence Parker, PhD
Thomas Jefferson Medical College
Philadelphia, PA

Ivor Pattison, RN, MscN
Boston College
Chestnut Hill, MA

Shelley-Rae Pehler, RN, MSN
Genesis Medical Center
Davenport, IA

Kathryn Richardson, MS, RN
New York Technical College
Brooklyn, New York

Sharon Ridgeway, RN, PhD
University of Minnesota
Minneapolis, MN

Assumpta Rigol, MS, Enf.
Universitat de Barcelona
Spain

Virginia K. Saba, EdD, RN, FAAN, FACMI
Georgetown University
Washington, DC

Shigemi Sato, PhD, RN
Nagano College of Nursing
Japan

Leann Scroggins, MS, RN, CRRN
Mayo Foundation
Rochester, MN

Sheila M. Sparks, DNSc, RN, CS
Shenandoah University
Winchester, VA

Harry John Tillman, RN, PhD
Naval Medical Center
Portsmouth, VA

Madeline Wake, PhD, RN, FAAN
Marquette University
Milwaukee, WI

Judith J. Warren, PhD, RN, FAAN
NANDA President

Donna Watson, RN, MSN, CNOR
Staff Nurse, St. Joseph Same Day Surgery
Gig Harbor, WA

Dickon Weir-Hughes, MA, RN
Chelsea Westminister Hospital
London, England

Bonnie Wesorick, MSN, RN
CPM Resource Center
Grand Rapids, MI

Georgia Griffith Whitley, EdD, RN
Northern Illinois University
DeKalb, IL

Kathy Wyngarden
Butterworth Hospital
Grand Rapids, MI

Yuko Yamamoto, MSN, RN
Osaka University
Japan

Poster Presentations

Cizone Maria Carneiro Acioly
E.P.L. Albersnagel-Thijssen
Iracema Alvim
Gina Anker
Elizabeth Archambault
E.A.M. Arcuri
Roel H. Bakker
Alba Lucia B.L. de Barros
Diane Berry
M. den Boer
Sonia Mara dos Santos Cardoso
Alorda Carmen
Emilia Campos de Carvalho
Tania Couto Machado Chianca
June Clarke
Marga S. Coler
Consuelo Garcia Correa
Mary J. Costa
M.P.G. Costa
Carol A. Craft
M. Crespf
Dina de A.L. Monteiro da Cruz
Marion Cont D'Hare
Niguir T.V. Donoso
Takako Egawa
Maria do Carmo Andrade Duarte
F.A.C. Farias

Maria de Oliveira Ferreira Filha
D. Forteza
Antonio Regina Furegato
G. Gallego
J. Garcia
Ana Gimenez
C.B. Solange Godoy
Marjory Gordon
Maria Gaby R. de Gutierrez
Diane Hanson
J.L. Van Der Heyden
P. Jaramillo
Dorothy A. Jones
P. Ferrer de Sant Jordi
Luiza Kanda
Marijke C. Kastermans
Geana P. Kurita
Kathia C. Leite
Maria H.B. de Moraes Lopes
Michelle Lyden
V.L.R. Maria
M. Marrugat
Ivete Martins
Mitsuko Matsuki
A. Maya
Rita do Socorro Periera Mendes
C.A.M. Mulder
Maria Miriam Lima da Nobrega

Chie Ogasawara
Yuko Ohno
Ana Claudia Oiveria
Jean A. O'Neil
Eiko Otani
Nico Oud
Antonia S. Paredes
Kathleen M. Parris
Dolores Pasini
Neuza Maria Correra Paula
M.S. Peixoto
Maria Auxiliadora Pereira
Cibele de Mattos Pimenta
Valdirene Polonio
E. Ponsell
Kathleen L. Powers
Lila Raamot
Stephanie J. Richardson
J.E. Schoemaker
Glaucia Borges Seraphim
Maria do Socorro M. Lins Silva
Sandra Regian Souza
H.A. Stallings
G.I.D.C.E. Urrutia
Iane Nogueira Do Vale
C. Vidal
Kathy Wyngarden
Yuko Yamamoto

Contents

Section 3: General Session Presentations

Section 3: General Session Presentations *(continued)*

Section 4: Paper Presentations

Nursing Diagnosis in Clinical Practice

Section 4: Paper Presentations *(continued)*

Section 4: Paper Presentations *(continued)*

Section 4: Paper Presentations (continued)

Section 4: Paper Presentations *(continued)*

Section 5: Poster Abstracts

Section 5: Poster Abstracts (continued)

Section 5: Poster Abstracts *(continued)*

Section 5: Poster Abstracts (continued)

Section 6: Workgroup Reports

Section 7: Business of the Organization

Appendix

Preconference Presentation

Advanced Practice and the Use of Nursing Diagnoses: A Population-Based Perspective

Mary Ann Lavin, ScD, RN, CS, FAAN

This report was funded in part through an ongoing three-year Rural Health Outreach Demonstration Program Grant of the Office of Rural Health Policy, Bureau of Primary Health Care, Health Resources and Services Administration. The federal government is contributing 62% of the project total program cost of $1,273,000 with the HOPE (Health Outreach and Preventive Education) Consortium contributing the remainder in in-kind services.

Introduction

The role of the advanced practice nurse in primary care is defined by more than the performance of delegated medical acts and prescriptive authority. It also includes the development and extension of primary care services, when needed. The primary objective of this presentation is to report on the community assessment and diagnoses that laid the foundation for HOPE (Health Outreach and Preventive Education), a federally funded rural health outreach demonstration program. The second objective flows from the first. It is to present an overview of the practice of two of HOPE's advanced practice nurses and their attempts to incorporate nursing diagnoses into their practice. The third objective is to analyze in depth one nursing diagnosis: noncompliance. The fourth objective is to engage participants in a retrospective analysis of noncompliance in an attempt to gain a new perspective. These four objectives are developed in the following Parts I through IV.

Part I. Developing a Health Outreach and Preventive Education System

There are at least two approaches used in developing a community-based extension of a primary care service. The first is a social planning approach, where leaders in the community and health care fields come together and plan a program. The second is a community development approach, where residents of the community organize themselves and plan a program (Lavin, 1973). HOPE used a hybrid community development/social planning method, consisting of five steps: (a.) studied serendipity, (b.) building a initial support base, (c.) conducting a population-based needs assessment, (d.) validating diagnoses, and (e.) building a consortium. Each of these steps is described below.

Step 1. Studied Serendipity

Studied serendipity means that advanced practice nurses interested in extending primary care services need to be aware of organizational opportunities that present themselves. Serendipity was abundant in 1995. The Vice-President of Saint Louis University Health Sciences Center, Dr. James Kimmey, called for the formation of a Task Force on Interdisciplinary Education and the author was appointed Chair. One of the charges given to the Task Force was to develop a primary care system appropriate for interdisciplinary clinical education. About the same, time a request for a proposal was released by the federal Office of Rural Health Policy for rural health outreach demonstration programs, with special emphasis on improving the delivery of primary care services to medically underserved rural areas

Table 1

Selected Demographic Comparisons Between County A and the State of Missouri			
Variable	County A	Missouri	Source
Income			
100% poverty level or less	28%	14%	CHART
200% poverty level or less	55%	21%	CHART
Illiteracy			
Estimated percent	18%	11%	CHART
Education			
Percent of residents over			
18 years who have completed			
12 years of school	52%	75%	OSEDA
Race			
Caucasian	98%	88%	OSEDA
Age			
Under 18 years	30%	19%	OSEDA
Sex			
Female	49%	52%	OSEDA

Source: United States Department of Commerce, Bureau of the Census, Missouri Office of Administration (1990). Available http://www.oseda.missouri.edu:70/00/reference/census/mo (January, 1996); Community Health Assessment Resource Team [CHART] (1992). 1995 Demographic Projections. Jefferson City: Bureau of Primary Care (1993). Primary Care Access Plan [PCAP], 1992-County Profile. Jefferson City: Missouri Department of Health.

Table 2

Selected Mortality Rate Comparisons Between County A and the State of Missouri

	Mortality Rates/100,000	
Causes of Death	**County A**	**Missouri**
Death from all causes	645.2	535.8
Motor vehicle crashes	40.0	20.1
Work injuries	7.1	4.7
Lung cancer	49.7	42.6
Breast cancer	24.2	22.2
Cardiovascular disease	261.5	204.6
Homicide	11.2	9.9
Infant deaths	11.9	9.8

Source: Center for Health Information Management and Epidemiology (1994). Missouri Vital Statistics. Jefferson City: Missouri Department of Health.

Note: Mortality rate statistics for County A were extrapolated based on 1990 county population statistics and the number of deaths within each category. Because the total population size of the county is small (20,380), the rates extrapolated are estimates only.

through the formation of consortia. Recognizing the fit between the Vice-President's objective and those of the Office of Rural Health Policy is an example of studied serendipity.

Step 2. Identifying Significant Players

Besides the members of the Task Force on Interdisciplinary Education, significant players included a family nurse practitioner in a rural county southwest of Saint Louis, the administrator of the county hospital, and a number of lay persons from within the community. The lat-

ter became HOPE's Citizens' Advisory Board. All players agreed that the HOPE proposal go forward.

Step 3. A Population-Based Needs Assessment

The third step was to perform a rural county needs assessment to diagnose community responses to actual or potential health problems (North American Nursing Diagnosis Association [NANDA], 1990). To assess county-wide health care needs and risks, demographic variables were examined (Table 1). These data indicated that the County's heavily Caucasian population is younger and less well educated than the population of the State as a whole. Its illiteracy rate of 18% means that a significant number of the population need health workers sensitive to the issue, willing to assist clients with completing forms, and ready to rely largely on verbal or visual presentations of health education content. The sizeable percentage of persons at or below the 100% and 200% poverty levels is a signal that the need for state-funded health care services will be high as will be the prevalence of poverty-related health care problems. Health status indicators examined were mortality, maternal and child health, mental health, and dental health statistics. Mortality data (Table 2) show that the County's population is less healthy overall than that of the State and that this trend covers the lifespan.

Table 3 examines maternal and child health indicators. The number of adolescent pregnancies, the proportion of pregnant women who lack prenatal care, and the percent of pregnant women who smoke are higher in County A than in the State. These factors may help explain the number of abnormal conditions found at birth and the number of children with special needs. While the County Health Department

Table 3

Maternal and Child Health Indicators			
Variable	County A	Missouri	Source
Adolescent pregnancy	10%	5%	CHART
No prenatal care	25%	19%	CHART
Abnormal conditions at birth	13%	7%	1994 Vital Statistics
Mothers who smoked during pregnancy	28%	22%	CHART
Children with special needs (estimated)	15%	3%	PC

Source: Community Health Assessment Resource Team [CHART] (1992). 1984-1993 Maternal and Child Health Indicators. Jefferson City: Missouri Department of Health; Center for Health Information Management and Epidemiology (1994). Missouri Vital Statistics. Jefferson City: Missouri Department of Health; personal community [PC] with County School Principals.

Note: Abnormal conditions include anemia, birth injury, fetal alcohol syndrome, respiratory distress syndrome, meconium aspiration, and assisted ventilation. Within and between observer reliability of this statistic is less than ideal as it depends upon the accuracy of birth certificate documentation with which the information is documented on the birth certificate; and quality of the data is dependent upon the skill level of the person completing the form (Land & Vaughan, 1984; Woolbright & Harsbarger, 1995). Also, consistency in reporting among institutions is lacking (Schoendorf, Parker, Batkhan, & Kiely, 1993).

addressed the issues of maternal health and while various agencies, for example, public schools, Head Start, and Parents as Teachers, are alert to and provide some treatment for developmental disorders, there was no Child Development Clinic in the County. Professional evaluation and the initiation of a child development treatment program often required travel to St. Louis, about 82 miles from the County seat.

The Missouri Department of Mental Health provides statistical data on the region rather than on specific counties. According to its Division of Comprehensive Psychiatric Services Report (1995), an estimated 30% have a psychiatric need in the region. This percent is comparable to the State as a whole. To obtain community validation for this figure, members of the Citizens' Advisory Board were asked to give their own estimate of the extent of mental health problems in the area. They stated that the prevalence is considerably higher than regional statistics indicate. When asked to identify the most prevalent problem, they unanimously agreed that poverty-related depression was widespread. In terms of services, they recommended individual as opposed to group therapy. They cited reluctance to talk about personal matters in groups in an area where "everyone knows everyone else."

Both the residents of County A and professionals cite dental health as one of the highest primary care priorities. City water supplies serve 3,850 persons, or 20% of the County's population. None of the three water supplies in the County are fluoridated. The remaining 80% of the population are dependent upon private well water, which may or may not contain an optimal level (1.0 ppm) of naturally occurring fluoride. Almost 100% of these wells were untested for fluoride content. In addition, the number of

state-funded dental sealant eligible children who did not receive dental sealants in 1995 was estimated to be 73% on the basis of the number of children who received dental sealants provided by L. Mouden (personal communication, March, 1996) and the number of eligible children enrolled in each school's subsidized lunch program in County A. The Citizens' Advisory Board confirmed the need and indicated that dental health is a top priority issue.

County A is federally designated as medically underserved. Health provider statistics (Community Health Assessment Resource Team, 1991) indicated there was one physician per 5,162 persons in County A. This compares with a global ratio of one physician to every 6,760 in low income economies and one per 420 population in globally defined high income economies (Robinson, 1995) In Missouri as a whole, the physician to population ratio in 1991 was 1/512.

Registered nurses fared better. The registered nurse per population ratio of one per 645 persons for County A fell between the one per 140 persons found globally in high income economies and the one per 980 persons found in economies defined as middle income (Robinson, 1995). For the State of Missouri, the registered nurse per population ratio was one for every 127 persons.

There were no health professional clinical education sites in the County, except for one rural health clinic, where HOPE's prospective Project Director, a family nurse practitioner, served as a preceptor for two or three nurse practitioner students per semester.

Selected state-provided health service utilization rates were examined. Prior to the initiation of HOPE in October, 1996, it was estimated that only 20% of the 2,000 eligible women in

County A had taken advantage of breast and cervical cancer control project (BCCCP) screens. Approximately 200 Healthy Children and Youth (HCY) screens had been performed. It was estimated that this represented about 16% of the children who were eligible. As previously indicated, less than one-fourth of the sealant-eligible children took advantage of the state's dental sealant program in 1995. Virtually no one in the county had their well water tested for fluoride content in a free program offered by the Missouri Department of Health. There was no child development clinic within the County and no systematic approach to health education.

Transportation is a problem for County A, which covers 760 square miles (United States [U.S.] Department of Commerce, 1998). Its two-lane state highways are not conducive to commerce, industry, nor safety in commuting to or from metropolitan areas. The closest interstate highway is about 55 miles away with another 27 miles of travel needed to reach midtown St. Louis. Bus transportation is provided by Southeastern Missouri Transportation System. It travels to St. Louis for medical purposes only two days of the week. In 1994, this round trip cost $10.00; within-county bus rides cost $3.00 round trip.The cost or the need for advance notification was problematic for some.

Step 4. Population-Based, Aggregate or Community Diagnoses

The following population-based diagnoses were derived from the assessment data:

1. Underutilization of state-funded services, secondary to transportation problems.
2. Diagnostic and child development treatment service deficit.
3. Mental health and social service deficit
4. Dental health primary prevention program deficit.
5. Lack of a systematic health education program.
6. Lack of health professional education.

After their confirmation by the Citizens' Advisory Board, these diagnoses served as the basis for establishing outcome-based goals and related primary care services, that is, community interventions or treatments.

Step 5. Building a Consortium

At this point in time, only two institutions were involved: Saint Louis University Health Sciences Center and Washington County Memorial Hospital. At Saint Louis University, the population based needs assessment and the diagnoses derived from it were presented to the Health Sciences Center Task Force on Interdisciplinary Education. The Task Force decided to request permission to go forward with the proposal from the Vice President and Deans of the Health Sciences Center and other interested Deans and Department Chairs. They approved.

The next step was to obtain the approval to proceed from the Administrator of County A Hospital. After his approval was obtained, the family nurse practitioner in County A and the author called a planning meeting of representatives of institutions with a stake in the health of County A. The threefold purpose of this meeting was: to present the population needs assessment, diagnoses, and suggested services; to decide whether or not to form a consortium; and to outline or plan for the services in greater detail.

There were a number of assumptions underlying this meeting. One was dictated by the funding agency, that is, the main applicant and the project director must be from the rural area. The assumptions of those taking a lead role in writing the proposal were: (a.) only by working together could the needs of the County be met or even addressed; (b.) interagency and interdisciplinary respect was essential; and (c.) a win/win situation for all involved was the outcome desired. At the conclusion of this planning meeting, nine organizations agreed to become members of HOPE (Health Outreach and Preventive Education), the consortium's name. Since then, one member, the County Health Department, withdrew from the consortium because the cost of membership seemed greater than the benefit obtained. Efforts at renegotiating a partnership are being made. Currently, the eight member consortium consists of the following organizations: County A Memorial Hospital, Saint Louis University Health Sciences Center, St. Louis Behavioral Medicine Institute, Healthline Management, Inc., Missouri Bureau of Dental Health, County A Board for the Handicapped, Potosi Family Dental, and Edward Lake, DDS. The diagnostic-specific service areas to be addressed by the demonstration program were identified as follows:

1. Nurse practitioner and physician outreach via the HOPE van to provide Healthy Children and Youth (HCY) screens, breast and cervical cancer screens, adult male and older adult screens.
2. Child development clinic services.
3. Mental health (with a telecommunication component) and social services.
4. Preventive dental health services.
5. County-wide health education.
6. Interdisciplinary clinical site

development for health professional education.

The grant proposal was submitted in March of 1996. Of more than 300 proposals submitted nationwide, HOPE was one of 35 funded in the fall of 1996.

Part II. Advanced Practice Nursing and Nursing Diagnoses Within HOPE

The second objective of this presentation is to present an overview of the practice of two of HOPE's advanced practice nurses and their attempts to incorporate nursing diagnoses into their practice. Dr. Ruth Murray, a certified psychiatric/mental health clinical nurse specialist on the faculty at Saint Louis University School of Nursing, provides weekly mental health services through HOPE in County A. The second advanced practice nurse (APN) is the author, a member of the faculty of Saint Louis University School of Nursing, Coordinator of HOPE Services for the University, and a certified adult nurse practitioner who provides HOPE's breast and cervical cancer screening services. A summary of their work follows.

Advanced practice: Mental health nursing. Ruth Murray, EdD, RN, CS, began providing mental health services September, 1997. As of March 31, 1998, she had conducted 98 sessions with 33 child/adolescent clients. Of these clients, 13 were referred by a school official (such as the social worker and principal), nine by a parent or guardian, four by the Department of Family Services, three by a nurse practitioner, one by the Health Department, two by juvenile officers, one by the hospital, and one by a physician. Nine clients came as a result of HOPE publicity. At intake and at a three month follow-up session, each client was assessed using the

Table 4

Human Response Pattern, Diagnoses, and Related Comments by Ruth Murray, EdD, RN, CS, in Her Faculty Practice with HOPE Program

Pattern 1. Exchanging

Altered nutrition, less than body requirements

Pattern 2. Communicating

Impaired verbal communication.

[Comment: Impaired communication is the relevant concept because, if communication is impaired, it is usually both a verbal and nonverbal impairment.

Pattern 3. Relating

Impaired social interaction, social isolation, altered role performance, ineffective family coping.

Pattern 4. Valuing

Spiritual distress.

Pattern 5. Choosing

Ineffective individual coping, impaired adjustment, defensive coping, ineffective family coping.

[Comment: In the opinion of Dr. Murray, people do not consciously choose to be ineffective or impaired. Thus, she is not convinced these diagnoses are appropriately categorized under a pattern named "choosing."]

Pattern 6. Moving

Fatigue, sleep pattern disturbance, altered growth and development.   [Comment: Instead of the label altered growth and development, Dr. Murray prefers Erikson's Epigenetic Theory and Piaget's Theory of Cognitive Development as she finds the latter provide for more diagnostic-specific interventions.]

Pattern 7. Perceiving

Negative self-concept, body image disturbance, self-esteem disturbance, identity disturbance, sensory/perceptual alterations, hopelessness.

[Comment: Dr. Murray finds that low self-esteem is a more diagnostically relevant term than self-esteem disturbance. Also, specifying the type of hallucination is more diagnostically usefull than the lable sensory/perceptual alteration.]

Pattern 8. Knowing

Altered thought processes, knowledge deficit. [Comment: Lack of knowledge or lack of understanding are more relevant diagnostic concepts than knowledge deficit.]

Pattern 9. Feeling

Chronic pain, grieving, potential for violence, directed toward self.

[Comment: It is important to distinguish between grief as a feeling and mourning as a process, which may be delayed, complicated, or unresolved, especially since the clinical usefulness of the diagnoses is a function of how well it specifies the response of the client. Also, the terms self-mutilation, suicidal ideation, and suicidal behavior are more relevant diagnostic concepts than potential for violence, directed toward self.]

Global Assessment of Functioning (GAF), documented in the fourth edition (1994) of the Diagnostic and Statistical Manual of Mental Disorders (DSM-IV). On average, there was an increase of 14 points in the GAF as assessed by the therapist.

Dr. Murray also saw 19 adult patients for a total of 57 visits. Of these three were referred by a nurse practitioner; three by the health department; three by a social worker; two by the Department of Family Services; and one each by a psychiatrist, a husband, and hospital staff; four were self-referred; and one either as a result of publicity about HOPE or because of contact by a community health worker. The average increase in GAF scores was 32 points. In caring for clients, Dr. Murray states that she organizes her nursing interventions around the human response patterns and diagnoses (NANDA, 1996) listed in Table 4. In the third column, she comments on how she adapts the diagnoses into concepts that are relevant for her own clinical practice.

Yet, Dr. Murray points out that she does not document these diagnoses in the chart; she formulates them in her mind only and organizes her interventions accordingly. It needs to be stated emphatically that Dr. Murray is an advocate of nursing diagnoses. She uses nursing diagnoses in her teaching at the undergraduate, master's, and doctoral levels. She incorporates nursing diagnoses into her professional writing (Murray & Huelskoetter, 1991; Murray & Zentner, 1997). She was a member of the planning committee of the First National Conference on the Classification of Nursing Diagnoses (Gebbie & Lavin, 1973). Still, Dr. Murray indicates there is insufficient time in practice to record them, given her full client caseload and need to organize her reporting, for reimbursement purposes, on the basis of psychiatric/mental health diagnoses, using the DSM IV classification system. She states that two possible solutions to this dilemma are to incorporate nursing diagnoses into DSM-IV or obtain insurance company recognition of nursing diagnoses. Recognition of nursing diagnoses in the International Classification of Diseases, version 10, Clinical Modification (ICD-10-CM) is a step forward in this direction (American Nurses Association, 1998).

Advanced practice nursing: Breast and cervical cancer screening. One of HOPE's services is to provide nurse practitioner/physician outreach for health prevention purposes. This outreach is provided by a nurse practitioner working in collaboration with a physician. Within HOPE, breast and cervical cancer screening outreach means providing services in church halls or community centers in the small rural towns outside of the county seat. Specifically, the service consists of a history and physical exam, a clinical breast exam accompanied by breast self-examination instructions, and a pelvic exam with a Papanicolaou test included. Specimens for saline slide preparations are collected and gonorrhea and chlamydia probes are obtained, as indicated. A bilateral screening mammogram is ordered. Opportunity is provided for health counseling and client education.

Tracking. Examination results are recorded for each client in a log book, designed to facilitate tracking. Essential features of this log book may be divided into the following categories: the client's name; identification number; normal or abnormal results of clinical breast examination, mammogram, pelvic examination, Papinicolau (Pap) test; dates mammogram and Pap test results were mailed to the client; and dates of return breast and pelvic/Pap appointments.

Categorizing clinical breast examination and mammogram results. Once a tracking system is in place, the data are used for client follow-up and program evaluation purposes. Clinical breast exam results when matched in a 2 x 2 table against normal and abnormal mammogram results in formation of the following groups:

1. Normal clinical breast examination and normal mammogram. Continue with routine annual screening.
2. Normal clinical breast exam and abnormal mammogram. Perform diagnostic mammography as indicated by radiologist and refer for surgical consult, if indicated.
3. Abnormal clinical breast exam and normal mammogram. If a discrete mass is noted, refer to surgeon for consult, even in the presence of a normal mammogram. If fibrocystic breast changes are the only abnormality, consider institution of clinical breast examinations every 4 - 6 months as detection of discrete masses becomes more difficult in presence of fibrocystic changes.
4. Abnormal clinical breast examination and abnormal mammogram. Perform diagnostic mammography as indicated by radiologist and refer to a surgeon for consult.

Dividing results into this kind of classification system is useful for overall evaluation purposes. Clinically, it is useful as it facilitates follow-up by community health workers, under the supervision of the advanced practice nurse.

Either because of the age of the client being too young for routine screening mammography or because of noncompliance with screening mammography, there are also clients with normal and abnormal clinical breast exams without a corresponding screening mammogram.

Total clinical breast examinations, percent compliant with screening mammogram recommendations, and related literature. During the first year of the HOPE program, there were a total of 105 exams. Of these, 62 were with mammograms and 43 were without mammograms. Of 67 screening mammograms prescribed, 62 were obtained, yielding a compliance rate of 92.5% and a noncompliance rate of 7.5%. None of the patients with abnormal clinical breast exams and for whom a screening mammogram was indicated were noncompliant with the recommendation.

How does this screening mammogram compliance rate data compare with the literature? In a Canadian study, Bryant (1996) reports a 66% screening mammogram compliance rate within a two month study period. Rosenberg (1996) reports an 82.8% compliance rate, with fear and not thinking the test was recommended being among the reasons for noncompliance. A study by Kreher, Hickner, Ruffin and Lin (1995) indicated that distance and time were not factors in mammogram compliance among rural women in Michigan.

Several compliance-related factors are identified in the literature. Foley, D'Amico and Merenstein (1990) found that compliance is facilitated by nurse identification of clients overdue for mammograms, a mammogram completion check-off list, and a back-up reminder system. Aiken, West, Woodward, Reno and Reynolds (1994) reported on the success of a theory based health promotion program. Burnett, Steakley, and Tefft (1995) found compliance with screening mammograms positively related to the influence of significant others and negatively related to uncaring health professionals. Friedman, et al. (1995) found compliance negatively related to perceived barriers and positively related to physician recommendation. Weber and Reilly (1997) reported that personalized education and case management tripled mammogram compliance among urban poor. The finding that many different kinds of interventions increase mammogram compliance raises a question: Is compliance increasing because the interventions are changing client behavior or because they reflect changes in provider or health care system behavior?

HOPE interventions intended to maximize compliance were: extension of personal invitation by community health workers to women in the laudromats, tanning parlors, and beauty salons; client-friendly health education at the time of the clinical breast exam; provider use of a log to track results; and encouragement through nurse practitioner follow-up telephone call or community health worker home visit, when indicated. In cases where fear or lack of transportation presented a barrier, community health workers volunteered to accompany clients to radiology.

In addition to the five clients with normal clinical breast exams but noncompliant with screening mammogram recommendations, there were also 38 women who had clinical breast exams but no mammograms. Of these 38:

1. Ten had abnormal clinical breast exams. (In 5, the only abnormality noted was fibrocystic breast changes and no mammogram was indicated. One client had an obvious cyst that was subsequently removed by a surgeon to whom she was referred. Another had a cyst and is now being followed by a surgeon. One had severe mastitis and mammography was postponed until the mastitis subsided. Two cases remained open at the time this presentation was made.)

2. Twenty-four had normal clinical breast exams and were under the age recommended for mammography.

3. Two had normal clinical breast exams along with mammograms within the past year and repeat mammography was not yet indicated.

4. Two decided for insurance or personal reasons to have their mammograms performed through their personal physicians and not under HOPE auspices.

Categorizing pelvic examination and Papanicolaou (Pap) results. Pelvic examination results when matched in a 2 x 2 table against Pap results in the formation of the following groups:

1. Normal pelvic examination and normal Pap results. Continue with routine annual screening.

2. Normal pelvic examination and abnormal Pap results. Institute appropriate treatment and repeat Pap test, if appropriate; or, if indicated, refer for colposcopy or LEEP procedures.

3. Abnormal pelvic examination and normal Pap results. Treat vaginal and/orpelvic inflammatory disease infections; refer if vaginal, uterine, ovarian, adnexal, or bladder masses are encountered. If cervical inflammation persists after treatment or if a suspicious abnormality is present, refer for colposcopy even in the presence of

a negative Pap test. Refer all suspicious vaginal, adenexal, pelvic, or bladder masses.

4. Abnormal pelvic examination and abnormal Pap results. Institute one or more of the recommendations given above.

Again, this kind of categorization facilitates both overall program evaluation and clinical follow-up. Total pelvic and Pap examinations, percent compliant with follow-up of abnormal Pap results, and related literature. During the first year of the HOPE program, there were a total of 90 pelvic/Pap index examinations. Of these, 11 had abnormal cellular findings. Of the 11, 8 were compliant with treatment and/or follow-up recommendations and 3 were noncompliant. Of these 3, one was noncompliant with follow-up appointments, one was lost to follow-up, and one, a cigarette smoker, chose an alternative medicine approach after being diagnosed with cancer in situ (II) of the cervix and after two lung masses were found upon computerized axial tomography. This yields a follow-up compliance rate of 73% or a noncompliance/lost-to-follow-up rate of 27%, despite follow-up phone calls, letters, and home visits by community health workers.

In a Canadian study, Alanen, Elit, Molinaro, and McLachlin (1998) report a 29% lost-to-follow-up rate but over a two-year follow-up period among clients with atypical cells of undertermined significance (ASCUS) or low grade squamous intraepithelial lesions (LSIL) who were scheduled for repeat Pap tests at six-month intervals or colposcopy. Among adolescents, Lavin, Goodman, Perlman, Kelly, and Emans (1997) report that of 76 patients in whom index Pap was the first abnormal Pap, 51

had a second Pap smear. This is a within clinic follow-up rate of 67%. Of the 60 adolescent clients scheduled for colposcopy, only 37 kept the appointment, despite outreach. The only significant factor between those who complied and those who did not was the scheduling of an appointment between notification of the abnormal Pap smear and the colposcopic procedure (P = .007).

Targeted interventions have also been designed to maximize follow-up treatment compliance among women with abnormal Pap tests. Stewart, Buchegger, Lickrish, and Sierra (1994) conducted a randomized trial among 108 women. The experimental group received an educational brochure dealing with information on the associated emotional distress and meaning of an abnormal Pap smear at the time of their booking for a colposcopy. The standard care group did not receive the booklet. A medical record review after 18 to 24 months showed a 30% (P = .002) increase in treatment compliance in the treatment group. Paskett, Phillips, and Miller (1995) studied the effect of a tracking system with and without an educational brochure that was mailed to clients with abnormal Pap tests along with their return appointment notification. Resuts indicated a significant increase in adherence for patients with dysplasia (P = .03) but not for patients with atypia (P = .23).

Although the numbers involved in the HOPE program evaluation data are too small to draw any conclusions, they did influence me. I now counsel clients with abnormal Pap tests that women may react differently to positive Pap and mammogram findings. In addition to exploring their concerns and fears, I include the following talking points:

1. There has been a lot of public

education about breast cancer.

2. Women may be more aware that early detection and treatment of breast cancer leads to a good probability of long-term survival.
3. Women may be less aware that early detection and treatment of cervical cancer also leads to a good chance of long-term survival.
4. Women may be more aware that suspicious mammograms do not necessarily mean cancer than they are aware that Pap tests that report atypia do not mean cancer is necessarily present.

I take this opportunity to encourage researchers to study the human responses of women to reports of an abnormal mammogram as compared with their responses to reports of abnormal Pap tests so that diagnostic- specific interventions may be applied.

Part III. Noncompliance (5.2.1.1), Related Literature, and Its Interpretation

Effective primary care, especially when it concerns compliance with preventive health measures, demands tracking of outcomes. For example, what is the screening mammography compliance rate? Or annual Pap compliance rate? Or positive Pap follow-up compliance rate? These compliance rates are outcome measures, reflecting program or practitioner effectiveness. Among nurses, they also evoke argument on philosophical, ideological, and ethical grounds and serve to generate scholarly discussion. The following is an initial attempt at the latter.

Noncompliance, as a nursing diagnosis (5.2.1.1), falls within NANDA's fifth diagnostic pattern called choosing. It is a subcategory of the diagnosis of *ineffective management of the therapeutic regimen* (5.2.1). Defined as a person's informed decision not to adhere to a therapeutic recommendation, it is related to the patient's value system, including health beliefs, cultural influences, spiritual values, and client-provider relationships. The diagnosis of non-compliance is made on the basis of: (a.) behavior (client or significant other statements or observation of noncompliance), (b.) objective tests (physiological measures, such as phenytoin levels or detection of markers, e.g. urine color changes that occur with phenazopyridine), (c.) complications, (d.) symptom exacerbations, (e.) failure to progress, and (f.) failure to keep appointments.

While NANDA lists evidence of development of complications, exacerbation of symptoms, and failure to progress as characteristics of non-compliance, these are both signs (characteristics) of noncompliance as well as outcomes. Noncompliance may have positive outcomes, such as fewer side effects and iatrogenic illness, or no deleterious effects at all as in the case of a client who does not appear for an unnecessary medical or nurse practitioner appointment. A review of recent nursing literature reveals that the diagnosis of noncompliance is used for research and clinical purposes. Four doctoral dissertations on the subject have been indexed in the Cumulative Index to Nursing and Allied Health Literature (CINAHL) since 1992. Poulin (1992) found that a health care behavior such as noncompliance may be a homeless person's response to stigma and oppression. Phillips (1993) addressed maternal noncompliance with three safety-belt behaviors during pregnancy. Portney (1994) examined noncompliance as a variable in an analysis of falls among elderly patients in acute care. Smith (1992) studied not patient but critical care nurse compliance with

Centers for Disease Control and Prevention (CDC) guidelines for wearing gloves as did the authors in three related articles also examining glove wearing, hand-washing, or infection control procedures in general (Hersey & Martin, 1995; Mayone-Ziomek, 1997; McPherson & Parris, 1997; Sulzbach-Hoke, 1996). While nurse compliance is not client compliance, it does make apparent a related issue, that is, that one connotation for compliance is obedience and for noncompliance, disobedience. The authors could have said they were studying nurses' obedience to glove wearing and infection control protocols and procedures as readily as they stated they were studying compliance. Such an obvious and easy substitution gives weight to the argument that compliance is a term used within authoritarian ("Do as I say"), paternalistic ("Father knows best"), or even maternalistic ("Be a good child") frameworks.

On the positive side, there are nonauthoritarian, nonpaternalistic, and nonmaternalistic nurses who use the term noncompliance. Their concerns center about the impact of noncompliance on client outcomes. For example, Putz, Lannon, and Satinsky (1996) studied compliance with guidelines for the prevention and treatment of sexually transmitted diseases among women at one sexual assault treatment center. They found higher than expected compliance rates but also found that noncompliance was associated with client misunderstanding related to the need for taking the medicine. The implications of their study for nursing are important: Nurses who directly interact with sexual assault victims are in the best position to enhance compliance by exploring client understanding. This includes allowing time for feedback, recognizing that the stress of the situation may interfere with attending to medication instructions, being willing to repeat content and provide reassurance as to medication efficacy, establishing a therapeutic alliance with the client, etc. Rather than being directed toward the client in an authoritarian, paternalistic, or maternalistic manner, these actions are reasoned recommendations for health care professionals interested in quality improvement.

Several authors advise caution or argue against the use of the term noncompliance. While continuing to use the term medication compliance, Forman (1993) points out that it is a joint responsibility of the health care professional and the patient, and that the latter must not be viewed as the guilty party. Bakker, Kastermans, and Dassen (1995) suggest that it be eliminated as a nursing diagnosis with the more comprehensive diagnosis of ineffective management of therapeutic regimen being used in its stead. Moore (1995) indicates that the term noncompliance exasperates professionals, induces worry about medical care outcomes, and results in labeling patients as "difficult" or "troublesome." Moore's concern about "medical" care outcomes may be blurred as more nurse practitioners become interested in care outcomes related to their own practices and as the term "medical" becomes replaced by terms such as health and human disease outcomes.

The diagnosis of noncompliance also brings up ethical concerns. Warren (1992) cites the work of Sackett and Haynes (1976) and Jonsen (1979). Sackett and Haynes hold that for compliance interventions to be ethical, the patient, after agreeing to treatment, enters into a parnership with the provider to select compliance-increasing interventions conditional upon an accurate (disease) diagnosis having been made and the probability that the benefit of prescribed therapy outweighs harm. Jonsen adds that compliance interventions are ethical when patient consent is free, based on mutual provider/patient understanding, and built on the assumption of mutual provider/patient responsibility for the outcomes achieved. However, Keeling (1993) argues that the nursing diagnosis of noncompliance is incongruent with nursing ethics as well as with nursing history, philosophy, and clinical utility, that is, its use does not lead to interventions appropriate to nursing.

Wuest (1993) reviewed 16 research studies on compliance. She makes a compelling argument that most studies conducted by nurses focused on compliance with physician recommendations. Only two investigated compliance with health promotion behavior and these were also the only two that suggested system changes to increase compliance. Using compliance/noncompliance research as a basis, she also points out several varieties of ethnic and gender bias influence in research questions asked, theoretical frameworks employed, and the knowledge base from which we operate. She concludes that noncompliance needs to be eliminated from our taxonomy.

For several authors, the word compliance (or noncompliance) presents no difficulty. They write on or study the subject of compliance without discussing the pros or cons of the term (Andrews, 1994; Ivey, 1995; Rose, 1993; Shell, 1995; Williams, 1994). Some authors deal with the compliance language problem by using another word as a substitute. For example, Hill and Berk (1995) use the term adherence and indicate it is the "newer" term for compliance.

Crespo-Fierro (1997) and Anastasio (1995) present sophisticated and discriminating approaches to the use of the term. They recognize its short-comings even as they use it and recommend interventions that are "person-spe-

cific and tailored" (Crespo-Fierro) or that advocate the development of "mutually participative nurse-patient relationships" (Anastasio). Their analyses, far from representing dichotomous thought, make a significant contribution to the compliance literature.

What seems apparent to this author is that the debate over the use or nonuse of the diagnosis is compliance is not clear cut but ambiguous. That the term noncompliance has authoritarian, paternalistic, and maternalistic overtones is true; but opposition to its use is sometimes expressed in overtones that are also authoritarian. Finally, that noncompliance is used as a term or as a diagnosis by some in a manner that is not authoritarian, paternalistic, nor maternalistic is also true. In brief, what we have is not an either/or situation but one with is more fluid, less rigid, even ambiguous in a complex world where exploration of ambiguous issues is an indicator of growth within the profession.

Having said that, it may also be true that a reconceptualization of compliance is needed. Perhaps the issue with which we are dealing is not compliance so much as health goal attainment, where the latter is a function of client, provider, treatment/diagnostic test, and system variables. Examples of client variables that influence health goal attainment are reading ability, acuity of hearing, the value attached to goal achievement, readiness, self-efficacy, family support. Examples of provider variables are expressed interest in the client, interpersonal competence, self-confidence. Examples of treatment/diagnostic test variables are pain/inconvenience associated with diagnostic tests, medication side effects, complexity of therapeutic regimen, cost. Examples of system variables affecting goal attainment are insurance, transportation, physical accessibility to agency/pharmacy.

The case for looking at health goal attainment rather than compliance takes the focus off of client behavior alone. Furthermore, it explains better the results of studies that show improvement in compliance behavior not when the client changed but when changes in provider behavior or in the health care system were made. To explore the possibility of reconceptualizing compliance in terms of a health goal attainment model, participants at the preconference were asked to divide into small groups to discuss the issue.

Part IV. Reconceptualizing Compliance and Noncompliance Background

At the conclusion of the presentation, participants were asked to form a small group or groups and discuss compliance, noncompliance, or health goal attainment. Fourteen participants remained (Table 5).

Group method. Group work proceeded in the manner similar to the process used at the First National Conference. One member volunteered to serve as a facilitator and another as the recorder, who was to remain silent. The diagnosis of noncompliance was to be reevaluated using retrospective analysis, that is, members, bringing to the group their knowledge and experience, were to share their professional reflections on the subject of noncompliance. There was no hidden agenda for the group to accomplish and no group outcomes were predetermined. Each person's input was considered equally valid. It was understood that even though the output of the group was not to be considered definitive, it was of value. A summa-

Table 5

Group Discussion Participants

Cecile Boisvert, MScN, RN, St. Aubin, France

Eleanor Borkowski, MSN, RN San Bernardino, California

Karen Cameron, BSN, RNC, Portland, Oregon

Lynda J. Carpenito, MSN, RN, CRNP, Clarksboro, New Jersey

Darlene Davis, BSN, MA, RN, Clearwater, Florida

Tina Durkowski, BSN, RN, ONC, CNOR, Plover, Wisconsin

Louise Flick, DrPH, RN, CS, Saint Louis, Missouri

Tatjana Ge, BSN, RN, Moribor, Slovenia

Dorothea Jakob, MA, RN, Toronto, Ontario

Alice F. Kuehn, PhD, RN, CS, FNP, GNP, Columbia, Missouri

Peggy McComb, MN, RN, CS, Portland, Oregon

Jeanette Nordorft, MSN, RN, Cuba City, Wisconsin

Annie Pascal, RN, Saint Etienne, France

Barbara Vassallo, EdD, RN, ANP, Willingboro, New Jersey

ry of the group's work was to be circulated among the participants for their approval and recommended changes, and reported in the Proceedings of the Conference.

Group results. The first question addressed was: Is noncompliance a diagnosis or an outcome? There was little discussion on this point. One member stated that noncompliance is both a diagnosis and an outcome. She went on to state that this is not unusual as many outcomes have diagnostic chains inherent in them. There was no disagreement on this point.

The remaining discussion centered about the legitimacy of noncompliance as a nursing diagnosis. Group members actively engaged in the discussion. Their contributions were thought-provoking. Member responses are categorized under the following headings: noncompliance or decisional control, noncompliance as a choice and a behavior, noncompliance as a dynamic not a static event, noncompliance as nonadherence, noncompliance renamed as potential for health-seeking behavior, noncompliance reframed as health goal attainment behavior, noncompliance as potential for harm reduction, and the problem with "at risk for" "potential for" terminology,

Noncompliance or decisional control. One participant indicated that in this group discussion two aspects of compliance were under consideration: its label and its definition. "I could," she said, "accept its label; I cannot accept its definition." She went on to say that the definition, that is, "a person's informed decision not to adhere to a therapeutic recommendation" (NANDA, 1997-1998), is not noncompliance but decisional control. To illustrate her point, she told a story about a woman who was severely burned and taken to an intensive care unit in a medical center in Spain (Allue, 1996). After

several weeks, the patient decided she wanted to transfer to a smaller town in Spain for the remainder of her rehabilitation. Predicting dire consequences, professional staff and her family opposed the move. Against their advice, the patient decided to move. Upon arrival in the small town, the patient met physical therapy staff who became very much involved with her care. They agreed with her that increased mobility was the therapeutic goal. Her recovery proceeded uneventfully and the degree of mobility she attained was greater than that predicted at the medical center; and, it was increased mobility that was the patient's goal from the beginning. This patient exhibited a high degree of decisional control; and this is the appropriate name or label of the behavior. To say that she made an informed choice not to adhere to a therapeutic recommendation and to label it noncompliance is to emphasize what she did not do. It is preferable to emphasize what she did positively for herself: She assumed decisional control of her health and future. The concept of decisional control needs to be considered when dealing with an individual's effective management of a therapeutic regimen.

Noncompliance as a choice and a behavior. Another group member indicated that the NANDA definition may be lacking in that noncompliance in not only a choice but a choice to do or not to do something. As such, it is also a behavior.

Noncompliance as a dynamic not a static nor singular event. Noncompliance, a group member noted, is not a singular event. If placed within the context of the transtheoretical model of behavior change (Prochaska & DiClemente, 1984), noncompliance may be a temporary behavior of a person within the precontemplation, contemplation, planning or preparation stages of change. For example, a person abusing drugs may not be willing to stop the abuse now but may be able to do so three months from now. The principle is that the nurse does not give up on people.

Another group member stated that when working with adolescents who are at risk of an unwanted pregnancy or who are considering birth control strategies, a clinician does not take a client decision made today as a definitive choice. Rather, the adolescent's initial interest may be called a "mild" health seeking behavior response or even a "desire" for health-seeking behavior. These responses may be further explored or built upon at subsequent appointments.

A third member indicated that while noncompliance may not be a fixed behavior, the client's current noncompliance may preclude the prescription of certain drugs. For example, one internist recommended that a particular patient noncompliant with therapy not be placed on protease inhibitors because sporadic or less than full compliance would induce resistance; whereas, by waiting a year, a cure for HIV may be available.

The point is not to penalize the patient, said another group member; and, she continued, if noncompliance is an informed choice, there should be no question of penalizing noncompliance. This statement concluded this segment of the discussion on noncompliance as a dynamic not a static event.

Noncompliance renamed as potential for or as desire for health-seeking behavior. Perhaps, one member stated, we should reframe the diagnosis of noncompliance and call it potential for or a desire for health-seeking behavior, albeit sometimes only a mild response. For example, one way of looking at a person,

who after three months, becomes noncompliant with a smoking cessation program is that the person is noncompliant. Another way of looking at the same behavior is that a person had a mild, positive response to a health-seeking behavior program. At least the person was interested in and tried to stop smoking. By reconceptualizing the behavior, the nurse refocuses his or her own vision of the client and leaves open the door to future exploration of the same or other smoking cessation behaviors. Also, relabeling a noncompliant response as a mild desire for health-seeking behavior eliminates the bind of labeling a client response in a manner that may place the patient at risk of being penalized financially by insurance companies or health maintenance organizations. This is no small consideration in today's health care system.

Noncompliance as non-health-seeking behavior. Because noncompliance often opposes health, one member suggested that, for precision's sake, noncompliance be relabeled an non-health-seeking behavior rather than as potential for health-seeking behavior.

Noncompliance as nonadherence. Several group members contributed to the notion that noncompliance is better named nonadherence. Reasons in favor of this position were that nonadherence did not imply an obedience/disobedience mindset as does compliance/noncompliance. Another stated that recent clinical studies in medicine have used the term nonadherence. This segment of the discussion concluded when a member stated that nonadherence has the same connotation as noncompliance and that using nonadherence as a substitute term is hair splitting.

Noncompliance reframed as health goal attainment behavior. Perhaps, then, we should look at health goal attainment as a model instead of the diagnosis on noncompliance because it looks more at the process involved in meeting the health objective. The group, however, did not pursue this avenue. Noncompliance as potential for harm reduction or potential for risk reduction. Still another group member suggested renaming noncompliance as potential for harm reduction because such terminology also frames the problem more positively while indicating that current behavior, such as, smoking, is harmful. It is more positive because it takes noncompliance out of an obedience/disobedience framework, which "reeks" of giving orders. Another indicated she preferred potential for risk reduction because it leaves room for negotiating over time and may be especially important in working with clients with alcohol abuse or compulsive gambling behaviors.

The problem with "at risk for" and "potential for" terminology. A concern was expressed that being "at risk" for developing a health-related problem and the related issue of having a "potential" for change or growth are not human "responses" and hence not true diagnostic statements. Two suggestions were made. The first was to label the behavior, such as, smoking cessation or smoking cessation attempts, as a risk reduction response. The second suggestion was to categorize such a response as a subtype of health-seeking behavior.

The need for quantifying levels of responses. One way of quantifying responses is in terms of mild, moderate, or severe. Another way is by establishing identifying phases or stages in the response being observed. Such methods may contribute greatly to diagnoses such as noncompliance, desire for health seeking behavior, decisional control, etc.

Conclusions. There are no definitive conclusions that can be drawn from this group dis-cussion regarding the diagnosis of noncompliance. What can be affirmed is that there were clinically sound reasons expressed for reexamining the diagnosis and/or generating new diagnoses to describe the wide variety of responses exhibited by clients and observed by nurses.

The high degree of enthusiasm among the group members for the group process can also be affirmed. Several concurred with a suggestion of forming an electronic group to continue the work. Others suggested specific research topics that could be pursued at multicenter sites. It was an intellectually stimulating and mutually satisfying collegial activity that may be used as a model to replicate at future conferences.

There are conclusions that can be reached in terms of advanced practice nursing and the use of nursing diagnoses. APNs are in an excellent position to assess and diagnose communities, plan and implement diagnostic-specific services, use nursing diagnoses effectively within their own practice, study one or more diagnoses in depth, engage others in dialogue regarding the appropriateness of diagnoses currently in use, and facilitate discussion aimed at refining current or supporting the research and development of new diagnoses. I look forward to seeing the progress to be made in this field.

References

Aiken L.S., West, S.G., Woodward, C.K., Reno, R.R., & Reynolds, K.D. (1994). Increasing screening mammography in asymptomatic women: Evaluation of a second-generation, theory-based program. *Health Psychology, 13*(6), 526-538.

Alanen, K. W., Elit, L.M., Molinaro, P.A., & McLachlin, C.M. (1998). Assessment of cytologic follow-up as the recommended management for patients with atypical squamous cells of undetermined significance or low grade squamous intraepithelial lesions. *Cancer, 84*(1), 5-10.

Allue, M. (1996). *Perder Piel.* Barcelona: Seix Barral Ed.

American Nurses Association (1998). *Developing ideas: Nursing diagnoses are part of ICD-9-CM and the new ICD-10-CM.* Available: http://www.nursingworld.org/pulse/idea2.htm (June 16, 1996).

American Psychiatric Association. (1994). *Diagnostic and statistical manual of mental disorders* (4th ed.). Washington, DC: Author.

Anastasio, C.J. (1995). HIV and tuberculosis: Noncompliance revisited. *Journal of the Association of Nurses in AIDS Care 6*(2), 11-23.

Andrews, C. (1994). Ulcer-healing drugs and their actions and side-effects. *Nursing Times 90*(33), 38-40.

Bakker, R.H., Kastermans, M.C., & Dassen, T.W. (1995). An analysis of the nursing diagnosis ineffective management of therapeutic regimen compared to noncompliance and Orem's self-care deficit theory of nursing. *Nursing Diagnosis 6*(4), 161-166.

Blair, A. (1997). Advice of counsel. Documenting noncompliance along with patient care. *R.N. 60*(5), 64.

Bryant, H. (1996). How should we interpret noncompliance with screening mammography? *Canadian Medical Association Journal, 154*(9), 1353-1355.

Burnett, C.B., Steakley, C.S., & Teft, M.C. (1995). Barriers to breast and cervical cancer screening in underserved women of the District of Columbia. *Oncology Nursing Forum, 22*(10), 1551-1557.

Community Health Assessment Resource Team (1991). *CHART: Physicians, nurses, and populations.* Jefferson City: Missouri Department of Health.

Crespo-Fierro, M. (1997). Compliance/adherence and care management in HIV disease. *Journal of the Association of Nurses in AIDS Care, 8*(4), 43-54.

Division of Comprehensive Psychiatric Services (1995). *Missouri's comprehensive mental plan: Table III-A, Missouri point prevalence estimates for different kinds of psychiatric need.* Jefferson City: Missouri Department of Mental Health.

Foley, E.C., D'Amico, F., & Merenstein, J.H. (1990). Improving mammography recommendation: A nurse-initiated intervention. *Journal of the American Board of Family Practice, 3*(2), 87-92.

Forman, L. (1993). Medication: Reasons and interventions for noncompliance. *Journal of Psychosocial Nursing and Mental Health Services, 31*(10), 23-25.

Friedman, L.C., Woodruff, A., Lane, M., Weinberg, A.D., Cooper, H.P., & Webb, J.A. (1995). Breast cancer screening behaviors and intentions among asymptomatic women 50 years of age and older. *American Journal of Preventive Medicine, 11*(4), 218-223.

Gebbie, K. & Lavin, M.A. (1975). *Classification of nursing diagnoses: Proceedings of the first national conference.* St. Louis: Mosby.

Hersey, J.C. & Martin, L.S. (1995). Infection control. Use of infection control guidelines by workers in health care facilities to prevent occupational transmission of HBV and HIV: Results from a national survey. *Today's OR-Nurse, 17*(3), 37-48.

Hill, M.N., & Berk, R.A. (1995). Psychological

barriers to hypertension therapy adherence: instrument development and preliminary psychometric evidence. *Cardiovascular Nursing, 31*(6), 37-43.

Ivey, J.B. (1997). The adolescent with pelvic inflammatory disease: Assessment and management. *The Nurse Practitioner, 22*(2), 78, 81-82, 84, Passim.

Jonsen, A.R. (1979). Ethical issues in compliance. In R.B. Haynes, D.W. Taylor, & D.L. Sackett (Eds.), *Compliance in health care* (pp. 113-120). Baltimore: Johns Hopkins University Press.

Keeling, A., Utz, S.W., Shuster, G.F., & Boyle, A. (1993). Noncompliance revisited: A disciplinary perspective of a nursing diagnosis. *Nursing Diagnosis, 4*(3), 91-98.

Kreher, N.E., Hickner, J.M., Ruffin, M.T., & Lin, C.S. (1995). Effect of distance and travel time on rural women's compliance with screening mammography: An Upper Peninsula Research Network study. *Journal of Family Practice, 40*(2), 143-147.

Land, G., & Vaughan, W. (1984). Birth certificate completion procedures and the accuracy of Missouri birth certificate data. *Journal of the American Medical Record Association, 55*(8), 31-34.

Lavin, C., Goodman, E., Perlman, S., Kelly, L.S., & Emans, S.J. (1997). Follow-up of abnormal Papanicolaou smears in a hospital-based adolescent clinic. *Journal of Pediatric and Adolescent Gynecology, 10*(3), 141-145.

Lavin, M. A. (1973). Cross-cultural identification and utilization of nursing approaches applicable to the delivery of health care. *International Nursing Review, 20*(3), 73-77.

Mayone-Ziomek, J.M. (1997). Best practice. Handwashing in critical care. *MEDSURG*

Nursing, 6(6), 364-369.

McPherson, D.C. (1997). Environmental rounds: What matters for infection prevention and control. *Journal of Gerontological Nursing 23*(11), 28-32.

Moore, K.N. (1995). Compliance or collaboration? The meaning for the patient. *Nursing Ethics: An International Journal for Health Care Professionals, 2*(1), 71-77.

Murray, R. & Huelskoetter, M. (1991). *Psychiatric/mental health nursing: Giving emotional care* (3rd ed.). Norwalk, CT: Appleton & Lange.

Murray, R. & Zentner, J. (1997). *Health assessment & promotion strategies through the life span* (6th ed.). Stamford, CT: Appleton & Lange.

NANDA (1996). *Nursing diagnoses: Definitions and classification 1997-1998*. Philadelphia: Author.

Paskett, E.D., Phillips, K.C., & Miller, M.E. (1995). Improving compliance among women with abnormal Papanicolaou smears. *Obstetrics and Gynecology, 86*(3):353-359.

Phillips, M.D. (1993). *Maternal knowledge, attitude, and practice of three motor vehicle safety belt behaviors during pregnancy* (Doctoral dissertation, University of Maryland).

Poulin, A.L. (1992). *Lower than a snake's belly: The role of stigma in the oppression of sheltered homeless families* (Doctoral dissertation, University of Utah).

Portney, L.G. (1994). *Falls among elderly patients in the acute care setting: methodological and administrative considerations* (Doctoral dissertation, Boston University).

Prochaska J.O. & DiClemente, C.C. (1984). *The transtheoretical approach: crossing*

traditional boundaries of change.
Homewood, IL: Dow Jones-Irwin.

Putz, M., Thomas, B.K., & Cowles, K.V. (1996). Sexual Assault victims' compliance with follow-up care at one sexual assault treatment center. *Journal of Emergency Nursing, 22*(6), 560-565.

Rose, M.A. (1993). Health concerns of women with HIV/AIDS. *Journal of the Association of Nurses in AIDS Care, 4*(3), 39-45.

Rosenberg, E. (1996). Primary-care quality improvement of mammography rates: a baseline study. *Connecticut Medicine, 60*(5), 259-262.

Robinson, J.(1995). The internationalization of professional regulation. *International Nursing Review, 42*(6), 183-186.

Sackett, D.L. and Haynes, R.B. (1976). *Compliance with therapeutic regimens.* Baltimore: Johns Hopkins University Press.

Schoendorf, K. C., Parker, J. D., Batkhan, L. Z., & Kiely, J. L. (1993). Comparability of the birth certificate and the 1988 Maternal and Infant Health Survey. *Vital and Health Statistics, 116*, 1-119.

Shell, R. (1995). Noncompliance in adolescent oral contraceptive users. *Nurse Practitioner, 20*(8), 7, 10.

Smith, M.A. (1992). *Variability of glove wearing by critical care nurses according to selected variables* (Doctoral dissertation, University of Alabama at Birmingham).

Stewart, D.E., Buchegger, P.M., Lickrish, G.M., & Sierra, S. (1994). The effect of educational brochures on follow-up compliance in women with abnormal Papanicolaou smears. *Obstetrics and Gynecology, 83*(4), 583-585.

Sulzbach-Hoke, L.M. (1996). Risk taking by health care workers. *Clinical Nurse Specialist, 10*(1), 30-37.

U. S. Department of Commerce, Bureau of the Census, Missouri Office of Administration (1998). *Available http://www.oseda.missouri.edu.historidata/ popsqmi/29221.htm* (June, 1998).

Warren, J.J. (1992). Ethical concerns about noncompliance in the chronically ill patient. *Progress in Cardiovascular Nursing 7*(4), 10-15.

Weber, B.E. & Reilly, B.M. (1997). Enhancing mammography use in the inner city: A randomized trial of intensive case management. *Archives of Internal Medicine, 157*(20), 2345-2349.

Woolbright, L. A. & Harshbarger, D. S. (1995). The revised certificate of live birth: Analysis of medical risk factor data from birth certificates in Alabama 1988-1992. *Public Health Reports, 110*(1), 59-63.

Williams, J.K. (1994). Behavioral characteristics of children with Turner syndrome and children with learning disabilities. *Western Journal of Nursing Research, 16*(1), 26-39.

Wuest, J. (1993). Removing the shackles: A feminist critique of noncompliance. *Nursing Outlook 41*(5), 217-224.

Pearls

Our Beginnings and Challenges: The First and Second National Conferences on the Classification of Nursing Diagnoses

Kristine M. Gebbie, DrPH, RN, FAAN

Mary Ann Lavin, ScD, RN, CS, FAAN
Contributing to this article:
Joan H. Carter, PhD, RN

Ann Becker, MSN, RN

These brief historical reviews have been titled "pearls," and it is an honor to be describing the first of those pearls to you. I am Kristine Gebbie, currently at Columbia University School of Nursing, and one of the co-conveners of the first nursing diagnosis conference 25 years ago. All analogies are dangerous and the one chosen for these presentations, pearls, is no exception. The image sought is one of the "string of pearls," the lovely piece of jewelry that captures the eye and pleases the imagination. And the opportunity to hear about a sequence of historical events from those who were there provides such a sequence of pleasures. However, the alternative imagery in this analogy is this: pearls grow from an irritant and they rarely grow in perfect symmetry. This, too, is valid analogy. Nursing diagnosis as a taxonomy and an association started from the irritant of information systems that did not capture what nurses identified in patients; and progress toward a complete, useful taxonomic system has been irregular over time and from place to place.

Background

Nursing as a discipline continuously struggles with contradictory and complementary identities. Is nursing an art or a science, and if both, how do they fit together? Is nursing practice a job or profession, and how does the choice between those affect practice? Should nursing develop qualitative or quantitative foundations, and if both, how do we relate these worlds?

Not only does nursing generally exist in a state of tension, so does nursing diagnosis. Nursing diagnosis, as an organized, national (or international) effort to identify and organize a professional terminology, began at a time of tension within nursing. A national commission on nursing and a substantial American Nurses Association-American Medical Association dialogue on joint practice was encouraging nursing to more clearly claim its intellectual basis for practice and to develop a research base for continued growth, while learning to collaborate more effectively with colleagues from other professions. Yet nursing generally was not clear on moving toward baccalaureate education even though higher education was needed for nursing's intellectual base to expand. Further, the distinctions among medical practice, nursing practice, and nurse practitioner practice were not clearly defined in many minds and caused extensive contention within nursing and between nursing and medicine.

1973 was also a time of a major surge toward computerization in health care settings, including efforts to develop computer-based diagnosis or problem lists. Institutions were encouraging automated systems for recording and tracking physician orders, supply orders, and pharmaceuticals, but the nursing data included was in narrative form, if it was included at all.

There was also substantial unrest throughout the system triggered by an surge in the costs of medical care in general and Medicare. The initial emergence of managed systems of care, diagnosis-related group reimbursement schemes and comprehensive health planning had both individual health professionals and hospitals anxious about the future and seeking changes to provide assurance about continuing viability.

Calling the First Conference

The major concern at St. Louis University School of Nursing about calling the first conference was a simple one: Would anyone come? This was at the top of the list because of the bold nature of the announced purpose and the lack of financial support for meeting or travel costs. In addition, we wondered if we could own a process rather than a product. That is, could we keep focus on finding a way for the profession as a whole to contribute to, "own" and use a taxonomy, rather than focus on the specific diagnostic

terms or the framework into which they were classified? This was difficult, given the clinical interests and investments of those of us involved with convening the meeting.

Further, we wondered if we could compress three to four hundred years into ten or twenty. Medicine had been developing its taxonomy, the International Classification of Diseases, over several centuries. Nursing probably did not have the luxury of that time, if it wished to have a diagnosis-based, practical, research-adaptable, and clinically useful computer-based records within the twentieth century.

There were more complex questions as well that had to be answered in order to structure the dialogue at that first meeting. We knew we could not satisfy everyone in the profession, yet we wanted the output to be intelligible to many nurses. Without that, the new nursing diagnosis terminology would quickly fade into the background along with other vocabulary or practice fads. This meant that compromises were needed and that whatever the results would be, they would probably be too empirical for the researcher, too inconsistent for the theorist, and too abstract for the clinician. In fact, achieving some measurable progress toward all of these "compromises" could be a sign of success for the gathering!

There would also be tension between detail and precision in contrast to breadth. It seemed most important that at least one diagnostic label be identified within each area of nursing practice to increase the taxonomy's breadth of interest in application and further development. That probably meant the first diagnostic labels would actually be labels for whole groups or clusters of conditions. At this first meeting, there would not be time to clarify the components of any one cluster.

A major struggle anticipated, and one that occurred, was that between re-invention and common sense. For example, there was serious debate about what to call the process that nurses engage in when comparing clinical observations with clinical concepts and when labeling the condition or state of the patient that demands nursing attention. A short time earlier the term "trophicognosis" had been proposed as a way of assuring ourselves as nurses and our medical colleagues that we were not trespassing into their world. The dictionary prevailed: Diagnosing is a process not unique to any discipline or field of endeavor and it is the right word for what was under discussion.

It took longer to sort out and clarify that nursing diagnosis labels were not intended to be new names for already known and labeled medical conditions, even for use in situations where the medical condition was identified by a nurse or nurse practitioner. There is no need (and in fact it would be inappropriate) to call otitis media something else within a nursing diagnosis taxonomy.

Finally, we had to decide how to start the process, given 5 days with 95 nurses, of whom 50% were clinicians, 25% educators, and 25% researchers. After extensive debate within the planning committee, we chose 10 "body systems" (e.g., gastrointestinal, genito-urinary) as the way to divide the group into working committees. Participants were asked to look at any nursing condition (that is, a condition identified by nurses, not conditions in nurses) related to that body system, whether from developmental, environmental, physiological, psychological, or sociological perspectives. Further, prevention, acute care, long-term care and rehabilitation were all appropriate foci, either collectively or individually. And these starting points worked:

Somewhere between 29 and 300 diagnoses, depending on how you count the application of modifiers, were labeled, defined and "classified" alphabetically that first week.

Diffusion of the Nursing Diagnosis Movement

Earlier, I mentioned that nursing was struggling with the relationship between quantitative and qualitative approaches to research and development. Perhaps one reason the process got off to a good start is that both were present: so far, you have heard from the qualitative half of the team. Mary Ann Lavin will now present some quantitative data about the diffusion of the nursing diagnostic movement.

Diffusion from a Rip Van Winkle Point of View

Muy bien venidos a la ciudad de San Luis y a la Conferencia de NANDA a todos los que hablan Castellano. An equally sincere welcome to all who speak English. I wish I could welcome everyone here in his or her own language, but know that you are all most welcome.

I am delighted and honored to be here today. As you know, my name is Mary Ann Lavin and I co-coordinated the First National Conference on the Classification of Nursing Diagnoses with Kristine Gebbie in 1973. At that time, I was enrolled at Harvard School of Public Health, working toward a master's of science degree in Health Services Administration. In 1974 I enrolled in the doctor of science degree program in health services administration. I completed my doctoral research in May of 1978, graduated from Harvard School of Public Health in June of 1978, and entered a cloistered, contemplative monastery the same month, where I remained for sixteen years.

Kris Gebbie and I kept in contact throughout those years. Although we discussed personal, national, and international events in our correspondence, we did not discuss nursing diagnoses. So, when I left the monastery in the fall of 1994, I had a most real Rip Van Winkle experience: The nursing diagnosis movement had spread worldwide. My interest in its diffusion began at that time. I had the good fortune of working on faculty with Dr. Joan Carter, whose doctoral research utilized Roger's Theory of Diffusion. With a few adaptations, we applied his thinking to the diffusion of the nursing diagnosis movement, and examined not only our beginnings but how far we have traveled in the ensuing years.

The Beginning

The idea for a First National Conference on the Classification of Nursing Diagnoses occurred in this way. In 1972 and 1973, Saint Louis University Hospital was beginning to computerize its patient information system. Its nursing department was interested in developing the capability of entering, accessing, and using nursing data in a manner that would best reflect nursing's contribution to patient well-being. When told that medicine planned on entering data by medical diagnosis, Kris and I suggested we enter data by nursing diagnosis. The fact that we had no list or classification of nursing diagnoses presented a "little" problem, however. At odd intervals, Kris and I discussed the notion of nursing diagnoses. Our discussion culminated around 4:30 or 5:00 p.m. one evening in our Cardiovascular Nursing Laboratory. As I recall, Kris said something to the effect that the idea of nursing diagnosis was good, but nurses do not diagnose — or at least nurses will argue they do not diagnose. I responded with the following

series of points: a.) nurses diagnose — in fact, they diagnose all the time; b.) a diagnosis is simply a conclusion flowing from nursing assessment; and c.) if nurses did not diagnose, they could not intervene, in coronary care units or elsewhere. "Great," Kris responded, "since we can't be the only ones having a problem with how to computerize nursing data, let's call a conference on classifying nursing diagnoses. We'll call it the First National Conference on the Classification of Nursing Diagnoses." Amazed at the leap in thought, I asked, "How can we do that? We are just two nurses without a national organization behind us. How can we call it a "national" conference? "Well," Kris said, "we will just invite nurse experts from every region of the United States. Then, the conference will be national."

Within a year and with the support of the Dean and Faculty of Saint Louis University, the First National Conference on the Classification of Nursing Diagnosis was held in the Jefferson Hotel in Saint Louis, Missouri. Ninety-five nurses attended from every region of the United States. Figure 1 illustrates the distribution of participants at the conference, and Table 1 presents a frequency count of the number of participants by state and region.

Part of the success of the First Conference may be due to its underlying assumptions (Table 2). The first dealt with the Conference's underlying theme, and the second the decision rules that guided our choice of participants from among the applicants. The latter was important because we needed national representation not only to legitimize naming it a national conference but to disseminate its outcomes nationally. We knew we needed theorists, educators, and researchers; but because diagnoses are clinical in nature, we decided to weigh participation in

Table 1

Frequency Count of 95 Participants at the First National Conference on the Classification of Nursing Diagnoses

South & Southwest (N=22)	Northeast (N=24)	Midwest (N=36)	West, & Hawaii (N=13)
Alabama (n=1)	Maine (n=1)	Illinois (n=6)	California (n=4)
Florida (n=2)	Maryland (n=1)	Iowa (n=3)	Hawaii (n=1)
Kentucky (n=2)	Massachusetts (n=6)	Kansas (n=7)	Oregon (n=1)
Oklahoma (n=2)	New Hampshire (n=3)	Michigan (n=3)	Utah (n=3)
North Carolina (n=1)	New Jersey (n=3)	Minnesota (n=1)	Washington (n=4)
South Carolina (n=3)	New York (n=6)	Missouri (n=10)	
Tennessee (n=2)	Pennsylvania (n=1)	Nebraska (n=1)	
Texas (n=8)	Rhode Island (n=3)	Ohio (n=2)	
Virginia (n=1)		South Dakota (n=1)	
		Wisconsin (n=2)	

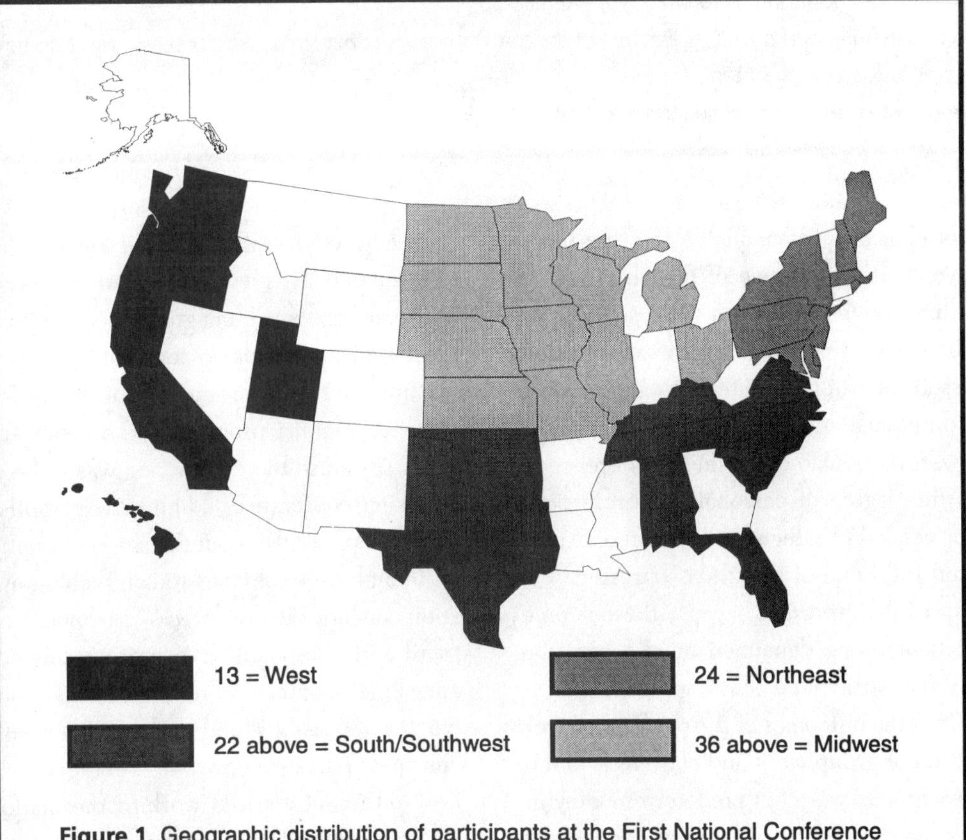

Figure 1. Geographic distribution of participants at the First National Conference on the Classification of Nursing Diagnoses.

Table 2

Assumptions Underlying the First National Conference on the Classification of Nursing Diagnoses

1. To compete in an increasingly computerized health care system, nursing must have a language capable of being computerized.
2. In addition to representing each region of the United States, participants need to represent each section of nursing: a.) practice, education, and research, with added weight given to nursing practice; b.) nursing theorists; c.) nursing specialties; and 4.) care and cure sides of the nursing continuum.
3. Every participant's viewpoint is a valid expression of that person's expert nursing experience.
4. All viewpoints are valid.
5. All participants are competent, committed professionals.
6. Conference outcomes are a function of the conference's group work and are not predetermined by its coordinators.
7. Conference outcomes demand consensus of participants. Diagnoses that do not achieve consensus are to be excluded from this round of consideration.
8. A successful group needs facilitators not for content purposes but to facilitate process, which in turn facilitates task accomplishment.
9. Administrative/secretarial support is critical.

favor of clinicians to encourage their participation even in the presence of theorists, such as Roy, King, and Orem.

The third through fifth assumptions addressed the intended interpersonal milieu of the Conference. As with all the assumptions, they were articulated at the Conference to insure the degree of personal and professional respect needed to safeguard freedom of expression and the value of the ideas expressed. This was especially important because the outcomes of the conference depended on the contributions of the participants (Assumption 6).

That the outcomes of the conference were a function of group work and consensus among participants and were not predetermined by the conference coordinators (Assumptions 7 and 8) needed frequent repetition by group facilitators in response to queries such as, "Are we doing this correctly? Is this what you had in mind?" Fortunately, Kris had spent many hours prior to the conference helping group facilitators to redirect such questions so that participants would assume control over and responsibility for conference content, progress, and outcomes.

Because the conference was to be a truly working conference, administrative and secretarial support was mandatory (Assumption 9). Although quite obvious today, such an assumption was not obvious in 1973. It meant moving staff and equipment (typewriters, mimeograph machines, copiers) from Saint Louis University to the Jefferson Hotel and renting a suite for business purposes only.

To continue the work of the conference, an economically self-sustaining organizational structure needed to be created (Assumption 10). Therefore, royalties from the Proceedings of the

Conference (Gebbie and Lavin, 1973) were used for this purpose. To create a structure to carry on the work (Assumption 11), the Saint Louis University Clearinghouse for Nursing Diagnoses was created and maintained by Ann Becker with the support of the Dean, Sister Mary Teresa Noth, until the North American Nursing Diagnosis Association (NANDA) came into its own 1982.

Diffusion Analysis

Rogers (1996) indicates that the important element in diffusion is not that the idea is new as much as that it be perceived as new. In 1973, nursing diagnosis was not a new idea. In 1972, the New York Nurse Practice Act was the first to define nursing as "diagnosing and treating human responses to actual or potential health problems through such means as case finding, health teaching and counseling" (Bullough, 1975, p. 160). In 1969, Abdellah wrote that the ability to make a nursing diagnosis and prescribe actions is fundamental to the development of a nursing science. While the idea of nursing diagnosis was not new at the time of the First National Conference, it was still perceived as new; and the notion of classifying nursing diagnoses was new.

Any innovation is diffused among members of a social system through its channels of communication over time. To analyze the diffusion of nursing diagnoses and their classification five indicators were employed: a.) conference participants, b.) state and international awareness, c.) publications, d.) regulatory inclusion, and e.) electronic media. Each indicator is analyzed below.

Conference Participants

The 1998 NANDA Conference is the thirteenth since 1973. Figure 2 shows the distribution of participants at the first twelve conferences. Conferences were open to all nurses with the exception of the first, which was invitational (personal communication with Ann Becker, July 16, 1998). All conference years, represented in this chart, were sponsored solely by NANDA except for the 1997 joint conference, which was sponsored by NANDA and the University of Iowa faculty involved in the development of Nursing Interventions Classification (NIC) and Nursing Outcomes Classification (NOC).

When speaking of the diffusion of an innovation, Rogers (1995) indicates that the frequency distribution of new adopters usually takes the shape of a normal bell-shaped curve, and a cumulative frequency distribution classically takes the an S-shape. While the distribution of NANDA conference participants speaks to the diffusion of the movement to classify nursing diagnoses, the data is neither discrete as in the case of new adopters only, nor is it cumulative because not all who attended one conference attended the next. Also, rather than being old and new adopters, NANDA conference participants were old and new opinion leaders of the nursing diagnosis movement and its classification, that is, nurses interested enough in the development, classification, and diffusion of nursing diagnoses to participate in its conferences. As a descriptive aid, imagine an S-curve superimposed on the distribution. Note that opinion leader participation began relatively slowly and was then followed by an upsurge of participation, not unlike the surge in a learning curve when a new content area is introduced. This was followed by an a return to a seemingly constant participation level. Thus, the more recent participation level is greater than the initial involvement but less than that which occurred during the years of surge. This initial

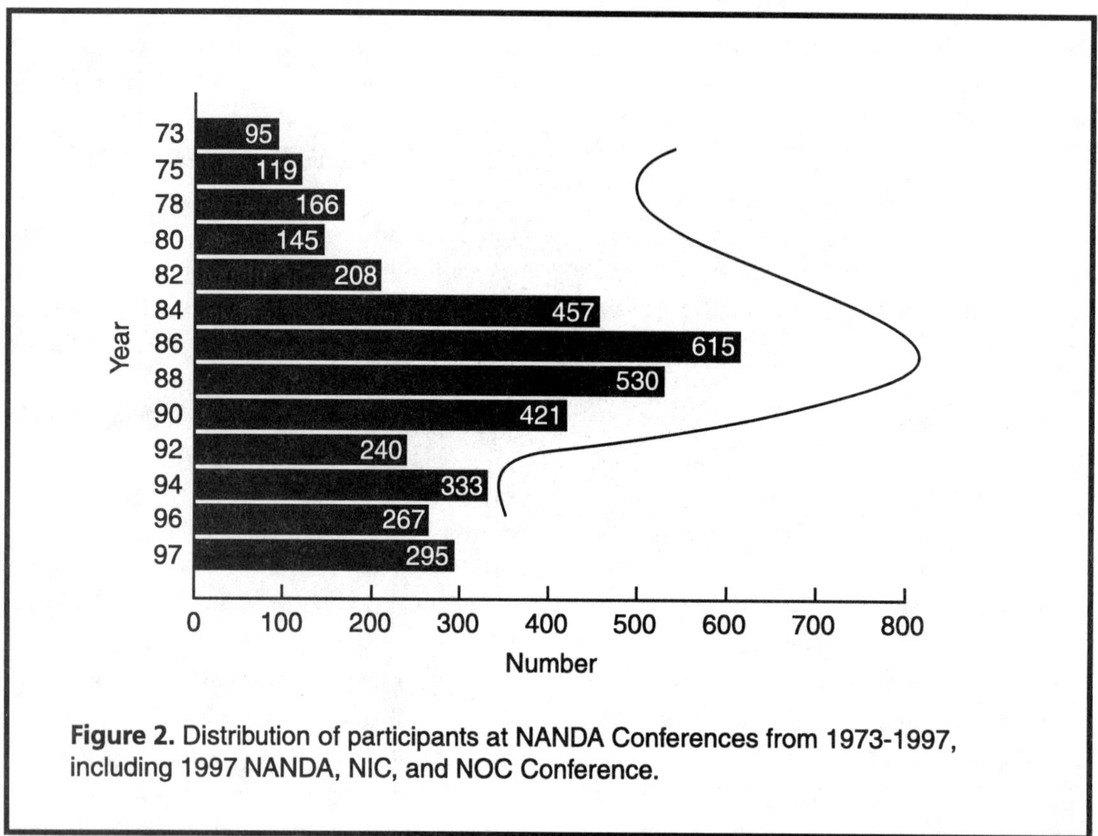

Figure 2. Distribution of participants at NANDA Conferences from 1973-1997, including 1997 NANDA, NIC, and NOC Conference.

upswing, surge, and subsequent stabilizing period is roughly S-shaped. This curve does not allow us to predict future trends, but it does provide us with a descriptive picture of the past with which to compare the future.

State and International Awareness

Figure 3 illustrates the number of states and countries represented at the NANDA conferences since 1973. Again, note the frequency distribution of the states represented. It does not represent states that are new adopters, as it too is a mix of old and new; it simply displays the total number of states represented at each conference. Although the distribution is somewhat flatter, it too is S-shaped, with a surge occurring in the years 1984 through 1994. It is too soon to tell whether the number of states represented will change. It is also too early to identify the shape of the developing frequency distribution curve representing countries in attendance. What is apparent is that interest in the development of nursing diagnoses and their classification is widespread nationally and growing internationally.

Publications

A CINAHL literature search between its first reference in November of 1981 to March 1998 reveals there were 2,021 publications when

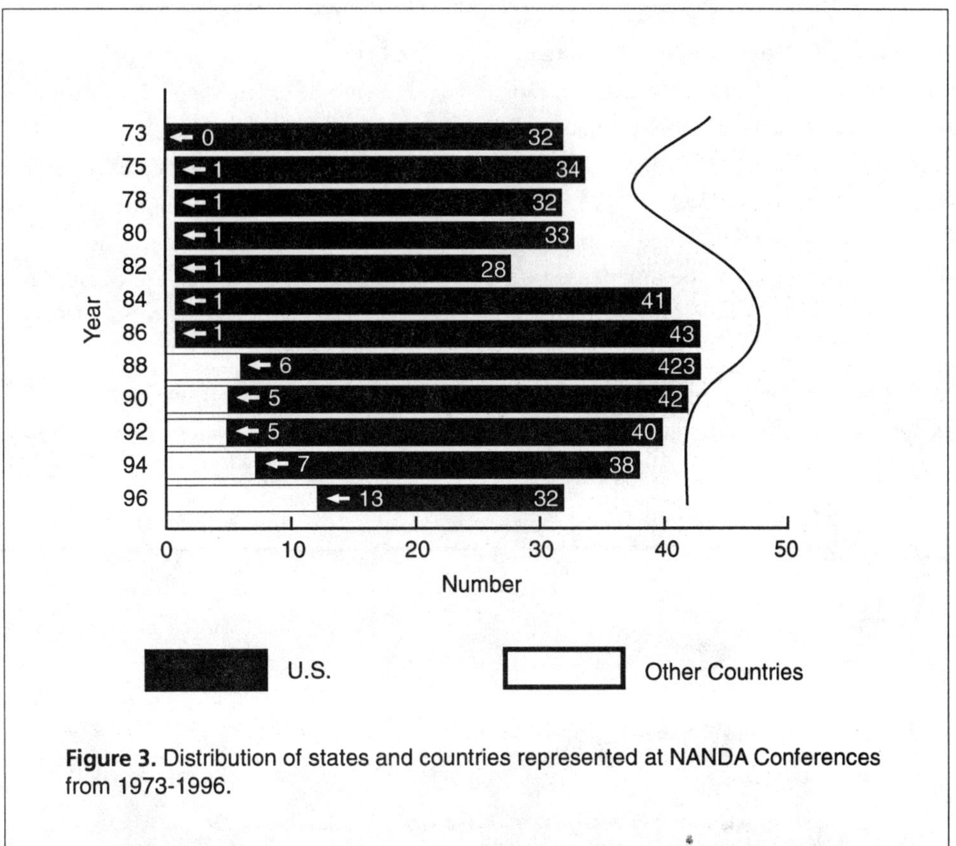

Figure 3. Distribution of states and countries represented at NANDA Conferences from 1973-1996.

combining the textword "nursing diagnosis" or "nursing diagnoses." This averages 129 publications/year during the 17-year period. When entering the same combination of textwords, a Medline search encompassing the years 1966 to April 1998 reveals 1300 publications or an average of 40/year over the 32-year period.

Regulatory Inclusion

Three indicators were used to evaluate the acceptance of nursing diagnoses by regulatory or official organizations that define or help define the practice of nursing. These indicators were acceptance of nursing diagnoses by: a.) the Joint Commission on the Accreditation of Health Care Organizations, b.) State Boards of Nursing in their Practice Acts, and 3.) the National Center for Health Statistics as related to the publication of the International Classification of Diseases, version 10, Clinical Modification (ICD-10-CM).

Although the Joint Commission on the Accreditation of Health Care Organizations (1996, p. Tx-2) speaks of diagnostic testing as part of the assessment process upon patient entry to a health care organization, it does not modify the term "diagnostic" by the words "medical" or "nursing." In its section on information management (1966, p. IM-2), it speaks generically of patient needs and clinical decision making. However, in the same section, it indicates that one example of appropriate management of nursing information would be "nursing care data related to patient assessment, nursing diagnosis or patient needs, nursing interventions and patient outcomes (that) are permanently integrated into the medical record" (1996, p. IM-21).

The second indicator of regulatory inclusion involves an evaluation of the practice acts of all 50 states (Lavin, Hegamin-Younger, Carlson, & Meyer, 1997). Operational definitions were developed to group practice acts in one of four ways, according to their:

1.) use of the two terms "nursing diagnoses" together;

2.) use of the term "diagnosis" without the modifier "nursing," but within a nursing context;

3.) defining the practice of registered nursing as including the performance of acts of "medical diagnosis".

4.) obvious avoidance or complete absence of reference to nursing diagnosis.

Figure 4 illustrates the distribution of states divided into each of these four categories. That the majority of states include nursing diag-

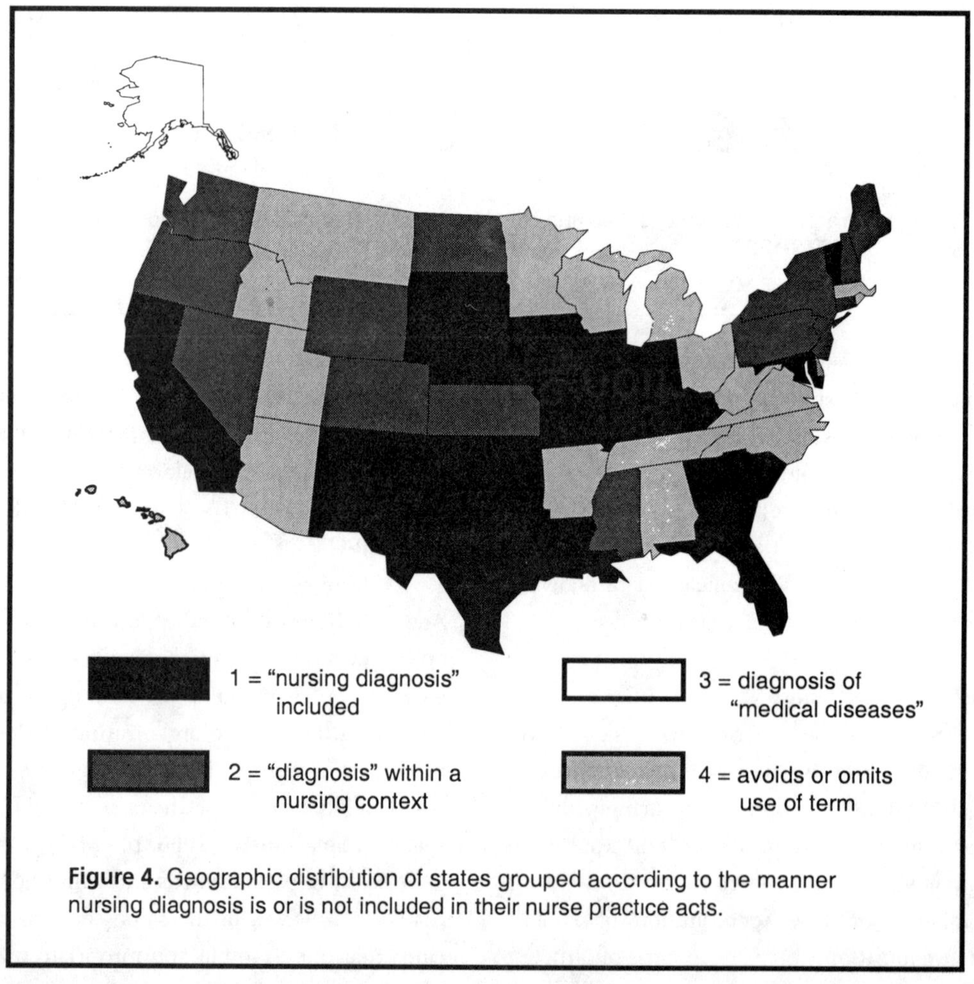

Figure 4. Geographic distribution of states grouped according to the manner nursing diagnosis is or is not included in their nurse practice acts.

nosis in their nurse practice acts is an example of regulatory acceptance of this nursing activity.

Acceptance of nursing diagnoses by regulatory groups within the larger health professional community is also evident. The International Classification of Diseases, version 9, Clinical Modification (ICD-9-CM) is used in the United States for reimbursement, epidemiological studies, and other purposes. According to an American Nurses Association electronic report of June 16, 1998, 90-95% of nursing diagnoses/problems from the NANDA list of nursing diagnoses, the Omaha System Problem List, and the Home Health Care Classification set of nursing diagnoses are already captured by the ICD-9-CM version. The "problematic" diagnoses are the "risk for" and "potential for" diagnoses, but staff at the National Center for Health Statistics believe that these problems may be solved by developing special coding guidelines for nursing diagnoses so that they, too, may be included in the ICD-10-CM version. This recognition gives further evidence of the successful diffusion of nursing diagnoses, legitimizes their use in the world of interdisciplinary and multidisciplinary practice, and has important reimbursement, policy, educational, and research implications.

Electronic Media

There is an abundance of information on the Internet. Although the amount of information on any one subject varies daily, it is possible to obtain insight into the diffusion of a concept by performing a search on any one day. An Alta Vista Simple Query, using the search words "nursing diagnosis" in all languages, performed on April 22, 1998, the evening before this presentation at the NANDA Conference, revealed more than 900,000 matches. Such searches of the electronic media document that the nursing diagnosis is a concept disseminated worldwide.

From the Past and Present into the Future

The purpose of this pearl is to show something of the beginnings of NANDA and the national and international impact of the nursing diagnosis movent during the past twenty-five years. I turn the podium back to Kristine Gebbie to discuss the challenges that the future presents.

The Challenges

The first of these challenges is the continuing confusion between a decision to develop or use nursing diagnostic terminology with something of a religious commitment to an absolute. While Mary Ann and I and the others involved in the early conferences support and encourage the use of nursing diagnosis, no one should be bound to use the proffered terms if they do not apply and every nurse involved in diagnosing should be thinking critically about improvements.

A second confusion is what appears to be the nursing diagnosis version of a recurrent nursing tendency to adopt products without process. In this case, it has taken the form in all too many practice sites or schools of nursing to push the use of some set of diagnostic labels without the prerequisite diagnostic thinking. "Get a label into the box on the care plan" takes precedence over thinking through the presenting signs and symptoms in order to draw a useful conclusion on which to plan care.

Moving On

The result of the first conference was that the stage was set for a continued effort on the part of the profession. The style of the publication from the proceedings of the second national conference was an attempt make the nature of the process as a "work in progress" visible: more a workbook than a conference proceedings.

There were also early efforts to develop support for research that would clarify and expand the taxonomy. Marge Gordon and I developed what I still believe is an elegant model of a multi-site epidemiological study of the incidence and prevalence of diagnoses. In 1974 and 1975 there was little understanding of the reason for the question, much less the validity of the design.

The profession continues to struggle with issues that were visible in the themes of the first conferences: Does a workable taxonomy demand allegiance to a single theory? How much research and of what kind is needed to allow entry of a diagnostic label into our vocabulary? And how do we take the need for breadth and common sense into account while moving toward a higher level of scientific clarity and purity? How do advanced practice nurses make use of this more traditional nursing line of thought while carrying out their roles that require use of a medical diagnostic label? These are just some of the challenges we face. It will be interesting to see how well we face them in the next twenty-five years.

It was and still is an honor to be associated with nursing diagnosis, and with Mary Ann Lavin, and to share these "pearls" with you.

References

Abdellah, F.G. (1969). The nature of nursing science. *Nursing Research, 18*(5), 390-393.

Alaska Statutes and Regulations (1996). *Nursing, Article 6, General Provisions, Section 4 1 0, Definitions, Sec. AS 08.68.410, 8(F).*

American Nurses Association (1998). *Developing ideas: Nursing diagnoses are part of ICD-9-CM and the new ICD-10-CM.* Available:http://www.nursingworld.org/pulse/idea2.htm (June 16, 1998).

Bullough, B. (1975). *The law and the expanding nursing role.* New York: Appleton-Century-Crofts.

Chetnik, T. (1969). Diagnoza pielegniarska. *Peilegniarka I Polozna, 2,* 14-15.

Colorado Board of Nursing (1995). *Nurse Practice Act, Article 12, Section 12-38-03, Definitions (10)(a).*

Gebbie, K. & Lavin, M.A. (1974).Classifying nursing diagnoses. *American Journal of Nursing, 74*(2), 250-253.

Gordon, M. (1973). Information processing strategies in nursing diagnosis. *Nursing Research Conference* (9), 387-406.

Horta, W. de A. (1967). Consideracoes sobre o diagnostico de enfermagem. *Revista Brasileira de Enfermagem, 20*(1), 7-13.

Joint Commission on Accreditation of Health Care Organizations (1996). *Comprehensive accreditation manual for hospitals: the official handbook.* Oakbrook Terrace, Illinois: author.

Kim, D.H. (1970). [Nursing diagnosis] Taehan Kanho. *Korean Nurse, 9*(5), 59-64.

Lavin, M. A., Hegamin-Younger, C., Carlson, J., & Meyer, G. (1997). *Unpublished presentation at the 24th Annual Research Conference,* Saint Louis University School of Nursing.

Lesnik, M.J. & Anderson, B.E. (1947). *Legal aspects of nursing.* Philadelphia: J. B. Lippincott Company.

Levine, M.E. (1965). Trophicognosis: An alternative to nursing diagnosis. *ANA Clinical Conferences, 2,* 55-70.

Mori, H., Koyama, K., Takaguchi, E., Furuya,

Y., &Nakanishi, H. (1972). Discussion: Approach to nursing diagnosis. *Kangogaku Zasshi, Japanese Journal of Nursing, 36*(5), 588-601.

Montana State Board of Nursing (1996). *Statutes and Rules Relating to Nursing, Chapter 8, Nursing, Part 1, Section 37-8-102, (5)(b).*

New Mexico Board of Nursing (1995). *State of New Mexico Nursing Practice Act, Chapter 61, Article 3, Section 2. Definitions.*

New Jersey Board of Nursing (1995). *Nursing Practice Act, 45:11-23. Definitions.*

Paz Sifuentes, M., Rodriguez, M.L., & De la Luz Rodriguez, M. (1974). Editorial: Diagnostico de enfermeria. *Archivos del Instituto de Cardiologia de Mexico, 44*(2), 169-171.

Rogers, E.M. (1995). *Diffusion of Innovations.* New York: The Free Press.

Pearl: The Fifth NANDA Conference

Marjory Gordon, PhD, RN, FAAN

In 1982, at the Fifth Conference for Classification of Nursing Diagnoses, NANDA was born. The nine years, 1973-1982, of the NANDA's "pre-natal" growth were exciting and challenging. It was the end of a developmental process when the North American Nursing Diagnosis Association evolved out of the National Group for Classification of Nursing Diagnoses in 1982.

Prior to 1982 there was a Task Force of the National Group and I was its chairperson; many of you were on its Steering Committee that year when NANDA was born: Ann Becker, Audrey Mc Lane, Trudy McFarland, Sylvia Weber, Dorothea Jakob, Kristine Gebbie, and others. Let me tell you how the Task Force that evolved into the NANDA came to be — we have Harriet Werley to thank for that. The story will be an all too familiar experience for many of you — you know, one suggests something and you end up being the chair of a committee. Allow me to go off on a tangent to describe the start of the National Task Force.

At the First Conference there was so much enthusiasm for the development and classification of nursing diagnoses. Everyone was very excited about the idea — in the 1970s there were not that many conferences that dealt with the content of practice. Toward the middle of the First Conference on Classification, one of the conference coordinators, Kristine Gebbie, asked four people to present some thoughts on the relevance of nursing diagnosis on the last day. I was asked to do 15 minutes on the relevance of nursing diagnosis to research. Callista Roy commented on education, Mary Duffy presented thoughts on legalities of practice, and Peggy Chinn talked about the relevance of nursing diagnosis to nursing practice. A few months before the conference I presented my dissertation entitled "Probabilistic Concept Attainment: A Study of Nursing Diagnoses" at an ANA Research Conference; I thought this was why I got an invitation to the first diagnosis conference but later found out it was because of a publication on assessment of activity tolerance.

I ended my speech on the relevance of nursing diagnosis to nursing research and the relevance of research to nursing diagnosis with a comment about the great enthusiasm we all felt at this first conference and that it must not be lost when we all departed. We needed to establish a committee. This committee could develop a mechanism for continuing the work that began at that first conference. Well you know what happens when you suggest a committee. Dr. Harriet Werley got up and, as only she can do, suggested that I do just that — organize a committee to plan another conference in two years. I did and this was the start of National Task Force in 1973. It grew and matured sufficiently well to develop the structure for the NANDA that was born nine years later in 1982.

The National Task Force

The new organization already had many things in place. Prior to 1982 the Task Force had spent nine years developing ways to promote the classification system and had established a clearinghouse for information on nursing diagnosis at St. Louis University. Dr. Ann Becker was the coordinator. In the early years the Clearinghouse played a major role in the dissemination and exchange of information both nationally and internationally. It served to inform many nurses of the developing diagnostic classification system and resources available for helping with implementation. The Task Force also established liaisons with national nursing organizations, planned biennial conferences, published a newsletter (*NDx*), stimulated education programs, and promoted the development of state and regional groups that would encourage implementation and research. Two of the early state groups were the one started in Massachusetts by Rosemary Harvey and the one

in Wisconsin in collaboration with the Wisconsin Nurses Association — Audrey McLane was in Wisconsin at that time.

The North American Nursing Diagnosis Association

The birth of the formal organization for classification in 1982 was a result of the commitment and perseverance of those early leaders. They donated their time and financed their attendance at meetings. There was no money for Task Force activities. The focus of the new organization that they created was to develop, refine, and promote a taxonomy of nursing diagnostic terminology of general use to professional nurses. This focus was evident in its working committees: Diagnosis Review, Taxonomy, Research, Program, Publications, Membership, Public Relations, and Nominations.

Driving forces that led to the establishment of NANDA were the growth of the development and classification effort and money. It took money to coordinate the development of a diagnostic classification system for North America. Federal funding was sought by Kristine Gebbie and I who met in a hotel room and wrote a grant one weekend. It was commended for its design but the topic, nursing diagnosis, was deemed too controversial. A few years later Mi Ja Kim submitted, without success as well. Thus, we thought that an incorporated association, such as NANDA, could attract private funding and donations to support the work of diagnosis review and classification. (It has taken 25 years to see that come to fruition with the NANDA Foundation.)

The Revolution/Evolution

In spite of the shortsightedness of some, nursing diagnosis was an idea that was about to revolutionize practice in the 1980s in two ways — the content of practice and its process. Consider for a moment the times. In the early 1970s most nurses focused on patient needs: need for teaching, need for emotional support. The needs described patients in terms of nurses' work or nurses' objectives such as those described by Abdellah's 21 Problems. Nurses talked about need for suctioning or need for teaching. The evolution in thought that nursing diagnosis stimulated was a focus on the patient's condition, as opposed to the caregiver's actions. This was a tremendous step for the profession and its clinicians, educators, and researchers to take.

Nursing diagnosis turned practice "on its head." It required that one identify why an intervention was selected. Now it was "why does the patient need suctioning?" and the answer: "because of ineffective airway clearance." Nursing diagnosis encouraged the focus of thinking to move from the notion of a work-task to a conceptualization of a health-related condition. The concept applied to patients, families, and communities. The tremendous transition in thinking that diagnostic concepts produced was that once the focus was on the patient's condition, many interventions "came to mind," not just suctioning. This served to improve the delivery of care. Nursing diagnosis was a tool for thinking at a time when documentation was characterized by statements such as "appears to be bleeding" or "appears to be dead."

In addition to the revolution in clinical focus was the revolution in process. Nurses began to realize that if they accepted the idea of nursing diagnosis to describe their practice, they also made a commitment to attend to their clinical reasoning and judgment skills. In 1970, when New York stated in its practice act that nursing was the diagnosis and treatment of

human responses and when Gebbie and Lavin called the first conference on classification of nursing diagnoses in 1973, and when ANA published the Standards of Practice in 1974, and the ANA Social Policy statement in 1980, it was clear that nurses made clinical judgments. The handmaiden era was dead! I don't believe that the influence of nursing diagnosis has been clearly described, particularly the effect on it has had on practice and on nursing science.

In 1982, nursing diagnosis was an exciting new concept that helped nurses talk about and think about their practice. Those in clinical practice recognized the usefulness of nursing diagnosis long before most educators and certainly long before most researchers — who, today, are still reticent to conceptualize their research in a more precise way using diagnostic concepts. It wasn't until the 1980s that most educators started to give nursing diagnosis a place in the curriculum and to purposefully teach clinical reasoning and judgment. From my observations at the time, the group that sustained the work on nursing diagnosis 1973-1982 were the nurses in practice. They were able to see the immediate benefits. It was also a benefit that in the early years there was a nice balance in the classification effort between clinicians and educators. Now just as a backdrop it is interesting to raise the question of what nurses were talking about in 1982. With the ANA Standards of Practice containing Standard II that "Nursing diagnoses are derived from health status data" and the ANA Social Policy Statement defining nursing as "the diagnosis and treatment of human responses" there was great interest in the identification and classification of nursing diagnoses. Controversy swirled around the definition of a nursing diagnosis and so there was interest in the paper presented by Joyce Shoemaker at the

Fifth Conference on a Delphi study to define nursing diagnosis. In later years when NANDA established its definition of nursing diagnosis much of her work was used. There was much discussion about a way of organizing the diagnoses in a classification system. By 1982 the question of do nurses diagnose had decreased in frequency and "what will the doctors say" was hardly heard at all. The major question was "How do you implement nursing diagnosis?" Many of the papers at the Fifth Conference were devoted to this topic in education and practice. At the Fifth Conference Callista Roy gave a paper summarizing the seven years work of the Theorist Group. From this work the NANDA taxonomy evolved under the direction of Phyllis Kritek who chaired the Taxonomy and Diagnosis committees.

NANDA has always been "pulled" by the call of the clinicians for more and more diagnoses on the one hand and on the other hand the call of the science for clear and precise diagnostic concepts. The years that we drifted more to science and research we encountered the ire of the clinicians for being exclusive and slow to approve diagnoses. In the years when we drifted toward the pragmatic, everyday needs we were criticized by the researchers and a number of nursing leaders. By 1982 we were starting to blend these two forces and have the confidence to find our own synthesis.

Three Conferences, Three Pearls: The Janus View, The Gateway to Scientific Practice, Clinical Judgement and Decision Making: The Future with Nursing Diagnosis

Winnifred C. Mills, RN MEd

To review conferences past requires sorting through personal notes made during those experiences and then rereading the proceedings emanating from each. What a pleasure that provides! There is a certain nostalgia attached to this exercise, as we revisit the authors of the papers, posters and dialogue therein. It is like spending time with a group of great NANDA friends, as each page reintroduces one to a past happy encounter. There is an element of subjectivity attached to such a review however — the author admits that with such a richness of material to choose from, biases occur — but efforts have been made to highlight that which is most significant for NANDA progress in the future.

How eagerly we awaited the publication of each volume! NANDA has been blessed by presenters representative of the very best minds in nursing in the 20th century. Some of these have openly challenged the beliefs of NANDA participants, engendering useful dialogue on issues, such as etiology, which continue to concern us. Also, we have benefited from the scholarly efforts of editors who are themselves NANDA participants and from publishers who have been supportive of our movement on the very frontier of modern nursing practice. They have given a second life — perhaps immortality — to the collection of work from each conference. We owe a debt of gratitude to each for their significant contribution to our history.

To prepare this paper a framework of three questions was used, against which the conference activities and proceedings were examined:

- What were the objectives for the conference?
- What happened?
- What did we learn?

The Janus View: The Sixth Conference, 1984

Objectives

The sixth conference was the first held under the auspices of the new North American Nursing Diagnosis Association (NANDA) since its inception in 1982. Accordingly, a Program

Committee, chaired by Audrey McLane, organized the event. It was planned to assist participants to review and appreciate the origins of the organization; and then to look forward to prepare for the future. The conference proceedings were ably compiled for publication by editor Mary Hurley.

What happened?

The conference was held in St Louis, at the Chase/Park Plaza Hotel, April 4-6, 1984. The largest group of participants to date — 460 nurses — gathered to discuss nursing diagnosis. For some participants, the numbers present may have seemed overwhelming. Original task force members were accustomed to familiar faces in small work groups where intense inductive generation of diagnoses was the pattern of activity directed towards achieving consensus. Bylaws of the new organization determined that a new approach to the approval of diagnoses was to be developed, precluding the previous approach. Although 25 new diagnoses had been submitted, no formal mechanism for their review or approval had as yet been submitted to the membership.

During the course of the conference 21 formal papers were presented and 18 posters were available for viewing. Regional groups from 16 areas met to discuss their needs and goals and 10 Special Interest Groups met for the first time. The first business meeting of the new NANDA was convened by President Marjorie Gordon and the first reports were received from eight committees named in the bylaws. The Publications Committee clarified NANDA's interest in having nursing diagnosis and the taxonomy in the public domain. The program committee announced an Awards Ceremony to honour five of the early initiators of nursing diagnosis work. Recipients of an award included Kristine Gebbie, Mary Ann Lavin (in absentia), Sister Theresa Noth, Sister Callista Roy and Marjorie Gordon.

What did we learn?

Mi Ja Kim, in her keynote address, looked back to the period of skepticism and criticism attendant upon the early use of the term "nursing diagnosis." Nurses' right and obligation to diagnose was established in the Social Policy Statement of the American Nurses' Association (ANA). It was, therefore, incumbent upon NANDA to fulfill its objectives and to identify valid, reliable diagnoses through adequate research and to build these into a scientifically acceptable taxonomy — an effort not without peril, she suggested. Developing standardized nomenclature would be imperative in the future, she stated, as would clarification of the concept of etiology as used in relation to nursing diagnosis.

Norma Lang reviewed the relationship of NANDA and ANA, particularly the ANA Committee on Nursing Practice Phenomena. Clearly, collaboration was of interest and potential benefit to both organizations in furthering the fulfilment of the Social Policy Statement. Productive outcomes were anticipated for the future.

Phyllis Kritek revisited the taxonomic work done to date. In pointing to tasks still to be accomplished she suggested that hierarchical partitions might be better replaced by "cover sets" in a revised taxonomy. This theoretical approach supports a multidimensional network of concepts, allowing some overlap in relationships — a possible advantage in future considerations of NANDA's classification task.

Marjory Gordon addressed the concern

arising from lack of refinement among the current 62 diagnostic categories. Absence of clear operational definitions and defining characteristics was paramount here. Users experienced difficulty in specifying etiologic factors and there was a need to differentiate between risk and cause for diagnoses described as potential.

Many other presenters challenged our thinking. Among them, Franklin Schaffer introduced us to Diagnostic Related Groups (DRG's), and Lucille Joel challenged us to recognize the potential and initiate efforts to determine nurse resource measurement based on nursing diagnoses related to specific DRG's. Margaret Grier left us with what she referred to as "big ideas," some of which included development of computerized nursing information systems. We've come a long way down that round in the ensuing 14 years!

Participants were tired but exuberant at the close of this conference. It was clear from evaluations that many previous conference participants wanted to see the small work group activity reinstated in the future. For others, this was a first time experience of a major conference on nursing diagnosis and it was an important learning experience. For the Board and the Program Committee, the conference was an organizational and financial success.

The Gateway to Scientific Practice: The Seventh Conference, 1986
Objectives
"The purpose of this conference is to examine developments in the evolution of a taxonomy for nursing diagnosis and its relevance for nursing practice. The conference will provide a forum for nurses to share information related to nursing diagnoses in the areas of practice, research and education." (NANDA Program Committee report to the Board, March 22, 23, 1985.) Six more specific objectives followed, including networking and exploration of etiologies.

What happened?
Over 600 participants were welcomed to the Omni International Hotel in St. Louis by President Marjory Gordon for the 7th Conference, March 9-12, 1986. Eleven invited papers were offered and an overwhelming response to the call for abstracts resulted in the choice of 47 scientific papers and 27 poster presentations. Representatives of 8 regional groups met twice during the conference, and 71 nurses participated in 11 Special Interest Groups.

The Diagnosis Review Committee conducted the first assembly review of submissions using the new Submission/Development Guidelines for new diagnoses, resulting in approval of 22 new diagnoses for inclusion in the approved list. The review cycle for new diagnoses was also explained to participants.

An historic achievement of this conference was the endorsement of the Human Response Patterns, first initiated by the nurse theorist group, as the organizing framework for Taxonomy 1. The process of organizing diagnoses coded numerically under patterns, rather than depicted graphically, was explained for the assembly.

What did we learn?
In the keynote address Myrtle Aydelotte reviewed the history of nursing knowledge. She reminded us of Bertha Harmer's contribution, in 1926, of a text directing us to a scientific process for nursing practice. The keynote differentiated between taxonomy and classification and emphasized the need for standardization of nomenclature, based on defined, clinically vali-

dated and reliable diagnostic data.

Marjory Gordon's address further emphasized this evident need for both quantitative and qualitative research, to establish the validity and reliability of individual diagnoses and also to identify the occurrence of diagnoses in various populations. She informed participants of efforts of ANA to seek inclusion of nursing elements in the next revised classification of diseases published by the World Health Organization (WHO).

Harriet Werley provided a thorough explanation of the work done to formulate a Nursing Minimum Data Set (NMDS). She discussed the importance of nursing diagnosis as part of that data set and explained the potential benefits of implementing the NMDS. She reiterated the importance of ANA's approach to WHO via the Center for Classification of Diseases in North America.

Kristine Gebbie provided a cogent, yet realistic overview of the challenges to nurses' possibilities for reimbursement based on nursing diagnoses. As a nurse grounded in the reality of clinical practice, she outlined obstacles in the present delivery system, including the disinclination of some nurses to use a system of documentation so cumbersome and so controversial as NANDA nursing diagnoses. As a manager, her awareness of public beliefs and political factors provided an objective view of nurses who 'diagnose'. This dose of reality was finely tempered by her enduring commitment to the belief that nursing diagnosis will be a valuable way to document practice for nurses who wish to clarify their contribution to reduced morbidity and mortality. From the beginning, Kristine Gebbie has functioned as the conscience of the nursing diagnosis movement. Her paper is as relevant today in its views of nursing as it was in

1986. Her words bear rereading as they continue to be a lesson in reality for us all.

The summary of the seventh conference, in the Proceedings prepared by editor Audrey McLane, provides a fascinating historical review of NANDA's accomplishments and of the threads she has perceived weaving throughout the fabric of the first seven conferences. Among these recurring themes the following issues were apparent: the pressing need for sufficient quality research to establish beyond scientific doubt the validity and reliability of the existing nursing diagnoses; clarification of the critical defining characteristics necessary to establish each diagnosis; simplification in the language of the taxonomy to enable general use of the diagnoses in clinical practice; and careful examination of the concept of etiology through research to establish the diagnosis/etiology relationships. Additional considerations include encouragement for the work of establishing a taxonomy of interventions and careful consideration of the impact future technology would have on documentation and the need for the Nursing Minimum Data Set.

Clinical Judgement and Decision Making: The Future with Nursing Diagnosis: Calgary, 1987

Shakespeare said 'There is a tide in the affairs of men which taken at its flood leads on to fortune, ...'' (Macbeth). Perhaps that is the view we might take of the original idea and planning for this conference, in which NANDA members played such a central part. A tripartite agreement between NANDA, a Canadian university faculty of nursing and a Canadian entrepreneurial group made the conference a reality. This was not without consternation on the part of some NANDA Board members, who believed the idea to be ill-conceived and financially too risky. Those NANDA members who participated have since noted that the opportunity to open the door to the world was an auspicious one.

What happened?

In Calgary, Alberta, Canada, May 27-29, 1997, more than 600 participants representing 32 countries and nursing worldwide came together in an international forum to exchange ideas and to dialogue about clinical decision making, clinical judgement, goals for the year 2000, and nursing diagnosis. The openness and friendliness of nurses from so many different backgrounds was inspiring. The sharing of common problems such as describing nursing for the public, for politicians, for physicians and for other nurses confirmed a belief among the sponsors that international nursing has more in common than it has differences worldwide — a notion supported by the International Council of Nurses (ICN). More than 100 papers were presented in six streams. These were clinical practice applications — community health and clinical practice applications; hospital settings; NANDA focus; nursing research; nursing education; and quality assurance/administration. In addition, 50 posters were presented. Proceedings were prepared by an editorial group and distributed to participants in the months following the conference.

What did we learn?

- Nurses around the world are more professionally alike than they are different.
- The problem of describing nursing practice transcends individual language differences.
- Direct translations of words do not always allow for conceptual clarity.

- The advent of computer technology is forcing the issue of standardized language for documentation.
- There is a worldwide interest in the work of NANDA.

Phyllis Kritek, in her closing address to this assembly, stated that "nurses need to create, implement, and perfect models of consensus... The health of the species as a whole depends on it" (Kritek, 1987 p587). Perhaps the Calgary conference was a beginning for that international endeavour.

References

Hannah, K., Reimer, M., Mills, W., & Letorneau, S.. (Eds.) (1997). *Clinical Judgement and Decision Making: The Future with Nursing Diagnosis*. Toronto: John Wiley and Sons.

Kritek, Phyllis. (1997). Risks and realities. In K. Hannah, M. Reimer, W. Mills, S. Letorneau, (Eds.) *Clinical judgement and decision making: the future with nursing diagnosis*, (p587). Toronto: John Wiley and Sons

North American Nursing Diagnosis Association.(1985). *Minutes of the meeting of the Board, May, 1985. Report of the program committee, attachment A1*. St. Louis: the Association

North American Nursing Diagnosis Association. (1986) *Classification of Nursing Diagnoses. Proceedings of the Sixth Conference. M. E. Hurley (Ed.)*. St. Louis: The C.V.Mosby Company

North American Nursing Diagnosis Association. (1988) *Classification of Nursing Diagnosis. Proceedings of the Seventh Conference. A. M. McLane (Ed.)*. St. Louis: The CV Mosby Company

Create the Vision: The Ninth NANDA Conference

Judith J. Warren, PhD, RN, C, FAAN

The theme of NANDA's ninth conference was "Create the Vision." The vision for this conference truly created some firsts for NANDA. A new decade, the 1990's, had begun and Jane Lancour was the second president. Ken Cianfrani was the program committee chairman for the first conference held outside of St. Louis, Missouri. The ninth conference was held in March at Orlando, Florida, with the biggest attendance ever. This conference marked a turning point in the maturity of NANDA. A definition of a nursing diagnosis was adopted, a proposed Taxonomy II was discussed, and a proposal for including nursing diagnoses in the 10th edition of the International Classification of Diseases was presented.

Between the eighth and ninth conferences the Board of Directors conducted a Delphi study to develop a definition of a nursing diagnosis that would provide criteria for accepting a nursing diagnosis for inclusion in the taxonomy. The work was presented by the Diagnosis Review Committee (DRC) chairman, Lynda Carpenito. This definition continues to guide the work of the DRC today. NANDA's official definition is "A nursing diagnosis is a clinical judgment about an individual, family, or community response to actual or potential health problems/life processes which provides the basis for definitive therapy toward achievement of outcomes for which the nurse is accountable" (Carpenito, 1991, p. 65).

The DRC also struggled with the concept of a nursing diagnosis syndrome as several had been submitted to them for consideration. The notion of what a nursing diagnosis syndrome would look like and how it would fit into the taxonomy was studied and debated. A syndrome was defined as a group or cluster of signs and symptoms that almost always occur together. While no official action was taken, the following are common characteristics of the syndromes that have been submitted: "syndromes represent a cluster of nursing diagnoses; their labels give clue to the cause; syndromes have initial and long-term phases; syndromes have emotional, social, and physical components; and syndromes represent complex, clinical conditions requiring expert nursing assessment and expert nursing interventions" (McCourt, 1991, p. 81). The diagnoses that began this discussion were rape trauma syndrome, translocation syndrome, and risk for disuse syndrome.

The Taxonomy Committee presented a proposal for Taxonomy II at the ninth conference in response to a membership request to reconsider the relevance of the human response patterns as an organizing framework. While the framework appeared to be relevant for organizing and developing nursing diagnoses, it was not perceived to be clinically relevant and was difficult to implement in a computerized nursing information system. After much study, the committee determined that the framework was still useful for the organization of the taxonomy and could become clinically relevant. Subsequently, the human response patterns were redefined for clarity and precision (Fitzpatrick, 1991, see page 25). Using these new definitions and the proposed definition of a nursing diagnosis, all nursing diagnoses were re-evaluated for location in the taxonomy and whether they were a nursing diagnosis. Several diagnoses needed to be reclassified into different human response patterns, e.g., *dysreflexia* moved to the communicating pattern. Some nursing diagnoses were found to not meet the criteria in the new proposed definition of a nursing diagnosis, e.g., *knowledge deficit* was recommended to be revised or deleted. Finally, the committee recommended that the taxonomy become multiaxial to increase flexibility of expression of diagnostic concepts. The axes proposed were unit of analysis (person, family, community, aggregate), age group, wellness, illness, acuity, and chronicity (Hoskins, 1991; Warren, 1991).

After much debate, the Taxonomy Committee was charged with conducting an impact and feasibility study concerning changing classification structures and coding formats. The committee was to develop a transition plan from the Taxonomy I framework to the Taxonomy II framework. The impact report and the transition plan, along with the Taxonomy II proposal, was to be presented to the membership at the tenth conference. During the time between the ninth and tenth conferences, the Board of Directors and the Taxonomy Committee determined that NANDA was not ready for a multi-axial classification.

Taxonomy I was revised through the addition of new diagnoses and published as "Taxonomy I, Revised, 1990." Within the following year, Taxonomy I, Revised became the first classification to be officially recognized by the American Nurses Association (there are now six recognized classifications and one recognized data set). This recognition contributed to the growing acceptance of NANDA in practice and education.

In 1988, the American Nurses Association (ANA) approached NANDA with an opportunity to collaborate on a submission of nursing diagnoses to the World Health Organization for inclusion in the 10th edition of the International Classification of Diseases (ICD-10). The Taxonomy Committee worked with a representative of the ANA, Virginia Saba, to develop a translation between NANDA and the classification framework of the ICD-10 (Fitzpatrick, 1991; Saba, 1991). This required limiting the classification of nursing diagnoses to three levels, instead of the six levels present in NANDA and a modification of the "potential" modifier to an "at risk" modifier. The proposal was submitted but did not meet all the requirements for inclusion into ICD-10 (author's note: in 1997, the United States decided to develop a clinical modification of the ICD-10 and negotiations are underway to include NANDA and other ANA recognized classifications in this edition, ICD-10-CM).

The last major "first" during the ninth conference was a panel from the Research Committee reporting on NANDA's invitational research conference held in 1989 in Palm Springs. The papers were published in a monograph by NANDA (the monograph is out of print). Selected methodology papers from the conference were presented to encourage nursing diagnosis research. The Research Committee presented three categories of research methods designed for nursing diagnosis development, validation, and clinical testing: qualitative methods (MacFarlane, 1991), quantitative methods (Schroeder, 1991), and integrated methods (Kim, 1991). The panel was well received by the attendees and the presenters agreed to consult with individuals during the conference.

In summary, the ninth conference was full of "firsts" and very exciting! There was animated discussion about the new nursing diagnosis definition and the proposed changes to the taxonomic structure. Consultations and debate on appropriate research methods to employ were abundant in every room and corridor. And as you visited NASA, Epcott, and Disneyland (yes, we did plan time to play), you could hear the enthusiastic discussions about nursing diagnoses, new research methods, and the papers being planned for submission to the tenth conference. This conference was truly a turning point in NANDA's development that lived up to the theme "Create the Vision" for the future.

References

Carpenito, L. J. (1991). The NANDA definition of nursing diagnosis. In R. M. Carroll-Johnson (Ed.). *Classification of nursing diagnoses: Proceedings of the ninth conference*, (pp. 65-71). Philadelphia: J. B. Lippincott.

Fitzpatrick, J. J. (1991). Taxonomy II: Definitions and development. In R. M. Carroll-Johnson. (Ed.). *Classification of nursing diagnoses: Proceedings of the ninth conference*, (pp. 23-29). Philadelphia: J. B. Lippincott.

Fitzpatrick, J. J. (1991). The translation of NANDA Taxonomy I into ICD code. In R. M. Carroll-Johnson (Ed.). *Classification of nursing diagnoses: Proceedings of the ninth conference*, (pp. 19-22). Philadelphia: J. B. Lippincott.

Hoskins, L. M. (1991). What is the focus of Taxonomy II: Nursing diagnosis axes. In R. M. Carroll-Johnson (Ed.). *Classification of nursing diagnoses: Proceedings of the ninth conference*, (pp. 35-37). Philadelphia: J. B. Lippincott.

Kim, M. J. (1991). Integrated methods for nursing diagnosis research. In R. M. Carroll-Johnson (Ed.). *Classification of nursing diagnoses: Proceedings of the ninth conference*, (pp. 201-208). Philadelphia: J. B. Lippincott.

McCourt, A. E. (1991). Syndromes in nursing: A continuing concern. In R. M. Carroll-Johnson (Ed.). *Classification of nursing diagnoses: Proceedings of the ninth conference*, (pp. 79-82). Philadelphia: J. B. Lippincott.

McFarlane, E. A. (1991). Qualitative methods for nursing diagnosis research. In R. M. Carroll-Johnson (Ed.). *Classification of nursing diagnoses: Proceedings of the ninth conference*, (pp. 185-191). Philadelphia: J. B. Lippincott.

Saba, V. K. (1991). The International Classification of Diseases (ICD); Classification of nursing diagnoses. In R. M. Carroll-Johnson (Ed.). *Classification of nursing diagnoses: Proceedings of the ninth conference*, (pp. 14-18). Philadelphia: J. B. Lippincott.

Schroeder, M. A. (1991). Quantitative methods for nursing diagnosis research. In R. M. Carroll-Johnson (Ed.). (1991). *Classification of nursing diagnoses: Proceedings of the ninth conference*, (pp. 192-200). Philadelphia: J. B. Lippincott.

Warren, J. J. (1991). Implications of introducing axes into a classification system. In R. M. Carroll-Johnson (Ed.). *Classification of nursing diagnoses: Proceedings of the ninth conference*, (pp. 38-44). Philadelphia: J. B. Lippincott.

Sailing the Course to Advance Professional Practice with Nursing Diagnosis: the Tenth and Eleventh Conferences

Lois M. Hoskins, PhD, RN, FAAN

The purposes of this paper are to present memorable events and relate pearls of wisdom that I have gleaned from my memories and from the proceedings of the 10th and 11th NANDA conferences. This effort will be influenced by my own perceptions, and those perceptions will be influenced by the different roles and responsibilities that I had in the organization at the time, as well as by my own values and human frailties.

The 10th conference was held in April 1992 off San Diego Bay at the time of the American Cup races. The theme of the meeting was "Sailing the Course, New Directions into the 21st Century." Kenneth Cianfrani, who is no longer with us, was Program Chairman and Jane Lancour was President. The 11th conference was held March 1994 in Nashville, Tennessee, land of the Grand Old Opry and country music. Lynda Carpenito was Chair of the Program and I was President. The theme of the conference was "Advancing Professional Practice with Nursing Diagnosis."

These two conferences had as a historical background the health care reform movement. Managed care was burgeoning. In 1976 , six million people, or 2.8% of the U.S. population, were enrolled in HMOs. By 1993, 45 million or 17.5% were covered (Zitter, 1996). We were moving from an unstructured system of health care with fee-for-service and episodic coverage to one of managed care competition with capitated payment. The goal of this new system was population-based health management. Two significant events occurred near the time of these conferences. The Agency for Health Care Policy and Research was established in 1989 to enhance the quality, appropriateness, and effectiveness of health care services. Among its activities were the development of clinical practice guidelines and the conduct of medical effectiveness research. In 1992, the National Institute of Nursing Research held a conference to examine the effectiveness of nursing practice. Among the recommendations from this conference was the need to facilitate the use and expansion of existing data sources and data bases, and the development of new ones for the evaluation of the effectiveness of nursing practice in outcomes research (NIH, 1993). The move to managed care and cost containment and the increasing emphasis on quality, effectiveness, and outcomes of care were forces affecting our work in NANDA.

From both the 10th and 11th conferences the most memorable events are the presentations of papers and posters describing diagnostic validation studies and taxonomic development. This is our reason for being. It must not be overshadowed by the wealth of presentations that provide us with information, consultation, and entertainment.

Among other memorable events at the 10th conference (1994), a symposium on validation models demonstrated our increasing sophistication in research design. A panel of specialty organizations, including the ANA Council of Nurses in Advanced Practice, the National Association of Orthopaedic Nurses, the American Holistic Nurses Association, and the American Association of Critical-Care Nurses discussed their use of nursing diagnosis. This effort provided affirmation of NANDA's desire to collaborate with specialty organizations. Ten new nursing diagnoses were added to our classification.

Among our speakers, Phyllis Kritek (1994) commented on persisting challenges for NANDA and of the need for us to seek balance in what she labeled as "our sometimes competing and conflicting vectors" (p. 6). She stated that NANDA's collective effort presents itself in human form:

> It is exhilarating, stimulating, concentrating, expanding, enlivening. It brings forth our best in intellect, in collaborative sharing, in common cause,

in discovery and release. It is also, at once, trivializing, petty, avaricious, cruel, confining, grandiose, confused, angry, proud, fearful, defensive. It is, in short, a human effort. And the persisting challenges are, thus, profoundly human challenges (pp. 6-7).

Kay Avant (1994) encouraged us to deal with misconceptions about theory and practice, and to be fully aware that we are involved in the definition and study of concepts that are the building blocks of theory. This activity, she said, requires producing scientists and working scientists. Producing scientists generate new knowledge and working scientists are responsible for using it. If the new knowledge does not work, the producing scientists must revise it. Their collective action is required for success. Ada Jacox (1994) identified the increasing interdependence and overlap among the activities of health care professionals. She urged us to be inclusive in our language development, including not only our nursing diagnoses but also those diagnoses that we share with others. She encouraged the use of a "loosely developed logical framework" (p. 25) to underlie our taxonomy so that it might accommodate new knowledge. Susan Dean-Baar (1994) stated that nursing must be able to name and label all that it does. In doing so it must expand the original definition of collaborative problems developed by Carpenito (1989 as cited by Dean-Baar). The definition must reflect a multidisciplinary focus on problems rather than being narrowly oriented to nursing and medical problems. She further emphasized the need to link nursing diagnoses, interventions and outcomes to be more effective in guideline development.

President Jane Lancour (1994) identified three specific issues that NANDA needed to address. First, she urged broadening the definition of nursing diagnosis so that it might "demonstrate the contribution of nursing in a changing health care delivery system" (p. 75). Second, the diagnosis review process needed to be revised, and finally the area of taxonomic development needed to address the emerging international perspective. She recognized that for NANDA these issues were overshadowed by its fiscal problems. Winifred Mills (1994) commented that we were "tacking through troubled waters toward desired outcomes" (p. 126).

The 11th Conference

There were a number of memorable events at the 11th conference (1995). We had an international panel of presenters from Brazil, France, Japan, Spain, and The Netherlands. Each presented the state of the use of nursing diagnosis in their respective countries. As a specialty forum the relationship between the American Organization of Operating Room Nurses and NANDA was presented.

For the first time in our history small groups of research and clinical experts met to refine or clarify 10 selected diagnoses that were in the NANDA classification. This step was a beginning to bring diagnoses accepted at an earlier time in our development into conformity with present day review criteria.

As pearls grow from irritants, a number of challenges were given to us and some I learned of in my role as your representative to the ANA Steering Committee on Databases to Improve Clinical Nursing Practice. It was the perception of this group that our process of diagnostic review made it difficult for specialty organizations to have their diagnoses added to our list. In response to this and our own concerns, a new diagnostic review process was launched. The procedure, fashioned after the process of review used by the American Psychiatric Association, incorporates developmental stages with criteria for acceptance at each of four stages. We also added 19 new diagnoses to the NANDA classification list.

At the 11th conference we announced the signing of an agreement, the Nursing Diagnosis Extension and Classification (NDEC) project, with a research team from the University of Iowa. Over time there had been concerns expressed about the differing levels of conceptual clarity and the research base of the nursing diagnoses (Creason, Camilleri & Kim, 1993). Among its recommendations for research the National Center for Nursing Research Priority Expert Panel on Nursing Informatics (1993) included "Conduct large-scale validation of existing sets of clinical terms and solicit proposals for validating sets of terms to be developed (as with the NANDA diagnosis list)" (p. 36-37). The NDEC project being reported at this conference (13th) has addressed the first level, the need for concept analysis and clarification, and it is now moving to expert validation of our approved list.

Also at the 11th conference, we welcomed Nursecom as the organization responsible for the management of our affairs and as publisher of our journal, *Nursing Diagnosis*. Along with this change was the move of our official office from St. Louis to Philadelphia, Pennsylvania.

Invited papers addressed the integration of nursing diagnosis into advanced practice nursing in long term care, acute care, the community, school nursing, and in nursing education. Validation papers reflected a diversity of research approaches including consensual validation, a phenomenological approach, bayesian methodology, and case control designs.

Among our speakers Joyce Fitzpatrick, in a paper with Renzo Zenotti, (1995) addressed nursing diagnosis internationally. Their survey of 33 countries showed demonstrable growth and support for NANDA and the use of nursing diagnosis. To extend our collaboration to other countries, they expressed the need for "a common language and common definitions of the phenomena of concern to our discipline" (p. 66). They urged NANDA to take a leadership role in international initiatives including conferences, clinical evaluation projects, and research. Jean Jenny (1995) reviewed taxonomic development and said, "the time has come for this organization to offer a new framework for diagnosis development, one that is timely, consistent with nursing's orientation, and intelligible to nurses in all practice areas" (p. 80). Kristine Gebbie (1995) spoke to us about politics, "politics as power distribution and politics as the art of the possible" (p. 86). Both of these facets, power and negotiation, are dynamic within NANDA, the nursing profession, nursing organizations, and other health care professions and organizations. Focusing upon health care reform, she said we are talking about a health system that is committed to outcomes and quality yet we do not have the data necessary to identify nursing's contribution. She urged us by whatever means necessary to be included among the power brokers that draft the legislation to identify the necessary information to be gathered from all enrollees in the health care system. If we want nursing diagnosis to be there, we will have to be pragmatic and adaptable. In her words, "if it's got to be purist or nothing, the odds are it will be nothing" (p. 92).

Summary and Conclusions

From my observations I extracted four recurring themes. These were reform, technology, globalization, and interdependence. These themes do not change the mission of this organization, which is to "develop, refine, disseminate and promote nursing diagnostic terminology as well as taxonomic structure for use by professional nurses" (NANDA Bylaws, Article I, Section 2, Rantz & LeMone, 1997, p. 481). These themes do not change the need for this continuing work, but I offer as a pearl of wisdom that if we are to sail the course successfully we must do some tacking to accommodate these factors. I found agreement on the need for a common nursing language with common definitions that can be used on a global basis, and a language that is easily interpretable to non-nurses. I also found agreement on the need for a taxonomic structure that is logical, adaptable to change, and easily related to nursing interventions, and outcomes.

In conclusion I offer a remark made by Rose Mary Carroll-Johnson in her editorial column in *Nursing Diagnosis* following the 10th conference.

> Alas, the journey we face will most likely not be smooth or uneventful, but we are experienced sailors, weathered by rough winds and battered by high seas, but afloat nonetheless. Afloat in large measure by virtue of two undeniable assets: a resilient, perceptive, and ingenious crew and a sturdy, seaworthy craft... the concept of nursing diagnosis and the wider implications of a taxonomy for professional nursing practice (1992, p. 47).

References

Avant, K. (1994). The link of theory to practice. In R.M. Carroll-Johnson & M. Paquette,

(Eds.), *Classification of nursing diagnoses: Proceedings of the Tenth Conference North American Nursing Diagnosis Association* (pp. 11-16). Philadelphia: Lippincott.

Carpenito, L. J. (1989). *Nursing diagnosis: Application to clinical practice* (3rd ed). Philadelphia: Lippincott.

Carroll-Johnson, R. M. & Paquette, M. (1994). *Classification of nursing diagnoses: Proceedings of the Tenth Conference North American Nursing Diagnosis Association.* Philadelphia: Lippincott.

Carroll-Johnson, R.M. (1992). Editorial. *Nursing Diagnosis, 3*(2), 47.

Creason, N.S., Camilleri, D. D., & Kim, M. J. (1993). Concept development in nursing diagnosis. In B. L. Rodgers & K. A. Knafl (Eds.), *Concept development in nursing: Foundations, techniques, and applications* (pp. 217-234). Philadelphia: Saunders.

Dean-Baar, S. (1994). Nursing diagnosis: New opportunities. In R.M. Carroll-Johnson & Paquette, M (Eds.), *Classification of nursing diagnoses: Proceedings of the Tenth Conference North American Nursing Diagnosis Association,* (pp. 27-33). Philadelphia: Lippincott.

Fitzpatrick, J., & Zanotti, R. (1995). Nursing diagnosis internationally. In M. J. Rantz & P. LeMone (Eds.) *Classification of nursing diagnoses: Proceedings of the Eleventh Conference North American Nursing Diagnosis Association* (pp. 66-72), Glendale, California: CINAHL Information Systems.

Gebbie, K. (1995). The politics of nursing diagnosis. In M. J. Rantz & P. LeMone (Eds.) *Classification of nursing diagnoses: Proceedings of the Eleventh Conference North American Nursing Diagnosis*

Association (pp. 85-96), Glendale, California: CINAHL Information Systems.

Jacox, A. (1994). Toward inclusiveness of scope in nursing diagnosis. In R.M. Carroll-Johnson & M. Paquette(Eds.), *Classification of nursing diagnoses: Proceedings of the Tenth Conference North American Nursing Diagnosis Association,* (pp. 17-26). Philadelphia: Lippincott.

Jenny, J. (1995). Advancing the science of nursing. In M. J. Rantz & P. LeMone (Eds.) *Classification of nursing diagnoses: Proceedings of the Eleventh Conference North American Nursing Diagnosis Association* (pp. 73-81), Glendale, California: CINAHL Information Systems.

Kritek, P. (1994). Diagnosis in action. In R.M. Carroll-Johnson & M. Paquette (Eds.), *Classification of nursing diagnoses: Proceedings of the Tenth Conference North American Nursing Diagnosis Association,* (pp. 5-10). Philadelphia: Lippincott.

Lancour, J. (1994). President's open forum: Present and future perspectives. *Classification of nursing diagnoses: Proceedings of the Tenth Conference, North American Nursing Diagnosis Association* (pp. 75-76). Philadelphia: Lippincott.

Mills, W. C. (1994). Tacking through troubled waters: Toward desired outcomes. In R.M. Carroll-Johnson & M.Paquette (Eds.), *Classification of nursing diagnoses: Proceedings of the Tenth Conference, North American Nursing Diagnosis Association* (pp. 126-130). Philadelphia: Lippincott.

North American Nursing Diagnosis Association (1997). North American Nursing Diagnosis Association Bylaws. In Rantz, M. J. & LeMone, P. (Eds.) (1997). *Classification of nursing diagnoses: Proceedings of the*

Twelfth Conference North American Nursing Diagnosis Association (pp. 481-486). Glendale, California: CINAHL Information Systems

National Institute of Nursing Research (1992). *Patient Outcomes Research: Examining the effectiveness of nursing practice.* (NIH Pub. No. 93-3411). Bethesda, MD: NIH, PHS, US DHHS.

National Center for Nursing Research (NCNR)(1993). *Defining and describing data and information for patient care. In Report of the NCNR Priority Expert Panel on Nursing Informatics, Nursing informatics: Enhancing patient care,* (NIH Pub. No. 93-2419, pp. 31-42). Bethesda, MD, NIH, PHS, US DHHS.

Rantz, M. J., & LeMone, P. (Eds.) (1995). *Classification of nursing diagnoses: Proceedings of the Eleventh Conference North American Nursing Diagnosis Association.* Glendale, California: CINAHL Information Systems.

Zitter, M. (1996). A new paradigm in health care delivery: Disease management. In W. E. Todd & D. Nash (Eds.), *Disease management: A systems approach to improving patient outcomes* (pp. 1-26). Chicago: American Hospital Publishing Inc.

NANDA and the Nurse Theorists:
The Truth of Theory

Sister Callista Roy, PhD, RN, FAAN

It is a pleasure to address the 25th Anniversary National Conference of the North American Nursing Diagnosis Association. I am delighted to have the opportunity to share with you about the six-year era of the Nurse Theorist Group of NANDA, some of the facts and some of the stories behind the work. As I look at nursing in the next century, I think of how quickly we are exploring our universe and understanding our place in relation to that magnificent environment. Nurses in the quest for describing and naming the universe of nursing are in an exciting adventure parallel with that of the astronauts and astrophysicists exploring space and the many universes. What I want to share with you in the brief time that I have for this Pearl in the string of NANDA accomplishments is the Nurse Theorists: a little history, a few stories, and some sample contributions of our alumnae. I will be highlighting our beginnings, our tasks and product, along with observations of the human processes and experience behind the work, at least from the point of this participant-observer.

Founding of the Nurse Theorist Group

When I heard the announcement in the early 1970s of the convening of the First National Conference on Nursing Diagnosis by Kristine Gebbie and Mary Ann Lavin, I immediately recognized the significance of this event for the development of nursing as a practice discipline, and equally important, the potential that it offered for providing a structure for the development of nursing knowledge. I waited eagerly to hear whether my application had been accepted for this invitational conference. The First National Conference was exceedingly productive and we came up with that first list of nursing diagnoses, derived inductively from the collective knowledge and experience represented by the members of assigned work groups. By the second national conference, I was asked to give the keynote address and among my remarks, made a plea to search for an organizing principle for the taxonomy, a structure for the tree on which to hang our labels. Many of you have heard me note that the alphabet is a good way to organize a telephone directory, but such a method of organization adds nothing to our understanding of the structure of the language of our discipline. I believe that NANDA's work is both the language and the structure for the language of the discipline.

When I did not see any particular movement to deal with the issue, I presented a proposal to the Nursing Diagnosis Task Force in 1977 to convene a group of nurse theorists to take on the challenge of creating a framework for the diagnoses. The Task Force, chaired by Marjorie Gordon, that served as the planning committee for the Third National Conference, enthusiastically endorsed the idea. The one word of caution was that the task force members did not want the Theorists to be an elite group, separated from the work of the conference. Thus, a major goal throughout the era of the Nurse Theorists was keeping the project integrated with the work of the National Conferences.

The early development of the Nurse Theorist Group involved two stages: first, inviting members to be part of the group, and second, an intensive period of homework prior to the next national conference. My colleague and friend, Dorothy E. Johnson, met with me in Los Angeles, California, to compose a list of potential members and to organize how the group would approach their task. We had 21 names on the original list and reviewing the list we came up with, Dorothy observed: "We sure have made a lot of noise for so few of us."

In the letter of invitation, it was clearly noted that what we needed was each person's skill of high level conceptualization, not each one's given approach to a framework for nursing. Further, we explained that we would all be self-supporting, traveling and working between con-

ferences at our own expense. Fourteen theorists responded positively to the invitation to join the group.

Our homework began with long worksheets in which we took the original 88 diagnostic labels and analyzed them to identify the order of knowledge of each and the conceptual scheme from which it was derived. This material was synthesized into another level of analysis in which the diagnostic label from the National Conference was paired with an identification of the nature of the problem implied. For example, the term "hypervigilance" was listed as a hypothetical construct derived from neurology and implied a problem of the need to watch out for dangers which prevent sleep. I admit I was somewhat surprised as these women began doing the homework, mailing their responses, and sometimes sending notes of apology for missing a deadline.

We came together for the first time at the Third National Conference in 1978 at the Sheraton Hotel in St. Louis, Missouri. Although we knew each other's work, for many of us it was the first time that we were to meet face to face. I remember well my feelings as I walked toward that meeting room; I said to myself, "This could be an historic moment; or this place could blow up from the sheer energy in the room." I would like to share with you the list of persons who came to that meeting, organized retrospectively into what emerged as a relevant typology:

Nurse Theorist Group Members Attending Third National Conference, 1978

Metatheorists

Andrea Bircher	Margaret Hardy
Rosemary Ellis	Rose McKay
Marjorie Gordon	Gertrude Torres

Grand Theorists (other than Rogers)
    Imogene King
    Dorothea Orem
    Sr. Callista Roy

Rogerians
    Martha Rogers
    Joyce Fitzpatrick
    Margaret Newman
    Rosemarie Parse
    Mary Jane Smith
    3 doctoral students from Wayne State University

Margaret Hardy was sitting next to me and she was making a tally sheet as each person introduced herself, and as Marg finished the list she turned to me and said, "We are outnumbered." What had happened was that people began to hear of the work of the group and called me to invite themselves, so unknown to me, the deck was being stacked.

In addition to this observation about our beginnings, I must say also that in spite of the common homework we had done (except for those who were added to the group later in the pre-conference process), and in spite of the pleas to bring one's best thinking skills, not one's prepared perspective, the meeting began with handouts being passed around. There were at least three sets of individual theorists' work that were offered as "the answer." The amazing fact is that over the next six years, we learned to listen to each other, to know and to respect each other, and even sometimes to make compromises. Dorothea Orem was the one who insisted that we include "goal-seeking," implying free will, in our characteristics of unitary persons as open systems. In one lunch break conversation at a midwestern cafe near the airport hotel where we were meeting in Chicago, I recall a momentous statement made by Martha Rogers. She was describing the difference between individual and group behavior and noted that, for example, there were things she would agree with for the sake of the group project that may not be her own opinion.

Task of the Nurse Theorists: Process

The task of the Nurse Theorists was twofold: (1) to develop a conceptual scheme to provide an organizing principle for the work of the conference and (2) to come up with recommendations on the order of generality of the diagnostic labels. The process included meeting about twice a year for six years; working both inductively and deductively; and using a dialectic that often meant agreeing, disagreeing, and coming to a synthesis. The characteristics of the process entered into by this extraordinary group of women can be described as one of commitment, scholarship, courage, commonality, and fun. The commitment and courage included the fact that the group kept coming, at their own expense, regardless of health concerns, travel and weather difficulties. Martha was often short of breath, Rosemary propped up her paralyzed side, I survived my first craniotomy. We worked hard at the meetings; we worked hard in between meetings, challenging each other to keep the scholarship of the group at the high level that was characteristic of each of us as individuals. The young ones, Joyce Fitzpatrick, Margaret Newman, and I, often stayed late after a meeting and borrowed a hotel secretary's typewriter to prepare the work for the meeting on the next day. Significant meetings between conferences were: New York, December 1978; Chicago, May 1979; St. Louis, September 1979 (with the National Task Force); St. Louis before the Fourth National Conference in 1980; and Chicago, November 1981.

It was a challenging and growing experience to Chair this group for the whole six years. Sometimes people would ask me why there was not more of my own thinking represented in the product of the Theorist Group. My response was simply that it took my entire energy to manage the group dynamics and to keep us working productively on the task. At times I tried to rotate the Chair of the group, but that movement was cut off by Martha's cryptic statement, "Now, Callista, you know that you are the only one that can hold us together." I admit that I used varying strategies to manage the diverse personalities and strengths within the group; for example, when someone got too overbearing, I asked that person to take the minutes. But for the most part, the spirit of commonality and fun prevailed. We enjoyed each other's company; we enjoyed interacting with the clinical nurse specialists and other conference participants; and we enjoyed some of the glorious settings we found ourselves in. For example, the Presidential Suite at the Hilton, kindness of the Nursing Theory Conference coordinators of the Nurse Educator journal, was a real contrast to our airport hotels. In fact, the work turned out in that suite became the cornerstone of our product.

Outcome of the Nurse Theorist Group Work

From the work of the theorists as a group, we developed an initial definition of nursing diagnosis: *nursing diagnosis is a concise phrase or term summarizing a cluster of empirical indicators representing patterns of unitary man* (Roy, 1982, 219). This definition was revised after the Fourth National Conference to read: *nursing diagnosis is a phrase or term which is a synthesis of a cluster of empirical indicators describing characteristics of unitary man (person)* (Roy, 1982, 240). Table 1 summarizes the conceptual schema developed by the Nurse Theorist Group and presented in April of 1980 to the National Conference as a framework for identifying and classifying nursing diagnoses.

Our recommendation about the order of generality of the labels was that in fact there were many orders of generality, from empirical indicators to abstract concepts, and this issue needed to be addressed in further taxonomy work.

Impact of the Work of the Nurse Theorists

The impact of the work of the nurse theorists as part of NANDA will be judged by history. However, I believe that the effects of working together upon each of us was significant. Likely the mutual influences could be examined in each theorist's work from the dates following our intense collaboration together on the task for NANDA. For our purposes, I want to review evidence of continuing impact of the theorists' work that comes from contributions of members of the Theorist Group after we presented the recommendations related to our twofold task.

First, an example of Joyce Fitzpatrick's work with the Taxonomy Committee is presented in Table 2. From the Human Response Pattern of Choosing, the committee developed the related structure of diagnoses concerning family coping, health seeking behavior, and individual coping. This work was published in major nursing journals, as well as in NANDA publications (Fitzpatrick, et. al, 1989a and 1989b).

At the Seventh National Conference, Dr. Fitzpatrick contributed to the dialogue about the conceptual concerns related to etiology, as related to the development of the discipline and

Table 1

**Framework for Identifying and Classifying Nursing Diagnoses
Nurse Theorist Group Report, April 10, 1980**

I. Conceptual schema

    A. Phenomena—unitary man—open system

    B. Characteristics of unitary man as an open system
        1. Developmental process
            a. Growing
            b. Evolutionary
            c. Negentropic
        2. Four-dimensional field
            a. Pattern
            b. Organization
            c. Unity
            d. Transaction
            e. Arbitrary boundaries
        3. Patterning of energy
            a. Rhythm
            b. Ordering
            c. Mutual simultaneous interaction
        4. Goal seeking

    C. Goal of nursing — to promote health

    D. Health — a rhythmic pattern of energy exchange which is mutually enhancing and expresses full life potential

    E. Service nursing provides — participation in this goal by the use of self and a body of nursing knowledge.

II. Characteristics of Unitary Man

    A. Factor I: Interaction
        Exchanging, Communicating, and Relating

    B. Factor II: Action
        Valuing, Choosing, and Moving

    C. Factor III: Awareness
        Waking, Feeling, and Knowing

(adapted from Roy, 1982)

Table 2

Example from NANDA Taxonomy I: Proposed ICD-10 Version

Human response pattern: Choosing

*Y00	Family coping, impaired	
	Y00.0	compromised
	Y00.1	disabled
Y01	Health seeking behavior	
	Y01.0-9	health seeking behaviors, (specify)
Y02	Individual coping, impaired	
	Y02.0	adjustment, impaired
	Y02.1	conflict, decisional
	Y02.2	coping, defensive
	Y02.3	denial, impaired
	Y02.4	noncompliance

(Fitzpatrick, et al., 1989a)

---

specifically the issues related to etiology of nursing diagnosis (Fitzpatrick, 1987). Dr. Fitzpatrick carried the message beyond the NANDA organization and also provided significant contributions through her work with the 1989 National Forum on Doctoral Education in Nursing in Indianapolis, Indiana in June 1989. She presented a conceptual basis for the organization and advancement of nursing knowledge called the nursing diagnosis taxonomy. In an early issue of *Nursing Diagnosis*, Dr. Fitzpatrick made the significant statement that: "With the inherent assumption of a need for development of clinical judgment as part of the process of diagnosis and the conceptual or theoretical emphasis on holistic human patterns, nursing diagnosis represents the most relevant conceptualization for immediate development of disciplinary content."

(Fitzpatrick, 1990).

Another example is the work done by Andrea Bircher through both her continued work within NANDA (Bircher, 1986) and her development of related knowledge for the discipline. In a book on implementing nursing diagnosis-based practice (Bircher, 1991), Dr. Bircher described nursing diagnosis as providing a bridge over the knowledge-practice gap. This is illustrated in Figure 1 where the steps of the nursing process are related to levels of theory, through an understanding of nursing diagnosis.

Dr. Margaret Newman was another alumnae of the Nurse Theorist Group who continued to contribute through the NANDA Conferences, as well as through the broader nursing literature. In 1984, she published a paper in the *American Journal of Nursing*,

Figure 1

Nursing Diagnosis: Bridge over the Knowledge Practice Grap (Bircher, 1991)

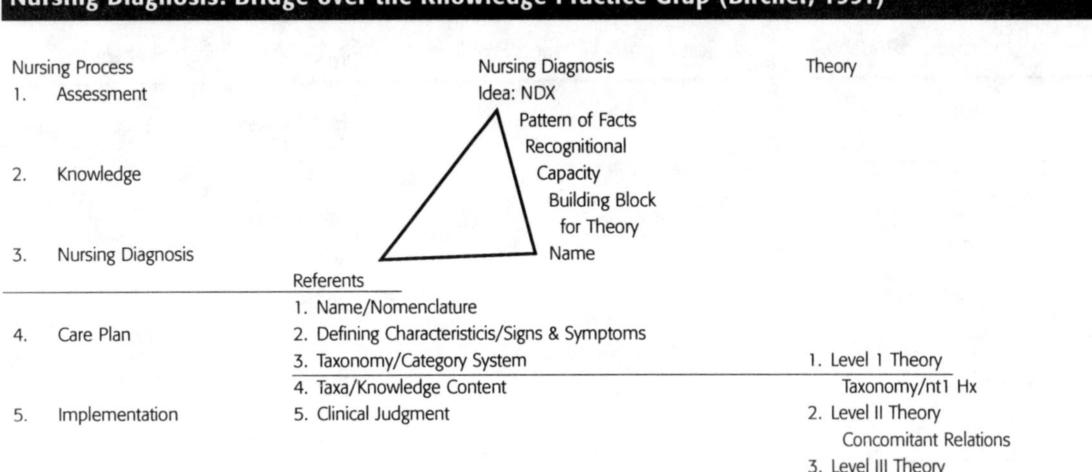

"Nursing Diagnosis: Looking at the Whole" (Newman, 1984), and at the Seventh Conference, Dr. Newman addressed the diagnosis of pattern in relation to nursing's emerging paradigm.

It is interesting to note retrospectively that it was one of the nurse theorists in the NANDA group who wrote one of the earliest publications on nursing diagnosis. Dorothea Orem was the first author on a paper in 1952, "Diagnosis of Hospital Nursing Problems" in the journal *Hospitals* (Orem & O'Malley, 1952). Finally, I will offer an example from my latest work on the Roy Adaptation Model (Roy & Andrews, 1999) in which each chapter on the adaptive modes includes a table comparing the Roy Adaptation Model positive indicators of adaptation and adaptation problems with the relevant NANDA diagnostic labels. Table 3 shows this comparison in relation to the Self Concept-Group Identity Mode of Adaptation.

Conclusion

In summary, let me change the image of space exploration that I started with and say I think the Nurse Theorists may have embarked on a venture like finding the Holy Grail. At least perhaps, we provided a cup of water for refreshment on this great venture and journey of organizing the language of knowledge for practice. Congratulations to NANDA on 25 years of contributions and best wishes for a wonderfully productive future.

References

Bircher, A. (1986). Nursing diagnosis: Where does the conceptual framework fit? (pp. 66-97). In Hurley, M. (Ed.). *Classification of nursing diagnoses: Proceedings of the sixth conference.* St. Louis: C.V. Mosby Co.

Bircher, A. (1991). Nursing diagnosis: An Overview. (pp. 3-31). In D'Argenio, C. (Ed.). *Implementing nursing diagnosis-based*

Table 3

Nursing Diagnostic Categories For Self Concept/Group Identity		
Positive Indicators of Adaptation:	Common Adaptation Problems:	NANDA Diagnostic Labels:
Positive body image	Body image disturbance	Body image disturbance
Effective sexual function	Sexual dysfunction	
Psychic integrity with physical growth	Rape trauma syndrome Loss	Ineffective denial Anticipatory grieving
Adequate compensation for bodily changes		Dysfunctional grieving
Effective coping strategies for loss		Rape trauma syndrome: compound reaction, silent reaction
Effective process of life closure		Altered sexuality patterns
Stable pattern of self consistency	Anxiety	Anxiety: powerlessness, hopelessness
Effective integration of self ideal	Powerlessness	
Effective processes of moral-ethical-spiritual growth	Guilt	Personal identity disturbance
	Low self esteem	Chronic low self-esteem
Functional self-esteem		Situational low self-esteem
Effective coping strategies for threats to self		Self-esteem disturbance Spiritual distress
Effective interpersonal relationships	Ineffective interpersonal relations	
Supportive culture	Oppressive culture	
Positive morale	Low morale	
Group acceptance	Stigma	
Principle-based relationships	Abusive relationships	
Value-driven relationships	Valueless relationships	

(Roy & Andrews, 1999)

practice: *Managing the change.* Gaithersburg, MD: Aspen Publications.

Fitzpatrick, J. et. al. (1989a April). Translating nursing diagnosis into ICD Code. *American Journal of Nursing*, 493-495.

Fitzpatrick, J., Kerr, M., Saba, V.K., Hoskins, L., Hurley, M., Mills, W., Rottkamp, B., & Warren, J. (1989b). NANDA Taxonomy 1: Proposed ICD-CD 10 Version. *Applied Nursing Research, 2*(2), 90-91.

Fitzpatrick, J. (1990). Conceptual basis for the organization and advancement of nursing knowledge: Nursing Diagnosis/taxonomy. *Nursing Diagnosis, 1*(3), 102-106.

Newman, M.A. (1984). Nursing Diagnosis: Looking at the whole. *American Journal of Nursing, 84,* 1496-1499.

Newman, M.A. (1987). Nursing's emerging paradigm: The diagnosis of pattern. In *Proceedings of the seventh conference* (pp. 53-60). St. Louis, MO: Mosby.

Orem, D. E., and O'Malley, M. (1952 August). Diagnosis of hospital nursing problems. *Hospitals, 26,* 63.

Roy, C. (1982). Theoretical framework for classification of nursing diagnoses (pp. 215-235.). In Kim, M.J. and D.A. Moritz (eds.) *Classification of nursing diagnoses: Proceedings of the third and fourth conferences.* New York: McGraw Hill, Inc.

Roy, C. (1982). Historical perspective of the Theoretical Framework for the classification of nursing diagnosis (p. 235-246). In Kim, M.J. and D.A. Moritz (eds.) *Classification of nursing diagnoses: Proceedings of the third and fourth conferences.* New York: McGraw Hill, Inc.

Roy, C. & Andrews, H. (1999). *The Roy Adaptation Model* (second edition). Norwalk, CT. Appleton & Lange.

Section 3

General Session Presentations

Nursing Diagnosis Extension Classification (NDEC): History, Methods, Completed Work, and Future Directions

Martha Craft-Rosenberg, PhD, RN, FAAN
Connie Delaney, Ph.D., RN, FAAN
Janice Denehy, PhD, RN
NDEC Research Team

Part I

Introduction, History, & Methods

The development of a language to capture health phenomena which nurses treat to reach desirable outcomes is essential to nursing science, practice, education, and policy development. Like all sciences, nursing identifies phenomena to be included in its domains of responsibility and study. These phenomena are described and become the knowledge base or subject matter for the discipline (Aydelotte & Peterson, 1986; Gebbie & Lavin, 1975; Jenny, 1994). The recognition of similarities and differences in phenomena is the first step in organizing knowledge. These recognized similarities and differences are the basis for classifications and for the criteria of category inclusion or exclusion (Fleishman, 1975). The concepts and their language then provide a standardized health language needed for communicating knowledge, enhancing the quality of nursing practice, and evaluating health care effectiveness.

Building on the recognition of the Nursing Minimum Data Set (NMDS), the classifications of NANDA (NANDA, 1996), the Nursing Interventions Classification (NIC) (Iowa Interventions Project, 1992), Nursing Outcomes Classification (NOC), Iowa Outcomes Project (1997), the Omaha System (Martin & Sheet, 1992), the Home Health Care Classification (Saba et al., 1991), and the Patient Care Data Set (PCDS) (Ozbolt, Fruchnight, & Hayden, 1994) have been recognized by the American Nurses Association Steering Committee on Databases to Support Clinical Practice (ANASCD). Moreover ANASCD has recommended these data elements and classifications for inclusion in national and international databases. A second minimum data set, the Nursing Management Minimum Data Set (NMMDS) (Delaney, 1996), is currently under review. All of ANASCD work underscores the critical need for nursing minimum data sets and standardized nursing languages to be included in local,

"

national, and international databases so that nursing can document care, test effectiveness of care, and submit nursing data for health policy analysis and health policy decisions.

The classification work of NANDA, a pioneering effort for nursing, was the first attempt on the part of nursing to develop and classify a language. This effort contributed to later work by the Nursing Interventions Classification (NIC) (Iowa Interventions Project, 1992) and Nursing Outcomes Classification (NOC) (Iowa Outcomes Project, 1997). However, the ongoing work of NANDA for over 25 years has been accomplished by predominantly voluntary effort. This situation contributed to inadequate systematic concept development and validation of the classification.

As nursing moves closer to the twenty-first century, problems with the existing NANDA taxonomy are being discussed openly, both within the organization and across the discipline. Kim (1989) noted the major weaknesses in nursing diagnosis validation research, including lack of established inter-rater reliability, little attention given to construct validity, and lack of replication studies for external validity. Kim and Camilleri (1994) summarized the theoretical and implementation criticisms for the NANDA taxonomy (See Table 1, What NDEC Will do to Address the Criticisms of NANDA). These criticisms speak to the problems of internal and external validity with individual diagnoses and with the entire taxonomy. Fehring (1986) has also noted that since the process for submission, review, and acceptance of diagnoses had been evolving, not all diagnoses have been reviewed and accepted consistently. Because of the way the diagnoses were approved and the paucity of studies which contribute to evidence of diagnostic validity, virtu-

ally every diagnostic label in this taxonomy needs to be validated. Leaders in NANDA have acknowledged this reality, writing that, "Within the discipline, there is sentiment held by some members that the nursing diagnosis taxonomy in current use is a poor classification of nursing diagnoses, and it may well be. However, questioning the validity of the nursing diagnoses as well as the organizing structure opens the horizon for growth and development" (Kerr et al., 1993).

According to Fleishman (1975), the criteria for evaluating classification systems are: a) internal validity, the extent to which the system is logical and parsimonious within itself; b) external validity, whether the system is capable of accomplishing its intended purpose of predicting a behavioral effect; and c) use rate, whether the system is actually used by scientists and technologists in the fields of interest. The current NANDA taxonomy does not appear to meet the criteria for internal validity and external validity.

In spite of the criticisms, the NANDA classification has been adopted within the United States and internationally. It is used widely in information systems, books, care maps, and curricula. Thus, the need for a valid taxonomy of diagnoses is most urgent. As noted by Warren (1994), the biggest roadblock to validation has been money and the resources to do the research.

It remains a challenge to continue the development and refinement of NANDA diagnoses to facilitate diagnosis refinement, development, expert validation, and clinical validation. After consultation with the NANDA board a collaborative agreement for a joint venture between a research team at The University of Iowa College of Nursing and NANDA was

Table 1

What NDEC will do to Address the Criticisms of NANDA

Problems	Actions
Lack of clarity in characteristics of diagnosis concepts	Characteristics of the diagnosis concept has been jointly clarified by NDEC and NANDA consultants at the invitation of the agreement
Need for guidelines for improving conceptual clarity	Concept analysis procedures have been developed and are being used by NDEC to refine the existing NANDA diagnosis
Inadequate scope, comprehensiveness, specificity, and clinical usefulness	Extension of scope to encompass generalist to specialist, and novice to expert practices, use of Satellite Diagnosis Work Groups which include Advanced Practice Nurses
Lack of an accepted means for differentiating among diagnoses	Diagnoses represent a select group of signs/symptoms to be identified through concept analysis and validated by nurses to provide differentiation
Lack of accepted means for differentiating among diagnosis labels, defining characteristics, and related factors	Differentiation methods have been developed using concept analysis with validation by experts
Need for development of definitions and decision rules for component parts for diagnoses	Have been completed (see Table 4)
Need to refine language and to increase clinical utility and linkage to other classifications in nursing and other disciplines	Guidelines for development of language have been developed. Clinical utility and linkage to refinement, expert validation, list extension, and linkage to other classifications at the end of the project.
Lack of a systematic approach for establishing reliability, validity, and external validity of diagnoses	Reliability and validity of the diagnoses will be conducted with a systematic approach. External the validity will be established through the use of a national sample of experts in specialties
Need for clinical testing	Is being conducted
Inadequate conceptual framework	NDEC uses inductive methods and validate with conceptual frameworks
Lack of aggregate and wellness diagnoses	NDEC has Diagnosis Work Groups addressing family, group, and community aggregates; wellness diagnoses are developed for all appropriate diagnostic concepts
Lack of fit between the nine Human Response Patterns and diagnoses that require both interdependent and independent nursing interventions	Nurses share domains with other disciplines; NDEC diagnoses include both nursing diagnoses that are the responsibility of nurses alone and those with responsibility shared with other disciplines.

Table 2

The Relationship of NANDA and NDEC

NDEC	NANDA
1. Will refine existing NANDA diagnoses and submit to NANDA	1. Will review using the same review process as used for all submissions
2. Complete research aims and publish research findings, such as refined diagnoses, new diagnoses and classification of diagnoses	2. Shall hold copyright on all diagnoses in the NANDA Taxonomy including revised diagnoses and new diagnoses that are products of the NDEC research

Collaborative NDEC/NANDA

1. NDEC's Advisory Board will include (but not be limited to) the President of NANDA, the Chairs of NANDA's Taxonomy Committee and Diagnostic Review Committee

2. NANDA will publicly recognize the collaborative relationship, and NDEC will include NANDA as a cooperative agency on all funding proposals

3. The NANDA Board will include NDEC on its regular agenda and will receive minutes and related documents from NDEC

4. NANDA Board representatives will complete an on-site visit of the NDEC Team once per year

5. The NDEC Co-PIs will attend at least one NANDA Board meeting per year

reached in 1994 (Hoskins, 1994; NANDA/NDEC, 1997; Craft-Rosenberg & Delaney, 1997) to extend the NANDA work. The goal of this collaborative agreement is to improve the comprehensiveness, scope, specificity, clinical usefulness, and clinical testing of the NANDA taxonomy (see Table 1).

The relationship of NANDA and NDEC is summarized in Table 2. The primary role of NDEC is research, while the primary role of NANDA is that of policy. Specific aims for NDEC are to: (1) identify and resolve conceptual and methodological issues; (2) evaluate and revise NANDA nursing diagnoses using criteria for the development of standardized languages; (3) develop and evaluate candidate concepts to extend the NANDA list of nursing diagnoses;

(4) examine the validity of revised and new diagnosis concepts; and (5) examine the clinical validity of the revised and new diagnosis concepts. The research team is currently working on aims three through five.

When the NANDA board and the NDEC team signed agreement, plans for continued discussion and decision making were made. The Principal Investigators at that time, Craft-Rosenberg and Delaney, met with the NANDA board in March, 1995, to present plans for addressing the limitations of the existing nomenclature. In the summer of 1995 the NANDA President, Lois Hoskins, the president-elect, Judy Warren, and another member of the NANDA board, Joan Fitzmaurice, came to The University of Iowa to assist the NDEC

Table 3

Definition of Terms (Adapted from NANDA, Nursing Diagnosis Definition & Classification, 1996)

Nursing diagnosis is a clinical judgment about individual, family or community responses to actual or potential health problems/life processes. Nursing diagnoses provide the basis for selection of nursing interventions to achieve desired outcomes

Actual nursing diagnoses describe human responses to health conditions/life processes that exist in an individual, family, or community. The diagnosis is supported by signs and symptoms (manifestations, defining characteristics) that cluster in a unique pattern.

Risk nursing diagnoses describe human responses to health conditions/life processes which may develop in a vulnerable individual, family, or community. The risk diagnosis is supported by risk factors that contribute to increased vulnerability.

Wellness nursing diagnoses describe human responses to levels of wellness in an individual, family, or community that have a potential for enhancement to a higher state.

The components (structure) of a nursing diagnosis include a label, definition, signs and symptoms, and related factors.

The label provides a name for a diagnosis. It is a concise term or phrase that represents a pattern of related signs and symptoms.

The definition provides a clear, precise description, delineates its meaning, and helps differentiate it from other diagnoses.

Signs and symptoms are observable or verifiable cues that cluster as manifestations of a nursing diagnosis or as manifestations of vulnerability to illness or decreased wellness.

Related factors are conditions/circumstances that contribute to the development/maintenance of an existing nursing diagnosis. A related factor can be a cause (etiology) or a co-existent, associated condition or circumstance that contributes to or influences the diagnosis.

Classification is the ordering or arranging of nursing diagnoses into groups or sets on the basis of their relationships and the assigning of labels and definitions to these groups.

Risk factors are environmental factors and physiological, psychological, genetic, or chemical elements that increase the vulnerability of an individual, family, or community.

team with the preparation of a research proposal for submission to the Nursing Institute for Nursing Research. During the deliberations it was decided that NDEC would use the same nursing diagnosis structure and definitions that are used by NANDA, with two exceptions. First, the definition of nursing diagnosis for NDEC eliminated the phrase "for which nurses are accountable" to increase the scope of diagnoses and recognize those diagnoses with shared responsibility with other disciplines. Second, the words "signs" and "symptoms" rather than "defining characteristics" were chosen by NDEC, with board approval, to describe the attributes of the diagnosis (see Table 3).

There is an immediate need for the findings from the NDEC research. The linkage of diagnoses, interventions, and outcomes is central to the structuring of nursing knowledge and the study of nursing effectiveness. Since the diagnoses statements frame the client phenomena, diagnoses determine outcomes and interventions. If the diagnoses are not reliable, valid, or accurate, the outcomes and interventions may be unnecessary or inaccurate. Refinement of the existing NANDA diagnoses using empirical findings from the literature will refine and update the diagnoses. This work should also increase the reliability and validity of the labels. Development of new diagnoses using systematic concept analysis methods will increase the scope of diagnoses as well as the reliability and validity of the diagnoses.

The NDEC research team consists of three Principal Investigators with differing responsibilities. In addition there is a large team of clinicians, academicians, and researchers representing all major clinical practice areas. The majority of investigators have doctoral degrees and most investigators are conducting research on nursing diagnosis. All faculty team members teach nursing diagnoses, interventions, and outcomes at the undergraduate and/or graduate levels. All team members are members of NANDA. Two team members have held or currently hold NANDA offices (Maas and Glick). Craft-Rosenberg is on Taxonomy Committee and Delaney is on the Diagnosis Review Committee. Several participants possess informatics and/or classification development expertise, including Craft-Rosenberg, Delaney, Denehy, Donahue, Glick, Clarke, Maas, and Schenfelder.

Even though two proposals have been submitted to the Nursing Institute Nursing Research, none have been funded. NDEC has received one grant from the University of Iowa Central Investment Fund for Research Enhancement in 1995, but the rest of the work has been donated by the investigators and members of diagnosis work groups.

Refinement of Existing NANDA Diagnoses

The first aim of the NDEC research has been to refine the existing NANDA diagnoses. The decision to begin with refinement was suggested by NANDA President, Lois Hoskins, and then President-elect Judy Warren in the summer of 1995. The research team recognized that the refinement work would enable us to develop, pilot, and use concept analysis, expert validation, and clinical validation procedures for continued use in diagnosis development and testing.

Concept Analysis

The purposes of concept analysis of the approved NANDA diagnoses were to: 1) evaluate the completeness of the diagnosis concepts and identify labels for missing concepts; 2) evaluate and refine the definition of the diagnostic concept; 3) evaluate and refine the signs and symptoms and related factors based on the literature; and 4) recommend the staging category. NDEC established the NANDA Stage 2.1 as the minimum acceptable level for refinement work.

A Concept Analysis Protocol was developed using the work of Waltz and Strickland (1991) in addition to the work of Rogers and Knafl (1993). All of the NANDA diagnoses were subjected to the same concept analysis processes. The concept analysis protocol (see Appendix A) includes six phases: (a) concept analysis by individuals; (b) review, discussion, and validation through consensus building in small groups of clinical experts (Diagnosis Work Groups [DWG]) chaired by doctorally prepared investigators; (c) critique for conformity to standardized language rules by the Rules Review Committee; and (d) review and validation by the large NDEC research team consisting of clinical experts representing most nursing specialties as well as care across the lifespan and settings. Expert validation and clinical validation follow.

The literature data base for concept analysis included these journals: (a) Western Journal of Nursing Research; (b) Advances in Nursing Science; (c) *Nursing Research*; (d) *Image-Journal of Nursing Scholarship*; (e) *Annual Review of Nursing Research*; (f) *Nursing Diagnosis*; and (g) *Proceedings of the North American Nursing Diagnosis Association*. Sources from other disciplines were used when needed to describe the phenomena. Reports of empirical studies were given priority. The quality of the articles was evaluated for diagnosis content and representation across health-illness diagnoses, units of care (individual, family, community), and stages of development (See Appendix B NDEC Diagnosis Work Group Source Rating Tool). If the quality of the article met the needs of the project, the article was selected for Concept Analysis. The diagnostic label, conceptual definition, signs and symptoms, related/risk factors, synonyms and related concepts were extracted from each article (See Appendix C NDEC Concept Analysis Worksheet). The problem statement, variables, method, sample, instruments, and findings were identified and critiqued for empirical studies (see Appendix D NDEC Concept Analysis Worksheet for Empirical Studies). Findings from all articles were compared and synthesized. To increase specificity of complex concepts, additional concepts were identified.

One concept analysis summary was completed for each label. This summary included the recommended diagnostic label, conceptual definition, signs/symptoms, related/risk factors, and any additional concepts (see Appendix E NDEC Completed Concept Analysis Form) The conceptual definition had to describe the complete meaning of the concept, be internally consistent, clear, simple, and refer to all signs/symptoms. Each related factor or sign and symptom had to be supported by the literature. All terms used in the signs and symptoms had to be measurable or verifiable. Additional concepts identified in the synthesis stage formed the foundation for development of new diagnostic labels. The concept analysis synthesis was then forwarded to the DWG for discussion.

Review, Discussion, and Validation by Diagnosis Work Groups (DWG)

A schedule was developed for presentation of the synthesis of the concept analysis to the

Appendix A

NDEC Concept Analysis Protocol

Walz & Strickland (1991); Rogers & Knafl (1993)

The purpose of the NDEC concept analysis is to generate or revise a nursing diagnosis. The finished product will include a recommendation for a diagnosis label, definition, signs and symptoms, and related factors or risk factors that reflect all dimensions of a concept (diagnosis). The following protocol will assist team members in proceeding through the concept analysis process in a consistent manner.
Diagnosis Group_________________________________Reviewer_________________________________

A.   Step 1--Identify key literature related to this concept.
   [] 1. Select 5-10 key sources that represent both conceptual and empirical bases.
   [] 2. Complete a Diagnosis Source Rating Tool for each source.

B.   Step 2--Develop a preliminary conceptual definition.
   Use the NANDA definition or one of your own.

Concept____
Definition____
____
____
____

C. Step 3--Critically analyze the elements of the concept identified in the literature and in NANDA (if revising a concept).
   [] 1. List all elements of the concept on the NDEC Concept Analysis Worksheet (one worksheet for each literature source). These elements include the conceptual definition, synonyms and definitions, related factors or risk factors, and signs and symptoms.
   [] 2. List related concepts and definitions on the NDEC Concept Analysis Worksheet.

D. Step 4--Develop a conceptual definition.
   [] 1. Select those parts of the conceptual definitions that are consistently present in the literature sources (critical elements) to revise the preliminary definition.
   [] 2. Begin to construct a conceptual map (an outline, table, or diagram) to represent the critical elements of the definition.
   [] 3. Evaluate the revised conceptual definition by answering the following questions:
       a. Is the definition too complex (needs to be divided)?   Y   N
       b. Are any elements of the definition missing?   Y   N
       c. Does the definition describe the complete meaning of the concept?   Y   N
       d. Is the definition as a whole internally consistent with the concept?   Y   N
       e. Is the definition clear and simple?   Y   N
       f. Does the definition refer to all signs and symptoms included with the concept?   Y   N
       g. Does the definition differ from or exclude the related concepts and definitions?   Y   N

   [] 4. Update the preliminary conceptual definition.

E. Step 5--Develop signs and symptoms for the concept.
[ ] 1. Remove redundancies in lists of signs/symptoms between the sources.
[ ] 2. Cluster the signs/symptoms if too numerous.
[ ] 3. Obtain additional sources if the list is too short.
[ ] 4. Evaluate the signs/symptoms by answering the following questions:
    a. Are the signs and symptoms precise?　　　　　　　　　　　　　　　Y　N
    b. Is their congruency between the diagnosis, related factors, and signs/symptoms?　Y　N
    c. Are the terms used in a consistent manner?　　　　　　　　　　　　Y　N
    d. Are the elements inclusive, representing all dimensions of the concept?　Y　N
    e. Are the signs and symptoms measurable?　　　　　　　　　　　　Y　N
    f. Are the terms sensitive and useful for nursing?　　　　　　　　　　Y　N

[ ] 5. Review and update the conceptual definition as needed.
[ ] 6. Add signs and symptoms to the conceptual map.

F. Step 6--Develop related factors or risk factors for the concept.
[ ] 1. Remove redundancies in lists of related factors/risk factors between the sources.
[ ] 2. Cluster the related factors/risk factors if too numerous.
[ ] 3. Obtain additional sources if the list is too short.
[ ] 4. Evaluate the related factors/risk factors by answering the following questions:
    a. Are the related factors/risk factors precise?　　　　　　　　　　Y　N
    b. Is their congruency between the diagnosis, related factors/risk factors, and signs/symptoms? Y　N
    c. Are the terms used in a consistent manner?　　　　　　　　　　　Y　N
    d. Are the elements inclusive, representing all dimensions of the concept?　Y　N
    e. Are the terms sensitive and useful for nursing?　　　　　　　　　Y　N

[ ] 5. Review and update the conceptual definition as needed.
[ ] 6. Add the related factors or risk factors to the conceptual map.

G. Step 7--Develop a label for the diagnosis definition. The label is a noun phrase that concisely summarizes the conceptual definition.
[ ] 1. Evaluate the label by answering the following questions:
    a. Is the label a 2-4 word phrase?　　　　　　　　　　　　　　　Y　N
    b. Does the label consist of a non-evaluative descriptive noun followed by an
       accepted NDEC/NANDA noun qualifier?　　　　　　　　　　　Y　N
    c. Is the label precise?　　　　　　　　　　　　　　　　　　　Y　N
    d. Is the label concise?　　　　　　　　　　　　　　　　　　　Y　N
    e. Is the label clear?　　　　　　　　　　　　　　　　　　　　Y　N
    f. Is the label non-synonymous?　　　　　　　　　　　　　　　　Y　N
    g. Is the label reliable?　　　　　　　　　　　　　　　　　　　Y　N
    h. Is the label meaningful?　　　　　　　　　　　　　　　　　　Y　N
    i. Is the label clinically useful?　　　　　　　　　　　　　　　　Y　N

continued on next page

H. Step 8--Connect the related factors to the new diagnosis label, then add the signs and symptoms associated with that label/related factor combination.
[ ] 1. Create distinct labels by associating each related factor to the diagnosis label.
[ ] 2. Connect the signs and symptoms or clusters of signs and symptoms associated with each label/related factor combination created in 8.1.

I. Step 9--Recommend the revised or developed nursing diagnosis to Rules Committee
[ ] 1 Submit a Completed Concept Analysis Form.
[ ] 2. Submit the supporting documentation.
  a. An NDEC Concept Analysis Worksheet for each literature source.
  b. A Diagnosis Source Rating Tool for each literature source.
  c. A conceptual map, if applicable.

Appendix B

NDEC Diagnosis Work Group Source Rating Tool

Title: _______________________ Rater: _______________________
Author: _______________________ Diagnosis Group: _______________________
Year: _______________________ Date: _______________________

Circle the number that corresponds to the extent you disagree or agree with the following statements
(1 = Strongly Disagree, 2 = Disagree, 3 = Unsure, 4 = Agree, 5 = Strongly Agree).

A. This source contains clear statements of health conditions, problems,   1   2   3   4   5
or needs (nursing diagnoses), signs and symptoms (defining
characteristics), etiologies or contributing factors (related factors),
and risk factors.

   A.1. The signs and symptoms are observable, measurable, 13or   1   2   3   4   5
verifiable.

   A.2. The related factors or risk factors can be modified through   1   2   3   4   5
interventions (nursing and others).

   A.3. The diagnoses, signs and symptoms, and related factors/risk   1   2   3   4   5
factors are easy to find within the text.

B. This source contains a comprehensive sample of diagnoses, signs   1   2   3   4   5
and symptoms, and related factors/risk factors that represents a
selected area of nursing practice.

C. This source contains diagnoses, signs and symptoms, and related   1   2   3   4   5
factors/risk factors that apply to current nursing practice.

D. The diagnoses in this source are empirically based (references cited).   1   2   3   4   5

E. This source includes diagnoses for which nurses are responsible for   1   2   3   4   5
treating.

   E.1. independently.   1   2   3   4   5
   E.2. dependently (under physician supervision).   1   2   3   4   5
   E.3. interdependently.   1   2   3   4   5

F. Refer to the Diagnosis Group Chart for clarification of possible   1   2   3   4   5
dimensions.

DEVELOPMENTAL PROCESS

INDIVIDUAL	FAMILY/GROUP	COMMUNITY
I-A: Infant/child/adolescent Ad: Adult Ag: Aging	C: Changing S: Stable O: Other	E: Emerging/pioneer M: Mature/industrious/productive R: Restructured/changing

NDEC DIAGNOSIS GROUP DEFINITION
Settting Care Environment

Unit of Care Health Illness Continuum	Client Work Site			Schools			Office/ Clinics			Hospitals			Homes			Supportive Living			Other		
INDIVIDUAL	I-A	Ad	Ag	I-A	Ad	Ag	I-A	Ad	Ag	I-A	Ad	Ag	I-A	Ad	Ag	I-A	Ad	Ag	I-A	Ad	Ag
Wellness																					
At risk																					
Illness -- Psychosocial																					
Illness -- Physiological																					
Dying																					
FAMILY/GROUP	C	S	O	C	S	O	C	S	O	C	S	O	C	S	O	C	S	O	C	S	O
Wellness																					
At risk																					
Illness -- Psychosocial																					
Illness -- Physiological																					
Dying																					
COMMUNITY/PUBLIC	E	M	R	E	M	R	E	M	R	E	M	R	E	M	R	E	M	R	E	M	R
Wellness																					
At risk																					
Illness -- Psychosocial																					
Illness -- Physiological																					
Dying																					

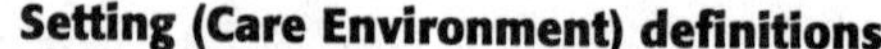

Setting (Care Environment) definitions

Client Work Site: Any setting in which people are employed. Examples include industries and shops.

Offices/clinics: Offices and clinics in which physicians and /or nurses provide care.

Schools: Educational settings including daycare settings, pre-schools, schools for children and colleges/universities.

Homes: Place of residence intended for single family dwelling.

Supportive Living: Homelike alternatives in which assistance and supervision may be provided for activities of daily living. Examples include long term care facilities of assisted living dwellings for the chronically mentally ill or retarded, shelters, and jail.

Hospitals: Hospitals of any size. Client conditions will include those seen in ambulatory, inpatient, emergency, operating room and rehabilitation.

Other: Please note the setting, client conditions diagnosed, and how setting and conditions differ from other setting categories.

Appendix C

NDEC Concept Analysis Worksheet

Complete this form for each article reviewed.

Reviewer: _______________________   Diagnosis Group: _______________________

Article #: _______________________   Date: _______________________

COMPLETE CITATION

____

____

____

____

TYPE: ___________ Concept Analysis/Lit Review _______________________ Empirical (see page 3)

DIAGNOSIS LABEL

____

____

____

CONCEPTUAL DEFINITION

____

____

____

____

SYNONYMS AND DEFINITIONS

____

____

____

____

SIGNS AND SYMPTOMS

____

____

____

RELATED FACTORS/RISK FACTORS

____

____

____

____

RELATED CONCEPTS AND DEFINITIONS

____

____

____

____

Appendix D

NDEC Concept Analysis Worksheet For Empirical Studies

Complete this form for each article reviewed.

Reviewer: _______________________   Diagnosis Group: _______________________
Article #: _______________________   Date: _______________________

1. PROBLEM STATEMENT:

____
____
____
____

2. VARIABLES (conceptual and operational definitions):

____
____
____
____

3. METHOD:

____
____
____
____

4. SAMPLE:

____
____
____
____

5. INSTRUMENTS (include validity and reliability summary):

____
____
____
____

6. FINDINGS

____
____
____
____

Appendix E

NDEC Completed Concept Analysis Form

Complete this form and submit to Marty Craft-Rosenberg and Connie Deleney when the concept analysis is finished.

Reviewer: _______________________________   Diagnosis Group: _______________________________

Article #: _______________________________   Date: _______________________________

DIAGNOSIS LABEL

CONCEPTUAL DEFINITION

SIGNS AND SYMPTOMS

RELATED FACTORS/RISK FACTORS

CANDIDATE DIAGNOSIS IDENTIFIED FOR CONSIDERATION

Table 4

NDEC Rules for the Development of Standardized Languages

Rule 1: A nursing diagnosis label is a noun phrase which describes a client health related state, behavior, response, or phenomena

Rule 2: A diagnosis label may or may not contain a qualifying term (placed following the core concept or "root"), which expresses:
   a. Place of the diagnosis label on the health-illness continuum, such as Risk or Enhancement Potential
   b. Deviation from benchmark (change from baseline, norm, expectation): from the NANDA list of qualifiers and other qualifiers.

Rule 3: A term acting as a "specifier," will preceed the core concept, or "root." Specifiers include words that describe a unit of care (family, community), severity (acute, chronic,) or timing of the diagnoses (intermittent). Diagnoses without the specifiers of family or community are diagnoses for the individual.

Rule 4: Each nursing diagnosis label will contain two-four words. It will be:
   a. exact, accurate (precision)
   b. compact, succinct (concision)
   c. clear in meaning, lacking ambiguity (clarity)
   d. dissimilar and distinct from other diagnoses (nonsynonymity)
   e. meaningful to the clinician

Rule 5: The NDEC format for presentation of a nursing diagnosis shall be: (a) Label (1-4 words); (b) Definition; (c) Signs and Symptoms, (d) Related/Risk Factors; (e) References, and (f) Recommended NANDA Staging.

Rule 6: All signs/symptoms and related factors will be referenced.

Rule 7: The words "Increased," or " Decreased" will be used to show variance, instead of specific values.

Rule 8: For each label and its' associated related factor it is anticipated that there must be at least one specific sign or symptom which distinguishes this diagnosis from all other diagnoses.

Rule 9: Actual and Risk diagnoses will be presented as a continuum, with the risk factors becoming related factors when signs/symptoms are present.

Rule 10: Risk and Related factors will be those factors that are associated directly with the diagnosis. For example, the related factor for Family Process Alteration: Alcoholism, is alcohol abuse, rather than genetic predisposition to alcohol abuse.

Rule 11: Punctuation will include the use of a colon between the diagnosis and related factor (i.e. Family Processes Alteration: Alcoholism). No commas will be used for clinical usage.

Rule 12: The root of the label will be placed first for indexing, using a comma to separate the root from the qualifier.

Rule 13: The structure and the words of the diagnosis will have clinical feasibility and be compatible with information systems and database design principles.

DWG for discussion and critique. If the concerns raised by the group were substantive, additional presentation(s) for further discussion were scheduled. When there was group consensus that the synthesis was supported by the literature, the concept analysis was forwarded to the Rules Committee for review.

Critique for Conformity to Rules for the Development of Standardized Languages

The purpose of the review process by the Rules Committee was to ensure that the synthesis completed in the DWG conformed to language and formatting rules developed and adopted for use by NDEC. When possible the review process included the person who completed the concept analysis so that questions could be answered directly. Modification suggestions were given to the DWG by the Rules Committee. The work was refined and returned to the Rules Committee for another review prior to going to the large team. Each concept synthesis was evaluated for consistency with the Rules for the Development of Standardized Languages outlined in Table 4. These rules were based upon existing recommendations (NANDA, 1994; Evans, 1994; Gillenson, 1985; Loucopoulos & Zicari (Eds.), 1992, and the ANA Steering Committee on Databases to Support Clinical Practice). In addition, they were developed in consultation with Colleen Prophet (an NDEC investigator), Director of Information Systems for the Department of Nursing the University of Iowa Hospitals, and her colleagues, Gloria Dorr and Teresa Gibbs, who are Advanced Practice Nurses and Nursing Informatics Specialists at the University of Iowa Hospitals and Clinics; and Mary Clarke, Nursing Informatics Specialist, Genesis Medical Center, Davenport, IA.

Review and Validation by Large Research Team

The NDEC research team completed the final review of each label. At the team meeting, the DWG member who conducted the concept analysis and the chair of the associated DWG were present to provide clarification and respond to questions. All refinement suggestions were incorporated following the meeting. Finally, the approved labels were added to the database, where they were formatted for submission to NANDA and prepared for external expert and clinical validation.

Part II
Completed Work

This part includes 96 revised and/or new labels. Two reference listings preceed the labels themselves. Listing one provides the name of each NDEC label and the corresponding NANDA label, if applicable. The labels are presented alphabetically by NDEC label. The second listing illustrates each NDEC label and the related indexing format for that label. In most instances the clinical label and indexing label are the same; "acute pain" represents one example of difference. Each revised/new label follows in alphabetical order. The label, NANDA label (if applicable), definition, signs and symptoms, related factors/risk factors, reference list, and recommended staging are stated for each label. All signs/symptoms, related factors/risk factors are referenced to published works. Every label is developed to a minimum recommend staging of 2.1; it is significant that a large number of labels are ready for clinical testing and/or have been developed beyond the highest currently defined stage.

ACUTE PAIN (NANDA Pain)

DEFINITION: Experience of unpleasant sensory and emotional sensations for a duration of less than six months. [1,2,5]

SIGNS AND SYMPTOMS (Observed or Reported):
Patients self report of pain [1,3,4,5,6]
Change in pulse rate [1,5,6]
Change in blood pressure [1,5,6]
Change in respiratory pattern, e.g. rate, depth [1,5,6]
Restlessness [5,6]
Diaphoresis [1,5,6]
Grimacing [2,4,5,6]
Increased muscle tension [2,4,5,6]
Whining [2,4,5]
Whimpering [2,4,5]
Crying [2,4,5,6]

RELATED FACTORS:
Physical injuring agent [1,2,3,4]
Psychological injuring agent [1,2,5]

REFERENCES:
1. Acute Pain Management Guideline Panel. (1993). <u>Acute pain management in adults: Operative procedures: quick reference guide for clinicians</u>. AHCPR Pub. No. 92-0019. Rockville, MD: Agency for Health Care Policy and Research, Public Health Service, U.S. Department of Health and Human Services.
2. Acute Pain Management Guideline Panel. (1993). <u>Acute pain management in infants, children and adolescents: Operative and medical procedures. Quick reference guide for clinicians</u>. AHCPR Pub. No. 92-0020. Rockville, MD: Agency for Health Care Policy and Research, Public Health Service, U.S. Department of Health and Human Services.
3. Jurf, J.B., & Nirschl, A.L. (1993). Acute postoperative pain management: A comprehensive review and update. <u>Critical Care Nursing Quarterly, 16</u>(1), 8-25.
4. Mahon, S.M. (1994). Concept analysis of pain: Implications related to nursing diagnosis. <u>Nursing Diagnosis, 5</u>(1), 14-25
5. McGuire, D.B. (1984). The measurement of clinical pain. <u>Nursing Research</u>, 33(3), 152-56.
6. Simon, J.M., Nolan, L., & Baumann, M.A. (1995). Validation of the nursing diagnoses acute pain and chronic pain. In M.J. Rantz & P. LeMone (Eds), <u>Classification of nursing diagnoses: Proceedings of the eleventh conference, North American Nursing Diagnosis Association</u> (pp.199-203). Glendale, CA: CINAHL Information Systems.

RECOMMENDED NANDA STAGING: 2.3

ADJUSTMENT IMPAIRMENT (NANDA Impaired Adjustment)

DEFINITION: Inability to modify life style/behavior in a manner consistent with a change in health status

SIGNS AND SYMPTOMS (Observed or Reported):
Failure to achieve optimal sense of control [4]
Denial of health status change [1,2,7]
Demonstration of non-acceptance of health status change [2]
Failure to take actions that would prevent further health problems [2]

RELATED FACTORS:
Disability/health status change requiring change in life style [1,2,3,4,5,6]
Absence of social support for changed beliefs and practices [7,1,5,6]
Multiple stressors
Lack of motivation to change behaviors [6,8]
Intense emotional states [1,3]
Negative attitudes toward health behavior [5,6,]
Low state of optimism [8,7]
Failure to intend to change behavior [5,6,]

REFERENCES:
1. Beach, E.K., Smith, A., Luthringer, L., Letz, S., Ahrens, S., & Whitmire, V. (1996). Self care limitations of persons after acute myocardial infarction, Applied Nursing Research, 9(1), 24-28.
2. DiIorio, C., & Henry, M. (1995). Self management with epilepsy, Journal of Neuroscience Nursing, 27(6), 338-343.
3. DeVon, H.A.,& Powers, M.J. (1984). Health beliefs, adjustment to illness, and control of hypertension, Research in Nursing and Health, 7(1), 10-16.
4. Miller, P., Wikoff, R., Garrett, M.J., McMahon, M., & Smith, T. (1990). Regimen compliance two years after myocardial infarction, Nursing Research, 39(6), 333-336.
5. Miller, P., Wikoff, R., & Hiatt, A. (1992). Fishbein's model of reasoned action and compliance behavior of hypertensive patients, Nursing Research, 41(2), 104-109.
6. Pender N., & Pender, A. (1986). Attitudes, subjective norms, and intentions to engage in health behaviors, Nursing Research, 35(1), 15-18.
7. Powers, M., & Jalowiec, A. (1987). Profile of the well-controlled, well-adjusted hypertensive patient, Nursing Research, 36(2), 106-110.
8. Taylor, S. (1983). Adjustment to threatening events: A theory of adaptation, American Psychologist, 11, 1161-1173.

RECOMMENDED NANDA STAGING: 2.1

AIRWAY CLEARANCE INEFFECTIVENESS (NANDA Airway Clearance, Ineffective)

DEFINITION: Inability to clear secretions or obstructions from the respiratory tract.

SIGNS AND SYMPTOMS (Observed or Reported):

Adventitious breath sounds e.g. crackles, gurgles, wheezes [1,3,7]

Reports chest congestion [1,3,7]

Reports difficulty with sputum [2,7]

Ineffective or absent cough [2,3,4,6,7]

RELATED FACTORS:

Obstructed Airway:

Airway spasm [8]

Retained secretions [6]

Exudate in the alveoli [2]

Secretions in the bronchi [2]

Excessive mucus [6]

Foreign body in airway [8]

Presence of artificial airway [4]

Pathophysiology Process:

Asthma [8]

Allergic airways [8]

Chronic obstructive pulmonary disease [5]

Hyperplasia of the bronchial walls [6]

Infection [5, 6]

Neuromuscular dysfunction [7]

Environmental Irritants:

Smoking [5]

Smoke inhalation [8]

Second hand smoke [5]

REFERENCES:

1. Burrell, L.O. (Ed.). (1992). Adult nursing in hospitals and community settings. East Norwalk, CT: Appleton & Lange.
2. Brukwitzki, G., Holmgren, C., & Maibusch, R.M. (1996). Validation of the defining characteristics of the nursing diagnosis ineffective airway clearance. Nursing Diagnosis, 7(2), pp. 63-69.
3. Capuano, T.A., Hitchings, K.S., & Johnson, S. (1990). Respiratory nursing diagnoses: practicing nurses' selection of defining characteristics. Nursing Diagnosis, 1(4), 169-174.
4. Dossey, B.M. Guzzetta, C.E., & Kenner, C.V. (Eds.). (1990). Essentials of critical care nursing: mind, body, spirit. Philadelphia: J. B. Lippincott.
5. Hanley, M.V., & Tyler, M L. (1987). Ineffective airway clearance related to airway infection. In M J. Kim (Vol. Ed.), The Nursing Clinics of North America: Vol. 22 (1). II. Ineffective breathing patterns (pp. 135-150). Philadelphia: W.B. Saunders Co.
6. Hastings, B. (1989). Alterations in respiration. In C. Malloy & J. Hartshorn (Eds.). Acute care nursing in the home. New York: J. B. Lippincott.
7. Hoffman, L.A. (1987). Ineffective airway clearance related to neuromuscular dysfunction. In M.J. Kim (Vol. Ed.), The Nursing Clinics of North America: Vol. 22 (1). II. Ineffective breathing patterns (pp. 151-166). Philadelphia: W.B. Saunders Co
8. Whaley, L.F. & Wong, D L. (Eds.) (1991). Nursing care of infants and children. (4th Ed.). St. Louis: Mosby.

RECOMMENDED NANDA STAGING: 2.3

AUTONOMIC DYSREFLEXIA (NANDA Dysreflexia)

DEFINITION: A life threatening uninhibited response of the sympathetic nervous system for an individual with a spinal cord injury/lesion at T6 or above, and having recovered from spinal shock.

SIGNS AND SYMPTOMS (Observed or Reported):
Individual with spinal cord injury T6 or above with:
- Paroxysmal hypertension[1, 2,4,5,6,7]
- Bradycardia or tachycardia[1, 2,3,4,5,6,7]
- Diaphoresis above the level of the injury/lesion [1,2,4,5,6,7]
- Flushing or patchy erythema above the injury/lesion[1,4,5,6,7]
- Pallor, cool skin below the level of the injury/lesion[1,2]
- Piloerection below the level of the injury/lesion[1,2,6,7]
- Headache[1, 2,4,5,7]
- Anxiety[1, 2,4,7]
- Conjunctival congestion[2]
- Nasal congestion[2, 6,7]
- Visual changes [6]
- Metallic taste in mouth[2]
- Shortness of breath[2]
- Chest pain[6]
- Nausea[2, 7]

RELATED FACTORS:
Injury/lesion T6 or above with any noxious stimulus including:

Urological Problems:
- Bladder distention[1, 2,6,7]
- Spasm[2], stones[2, 7]
- Instrumentation or surgery[2]
- Epididymitis[2]
- Infection[1, 6]

Gastrointestinal Problems:
- Impaction[1,2,6,7]
- Enemas, stimulation, e.g. digital, instrumentation, surgery[1,2,6,7]
- GI system pathology[1, 2]

Integumentary Problems: [1,6,7]
- Cutaneous stimulation, e.g. pressure ulcer, ingrown toenail, dressings, burns

Situational Problems: [1,2,4,6,7]
- Positioning
- Range of motion exercise
- Pelvic pathology
- Pregnancy
- Labor delivery
- Drug reaction, e.g. decongestants, sympathomimetic, vasoconstrictors, narcotic withdrawal
- Esophageal reflux

REFERENCES:
1. Braddom, R.L., & Rocco, J.F. (1991). Autonomic dysreflexia; a survey of current treatment. *American Journal of Physical Medicine and Rehabilitation, 70*(5), 234-241.
2. Dunn, K.L. (1991). Autonomic dysreflexia: A nursing challenge in the care of the patient with a spinal cord injury. *Journal of Cardiovascular Nursing, 5*(4), 57-64.
3. Pine, Z.M., Miller, S.D., & Alonso, J.A. (1991). Atrial fibrillation associated with autonomic dysreflexia. *American Journal of Physical Medicine and Rehabilitation, 70*(5), 271-273.
4. Kumar, V.N. & Mullican, C.N. (1989). Ovarian cyst and autonomic dysreflexia. *Archives of Physical Medicine and Rehabilitation, 70*(7), 547-548.
5. Finestone, H.M., & Teasell, R.W. (1993). Autonomic dysreflexia after brainstem tumor resection: A case report. *American Journal of Physical Medicine and Rehabilitation, 72*(6), 395-397.
6. Colachis, S.C. (1991). Autonomic hyperreflexia in spinal cord injury associated with pulmonary embolism. *Archives of Physical Medicine and Rehabilitation, 72*(12), 1014-1016
7. Hickey, J.V. (1992). *The clinical practice of neurological and neurosurgical nursing* (3rd Ed.). Philadelphia: J.B. Lippincott Co.

RECOMMENDED NANDA STAGING: 2.1

AUTONOMIC DYSREFLEXIA RISK (NANDA None)

DEFINITION: A life threatening uninhibited response of the sympathetic nervous system for an individual with a spinal cord injury/lesion at T6 or above, and having recovered from spinal shock.

RISK FACTORS:

An injury/lesion at T6 or above with any noxious stimulus including:

Cardiac/Pulmonary Problems: [2]
  Pulmonary emboli

Gastrointestinal Problems: [1,3,7,8]
  Distention
  Constipation
  Enemas
  Stimulation, (e.g. digital, instrumentation
    surgery)
  GI system pathology
  Gastric ulcers
  Esophageal reflux

Neurological Problems: [2]
  Painful/irritating stimuli below level of injury

Regulatory Problems: [2]
  Temperature fluctuations

Reproductive Problems: [2]
  Menstration
  Sexual intercourse
  Ejaculation

Skeletal Integumentary Problems:
  Cutaneous stimulation, (e.g. pressure ulcer,
    ingrown toenail, dressings, burns, rash) [1,7,8]
  Heterotropic bone [2]

Situational Problems: [1,3,5,7,8]
  Positioning
  Range of motion exercises
  Pregnancy
  Labor/delivery
  Drug reaction, e.g. decongestants,
    sympathomimetics, vasoconstrictors, narcotic
    withdrawal
  Constrictive clothing
  Fractures
  Deep vein thrombosis
  Ovarian cyst
  Surgical procedure

Urological Problems: [1,3,7,8]
  Bladder distention
  Spasm
  Instrumentation or surgery
  Epididymitis
  Urethritis
  Infection

REFERENCES:

1. Braddom, R.L., & Rocco, J.F. (1991). Autonomic dysreflexia; A survey of current treatment. American Journal of Physical Medicine and Rehabilitation, 70(5), 234-241.
2. Consortium for Spinal Cord Medicine. (1997). Clinical practice guidelines: spinal cord medicine. Acute management of autonomic dysreflexia: Adults with spinal cord injury presenting to health-care facilities. Journal of Spinal Cord Medicine, 20(3), 284-308.
3. Dunn, K.L. (1991). Autonomic dysreflexia: A nursing challenge in the care of the patient with a spinal cord injury. Journal of Cardiovascular Nursing, 5(4), 57-64.
4. Pine, Z.M., Miller, S.D., & Alonso, J.A. (1991). Atrial fibrillation associated with autonomic dysreflexia. American Journal of Physical Medicine and Rehabilitation, 70(5), 271-273.
5. Kumar, V.N. & Mullican, C.N. (1989). Ovarian cyst and autonomic dysreflexia. Archives of Physical Medicine and Rehabilitation, 70(7), 547-548.
6. Finestone, H.M., & Teasell, R.W. (1993). Autonomic dysreflexia after brainstem tumor resection: A case report. American Journal of Physical Medicine and Rehabilitation, 72(6), 395-397.
7. Colachis, S.C. (1991). Autonomic hyperreflexia in spinal cord injury associated with pulmonary embolism. Archives of Physical Medicine and Rehabilitation, 72(12), 1014-1016
8. Hickey, J.V. (1992). The clinical practice of neurological and neurosurgical nursing (3rd Ed.). Philadelphia: J.B. Lippincott Co.

RECOMMENDED NANDA STAGING: 2.1

BATHING/HYGIENE SELF CARE DEFICIT (NANDA Self Care Deficit: Bathing/Hygiene)

DEFINITION: Impaired ability to perform or complete bathing/hygiene activities for oneself.

SIGNS AND SYMPTOMS (Observed or Reported):

Inability to:
Get in & out of bathroom[9]
Get bath supplies[9]
Dry body[9]
Wash body or body parts[1,4,5,6]
Obtain or get to water source[1,4,5,6]
Regulate temperature or flow [4,5,6]
Discomfort [2,5,6]

Suggested Functional Level Classification: [3]
 0=Completely independent.
 1=Requires use of equipment or device.
 2=Requires help from another person for
   assistance, supervision, or teaching.
 3=Requires help from another person and
   equipment device.
 4=Dependent, does not participate in activity.

RELATED FACTORS:

Weakness & tiredness[5,6,7]
Pain[2,5,6]
Perceptual or cognitive impairment[5,6]
Neuromuscular impairment[5,6]
Musculoskeletal impairment[5,6]
Severe anxiety[5,6]
Inadequate information regarding body part or
 spatial relationship[5,6]
Environmental barriers[5,6]
Decreased/lack of motivation[8]

REFERENCES:

1. Baer, C.A., Delorey, M., & Fitzmaurice, J.B. (1984). A study to evaluate the validity of the rating system for self-care deficit. In Kim, M.J., McFarland, G.K., & McLane, A.M. (Eds.). Classification of nursing diagnoses: Proceedings of the fifth national conference. St. Louis,MO: The C.V. Mosby Company.
2. Chang, B. (1994). Validity of concepts for selecting nursing diagnoses. Clinical Nursing Research, 3(3), 183-208.
3. Jones, E. (1974). Patient Classification for Long-Term Care: Users' Manual (Adapted from). HEW, Publication No. HRA-74-3107.
4. Levin, R.F., Krainovitch, B.C., Bahrenburg, E., & Mitchell, C.A. (1989). Diagnostic content validity of nursing diagnoses. Image: Journal of Nursing Scholarship, 21(1), 40-44.
5. McKeighen, R.J., Mehmert, P.A., & Dickel, C.A. (1990). Bathing/hygiene self-care deficit: Defining characteristics and related factors across age groups and diagnosis-related groups in an acute care setting. Nursing Diagnosis, 1(4), 155-161.
6. McKeighen, R.J., Mehmert, P.A., & Dickel, C.A. (1991). Self-care deficit, bathing/hygiene: Defining characteristics and related factors utilized by staff nurses in an acute care setting. In Carroll-Johnson, R.M. (Ed.). Classification of nursing diagnoses: Proceedings of the ninth national conference. Philadelphia, PA: J.B. Lippincott Company
7. Rhodes, V.A., Watson, P.M., & Hanson, B.M. (1988). Patients' descriptions of the influence of tiredness and weakness on self-care abilities. Cancer Nursing, 11(3), 186-194.
8. Waters, K.R. (1994). Getting dressed in the early morning: Styles of staff/patient interaction on rehabilitation hospital wards for elderly people. Journal of Advanced Nursing, 19(2), 239-248.
9. Johnson, M. & Maas, M. (Eds.). (1997). Nursing outcomes classification (NOC). St. Louis: The C.V.Mosby Company.

RECOMMENDED NANDA STAGING: 2.3

BOWEL INCONTINENCE (NANDA Bowel Incontinence)

DEFINITION: Change in normal bowel habits characterized by involuntary passage of stool.

SIGNS AND SYMPTOMS (Observed or Reported):
Inability to delay defecation [1]
Constant dribbling of soft stool [4]
Fecal odor [4]
Fecal staining of clothing/bedding [4]
Red perianal skin [1]
Urgency [3,4]
Inattention to urge to defecate [3]
Inability to recognize urge to
  defecate [3]
Self report of inability to feel rectal fullness [3]
Recognizes rectal fullness but reports inability
  to expel formed stool [3]

RELATED FACTORS:
Environmental factors, e.g. inaccessible bathroom [2]
Stress [2]
Cognitive impairment [3]

Abnormally high abdominal/intestinal pressure
  (from gas) [4]
Laxative abuse [2]
General decline in muscle tone, e.g. abdominal,
  perineal, sphincter [2]
Impaction [3]
Incomplete emptying of bowel [4]
Chronic diarrhea [2]
Rectal sphincter abnormality [4]
Colerectal lesions [2]
Impaired reservoir (bowel) capacity [1]
Medications [2]
Upper motor nerve damage [1,2,3]
Lower motor nerve damage [1,2,3]
Immobility [3]
Self care deficit - toileting [3]
Dietary habits [3,4]

REFERENCES:
1. Hogstel, M.O., & Nelson, M. (1992). Anticipation and early detection can reduce bowel elimination complications. Geriatric Nursing: American Journal of Care for the Aging, 13(1), 28-33.
2. Lueckenotte, A.G. (Ed.). (1996). Gastrointestinal function. In Gerontologic nursing (pp. 644-692). St. Louis: C.V. Mosby.
3. Maas, M., & Specht, J. (1991). Bowel incontinence. In M. Maas, K. Buckwalter & M. Hardy (Eds.), Nursing diagnoses and interventions for the elderly (pp. 181-204). Redwood City, CA: Addison-Wesley.
4. Poulton, S. (1998). Bowel incontinence management: Encopresis. In M. Craft-Rosenberg & J. Denehy, Nursing interventions for childbearing and childrearing families. Thousand Oaks, CA: Sage Publishing Company.

RECOMMENDED NANDA STAGING: 2.1

BREASTFEEDING DIFFICULTY (NANDA Ineffective Breastfeeding)

DEFINITION: Problems experienced and/or reported by a mother, infant, or child during initiating and/or continuing of breastfeeding.

SIGNS AND SYMPTOMS (Observed or Reported):
Maternal:
Reluctance to put infant to breast [4]

Infant/Child:
Decreased urinary output [1]
Failure to gain weight [3]
Inability to latch on to the nipple [3]
Resistance to latch on to the nipple [3]
Infant arching of head and neck [1]
Crying [3]
Failure to suck [3]

RELATED FACTORS:
Maternal:
Sore nipples [1]
Engorgement [1]
Inverted/flat nipples [1]
Inadequate milk supply [3]

Inhibited let down reflex [1]
Inadequate knowledge [2]
Lack of support [2]
Fatigue [4]
Return to work [4]
Anxiety [2]
Positioning [1]
Sedation [1]
Drugs [1]
Separation [2]

Infant/Child:
Weak suck reflex [3]
Oralpharyngeal anomaly [1]
Prematurity [3]
Positioning [1]
Sedation [1]
Separation [2]

REFERENCES:
1. Lethbridge, D., McClurg, V., Henrikson, M., & Wall, G. (1993). Validation of the nursing diagnosis of ineffective breastfeeding. <u>JOGNN: Journal of Obstetric, Gynecologic, and Neonatal Nursing, 22</u>(1), 57-63.
2. Meier, P., Engstrom, J., Mangurten, H., Estrada, E., Zimmerman, B., & Kopparthi, R. (1993). Breastfeeding support services in the neonatal intensive-care unit. <u>JOGNN: Journal of Obstetric, Gynecologic, and Neonatal Nursing, 22</u>(4), 338-347.
3. Kavanaugh, K., Mead, L., Meier, P., & Mangurten, H. (1995). Getting enough: Mothers' concerns about breastfeeding a preterm infant after discharge. <u>JOGNN: Journal of Obstetric, Gynecologic, and Neonatal Nursing, 24</u>(1), 23-32.
4. Richardson, V., & Champion, V. (1992). The relationship of attitudes, knowledge, and social support to breast-feeding. <u>Issues in Comprehensive Pediatric Nursing 15</u>(3), 183-197.

RECOMMENDED NANDA STAGING: 2.3

BREASTFEEDING EFFECTIVENESS (NANDA Effective Breastfeeding)

DEFINITION: Establishment and maintenance of maternal/infant proficiency and satisfaction with the lactation process.

SIGNS AND SYMPTOMS (Observed or Reported):

Maternal:
- Freedom from nipple soreness [6]
- Freedom from breast tenderness [6]
- Flexible or demand feeding schedule [7]
- Continuation of breastfeeding upon return to work/school [4]
- Arrangements for feeding during work hours [4]
- Satisfaction with breastfeeding process [3]
- Satisfaction with available support for breastfeeding [4]
- Positive attitude about breastfeeding experience [3]
- Development of reciprocal relationship/attachment to infant [6]

Infant:
- Eager to initiate feeding [6]
- Content after feeding [6]
- Appropriate weight gain [5]
- Minimum of 8 feedings per day on demand [7]
- Six or more urinations per day [7]
- Two or more soft, yellow stools per day [7]

RELATED FACTORS:

Maternal:
- Comfortable/correct position during nursing [7]
- Milk ejection (letdown) reflex [5]
- Adequate milk production/supply [1,5]
- Recognition of infant's hunger and satiation cues [7]
- Family, health care provider, employer and community support of breastfeeding [4,1]
- Knowledge of breastfeeding process [5]
- Knowledge of benefits of continued breastfeeding [5]
- Commitment to lactation [3] universal
- Adequate sleep [6]
- Adequate nutrition and liquid intake [6]
- Confidence in ability to successfully breastfeed [3]
- Customizing feeding strategies based on infant's temperament [2]

Infant:
- Comfortable/correct position during nursing [7]
- Effective suck reflex [7]
- Effective latch on to breast [7]
- Correct tongue placement [7]
- Coordinated suck, swallow and breathing [7]
- Audible swallow [7]

REFERENCES:
1. Bear, K., & Tigges, B.B. (1993). Management strategies for promoting successful breastfeeding. Nurse Practitioner: American Journal of Primary Health Care, 18(6), 50, 53-4, 56-8, 60.
2. Hughes, R.B., Townsend, P.A., & Branum, Q.K. (1988). Relationship between neonatal behavioral responses and lactation outcomes. Issues in Comprehensive Pediatric Nursing, 11(5/6), 271-81.
3. Leff, E., Gagne, M., & Jefferis, S. (1994). Maternal perceptions of successful breastfeeding. Journal of Human Lactation, 10(2), 99-104.
4. McNatt, M.H., & Freston, M.S. (1992). Social support and lactation outcomes in postpartum women. Journal of Human Lactation, 8(2), 73-7.
5. Rentschler, D.D. (1991). Correlates of successful breastfeeding. Image: the Journal of Nursing Scholarship. 23(3), 151-4.
6. Riordan, J., & Auerbach, K.G. (1993). Breastfeeding and human lactation. Boston: Jones and Bartlett.
7. Shrago. L, & Bocar, D. (1990). The infant's contribution to breastfeeding. JOGNN: Journal of Obstetrical, Gynecologic, and Neonatal Nursing, 19(3), 209-215.

RECOMMENDED NANDA STAGING: 2.3

BREATHING PATTERN INEFFECTIVENESS (NANDA Breathing Pattern, Ineffective)

DEFINITION: Inspiration and/or expiration which does not provide adequate ventilation.

SIGNS AND SYMPTOMS (Observed or Reported):

Abnormal rate, rhythm, depth of
  breathing [1,2,3,4]
Decreased vital capacity [7]
Decreased inspiratory/expiratory pressure [7]
Decreased minute ventilation [7]
Use of accessory muscles [2,4]
Altered chest excursion [2]
Prolonged expiratory phase [2]
Purse lip breathing [2]
Increased anteroposterior diameter of chest [2]
Nasal flaring (infants) [2]
Three point position (hands on knees) [2]
Orthopnea [9]
Dyspnea [2]
Shortness of breath [2,6]
Cyanosis [2]
Anxiety [2]

RELATED FACTORS:

Hyperventilation [3]
Neurological immaturity [8]
Spinal cord injury [4]
Neuromuscular dysfunction [4]
Chest wall deformity [4]
Bony deformity [4]
Body position [8]
Obesity [4,5]
Hypoventilation syndrome [5]
Respiratory muscle fatigue [4,7]

REFERENCES:

1. Brukwitzki, G., Holmgren, C., & Maibusch, R. M. (1996). Validation of the defining characteristics of the nursing diagnosis ineffective airway clearance. Nursing Diagnosis, 7(2), pp. 63-69.
2. Capuano, T.A., Hitchings, K.S., & Johnson, S. (1990). Respiratory nursing diagnoses: practicing nurses' selection of defining characteristics. Nursing Diagnosis, 1(4) 169-174.
3. Hastings, B. (1989). Alterations in respiration. In C. Malloy & J. Hartshorn (Eds.). Acute care nursing in the home. New York: J. B. Lippincott.
4. Hoffman, L.A. (1987). Ineffective airway clearance related to neuromuscular dysfunction. In M. J. Kim (Ed.), The Nursing Clinics of North America: Vol. 22 (1). II. Ineffective breathing patterns (pp. 151-166). Philadelphia: W.B. Saunders Co.
5. Hopp, L.J., & Williams, M. (1987). Ineffective breathing pattern elated to decreased lung expansion. In M. J. Kim (Ed.), The Nursing Clinics of North America: Vol. 22 (1). II. Ineffective breathing patterns (pp. 193-206). Philadelphia: W.B. Saunders Co.
6. Lareau, S., & Larson, J. L. (1987). Ineffective breathing pattern related to airflow limitation. In M. J. Kim (Ed.), The Nursing Clinics of North America: Vol. 22 (1). II. Ineffective breathing patterns (pp. 179-191). Philadelphia: W.B. Saunders Co.
7. Larson, J.L., & Kim, M.J. (1987) Ineffective breathing pattern related to respiratory muscle fatigue. In M. J. Kim (Ed.), The Nursing Clinics of North America: Vol. 22 (1). II. Ineffective breathing patterns (pp. 207-223). Philadelphia: W.B. Saunders Co.
8. Whaley, L F., & Wong, D.L. (Eds.) (1991). Nursing care of infants and children. (4th Ed.). St. Louis: Mosby.

RECOMMENDED NANDA STAGING: 2.3

CARDIAC OUTPUT ALTERATION (NANDA Decreased Cardiac Output)

DEFINITION: A decrease or reduction in the amount of blood pumped by the heart. [1,7,8]

SIGNS AND SYMPTOMS (Observed or Reported):

Altered Heart Rate/Rhythm:
Arrhythmias (tachycardia, bradycardia)[1,2,4,5,6,8]
Palpations [1,2,7]

Altered Preload:
Jugular Vein Distention (JVD), [1,4,6,7]
Fatigue, [2,4,5,6,7,7]
Edema, [2,5,6,7]
Murmurs [6,7,7]
Altered Central Venous Pressure (CVP)[1,6,8]
Altered Pulmonary Artery Wedge Pressure
   (PAWP)[1,6,8]

Altered Afterload:
Cold/clammy skin, [1,4,6,7,8]
Shortness of breath/dyspnea, [1,2,4,5,6,7,8]
Oliguria, [2,4,5,6,7,8]
Decreased capillary refill [6,7]
Decreased peripheral pulses [1,2,4,5,6,8]
Variations in blood pressure readings, [1,2,4,5,6,8]
Increased/decreased systemic vascular resistence
   (SVR)[1,6,8]

Increased/decreased Pulmonary Vascular Resistence
   (PVR) [1,6,8]

Altered Contractility:
Rales, [1,2,3,5,6,7]
Cough [2,5,6]
Anxiety [2,7,8]
Orthopnea/paroxysmal nocturnal dyspnea, [2,3,6,8]
Cardiac Output <4.0L/min [1,2]
Cardiac Index <2.5L/min [6,8]
Restlessness, [4,5,7,8]
Decreased ejection fraction, Stroke Volume Index
   (SVI), Left Ventricular Stroke Work Index
   (LVSWI),[1,6,8]

RELATED FACTORS:
Altered heart rate/rhythm [1,2,6,7,8]

Altered stroke volume: [1,2,4,7,8]
   Altered preload
   Altered afterload
   Altered contractility

REFERENCES:
1. Kern, L & Omery, A. (1992). Decreased cardiac output in the critical care setting. Nursing Diagnosis, 3(3), 94-106.
2. Dougherty, C. (1986). Decreased cardiac output: Validation of a nursing diagnosis. DCCN: Dimensions of Critical Care Nursing, 5(3), 182-188.
3. Dougherty, C., Lee, C.M., & Helms, J. (1997). Decreased cardiac output: Update and recommendations from the 1994 NANDA small group. In M. Rantz & P. LeMone (Eds.). Classification of nursing diagnoses: Proceeding of the twelfth conference, (pp 268-276). Glendale, CA: CINAHL Information Systems.
4. Dalton, J. (1985). A descriptive study: defining characteristics of the nursing diagnosis cardiac output, alterations in: decreased. Image: The Journal of Nursing Scholarship, 17(4), 113-117.
5. Scanlon, L.M. (1991). 1991 Mary J. Nielubowicz Award recipient. The nursing diagnosis: decreased cardiac output – a clinical diagnosis validation study. Military Medicine, 157(4), 166-168.
6. Bumann, R., & Speltz, M. (1989). Decreased cardiac output: a nursing diagnosis. DCCN: Dimensions of Critical Care Nursing, 8(1), 6-15.
7. Dougherty, C.M. (1997). Reconceptualization of the nursing diagnosis decreased cardiac output. Nursing Diagnosis, 8(1), 29-36.
8. Futrell, A. G. (1990). Decreased cardiac output: Case for a collaborative diagnosis. DCCN: Dimensions of Critical Care Nursing, 9(4), 202-209).

RECOMMENDED NANDA STAGING: 2.2

CAREGIVER ROLE STRAIN (NANDA Caregiver Role Strain)

DEFINITION: A caregiver's felt or exhibited difficulty in performing the family caregiver role.[1,4,12]

SIGNS AND SYMPTOMS (Observed or Reported):

Altered Caregiving Activities:

Current:
  Difficulty performing required activities [4,7]
  Inability to complete caregiving tasks[12]
  Preoccupation with care routine [12]
Anticipated:
  Apprehension about the future
    regarding care receiver's health and
    the caregiver's ability to provide care [5]
  Apprehension about care receiver's care when
    caregiver is ill or deceased [5]
  Apprehension about possible
    institutionalization of care receiver [4]

Altered Caregiver Health Status:
  Physical: [2,8,18]
  GI upset e.g. mild stomach cramps,
    vomiting, diarrhea, recurrent gastric ulcer
    episodes[2,8,14]
  Weight change[2,8,14,15]
  Rash[1,7]
  Hypertension [2,8]
  Cardiovascular disease [2, 8]
  Diabetes [2,8]
  Headaches [2,8]
  Emotional:
  Impaired individual coping [9]
  Feeling depressed [2,5,8,9,12,15,17]
  Disturbed sleep [17]
  Anger [8,15,17,19]
  Somatization [19]
  Increased nervousness [8,12,19]
  Increased emotional lability [2,12,17,19]
  Impatience [2]
  Frustration [17]
  Socioeconomic:
  Withdrawals from social life [2,8,12,13,17]
  Changes in leisure activities [2,8,12,13,17]
  Low work productivity [2,5,7,17]
  Refuses career advancement [2,5,7,17]

Altered Caregiver-Care Receiver Relationship:
  Feeling loss of past relationship with care
    receiver [7,8,12]
  Feeling loss of anticipated relationship with care
    receiver [7,8,12]
  Feeling uncertainty with changed
    relationship[8,10,12]
  Difficulty watching the care receiver go through
    the illness [17]

Altered Family Processes:
  Lack of privacy [2,7,8,12,13,17]
  Family conflict [2,7,8,12,13,17]
  Concerns about marriage [2,7,8,12,13,17]

Inadequate resources:
  Time [2,5,7, 12,14,17]
  Emotional strength [2,5,7, 12,14,17]
  Physical energy [2,5,7, 12,14,17]
  Assistance and support (informal and
    formal) [2,5,7, 12,14,17]
  Finances [2,5,7, 12,14,17]

RELATED FACTORS:

Care Receiver Health Status:
  Illness severity [4,6,12]
  Illness chronicity [14]
  Increasing care needs/dependency [2,3,12]
  Unpredictability of illness course[4,5,6]
  Instability of care receiver's health[4,5,6]
  Problem behaviors [13]
  Psychological or cognitive problems [4,5,6]
  Addiction or codependency [4,6,12]

Caregiving Activities:
  Current:
  Amount of activities [4,6]
  Complexity of activities [4,6]
  24 hours care responsibilities [4,5,6]
  Ongoing changes in activities [4]
  Discharge of family member to home
    with significant care needs[4,6]
  Years of caregiving [18]
Anticipated:
  Unpredictability of care situation[5]

Caregiver Health Status:
  Physical problems [4,5,6,12,18]
  Psychological or cognitive problems [7]
  Addiction or codependency [4,6,12]
  Marginal coping patterns [4,5,6,12]
  Unrealistic expectations of self [5]
  Inability to fulfill one's own or other's
    expectations [5]

Socioeconomic:
  Isolation from others [2,4,5,6]
  Competing role commitments [4,6,12]
  Alienation from family, friends, & coworkers[5]
  Insufficient recreation [5]

Caregiver-Care-Receiver Relationship:
  History of poor relationship [5]
  Presence of abuse or violence[4,6,7]
  Unrealistic expectations of caregiver
    by care receiver [5]
  Caregiver female status [11,16]
  Change in relationship [7,8,12]
  Mental status of elder [18]

Family Processes:
  History of marginal family coping [4,6]
  History of family dysfunction [4,6]

Resources:
  Inadequate physical environment
    for providing care e.g. housing,
    temperature, safety [4,6]
  Inadequate equipment for providing
    care [4,6]
  Inadequate transportation [4,6]
  Inadequate community services [4,6]
  Lack of respite resources [4,5,6]
  Lack of recreational resources [5]
  Insufficient finances [5]
  Lack of support from significant
    others [5,17]
  Insufficient information [2]
  Caregiver is not developmentally
    ready for caregiver role e.g. young
    adult needing to provide for a middle
    aged parent [4,6,12]
  Inexperience with caregiving [4,6,12]

REFERENCES:
1. Archbold, P., Stewart, B., Greenlick, M., & Harvath, T. (1990). Mutuality and preparedness as predictors of caregiver role strain. Research in Nursing & Health. 13(6), 375-384.
2. Baldwin, B., Kleeman, K., Stevens, G. & Rasin, J. (1989). Family caregiver stress: Clinical assessment and management. International Psychogeriatrics, 1(2), 185-194.
3. Bowers, B.J. (1987). Intergenerational caregiving: Adult caregivers and their aging parents. Advances in Nursing Science, 9(2), 20-31.
4. Burns, C., Archbold, P., Stewart, B., & Shelton, K. (1993). New diagnosis: Caregiver role strain. Nursing Diagnosis, 4(2), 70-76.
5. Carpenito, L. (1995). Nursing diagnosis: Application to clinical practice (6th ed.). Philadelphia, PA: Lippincott.
6. Carroll-Johnson, R. & Paquette, M. (1994). Classification of nursing diagnosis: Proceedings of the tenth conference held on April 25-29, 1992 in San Diego, CA. Philadelphia, PA: Lippincott.
7. Given, G., Kozachik, S., Collins, C., DeVoss, D., & Given, C. (in press). Caregiver role strain: A nursing diagnosis. In M.L. Maas, K. Buckwalter, M.A. Hardy, T. Tripp-Reimer, & M. Titler (Eds.), Nursing Diagnoses, interventions, and outcomes for the elderly (2nd ed.).
8. Kelley, L. & Lakin, J. (1988). Role supplementation as a nursing intervention for Alzheimer's disease: A case study. Public Health Nursing, 5(3), 146-152.
9. Kuhlman, G., Wilson, H., Hutchinson, S., & Wallhagen, M. (1991). Alzheimer's disease and family caregiving: Critical synthesis of the literature and research agenda. Nursing Research. 40(6), 331-7.
10. McFarland, G., & McFarlane, (1993). Nursing diagnosis & intervention. St. Louis: Mosby.
11. Miller, B. & Cafasso, L. (1992). Gender differences in caregiving: Fact or artifact? Gerontologist, 32(4), 498-507
12. Nolan, M., Grant, G., & Ellis, N. (1990). Stress is in the eye of the beholder: Reconceptualizing the measurement of carer burden. Journal of Advanced Nursing. 15(5), 544-555.

13. O'Neill, C., & Sorensen, E. (1991). Home care of the elderly: A family perspective. <u>Advances in Nursing Science, 13</u>(4), 28-37.

14. Rankin, S., (1992). Psychosocial adjustments of coronary artery disease patients and their spouses: Nursing implications. <u>Nursing Clinics of North America, 27</u>(1), 271-284.

15. Romeis, J. (1989). Caregiver strain: Toward an enlarged perspective. <u>Journal of Aging and Health, 1</u>(2), 188-208.

16. Rose-Rego, S.K., Strauss, M.E., & Smyth, K.A. (1998). Differences in the perceived wellbeing of wives and husbands caring for persons with Alzheimer's disease. <u>Gerontologist, 38</u>(2), 224-30.

17. Stetz, K., & Hanson, W. (1992). Alterations in perceptions of caregiving demands in advanced cancer during and after the experience. <u>The Hospice Journal – Physical, Psychosocial, & Pastoral Care of the Dying, 8</u>(3), 21-34.

18. Vrabec, N.J. (1997). Literature review of social support and caregiver burden. 1980-1995. <u>Image: the Journal of Nursing Scholarship, 29</u>(4), 383-388

19. Wallhagen, M. (1992). Caregiving demands: Their difficulty and effects on the well-being of elderly caregivers. <u>Scholarly Inquiry for Nursing Practice. 6</u>(2):111-127, 129-133.

<u>RECOMMENDED NANDA STAGING</u>: 2.2

CHRONIC LOW SELF-ESTEEM (NANDA Self-Esteem Disturbance)

DEFINITION: Negative or unrealistic self evaluation/feelings which are long-standing.

SIGNS AND SYMPTOMS (Observed or Reported):

Physical:
Anorexia or obesity [6]
Decrease in sexual drive
Frequent expression of somatic aches and pains [6]
Self-neglect [6,9]
Developmental changes [9]

Behavorial:
*Frequent ruminations about past problems over time [6]
*Excessively seeks reassurance [8]
Decreased problem solving [9]
Difficulty in defining own needs [2]
Unable to initiate, follow through, or complete a task in a timely fashion [6,8]
Difficulties in job performance [6]
Perfectionism [6]
Perception of minimum strengths/assets [6]
Inability to accept and/or extremely sensitive to feedback [6,8]
Timid, seclusive, unassertive [6,8]
Lack of eye contact [6]
Verbalizations of unworthiness [2,6,8,9]
Resentment of others [6]
Fear e.g. change, taking risks, expressing anger. relating to others, rejection [6,8]
Abuse tolerance [9]
Self-destructive behavior [6,9]
Negative and distorted thinking e.g. helplessness, hopelessness, powerlessness, shame [2,6,8,9]
Increased anxiety [9]
Deviant behavior [9]
Projection of blame/responsibility for problems [8]
Rationalizing personal failures [8]
Grandiosity [6,8]

Social:
*Frequent lack of success in work or other life events [8]
*Overly conforming, dependent on other's opinions [8]
Decrease in sexual relationships [6]
Emotional distancing from significant others, activities and interpersonal relationships [6]
Lack confidence in social situations [6]

RELATED FACTORS:

Physical:
Physical illness/loss [2,6]
Cognitive/perceptual problems [6,9]

Psychological:
*Long-standing negativity as a fixated life response[6]
Psychiatric illness e.g. depression [6,9]
Loss of control [6]

Social:
*Isolated lifestyle [6]
Lack of adequate positive feedback [6]
Repeated negative interpersonal experiences [6]
Inadequate social support [6]
Ineffective social functioning [9]
Past or present neglect or abuse [6,9]

* Unique to this self-esteem label

REFERENCES:

1. Carroll-Johnson, R.M. (Ed.). (1991). Classification of Nursing Diagnoses: Proceedings of the Ninth Conference. Philadelphia: J.B. Lippincott Co.
2. Gibb, B., Kraynick,P.,& Biebel, M. (1987). Validating a nursing diagnosis, disturbance in self-esteem: A comparison of studies. In A.M. McLane, Classification of Nursing Diagnosis: Proceedings of the Seventh Conference. St. Louis: C. V. Mosby Co.
3. Juhasz, A.M. (1989). Significant others and self-esteem: Methods for determining who and why. Adolescence, 24(95), 5 81-594.
4. LeMone, P. (1991). Analysis of a human phenomenon: Self-concept. Nursing Diagnosis, 2(3), 126-130.
5. McCloskey, J.C. & Bulechek, G.M. (Eds.). (1996). Nursing Interventions Classification (NIC), (2nd ed.). St. Louis: Mosby-Year Book, Inc.

6. McFarland, G.K. & McFarlane, E.A. (1993). <u>Nursing Diagnosis and Intervention: Planning for Patient Care</u>. (2nd ed.). St. Louis: C.V. Mosby Co.

7. Morris, C.A. (1985). Self-concept as altered by the diagnosis of cancer. <u>Nursing Clinics of North America</u> 20(4), 611-630.

8. NANDA. (1994). <u>Nursing Diagnoses: Definitions and Classification 1995-1996.</u> (pp. 73-74). Philadelphia: North American Nursing Diagnosis Association.

9. Norris, J. (1992). Nursing intervention for self-esteem disturbances. <u>Nursing Diagnosis</u> 3(2), 48-53.

10. Norris, J. & Kunes-Connell, M. (1988). A multimodal approach to validation and refinement of an existing nursing diagnosis. <u>Archives of Psychiatric Nursing, 2</u>(2), 103-109.

11. Norris, J. & Kunes-Connell, M. (1987). Self-esteem disturbance: A clinical validation study, In A.M. McLane (Ed.), <u>Classification of Nursing Diagnosis: Proceedings of the Seventh Conference</u> (pp. 121-128). St. Louis: C.V. Mosby.

12. Zauszniewski, J.A. (1994). Nursing diagnosis and depressive illness. <u>Nursing Diagnosis, 5</u>(3), 106-114.

<u>**RECOMMENDED NANDA STAGING**</u>: 2.3

CHRONIC PAIN (NANDA Chronic Pain)

DEFINITION: An unpleasant sensory and emotional experience, duration greater than six months.[4,5,6,7,8,9]

SIGNS AND SYMPTOMS (Observed or Reported):

Physical:
Reports pain is present, [7,9]
Functional limitations [4,5,6,7,8,9]
Decreased activity [1,2,5,6,7,8,9]
Appetite changes [2,3,4,6]
Sleep pattern changes [2,3,4,6,7,9]
Rubbing painful area [1,2,7,9]
Moaning [1,2,9]
Grimacing [1,2,3,9]
Fatigue [6,7]
Guarded behavior [2,3,6,7]

Psychological:
Irritability [2,6,7,9]
Restlessness [6,7]
Increased anxiety [4,5,7,8]

Depressed mood [2,5,6,7,8,9]
Somatic preoccupation [4,5,7]
Difficulty concentrating [4,6,8]
Hopelessness [2,5,8]
Loss of control [4]
Altered meaning of life [4]

Social:
Social function changes [3,4,6,7,8,9]
Decreased sexual function [2,4,7]
Interference with family function [7,8,9]

RELATED FACTORS:
Physiologic insult [1,2,3,4]
Psychological insult [1,3,8,9]

REFERENCES:
1. Bigos, S., Bowyer, O., Braen, G, et al. (1994) <u>Acute low back problems in adults: Clinical practice guideline</u> No. 14. AHCPR Publication No. 95-0642. Rockville, MD: Agency for Health Care Policy and Research, Public Health Service, U.S. Department of Health and Human Services.
2. Burckhardt, C.S. (1990). Chronic pain. <u>Nursing Clinics of North America, 25</u>(4), 863-870.
3. Clinton, P., & Elans, J. (19). Pain. In M. Mass, K. C. Buckwalter, & M. Hard. <u>Nursing diagnosis and interventions for the elderly</u>. Benjamin/Cummings Publishing Co., Inc. Redwood City, CA.
4. Jacox, A., Carr, D.B., Payne, R., et al. (1994). <u>Management of cancer pain: Clinical practice guideline</u> No.9. AHCPR Publication No. 94-0592. Rockville, MD. Agency for Health Care Policy and Research, U.S. Department of Health and Human Services, Public Health Service.
5. Schwartz, D. P., DeGood, D.E., & Shutty, M.S. (1985). Direct assessment of beliefs and attitudes of chronic pain patients. <u>Archives of Physical Medicine and Rehabilitation, 66</u>(12), 806-809.
6. Sieggreen, M., Moorhouse, M.F., Judge, M.K.M., Boisvert, C., Goehner, E., & Fendrich, L. (1995) Pain. In M. J. Rantz & P. LeMone (Eds.), <u>Classification of nursing diagnoses: Proceedings of the eleventh conference North American Nursing Diagnosis Association</u> (pp.424-426). Glendale, CA: CINAHL Information Systems.
7. Simon, J.M., Nolan, L., & Baumann, M.A. (1995). Validation of the nursing diagnoses acute pain and chronic pain. In M. J. Rantz & P. LeMone (Eds.), <u>Classification of nursing diagnoses: Proceedings of the eleventh conference,</u> (pp.199-203). Glendale, CA: CINAHL
8. Taylor, A.G. (1988). Chronic pain: A guide to nursing intervention. <u>Applied Nursing Research, 1</u>(1), 8-13.
9. Turk, D.C., Rudy, T.E., & Boucek. (1993) Psychological Aspects of Pain. In C. A. Warfield, <u>Principles and practice of pain management</u> (pp. 43-52). New York: McGraw-Hill, Inc.

RECOMMENDED NANDA STAGING: 2.3

COMMUNITY COPING INEFFECTIVENESS (NANDA Ineffective Community Coping)

DEFINITION: A pattern of community activities for adoption and problem solving that is unsatisfactory for meeting the demands or needs of the community. [3,4]

SIGNS AND SYMPTOMS (Observed or Reported):

Community does not meet its own expectations [3]
Deficits in community participation [3]
Excessive community conflicts [3]
Expressed vulnerability [3]
Expressed community powerlessness [3]
High illness rates [3]
Stressors perceived as excessive [3]
Increased social problems, e.g. homicides, vandalism, arson, terrorism, robbery, infanticide, abuse, divorce, unemployment, poverty, militancy, mental illness [1]

RELATED FACTORS:

Deficits in community social support services, resources [3]
Inadequate resources for problem solving [3]
Natural or man-made disasters [2]
Ineffective or non-existent community systems, e.g. lack of emergency medical system, transportation systems, disaster planning systems [2]

REFERENCES:
1. Madela, E.N., & Poggenpoel, M. (1993). The experience of a community characterized by violence: Implications for nursing. Journal of Advanced Nursing, 18(5), 691-700.
2. Kalayjian, A.S. (1994). Mental health outreach program following the earthquake in Armenia: Utilizing the nursing process in developing and managing the post-natural disaster plan. Issues in Mental Health Nursing, 15(6), 533-550.
3. NANDA. (1994). Nursing diagnoses: Definitions and classification, (pp. 55-56). Philadelphia: NANDA.
4. Axelrod, C., Killam, P.P., Gaston, M.H., & Stinson, N. (1994). Primary health care and the Midwest flood disaster. Public Health Reports, 109(5), 601-605.

RECOMMENDED NANDA STAGING: 2.1

CONSTANT URINARY INCONTINENCE (NANDA Total Incontinence)

DEFINITION: Continuous involuntary flow of urine in the presence of normal voiding pattern.

SIGNS AND SYMPTOMS (Observed or Reported):
Constant wetness [3]
Leakage with no evidence of bladder distention [3]
Voiding normal amounts of urine at regular intervals [1,3]
Voiding normal amounts of urine at regular intervals [2]
Leaking increases when in erect or sitting positions [3]

RELATED FACTORS:
Ectopic ureter (females) [1,3]
Anatomic fistula [2,3]
Surgical trauma, e.g., post prostatecomy with wide open external sphincter caused by scar tissue. [3]
Congenital ectopic urethral, bladder or ureteral orifice that circumvents the normal sphincter mechanism [3]
Severe sphincter deficiency [3]

REFERENCES:
1. Lapides, J. (1971). Urinary incontinence. In A.K. Kendall & L. Karafin (Eds.), Practice of surgery (p. 1629-1644). Hagerstown, MD: Harper & Row.
2. Specht, J., Tunink, P.M., Maas, M., & Bulechek, G. (1991). Alterations inelimination:Urinary incontinence. In M. Maas, K. Buckwalter, & M. Hardy (Eds.). Nursing diagnoses and interventions for the elderly (p. 181-204). Menlo Park, CA: Addison-Wesley.
3. Wheatley, J.K. (1982). Bladder incontinence: Four types and their control. Postgraduate Medicine, 71(1), 75-82.

RECOMMENDED NANDA STAGING: 2.1

CONSTIPATION (NANDA Colonic Constipation)

DEFINITION: A decrease in a person's normal frequency of defecation accompanied by difficult or incomplete passage of stool and/or passage of excessively hard, dry stool.

SIGNS AND SYMPTOMS (Observed or Reported):
Unable to pass stool [3,4]
Decreased frequency [2,5]
Dry, hard, formed stool [2,3,4,5]
Decreased volume of stool [3,4,5]
Severe flatus [2]
Rectal fullness/pressure [2,3,4]
Hypo or hyperactive bowel sounds [2,3,4]
Distended abdomen [1,2,3,4]
Increased abdominal pressure [3,4]
Change in abdominal growling (borborygmi) [3,4]
Strain with defecation [2,3,4]
Pain with defecation [1,2,3,4]
Oozing liquid stool [3,4]
Bright red blood with stool [1,3,4]
Dark or black or tarry stool [1]
Palpable rectal mass [3,4]
Percussed abdominal dullness [1]
Abdominal tenderness with or without palpable
   muscle resistance [1,3,4]
Palpable abdominal mass (LLQ) [1,2,3,4]
Indigestion [3,4]
Anorexia [2,3,4]
Nausea/vomiting [2,3,4]
Generalized fatigue [2]
Abdominal pain [1,3,4]
Headache [2,3,4]
Change in bowel pattern [1,5]
Presence of soft paste-like stool in rectum
Atypical presentations in older adults [1]
   change in mental status
   urinary incontinence
   unexplained falls
   elevated body temperature

RELATED FACTORS:
Psychological Factors: [1,2,3,5]
  Depression [1,2,3,5]
  Emotional Stress [1,2,3,5]
  Mental confusion [1,2,3,5]

Pharmacological Factors: [1,2,3]
  Aluminum-containing antacids [1,2,3]
  Anticholinergics [1,2,3]
  Anticonvulsants [1,2,3]
  Antidepressants [1,2,3]
  Antilipemic agents [1,2,3]
  Bismuth salts [1,2,3]
  Calcium carbonate [1,2,3]
  Calcium channel blockers [1,2,3]
  Diuretics [1,2,3]
  Laxative overuse [1,2,3]
  Iron salts [1,2,3]
  Nonsteroidal anti-inflammatory agents [1,2,3]
  Opiates [1,2,3]
  Phenothiazides [1,2,3]
  Sedatives [1,2,3]
  Sympathomimetics [1,2,3]

Physiological Factors:
  Dehydration [1]
  Insufficient fiber intake [1]
  Poor eating habits [1,2,5]
  Change in usual foods and eating patterns [3]
  Decreased motility of gastrointestinal tract [2]
  Inadequate dentition or oral hygiene [1,2,5]
  Insufficient fluid intake [2]

Functional Factors:
  Insufficient physical activity [1,2,5]
  Inadequate toileting, e.g., timeliness,
    positioning for defecation, privacy [1,2]
  Irregular defecation habits [1]
  Abdominal muscle weakness [1,2]
  Habitual denial/ignoring of urge to
    defecate [1]
  Recent environmental changes [1]

Mechanical Factors: [1]
  Obesity [1]
  Pregnancy [1]
  Postsurgical obstruction [1]
  Prostate enlargement [1]
  Rectal prolapse [1]
  Rectocele [1]
  Rectal, anal stricture [1]
  Tumors [1]
  Neurological impairment, e.g., CVA [1]
  Rectal abscess or ulcer [1]
  Electrolyte imbalance [1]
  Rectal, anal fissures [1]
  Hemorrhoids [1]
  Megacolon (Hirschsprung's disease) [1]

REFERENCES:
1. Allison, O.C., Porter, M.E., & Briggs, G.C. (1994). Chronic constipation: assessment and management in the elderly. <u>Journal of the American Academy of Nurse Practitioners, 6</u>(7), 311-317.
2. Hogstel, M.O., & Nelson, M. (1992). Anticipation and early detection can reduce bowel elimination complications. <u>Geriatric Nursing – American Journal of Care for the Aging, 13</u>(1), 28-33.
3. McLane, A.M., & McShane, R.E. (1986). Empirical validation of defining characteristics of constipation: a study of bowel elimination practices of healthy adults. In M.E. Hurley (Ed.). <u>Classification of nursing diagnoses: Proceedings of the sixth conference</u> (pp. 448-455). St. Louis: C.V. Mosby.
4. McShane, R.E., & McLane, A.M. (1985). Constipation: consensual and empirical validation. <u>Nursing Clinics of North America, 20</u>(4), 801-808.
5. Meeroff, J.C. (1985). Approach to the patient with constipation. <u>Hospital Practice, 20</u>(1), 148, 152-3.

RECOMMENDED NANDA STAGING: 2.3

CONSTIPATION RISK (NANDA Perceived Constipation)

DEFINITION: At risk for a decrease in a person's normal frequency of defecation accompanied by difficult or incomplete passage of stool and/or passage of excessively hard, dry stool.

RISK FACTORS:

Psychological Factors:
Depression [1,2,3,5]
Emotional Stress [1,2,3,5]
Mental confusion [1,2,3,5]

Pharmacological Factors:
Aluminum-containing antacids [1,2,3]
Anticholinergics [1,2,3]
Anticonvulsants [1,2,3]
Antidepressants [1,2,3]
Antilipemic agents [1,2,3]
Bismuth salts [1,2,3]
Calcium carbonate [1,2,3]
Calcium channel blockers [1,2,3]
Diuretics [1,2,3]
Laxative overuse [1,2,3]
Iron salts [1,2,3]
Nonsteroidal anti-inflammatory agents [1,2,3]
Opiates [1,2,3]
Phenothiazides [1,2,3]
Sedatives [1,2,3]
Sympathomimetics [1,2,3]

Physiological Factors:
Dehydration [1]
Insufficient fiber intake [1]
Poor eating habits [1,2,5]
Change in usual foods and eating patterns [3]

Decreased motility of GI tract [2]
Inadequate dentition or oral hygiene [1,2,5]
Insufficient fluid intake [2]

Functional Factors:
Insufficient physical activity [1,2,5]
Inadequate toileting, e.g., timeliness, positioning for defecation, privacy [1,2]
Irregular defecation habits [1]
Abdominal muscle weakness [1,2]
Habitual denial/ignoring of urge to defecate [1]
Recent environmental changes [1]

Mechanical Factors:
Obesity [1]
Pregnancy [1]
Postsurgical obstruction [1]
Prostate enlargement [1]
Rectal prolapse [1]
Rectocele [1]
Rectal, anal stricture [1]
Tumors [1]
Neurological impairment, e.g., cerebral vascular accident [1]
Rectal abscess or ulcer [1]
Electrolyte imbalance [1]
Rectal, anal fissures [1]
Hemorrhoids [1]
Megacolon (Hirschsprung's disease) [1]

REFERENCES:
1. Allison, O.C., Porter, M.E., & Briggs, G.C. (1994). Chronic constipation: assessment and management in the elderly. Journal of the American Academy of Nurse Practitioners, 6(7), 311-317.
2. Hogstel, M.O., & Nelson, M. (1992). Anticipation and early detection can reduce bowel elimination complications. Geriatric Nursing – American Journal of Care for the Aging, 13(1), 28-33.
3. McLane, A.M., & McShane, R.E. (1986). Empirical validation of defining characteristics of constipation: a study of bowel elimination practices of healthy adults. In M.E. Hurley (Ed.). Classification of nursing diagnoses: Proceedings of the sixth conference (pp. 448-455). St. Louis: C.V. Mosby.
4. McShane, R.E., & McLane, A.M. (1985). Constipation: consensual and empirical validation. Nursing Clinics of North America, 20(4), 801-808.
5. Meeroff, J.C. (1985). Approach to the patient with constipation. Hospital Practice, 20(1), 148, 152-3.

RECOMMENDED NANDA STAGING: 2.3

COPING INEFFECTIVENESS (NANDA Coping, Ineffective Individual)

DEFINITION: Inability to form a valid appraisal of the stressors, inadequate choices of practiced responses, and/or inability to use available resources. [7, 8]

SIGNS AND SYMPTOMS (Observed or Reported):

Verbalization of inability to cope [13]
Change in usual communication patterns [13]
  eg. (verbal and nonverbal) angry outbursts,
  increasing demands, aggressive gestures, frequent
  criticism, suspiciousness, irritable behaviors,
  tense body, explosive speech
Inadequate problem solving [5]
Poor concentration [6]
Lack of goal directed behavior/resolution of
  problem including: inability to attend
  difficulty with organizing information [6]
Inability to meet role expectations [1]
Inability to meet basic needs [1]
Destructive behavior toward self or others [1]
Sleep disturbance [11]
Fatigue [3]
Decrease in use of social support [2,5,11]
Use of forms of coping that impede adaptive
  behavior [3] eg. avoidant behaviors, denial
Risk taking [3]
High illness rate [4]
Abuse of chemical agents [3]

RELATED FACTORS:

Situational or maturational crises [1, 2, 3, 4, 5]
Uncertainty [1, 6]
Disturbance in pattern of tension release [5, 13]
Disturbance in pattern of appraisal of threat [9,14]
Inadequate level of confidence in ability to
  cope [5, 6,14]
Inadequate level of perception of control [5, 6,14]
High degree of threat [14]
Inadequate social support created by
  characteristics of relationships [10, 14]
Inadequate opportunity to prepare for
  stressor [1,9]
Inability to conserve adaptive energies [13]
Inadequate resources available (social support,
  financial) [4,6, 11]
Gender differences in coping startegies [2, 14]

REFERENCES:

1. Becket, N. (1990). Clinical nurses' characterizations of patient coping problems. Nursing Diagnosis, 2(2), 72-78.
2. Damrosch, S.P., & Perry, L. (1989). Self-reported adjustment, chronic sorrow, and coping of parents of children with Down's Syndrome. Nursing Research, 38(1), 25-30.
3. Folkman, S., Lazarus, R.S., Gruen, R.J., & DeLongis, A. (1986). Appraisal, coping, health status, and psychological symptoms. Journal of Personality and Social Psychology, 50(3), 571-579.
4. Gass, K. (1987). The health of conjugally bereaved older widows: The role of appraisal, coping, and resources, Research in Nursing and Health, 10(1), 39-47.
5. Gulesserian, B., & Warren, C. (1987). Coping resources of depressed patients. Archives of Psychiatric Nursing, 1(6), 392-398.
6. Johnson, J.E., & Lauver, D.R. (1989). Alternative explanation of coping with stressful experiences associated with physical illness. Advances in Nursing Science, 11(2), 39-52.
7. King, F., Figge, J., & Harman, P. (1986). The elderly coping at home: A study of continuity of nursing care. Journal of Advanced Nursing, 11(1), 41-46.
8. LaMontagne, L., Hepworth, J., Johnson, B., & Cohen, F. (1996). Children's preoperative coping and its effects on postoperative anxiety and return to normal activity. Nursing Research, 45(3), 141-147.
9. McHaffie, H. (1992). The assessment of coping, Clinical Nursing Research, 1(1), 67-69.
10. McNett S. (1987). Social support, threat, and coping responses and effectiveness in the functionally disabled. Nursing Research, 36(2), 98-103.
11. Nyamathi, A.M. (1987). The coping responses of female spouses of patients with myocardial infarction. Heart and Lung, 16(1), 86-92.
12. Ryan-Wenger, N. (1994). Coping behavior in children: Methods of measurement for research and clinical practice. Journal of Pediatric Nursing, 9(3), 183-195.

13. Smyth, K.A., & Yarandi, H.N. (1992). A path model of type A and type B responses to coping and stress in employed Black women, <u>Nursing Research, 41</u>(5), 260-265.
14. Van Cleve, L. (1989). Parental coping in response to their child's spinal bifida, <u>Journal of Pediatric Nursing, 4</u>(3), 172-176.

<u>RECOMMENDED NANDA STAGING</u>: 2.1

DECREASED INTRACRANIAL ADAPTIVE CAPACITY (NANDA Decreased Adaptive Capacity: Intracranial)

DEFINITION: Failure of normal compensatory mechanisms for changes in intracranial volume or pressure. [2]

SIGNS AND SYMPTOMS (Observed or Reported):

Monitored patient:
- Repeated increases in ICP of greater than 10 mmHg for more than 5 minutes in response to various stimuli [5]
- ICP greater than 15-20 mmHg [1, 2,3,4]
- Wide amplitude ICP waveform [2, 4]
- Decreased cerebral perfusion pressure (less than 60 mmHg) [1,2,3]

Non-monitored patient:
- Cushing's triad [5]
- Decreased level of consciousness [5]
- Decorticate or decerebrate posturing [5]
- Altered breathing pattern [5]
- Increased severity of headache (in adults) [5]
- Visual field deficits [5]
- Changes in extraocular movements [5]

RELATED FACTORS:
- Cerebral edema [1, 2, 4, 5]
- Cerebral hemorrhage [1, 2, 4, 5]
- Cerebral vasodilation [1, 2, 4, 5]
- Hyperplasia/Tumor [1, 2, 4, 5]
- Hydrocephalus [1, 2, 4, 5]
- Decreased cerebral perfusion pressure [4]
- Systemic hypotension with intracranial hypertension [3]

REFERENCES:

1. Andrus, C. (1991). Intracranial pressure: Dynamics and nursing management. Journal of Neuroscience Nursing, 23(2), 85-92.
2. Mitchell, P.H. (1986). Decreased adaptive capacity, intracranial: A proposal for a nursing diagnosis. Journal of Neuroscience Nursing, 18(4), 170-175.
3. Eisenhart, K. (1994). New perspectives in the management of adults with severe head injury. Critical Care Nursing Quarterly, 17(2), 1-12.
4. Rauch, M.E., Mitchell, P.H., & Tyler, M.L. (1990). Validation of risk factors for the nursing diagnosis decreased intracranial adaptive capacity. Journal of Neuroscience Nursing, 22(3), 173-178.
5. Wall, B.M., Philips, J.P., & Howard, J.C. (1994). Validation of increased intracranial pressure and high risk for increased intracranial pressure. Nursing Diagnosis, 5(2), 74-81.

RECOMMENDED NANDA STAGING: 2.3

DECREASED INTRACRANIAL ADAPTIVE CAPACITY RISK (NANDA Decreased Adaptive Capacity: Intracranial)

DEFINITION: Risk for failure of normal compensatory mechanisms for changes in intracranial volume or pressure. [2]

RISK FACTORS:
Cerebral edema [1]
Cerebral hemorrhage [1]
Cerebral vasodilation [1]
Tumor/ hyperplasia [1]
Hydrocephalus [5]

REFERENCES:
1. Andrus, C. (1991). Intracranial pressure: Dynamics and nursing management. Journal of Neuroscience Nursing, 23(2), 85-92.
2. Mitchell, P.H. (1986). Decreased adaptive capacity, intracranial: A proposal for a nursing diagnosis. Journal of Neuroscience Nursing, 18(4), 170-175.
3. Eisenhart, K. (1994). New perspectives in the management of adults with severe head injury. Critical Care Nursing Quarterly, 17(2), 1-12.
4. Rauch, M.E., Mitchell, P.H., & Tyler, M.L. (1990). Validation of risk factors for the nursing diagnosis decreased intracranial adaptive capacity. Journal of Neuroscience Nursing, 22(3), 173-178.
5. Wall, B.M., Philips, J.P., & Howard, J.C. (1994). Validation of increased intracranial pressure and high risk for increased intracranial pressure. Nursing Diagnosis, 5(2), 74-81.

RECOMMENDED NANDA STAGING: 2.3

DEFENSIVE SELF-ESTEEM (NANDA Defensive Coping/ Self-esteem Disturbance)

DEFINITION: Protective mechanism that attempts to shield self from presumed gaps between the idealized self and positive self-regard and real accomplishments if gaps pose a significant threat.

SIGNS AND SYMPTOMS (Observed or Reported):
Denial of negative information through grandiosity, arrogance, or projecting blames/responsibility [2,3]
Superior attitude, one-ups-manship, insensitivity [3]
Cannot accept responsibility for decisions/behavior[3]
Denial of previous problems [3]
Hypersensitive to criticism [3]
Rationalizes failures [3]
Difficulty in relationship [3]
Hostile laugh/ridicules others [3]
Difficulty in reality testing [3]
Lack of participation in therapy [3]

RELATED FACTORS:
Situational stressors, e.g., functional impairment, loss of significant roles, objects, relocation [1,2,3,4]
Social role changes, e.g., unemployment, divorce, hospitalization, relocation [3]

REFERENCES:
1. Norris, J. (1992). Nursing intervention for self-esteem disturbances. Nursing Diagnosis, 3(2), 48-53.
2. Norris, J. & Kunes-Connell, M. (1985). Self-esteem disturbance. Nursing Clinics of North America, 20(4), 745-761.
3. Norris, J. & Kunes-Connell, M. (1988). A multimodal approach to validation & refinement of an existing nursing diagnosis. Archives of Psychiatric Nursing, 2(2), 103-109.
4. Turkat, D. (1983). Defensiveness in self-esteem research. Psychological Record, 28, 129-135.

RECOMMENDED NANDA STAGING: 2.3

DENTITION ALTERATION (NANDA None)

DEFINITION: Disruption in tooth development/eruption patterns or structural integrity of individual teeth.

SIGNS AND SYMPTOMS (Observed or Reported):
Excessive plaque[7]
Crown or root caries[2,4]
Halitosis[2]
Tooth enamel discoloration[7]
Toothache[2]
Loose teeth[2,5]
Excessive calculus[7]
Incomplete eruption for age (may be primary or permanent teeth)[2]
Malocclusion or tooth misalignment[5]
Premature loss of primary teeth[2]
Worn down or abraded teeth [2,5]
Tooth fracture(s) [2,5]
Missing teeth (or complete absence)[1,4,6]
Erosion of enamel[7]
Asymmetrical facial expression[2]
Teeth grinding [5]

RELATED FACTORS:
Related Factors:
Ineffective oral hygiene, sensitivity to heat or cold [1,4]
Barriers to self-care[1,4]
Access or economic barriers to professional care[1]
Nutritional deficits[1,4]
Dietary habits[1,4]
Genetic predisposition[1,4]
Selected prescription medications[1,4]
Excessive intake of fluorides[1,4]
Chronic vomiting[1,4]
Chronic use of tobacco, coffee or tea, red wine[4]
Lack of knowledge regarding dental health[1]
Excessive use of abrasive cleaning agents[1,4]

REFERENCES:
1. Coulter, I.D., Marcus, M., & Atchison, K.A. (1994). Measuring oral health status: Theoretical and methodological challenges. Social Science and Medicine, 38(11), 1531-1541.
2. Eldredge, J.B. (1991). Altered oral mucous membrane. In M. Maas, K. Buckwalter and M. Hardy (Eds.). Nursing diagnoses and interventions for the elderly (pp. 117-130). Fort Collins: Addison-Wesley.
3. Eilers, J., Berger, A., & Peterson, M. (1988). Development, testing and application of the Oral Assessment Guide. Oncology Nursing Forum, 15(3), 325-330.
4. Jette, A., Feldman, H., & Tennstedt, S. (1993). Tobacco use: A modifiable risk factor for dental disease among the elderly. American Journal of Public Health, 83(9), 1271-1276.
5. Kronmiller, J.E. (1987). Oral soft tissue abnormalities in children. Pediatric Nursing, 13(3), 161-165.
6. Ofstehage, J., & Magilvy, K. (1986). Oral health and aging. Geriatric Nursing, 7(5), 238-241.
7. Ransier, A., Epstein, J., Lunn, R., & Spinelli, J. (1995). A combined analysis of a toothbrush, foam brush and a chlorhexidine-soaked foam brush in maintaining oral hygiene. Cancer Nursing, 18(5), 393-396.
8. Woodtli, M., & Van Ort, S. (1993). Nursing diagnosis and functional health patterns in patients receiving external radiation therapy: Cancer of the digestive organs. Nursing Diagnosis, 4(1), 15-25.

RECOMMENDED NANDA STAGING: 2.1

DEVELOPMENT ALTERATION (NANDA Altered Growth and Development)

DEFINITION: A delay in one or more of the areas of social or self-regulatory behavior, or cognitive, language, gross or fine motor skills.

SIGNS AND SYMPTOMS (Observed or Reported):
Delay of 25% or more or failure to achieve developmental milestones [1-15]
Permanent loss of skills [1,5,10]

RELATED FACTORS:
Prenatal factors:
   Maternal age <15 > 35 years [4]
   Substance abuse [1,4,8,11,12,13]
   Infections [1,4,8,11,12,13]
   Genetic/endocrine disorders [1,4,8,9,12]
   Unplanned/unwanted pregnancy [8]
   Lack of/late/poor prenatal care [3,4,6, 8, 9]
   Inadequate nutrition [6,8]
   Illiteracy [6,7,9]
   Poverty [4,6,8,9,12,14]

Individual Factors:
   Prematurity [1,4,8,9,11,12,13]
   Seizures [1,5,6,8,9,12,14]
   Congenital/genetic disorders [1,4,5,8,9,11]
   Positive drug screening test [8]
   Brain damage, e.g., hemorrhage in postnatal period, shaken baby, abuse, accident, infection [4,5,8,9,10]

Vision impairment [1,4,6,8,14]
Hearing impairment frequent otitis media [1,4,6,8,9]
Chronic illness [1,4,6,8,9,12]
Technology dependent [1,3,4,8,9]
Failure to thrive inadequate nutrition [1,4,8,11,12]
Foster or adopted child [2]
Behavior disorders [2,3,6,7,10,15]
Substance abuse [4]

Caregiver Factors:
   Abuse [3,4,6,8]
   Mental illness [3,6,8,9]
   Mental retardation or severe learning disability [1,3,4,6,8,9]

Environmental Factors:
   Poverty [4,6,8,9]
   Violence [8,9,12]
   Lead poisoning [4,8]
   Radiation [4]
   Chemicals [4]

REFERENCES:
1. Batshaw, M.L., & Perret, Y.M. (1992). Children with handicaps: a medical primer -3rd Edition. Baltimore: Paul H. Brookes.
2. Brodzinsky, D.M., & Steiger, C. (1991). Prevalence of adoptees among special education populations. Journal of Learning Disabilities, 24(8), 484-489.
3. Child, A.A., Murphy, C.M., & Rhyne, M.C. (1980). Depression in children: Reasons and risks. Pediatric Nursing, 6(4), 9-13.
4. Curry, D.M., & Duby, J.C. (1994). Developmental surveillance by pediatric nurses. Pediatric Nursing, 20(1), 40-44.
5. Dam, M. (1994). Children with epilepsy: The effect of seizures, syndromes, and etiological factors on cognitive functioning. Epilepsia, 31(Supp. 4), S26-S29.
6. Davidhizar, R., & Frank, B. (1992). Understanding the physical and psychosocial stressors of the child who is homeless. Pediatric Nursing, 18(6), 559-562.
7. Glascoe, F.P., Altemeier, W.A., & MacLean, W.E. (1989). The importance of parents' concerns about their child's development. American Journal of Diseases in Children, 143(8), 955-958.
8. Kimmel, S.R., Quinn, E.A., & Phelps, K.A. (1994). Assessing child development. Primary Care, 21(4), 673-692.
9. King, E.H., Logsdon, E.A., & Schroeder, S. (1992). Risk factors for developmental delay among infants and toddlers. Children's Health Care, 21(1), 39-52.
10. Koskiniemi, M. , Kyykka, T., & Jarho, L. (1995). Long-term outcome after severe brain injury in preschoolers is worse than expected. Archives of Pediatric and Adolescent Medicine, 149(3), 249-254.
11. Little, B.B., Snell, L.M., Rosenfeld, C.R., Gilstrap, L.C., & Gant, N. (1990). Failure to recognize fetal alcohol syndrome in newborn infants. American Journal of Diseases in Children, 144(10), 1142-1146.

12. Lipsi, K., Clements-Shafer, K., & Rushton, C.H. (1991). Developmental rounds: An intervention strategy for hospitalized infants. <u>Pediatric Nursing, 17</u>(5), 433-7, 468, 452-3.
13. Singer, L., Arendt, R., Song, L.Y., Warshawsky, E., & Kiegman, R. (1994). Direct and indirect interactions of cocaine with childbirth outcomes. <u>Archives of Pediatric and Adolescent Medicine, 148</u>(9), 959-964.
14. Sran, S.K., & Baumann, R.J. (1988). Outcome of neonatal strokes. <u>American Journal of Diseases in Children, 142</u>(10), 1086-1088.
15. Stone, W.L., Hoffman, E.L., Lewis, S.E., & Ousley, O.Y. (1994). Early recognition of autism. Parental reports vs. clinical observation. <u>Archives of Pediatric and Adolescent Medicine, 148</u>(2), 174-179.

<u>RECOMMENDED NANDA STAGING</u>: 2.1

DEVELOPMENT ALTERATION RISK (NANDA None)

DEFINITION: At risk for delay of 25% or more in one or more of the areas of social or self-regulatory behavior, or cognitive, language, gross or fine motor skills.

RISK FACTORS:

Prenatal factors:
Maternal age <15 > 35 years [4]
Substance abuse [1,4,8,9,11,12]
Infections [1,4,8,9,11,12,13]
Genetic/endocrine disorders [1,4,8,9,12]
Unplanned/unwanted pregnancy [8]
Lack of/late/poor prenatal
  care [3,4,6, 8,9]
Inadequate nutrition [6,8]
Illiteracy [6,7,9]
Poverty [4,6,8,9,12,14]

IndividualFactors:
Prematurity [1,4,8,9,11,12,13]
Seizures [1,5,6,8,9,12,14]
Congenital/genetic disorders [1,4,5,8,9,11]
Positive drug screening test [8]
Brain damage, e.g., hemorrhage in postnatal
  period, shaken baby, abuse, accident [4,5,8,9,10]
Vision impairment [1,4,6,8,14]

Hearing impairment or frequent otitis
  media [1,4,6,8,9]
Chronic illness [1,4,6,8,9,12]
Technology dependent [1,3,4,8,9]
Failure to thrive inadequate nutrition [1,4,8,11,12]
Foster or adopted child [2]
Lead poisoning [4,8]
Behavior disorders [2,3,6,7,10,15]
Substance abuse [4]

Caregiver Factors:
Abuse [3,4,6,8]
Mental illness [3,6,8,9]
Mental retardation or severe learning
  disability [1,3,4,6,8,9]

Environmental Factors:
Poverty [4,6,8,9]
Violence [8,9,12]

REFERENCES:

1. Batshaw, M.L., & Perret, Y.M. (1992). Children with handicaps: a medical primer -3rd Edition. Baltimore: Paul H. Brookes.
2. Brodzinsky, D.M., & Steiger, C. (1991). Prevalence of adoptees among special education populations. Journal of Learning Disabilities, 24(8), 484-489.
3. Child, A.A., Murphy, C.M., & Rhyne, M.C. (1980). Depression in children: Reasons and risks. Pediatric Nursing, 6(4), 9-13.
4. Curry, D.M., & Duby, J.C. (1994). Developmental surveillance by pediatric nurses. Pediatric Nursing, 20(1), 40-44.
5. Dam, M. (1994). Children with epilepsy: The effect of seizures, syndromes, and etiological factors on cognitive functioning. Epilepsia, 31(Supp. 4), S26-S29.
6. Davidhizar, R., & Frank, B. (1992). Understanding the physical and psychosocial stressors of the child who is homeless. Pediatric Nursing, 18(6), 559-562.
7. Glascoe, F.P., Altemeier, W.A., & MacLean, W.E. (1989). The importance of parents' concerns about their child's development. American Journal of Diseases in Children, 143(8), 955-958.
8. Kimmel, S.R., Quinn, E.A., & Phelps, K.A. (1994). Assessing child development. Primary Care, 21(4), 673-692.
9. King, E.H., Logsdon, E.A., & Schroeder, S. (1992). Risk factors for developmental delay among infants and toddlers. Children's Health Care, 21(1), 39-52.
10. Koskiniemi, M., Kyykka, T., & Jarho, L. (1995). Long-term outcome after severe brain injury in preschoolers is worse than expected. Archives of Pediatric and Adolescent Medicine, 149(3), 249-254.
11. Little, B.B., Snell, L.M., Rosenfeld, C.R., Gilstrap, L.C., & Gant, N. (1990). Failure to recognize fetal alcohol syndrome in newborn infants. American Journal of Diseases in Children, 144(10), 1142-1146.
12. Lipsi, K., Clements-Shafer, K., & Rushton, C.H. (1991). Developmental rounds: An intervention strategy for hospitalized infants. Pediatric Nursing, 17(5), 433-7, 468, 452-3.

13. Singer, L., Arendt, R., Song, L.Y., Warshawsky, E., & Kiegman, R. (1994). Direct and indirect interactions of cocaine with childbirth outcomes. <u>Archives of Pediatric and Adolescent Medicine, 148</u>(9), 959-964.

14. Sran, S.K., & Baumann, R.J. (1988). Outcome of neonatal strokes. <u>American Journal of Diseases in Children, 142</u>(10), 1086-1088.

15. Stone, W.L., Hoffman, E.L., Lewis, S.E., & Ousley, O.Y. (1994). Early recognition of autism. Parental reports vs. clinical observation. <u>Archives of Pediatric and Adolescent Medicine, 148</u>(2), 174-179.

<u>**RECOMMENDED NANDA STAGING:**</u> 2.1

DIARRHEA (NANDA Diarrhea)

DEFINITION: Passage of loose, unformed stools. [2,3]

SIGNS AND SYMPTOMS (Observed or Reported):

At least three liquid, loose stools per day [6]
Hyperactive bowel sounds [3,5]
Urgency [3,5]
Abdominal pain [1,2,3,5,6]
Cramping [1,3,4,5]

RELATED FACTORS:

Pathophysiological:
Infectious processes [2,4,5,6]
Parasites [1,3]
Inflammation [3,5]
Irritation [3,5,6]
Malabsorption [1,3,5]

Situational:
Medications [1,2,3,4,5,6]
Toxins [3]
Contaminants [3,4]
Radiation [3,5]
Alcohol abuse [2,5]
Laxative abuse [5]
Tube feedings [4]
Travel [3,4]

Psychological:
Stress and anxiety [5]

REFERENCES:

1. Anderson, K., Anderson, L.E., & Glanze, W.D. (1994). Mosby's medical, nursing, and allied health dictionary. (4th Ed.). St. Louis: Mosby Inc.
2. Wadle, K. (1990). Diarrhea. Nursing Clinics of North America, 25(4), 901-908.
3. Watson, A.J.M., (1992). Diarrhea (abc of colorectal diseases). British Medical Journal, 304, 1302.
4. Ives C., & Hines, C. (1993). Common causes commonly not considered (diarrhea). Consultant, 93, 33, 95.
5. Cohen, M., & Moss, H. (1994). Severe vomiting and diarrhea: Initial measures emergency handbook. Patient Care, 28, 92.
6. Vines, S., Arnstein, P., Shaw, A., Buchholz, S., & Jacobs, J. (1992). Research utilization: an evaluation of the research related to causes of diarrhea in tube-fed patients. Applied Nursing Research, 5(4), 164-173.

RECOMMENDED NANDA STAGING: 2.1

DISORGANIZED INFANT BEHAVIOR (NANDA Disorganized Infant Behavior)

DEFINITION: Disintegrated physiological and neurobehavioral responses to the environment.

SIGNS AND SYMPTOMS (Observed or Reported):

Physiological/Autonomic System: [4]
 Heart rate (e.g., bradycardia, tachycardia, arrhythmias)
 Respiratory rate (e.g. bradypnea, tachpnea, apnea)
 Color (e.g., pale, cyanotic, mottled, flushed)
 Oximeter desaturation
 Feeding intolerance (e.g., aspiration, emesis)
 "Time-out signals" (e.g., gaze, grasp, hiccough, cough, sneeze, yawn, sigh, slack jaw, open mouth, tongue thrust)

Motor System: [3,4]
 Tone (e.g. increased, decreased, limpness)
 Movement (e.g., tremor, startle, twitch, jittery, jerky, uncoordinated)
 Posture (e.g., hyperextension, finger splay, fisting, hands to face, altered primitive reflexes)

State-Organization System: [4]
 Sleep: diffuse, state oscillation
 Quiet-awake: staring, gaze aversion
 Active-awake: fussy, worried gaze
 Crying: irritable, panicky

Regulatory State: [4]
 Irritability
 Inability to inhibit

Attention-Interaction System: [4]
 Abnormal response to sensory stimuli (e.g., difficult to soothe; inability to sustain alert state)

RELATED FACTORS:

Prenatal: [8]
 Congenital/genetic disorders
 Teratogenic exposure

Postnatal: [5,8]
 Prematurity
 Malnutrition
 Feeding intolerance
 Oral/motor problems
 Invasive/painful procedure
 Pain

Individual Factors: [1,5,6,7,8]
 Gestational age
 Postconceptual age
 Immature neurological system
 Illness

Caregiver Factors: [6,7]
 Cue misreading
 Cue knowledge deficit
 Environmental stimulation contribution

Environmental Factors: [1,2,3,5,6,7,9,10]
 Sensory deprivation
 Sensory overstimulation
 Sensory inappropriateness
 Physical environment inappropriateness

REFERENCES:

1. Als, H., Lawhon, G., Duffy, F.H., McAnulty, G.B., Gibes-Grossman, R., & Bleckman, J.G. (1994). Individual developmental care for the very low birth weight premature infant. Journal of the American Medical Assn, 272, 11, 853-858.
2. Blackburn, S. (1978). Sleep and wake states of the newborn. In KE Barnard et al. (Eds.). Early parent-infant relationships- module 3- A staff development program in perinatal nursing. The National Foundation: March of Dimes, 17-21.
3. Blackburn, S. (1978). State-related behaviors and individual differences. In KE Barnard et al. (Eds.). Early parent-infant relationships- module 3- A staff development program in perinatal nursing, (pp. 22-32). The National Foundation: March of Dimes.
4. Blackburn, S.T., & Vanderberg, K.A. (1993). Assessment and management of neurodevelopmental behavioral development. In C Kenner, A Brueggenmeyer & LP Gunderson (Eds.). Comprehensive neonatal nursing. Philadelphia: WB Saunders Co, 1094-1121.
5. D'Apolito K. (1991). What is an organized infant? Neonatal Network, 10(1), 23-33.
6. Lawhon, G. (1986). Management of stress in premature infants. In DJ Angeline, CM Whalen-Knapp, & RM Gibes (Eds.). Perinatal and neonatal nursing: A clinical handbook. Boston: Blackwell Scientific Publications, 30-31.

7. Lawhon, G., & Melzer, A. (1988). Developmental care of the very low birthweight infant. <u>Journal of Pediatric and Neonatal Nursing, 2</u>(1), 56-65.

8. Lott, J.W. (1989). Developmental care of the preterm infant. <u>Neonatal Network, 7</u>(4), 21-28.

9. National Association of Neonatal Nurses. (1993). Infant Developmental Care Guidelines. Petaluma, <u>CA: National Association of Neonatal Nurses,</u> 1-16.

10. Oehler, J. (1983). Sensory processing abilities of the preterm infant. <u>Journal of the California Perinatal Association, 3,</u> 6, 55-63.

<u>**RECOMMENDED NANDA STAGING:**</u> 2.1

DISORGANIZED INFANT BEHAVIOR RISK (NANDA Risk for Disorganized Infant Behavior)

DEFINITION: Potential for altered physiological and neurobehavioral responses to the environment.

RISK FACTORS:

Prenatal: [7]
  Congenital/genetic disorders
  Teratogenic exposure

Postnatal: [4,7]
  Prematurity
  Malnutrition
  Feeding intolerance
  Oral/motor problems
  Invasive/painful procedure
  Pain

Individual Factors: [1,4,5,6,7]
  Gestational age
  Postconceptual age
  Immature neurological system
  Illness

Caregiver Factors: [5,6]
  Cue misreading
  Cue knowledge deficit
  Environmental stimulation contribution

Environmental Factors: [1,2,3,4,5,6,7,8]
  Sensory deprivation
  Sensory over stimulation
  Sensory inappropriateness
  Physical environment inappropriateness

REFERENCES:
1. Als, H., Lawhon, G., Duffy, F.H., McAnulty, G.B., Gibes-Grossman, R., & Bleckman, J.G. (1994). Individual developmental care for the very low birthweight premature infant. Journal of the American Medical Assn, 272(11), 853-858.
2. Blackburn, S. (1978). Sleep and awake states of the newborn. In KE Barnard et al.(Eds.). Early parent-infant relationships-module 3- a staff development program in perinatal nursing care, (pp 17-21). The National Foundation: March of Dimes.
3. Blackburn, S. (1978). State related behaviors and individual differences. In K.E. Barnard et al. (Eds) Early parent-infant relationships-module 3- a staff development program in perinatal nursing care. The National Foundation: March of Dimes, 22-32.
4. D'Apolito, K. (1991). What is an organized infant? Neonatal Network, 10(1), 23-33.
5. Lawhon, G. (1986). Management of stress in premature infants. In DJ Angeline, CM Whalen-Knapp & RM Gibes (Eds.). Perinatal and neonatal nursing: A clinical handbook, (pp 30-31). Boston: Blackwell Scientific Publications.
6. Lawhon, G., & Melzer, A. (1988). Developmental care of the very low birth weight infant. Journal of Perinatal and Neonatal Nursing, 2(1), 56-65.
7. National Association of Neonatal Nurses. (1993). Infant Developmental Guidelines, (pp 1-16). Petaluma, CA: National Association of Neonatal Nurses.
8. Oehler, J. (1983). Sensory processing abilities of the preterm infant. Journal of the California Perinatal Association, 3(6), 55-63.

RECOMMENDED NANDA STAGING: 2.3

DRESSING/GROOMING SELF CARE DEFICIT (NANDA Self Care Deficit: Dressing/Grooming)

DEFINITION: An impaired ability to perform or complete dressing and grooming activities for oneself.

SIGNS AND SYMPTOMS (Observed or Reported):
Inability to:
Choose clothing [9]
Pick up clothing [9]
Put on clothing on upper body [9]
Put on clothing on lower body [9]
Use zippers [9]
Put on socks [9]
Put on shoes [9]
Remove clothes [9]
Put on or take off necessary items of clothing [3,6,7,8]
Obtain or replace items of clothing [3,6,7,8]
Fasten clothing [3,6,7,8]
Maintain appearance at a satisfactory level [3,6,7,8]
Discomfort [1,4,5]

Suggested Functional Level Classification: [2]
0=Completely independent.
1=Requires use of equipment or device.
2=Requires help from another person for assistance, supervision, or teaching.
3=Requires help from another person and equipment device.
4=Dependent, does not participate in activity.

RELATED FACTORS:
Weakness/tiredness [4,5,6]
Severe anxiety [4,5]
Decreased/lack of motivation [7,8]
Pain [1,4,5]
Perceptual or cognitive impairment [4,5]
Neuromuscular impairment [4,5]
Musculo-skeletal impairment [4,5]
Use assistive device [9]
Environmental barriers [4,5]

REFERENCES:
1. Chang, B. (1994). Validity of concepts for selecting nursing diagnoses. Clinical Nursing Research, 3, 3, 183-208.
2. Jones, E. (1974). Patient Classification for Long-Term Care: Users' Manual (Adapted from). HEW, Publication No. HRA-74-3107.
3. Levin, R.F., Krainovitch, B.C., Bahrenburg, E., & Mitchell, C.A. (1989). Diagnostic content validity of nursing diagnoses. Image: Journal of Nursing Scholarship, 21(1), 40-44.
4. McKeighen, R.J., Mehmert, P.A., & Dickel, C.A. (1990). Bathing/hygiene self-care deficit: Defining characteristics and related factors across age groups and diagnosis related groups in an acute care setting. Nursing Diagnosis, 1,4,155-161.
5. McKeighen, R.J., Mehmert, P.A., & Dickel, C.A. (1991). Self-care deficit, bathing/hygiene: Defining characteristics and related factors utilized by staff nurses in an acute care setting. In Carroll-Johnson, R.M. (Ed.). Classification of nursing diagnoses: Proceedings of the ninth national conference. Philadelphia, PA: J.B. Lippincott Company.
6. Rhodes, V.A., Watson, P.M., & Hanson, B.M. (1988). Patients' descriptions of the influence of tiredness and weakness on self-care abilities. Cancer Nursing, 11, 3,186-194.
7. Smits, M.W. & Kee, C.C. (1992). Correlates of self-care among the independent elderly: Self-concept affects well-being. Journal of Gerontological Nursing, 18(9), 13-18.
8. Waters, K.R. (1994). Getting dressed in the early morning: Styles of staff/patient interaction on rehabilitation hospital wards for elderly people. Journal of Advanced Nursing, 19, 239-248.
9. Johnson, M. & Maas, M. (Eds.). (1997). Nursing outcomes classification (NOC): Iowa outcomes project. St. Louis: The C.V. Mosby Company.

RECOMMENDED NANDA STAGING: 2.3

EATING DIFFICULTY (NANDA Ineffective Infant Feeding Pattern)

DEFINITION: Inability to orally consume or retain adequate nutrients and fluids.

SIGNS AND SYMPTOMS (Observed or Reported):

Physiological:
- Inadequate suck [1]
- Inappropriate feeding reflexes for developmental age [1]
- Hypersensitivity to oral stimulation [1]
- Poor tongue control [1]
- Swallowing dysfunction [1,5]
- Gagging [3]
- Vomiting/regurgitation during or after feedings [1]
- Diminished desire to eat [2]

- Neuromuscular impairment [1]
- Limited wrist/hand range of motion [5]
- Dysfunctional sensory system [1]
- Disordered gastrointestinal transit [2]
- Oral-motor defects [3]
- Swallowing problems [1,5]
- Uncoordinated suck-swallow-breath cycles [6]
- Maturational changes in anatomy & physiology [1]
- Cognitive impairment (dementia) [4]
- Gastric problems-delayed emptying [1]
- Persistent vomiting from gastroesophegeal reflux [3]
- Respiratory problems-aspiration, fatigue, hypoxia [1]
- Oral pain [6]

Behavioral:
- Excessive slowness [3,6]
- Negative reaction to food/food source [1]

RELATED FACTORS:

Physiological:
- Prematurity [1]
- Developmental delay [1]

Behavioral:
- Past negative feeding experience [1]

REFERENCES:

1. Bottei, K. (1995). Feeding dysfunction: A nursing diagnosis for infants who resist oral feeding. Nursing Diagnosis, 6(2), 80-88.
2. Clarkston, W.K., Pantano, M.M., Morley, J.E., Horowitz, M., Littlefield, J.M. & Burton, F.R. (1997). Evidence for the anorexia of aging: Gastrointestinal transit and hunger in healthy elderly vs. young adults. American Journal of Physiology, 272(1 Pt 2), 243-248.
3. Sanders, M.R., Patel, R.K., Le Grice, B., & Shepherd, R.W. (1993). Children with persistent feeding difficulties: An observational analysis of the feeding interaction of problem and non-problem eaters. Health Psychology, 12(1) 64-73.
4. Wagner, M.B., Vignos, P.J., Carlozzi, C., & Hull, A.L. (1993). Assessment of hand function in Duchenne muscular dystrophy. Archives of Physical Medicine & Rehabilitation, 74(8), 801-804.
5. Watson, R. (1993). Measuring feeding difficulty in patients with dementia: Perspectives and problems. Journal of Advanced Nursing, 18(1), 25-31.
6. Zickler, C.F., & Dodge, N.N. (1994). Office management of the young child with cerebral palsy and difficulty in growing. Journal of Pediatric Health Care, 8(3), 111-120.

RECOMMENDED NANDA STAGING: 2.3

EATING RELUCTANCE (NANDA None)

DEFINITION: Unwillingness to orally consume or retain adequate nutrients and fluids.

SIGNS AND SYMPTOMS (Observed or Reported):
Refusal to eat [9]
Lack of cooperation [8,12]
Refusal to follow commands [8]
Highly selective eating practices [8]
Consumes only small amounts of food [8]
Passivity [11]
Excessive slowness in eating [8]
Holds food in hand or mouth [8]
Plays with food [12]
Allows food to drop out of mouth [9]
Spitting [8,10]
Loss of appetite [4]

RELATED FACTORS:
Unrestrained access to food between meals [8]
Unpredictable mealtime schedule [8]
Abnormal eating attitudes and behaviors [3]
Caregiver mismanagement of food refusal episodes [8]
Negative comments about eating by caregiver [8]
Dysfunctional interactions [12]
Emotional entrapment in battle over food [8]
Coercive family processes/power struggles [8]
Inappropriate social attention [8]
Negative or absent instruction [8]
Anticipitory nausea and vomiting [2,5]
Fear/paranoia of food risk, e.g., pesticides [1]
Depression [4]

REFERENCES:
1. Bidlack, W.R. & Taylor, S. (1992) The fear of healthy eating: Understanding the paranoia. Journal of Pediatric Health Care, 6(6), 335-360.
2. Duigon, A. (1986). Anticipatory nausea, vomiting associated with cancer chemotherapy. Oncology Nursing Forum, 13(1), 35-40.
3. Fisher, M., Pastore, D., Schneider, M., Pegler, C., & Napolitano, B. (1994). Eating attitudes in urban and suburban adolescents. International Journal of Eating Disorders, 16(1), 67-74.
4. Kazes, M., Danion, J.M., Grange, D., Pardignac, A., & Schlienger, J.L. (1993). The loss of appetite during depression with melancholia: A qualitative and quantitative analysis. International Clinical Psychopharmacology, 8(1), 55-59.
5. King, C.R. (1997). Nonpharmacologic management of chemotherapy-induced nausea and vomiting. Oncology Nursing Forum, 24(7) Suppl, 41-8.
6. Norberg, A., Backstrom, A., Athlin, E., & Norberg, B. (1987). Food refusal amongst nursing home patients as conceptualized by nurses' aids and enrolled nurses: An interview study. Journal of Advanced Nursing, 13(4), 478-483.
7. Phillips, L.R. & VanOrt, S. (1993). Measurement of mealtime interactions among persons with dementing disorders. Journal of Nursing Measurement, 1(1), 41-55.
8. Sanders, M.R., Patel, R.K., Le Grice, B. & Shepherd, R.W. (1993). Children with persistent feeding difficulties: An observational analysis of the feeding interactions of problem and non-problem eaters. Health Psychology, 12(1), 64-73.
9. Watson, R. (1993). Measuring feeding difficulty in patients with dementia: Perspectives and problems. Journal of Advanced Nursing, 18(1), 25-31.
10. Watson, R. (1994). Measuring feeding difficulty in patients with dementia: Developing a scale. Journal of Advanced Nursing, 19(2), 257-263.
11. Watson, R. & Deary, I.J. (1994) Measuring feeding difficulty in patients with dementia: Multivariate analysis of feeding problems, nursing intervention and indicators of feeding difficulty. Journal of Advanced Nursing, 20(2), 283-287.
12. Zickler, C.F. & Dodge, N.N. (1994) Office management of the young child with cerebral palsy and difficulty in growing. Journal of Pediatric Health Care, 8(3), 111-120.

RECOMMENDED NANDA STAGING: 2.3

ENERGY FIELD DISTURBANCE (NANDA Energy Field Disturbance)

DEFINITION: An impedance in the flow of universal energy that creates disorganization between the mind, body, and spirit.

SIGNS AND SYMPTOMS (Observed or Reported):
Differences in energy field areas felt as:
Heat [5, 6, 10]
Thickness [5, 6]
Pressure [5, 6]
Heaviness [5, 6]
Fullness [5]
Coldness [5, 6, 10]
Void [6]
Drawing or pulling sensation [5, 6]
Tingling [5, 6, 10]
Dysrythmias or random pulsations of flow [5]

RELATED FACTORS:
Pain [2,10]
Anxiety [1,7,8,9]
Tension headache [3]
Stress [4]
Fatigue [10]
Depression [8,10]

REFERENCES:
1. Gagne, D. & Toye, R. C. (1994). The effects of therapeutic touch and relaxation therapy in reducing anxiety. Archives of Psychiatric Nursing, 8(3),184-189.
2. Heidt, P. R. (1991). Helping patients to rest: Clinical studies in therapeutic touch. Holistic Nursing Practice, 5(4), 57-66.
3. Keller, E. & Bzdek, V. M. (1986). Effects of therapeutic touch on tension headache pain. Nursing Research, 35(2), 101-106.
4. Kramer, N. A. (1990). Comparison of therapeutic touch and casual touch in stress reduction of hospitalized children. Pediatric Nursing, 16(5), 483-485.
5. Krieger, D. (1993). Accepting your power to heal: The personal practice of therapeutic touch. Santa Fe, New Mexico: Bear & Company Publishers.
6. Macrae, J. (1987). Therapeutic touch: A practical guide. New York: Knof.
7. Olson, M. & Sneed, N. (1995). Anxiety and therapeutic touch. Issues in Mental Health Nursing, 16(2), 97-108.
8. Quinn, J. F. & Strelkauskas, A. J. (1993). Psychoimmuniologic effects of therapeutic touch on practitioners and recently bereaved recipients: A pilot study. Advances in Nursing Science, 15(4), 13-26.
9. Simington, J. A. & Laing, G. P. (1993). Effects of therapeutic touch on anxiety in the institutionalized elderly. Clinical Nursing Research, 2(4), 438-450.
10. Wright, S. M. (1991). Validity of the human energy field assessment form. Western Journal of Nursing Research, 13(5), 635-647.

RECOMMENDED NANDA STAGING: 2.3

FAMILY COPING ENHANCEMENT POTENTIAL (NANDA Family Coping: Potential for Growth)

DEFINITION: Family unit seeking growth in passive and active behaviors used to deal with anxieties and tensions from stressor events. [2]

SIGNS AND SYMPTOMS (Observed or Reported):

Belief that problems can be mastered [2,6]

Cohesion or a sense of family pulling together [4,7,8]

Financial stability [8]

Seeking of help and assistance [6]

Adaptability, e.g., flexibility in discussion/decision making [2,8]

Family integration, e.g., family's common interest, affection, sense of economic interdependence, and other bonds of unity [2,4]

Family is healthy [8]

Conflict management or reduction [8]

Seeks spiritual comfort [6]

Controls meaning of potential stressors before they become a threat [1,3]

Role flexibility [2,4]

Confrontation of problems [6]

Seeks social support [7]

Expresses feelings & emotions [7]

Diverts attention [7]

Maintains a positive healthy dependence on others [4,7]

RELATED FACTORS:

Life transitions [6]

Perception of threat, harm, or loss [2,5]

Financial stability [2]

Numerous family social support systems [2]

Ability to use defense mechanisms [2]

Use of spiritual comfort [6]

REFERENCES:

1. Beutel, M. (1985). Approaches to taxonomy and measurement of adaptation in chronic disease. Psychotherapy & Psychosomatics, 43(4), 177-185.

2. Boss, P. (1987). Family stress. In M.B. Sussman, & S.K. Steinmetz (Eds). Handbook of marriage and family. New York, N.Y: Plenum Press.

3. Bouchard, G., Sabourin, S., Lussier, Y., Wright, J., & Richer, C. (1997). Testing the theoretical models underlying the ways of coping questionnaire with couples. Journal of Marriage and the Family, 59, 409-418.

4. Johnson, S.K., Craft, M., Titler, M, Halm, M., Kleiber, C, Montgomery, LA, Megivern, K. Nicholson, A. & Buckwalter, K. (1995). Perceived changes in adult family members' roles and responsibilities during critical illness. Image-The Journal of Nursing Scholarship, 27(3):238-43.

5. Lazarus, R.S. & Folkman, S. (1984). Stress appraisal and coping. New York: Springer.

6. McCubbin, H.I (1987). Family Coping Inventory. In H.I. McCubbin, & A.I. Thomson (Eds). Family assessment research and practice. Madison, WI: University of Wisconsin-Madison.

7. Miller, J.F. (1992). Coping with chronic illness: Overcoming powerlessness (2nd. Ed). Philadelphia, PA: F.A. Davis Company.

8. Stetz, K.M., Lewis, F.M., & Houck, G.M. (1994). Family goals as indicants of adaptation during chronic illness. Public Health Nursing, 11(6), 385-391.

RECOMMENDED NANDA STAGING: 2.2

FAMILY COPING INEFFECTIVENESS (NANDA Ineffective Family Coping: Compromised)

DEFINITION: Family unit's use of inadequate passive and active behaviors when dealing with anxieties and tensions emerging from stressor events. [4]

SIGNS AND SYMPTOMS (Observed or Reported):
Belief that problems are overwhelming [1,5]
Blame imposed on family members [6]
Expressions of pervasive, inappropriate guilt [1,3]
Generalized anger [1,3]
Social isolation [1,3]
Shared shame and embarrassment [1]
Pervasive sadness [1]
Distancing/avoidance of problems [2]
Feelings not expressed [6]
Problems are minimized [6]
Decision-making is delayed [6]
Does not actively seek help [6]
Lack of family cohesion [6]
Lack of flexibility [1]

RELATED FACTORS:
Life transitions [3,5]
Perception of threat, harm, or loss [1,3,4]
Financial instability [1]
Few family support systems [1]
Family inability to use defense
 mechanisms [1]
Lack of spiritual comfort [5]

REFERENCES:
1. Boss, P. (1987). Family stress. In M.B. Sussman, & S.K Steinmetz (Eds). Handbook of marriage and family. New York, N.Y: Plenum Press.
2. Bouchard, G., Sabourin, S., Lussier, Y., Wright, J., & Richer, C. (1997). Testing the theoretical models underlying the ways of coping questionnaire with couples. Journal of Marriage and the Family 59, 409-418.
3. Johnson, S.K., Craft, M., Titler, M, Halm, M., Kleiber, C, Montgomery, LA, Megivern, K. Nicholson, A. & Buckwalter, K. (1995). Perceived changes in adult family members' roles and responsibilities during critical illness. Image - The Journal of Nursing Scholarship, 27(3), 238-43.
4. Lazarus, R.S. & Folkman, S. (1984). Stress appraisal and coping. New York: Springer.
5. McCubbin, H.I (1987). Family Coping Inventory. In H.I. McCubbin & A.I. Thomson (Eds). Family assessment research and practice. Madison, WI: University of Wisconsin-Madison.
6. Miller, J.F. (1992). Coping with chronic illness: Overcoming powerlessness (2nd. Ed). Philadelphia, PA: F.A. Davis Company.

RECOMMENDED NANDA STAGING: 2.2

FAMILY COPING INEFFECTIVENESS RISK (NANDA None)

DEFINITION: Risk for the family unit's inadequate use of behaviors when dealing with the anxieties and tensions emerging from stressor events and changes. [3]

RISK FACTORS:
Life Transitions [3]
Perception of threat, harm, or loss [1,2]
Financial Instability [1]
Few family Social Supports Systems [1]
Family inability to use defense mechanisms [1]
Lack of Spiritual Comfort [3]

REFERENCES:
1. Boss, P. (1987). Family stress. In M.B. Sussman, & S.K. Steinmetz, Handbook of marriage and family. New York, N.Y: Plenum Press.
2. Johnson, S.K., Craft, M., Titler, M, Halm, M., Kleiber, C, Montgomery, LA, Megivern, K. Nicholson A. & Buckwalter K. (1995). Perceived changes in adult family members' roles and responsibilities during critical illness. Image-The Journal of Nursing Scholarship, 27(3), 238-43.
3. Lazarus, R.S. & Folkman, S. (1984). Stress appraisal and coping. New York: Springer.

RECOMMENDED NANDA STAGING: 2.2

FAMILY DECISIONAL CONFLICT (NANDA Decisional Conflict (Specify))

DEFINITION: Family unit's inability to move productively toward effective resolution.

SIGNS AND SYMPTOMS (Observed or Reported):
Inadequate problem-solving processes:
Lack of awareness of process of decision making[3]
Wishful thinking[4]
No search for information[1,5]
Ignoring correct information[2]
Ignoring information about risks[2]
No recognized options.... information overload[1,4]
Failure to recognize that a decision is needed[3]
Failure to explore alternatives[1,5]
Failure to perceive options[1,5]
Difficulty evaluating possible outcomes associated
    with each option[3,4,5]
Inability to assess consequences[1,3,5]
Rushing into decision....instantaneous decision[1,2]
Failure to reach solution[3]
Delay in reaching consensus[3]
Avoid speaking about decision[3]
Lack of planning for implementation and
    contigencies[1,2]

Conflict:
Competition.....power struggles[3]
Lack of cooperation.....lack or reciprocity[3,4]
Unresolved conflict....no mutual justice[3,4]
Lack of freedom to implement a choice[3]

Paternalism:
Participants not included [4,5]
Participant preferences not reflected in decision [4,5]

Emotions:
Anger.....depression[3,4]
Guilt.....jealousy[3,4]

Fear/anxiety[3]
Post decision regret[4]
Hopelessness

RELATED FACTORS:
Family:
Resources[1,2,3]
Insufficient social support[3,4]
Values/myths[1,2]
Communication patterns[3]
Cultural background [4]
Prior decision making pattern/distribution of
    power [3]
Discordant perceptions or values among members[3]

Individual:
Age[2]
Cognitive ability[1,3]
Gender roles[2]
Personality/self esteem[3]
Coping style[4,5]
Bias[1,2]

Situational:
Ethical implications[4]
Social pressures[3,5]
Unfamiliar situation with no prescribed solution-
new medical procedure/technology[1,3]
Crisis/firm deadline for decision[1,2]
Amount and type of information available[3]

REFERENCES:
1. Beckingham, A.C., & Baumann, A. (1990). The ageing family in crisis: Assessment and decision-making models, Journal of Advanced Nursing, 15(7), 782-787.
2. Coulton, C.J. (1990). Research in patient and family decision making regarding life sustaining and long term care. Social Work in Health Care, 15(1), 63-78.
3. Haber, L. C., & Austin, J.A. (1992). How married couples make decisions. Western Journal of Nursing Research, 14(3), 322-342.
4. Hilton, B.A., & Starzomski, R.C. (1994). Family decision making about living related kidney donation. ANNA Journal, 21(6), 346-55.
5. Russell, S., & Jacob, R.G. (1993). Living-related organ donation: The donor's dilemma. Patient Education and Counseling, 21(1/2), 89-99.

RECOMMENDED NANDA STAGING: 2.1

FAMILY NONADHERANCE (NANDA Ineffective Management of Therapeutic Regimen: Family)

DEFINITION: Family unit's inadequate support of and/or participation in the client's efforts to follow a health (care) plan.

SIGNS AND SYMPTOMS (Observed or Reported):
Worsening of health status [1,2,3,4,5,6]
Complications [1,2,3,4,5,6]
Verbalize difficulty in carrying out health care plan [1,2,3,4,5,6]
Failure to follow health care plan [1,2,3,4,5,6]
Family not participating in client efforts to follow a health care plan as evidenced by self report, observation, or physiological measures [1,2,3,4,5,6]

RELATED FACTORS:
Complexity of therapeutic regimen [1,2,3,4,5,6]
Health system barriers [1,2,3,4,5,6]
Inappropriate recommendations [1,2,3,4,5,6]
Ineffective communication [1,2,3,4,5,6]

Limited family resources [1,2,3,4,5,6]
Financial [1,2,3,4,5,6]
Lack of knowledge regarding health care plan [1,2,3,4,5,6]
Caregiver burden [1,2,3,4,5,6]
Limited family coping [1,2,3,4,5,6]
Ineffective planning [1,2,3,4,5,6]
Ineffective communication among family members [1,2,3,4,5,6]
Family conflict [1,2,3,4,5,6]
Ineffective decision making [1,2,3,4,5,6]
Limited community resources [1,2,3,4,5,6]
Client's needs exceed and/or are in conflict with family's resources or beliefs [1,2,3,4,5,6]
Needs exceed and/or are in conflict with family's beliefs [1,2,3,4,5,6]

REFERENCES:
1. Bakker, R.H., Kastermans, M.C. & Dassen, T.W.N. (1995). An analysis of the nursing diagnosis ineffective management of therapeutic regimen compared to noncompliance and Orem's self-care deficit theory of nursing. Nursing Diagnosis, 6(4), 161-166
2. Evans, R.L., Hendricks, R.D., Haselkorn, J.K., Bishop, D.S. & Baldwin, D. (1992). The family's role in stroke rehabilitation: A review of the literature. American Journal Physical Medicine & Rehabilitation, 71(3), 135-139.
3. Feigelman, S., Stanton, B., Rubin, J., & Carteli, N.A. (1993). Effectiveness of family notification efforts and compliance with measles post-exposure prophylaxis. Journal of Community Health, 18(2), 83-93.
4. Fujita, L.Y. & Dugan, J. (1994). High risk for ineffective management of therapeutic regimen: A protocol study. Rehabilitation Nursing, 19(2), 75-79.
5. Kontz, M. (1989). Compliance redefined and implications for home care. Holistic Nursing Practice 3(2), 54-64.
6. Miller, S.P., Wikoff, R., Garrett, M.J., McMahon, M., & Smith, T. (1990). Regimen compliance two years after myocardial infarction. Nursing Research, 39(6), 333-336.

RECOMMENDED NANDA STAGING: 2.3

FAMILY PROCESS ALTERATION (NANDA Altered Family Process)

DEFINITION: A change in family relationships and/or functioning of the family unit.

SIGNS AND SYMPTOMS (Observed or Reported):

Participation in decision making[4, 6]
Participation in problem solving[4, 6]
Communication patterns[2, 5, 6]
Assigned tasks[2, 3, 5]
Effectiveness in completing assigned tasks[4, 6]
Power alliances[4, 6]
Availability for emotion support[2]
Availability for affective responsiveness and intimacy[2, 4, 6]
Expressions of conflict within family[4, 6]
Expressions of conflict with and/or isolation from community resources[5][4, 5, 6]
Satisfaction with family[5]

Mutual support[5]
Patterns and rituals[1, 4, 6]
Somatic complaints[2]
Stress-reduction behaviors[2]

RELATED FACTORS:

Situational life transition[4, 5, 6]
Shift in health status of a family member[1, 2, 3]
Modification in family finances[4, 6]
Modification in family social status[4, 6]
Power shift of family member[4, , 6]
Developmental transitions[5]
Family roles shift[2, 4, 6]
Informal/formal interaction with community[3, 5]

REFERENCES:

1. Brewer, N.W. & Warren, A.M. (1994). Altered family processes related to an ill family member: a validation study. Nursing Diagnosis, 5(3), 115-120.
2. Cohen, M., Titler, M. & Craft, M.J. (1989). Validation of alterations in family processes: Perceptions of critical care hospitalization. In Carroll-Johnson, R. (Ed.). Classification of nursing diagnoses: Proceedings of the eighth conference. Philadelphia: Lippincott.
3. Decker, S.D. & Young, E. (1991). Self-perceived needs of primary caregivers of home-hospice clients. Journal of Community Health Nursing, 8(3), 147-154.
4. Grotevant, H.D., & Carlson, C.I. (1989). Family assessment: A guide to methods & measures. New York: Guilford Press.
5. Lipman, T.H. (1989). Assessing family strengths to guide plan of care using Hymovich's framework. Journal of Pediatric Nursing: Nursing Care of Children & Families, 4(3), 186-196.
6. Touliatos, J., Perlmutter, B.F. & Straus, M.A. (1990). Handbook of family measurement techniques. Newbury Park, CA. Sage Publishing Company.

RECOMMENDED NANDA STAGING: 2.3

FAMILY PROCESS ALTERATION: ALCOHOLISM (NANDA None)

DEFINITION: The chronic disorganization of psychosocial, spiritual, and or physical functions of the family unit related to the use of alcohol.

SIGNS AND SYMPTOMS (Observed or Reported):

Feelings of Family Members:
  Decreased self-esteem[3, 4]
  Anger[3, 4]
  Repressed emotions[3, 4]
  Shame/embarassment[3, 4,5]
  Depression [3, 4]
  Hostility [2,4]
  Abandonment[2, 4]

Roles and Relationships in the Family Change:
  Deterioration in family relationships [3, 4]
  Ineffective spouse communication/marital
    problems [3,4]
  Inconsistent parenting[4]
  Family denial[4, 5,6]
  Closed communication systems [4]
  Disruptive and unpredictable communication[4,5]
  Chronic family problems [3, 5]
  Intimacy dysfunction [4]
  Triangulating family relationships[4]
  Disrupted or lack of family rituals[2, 4]
  Lack family relationship skills [3]
  Enables alcoholic behavior [4]
  Role reversal[2, 3,4,5]

Behavior of Family Members:
  Difficulty with intimate relationships [3]
  Alcohol abuse by other family members[2, 3,4]
  Lack of understanding or knowledge of
    alcoholism [3, 5]
  Refusal to get help/inability to receive help[4]
  Inability to use problem-solving skills [2, 4]

Over dependency on family members e.g. unable
    to make independent decisions [4]
Unpredictable behavior of the alcoholic[3,5]
Life is alcohol centered [4]
Stress-related physical illness occur in family
    members [4, 5]
Disturbances in behavior of family members e.g.
    acting out [3]
Substance abuse other than alcohol in family
    members [1, 3, 4]
Conflict with alcoholic, among family members,
    and community [4]
Conspiracy of silence[5]
Orientation toward tension relief rather than
    achievement of long-term goals with related
    lowered stress [4]
Immaturity [4]
Seek approval and affirmation [4]

Environment:
  Anger [3]
  Fear [3]
  Frustration [3, 4]
  Unpredictable [3, 4]
  Inconsistent [3, 4, 5]
  Violence [3]

RELATED FACTORS:
Abuse of alcohol [3]
Experimentation with alcohol and drugs by
    children[1, 3]

REFERENCES:
1. Brody, G.H., & Forehand, R. (1993). Prospective associations among family form, family processes, and adolescents' alcohol and drug use. Behavioral Research and Therapy, 31(6), 587-593
2. Friedemann, M-L., & Musgrove, J.A. (1994). Perceptions of inner city substance abusers about their families. Archives of Psychiatric Nursing, 8(2), 115-123.
3. Heatherington, S.E. (1988). Children of alcoholics: An emerging mental health issue. Archives of Psychiatric Nursing, 2(4), 251-255.
4. Lindeman, M., Hawks, J.H., & Bartek, J.K. (1994). The alcoholic family: A nursing diagnosis validation study. Nursing Diagnosis, 5(2), 65-73.
5. Norton, J.H. (1994). Addiction and family issues. Alcohol, 11(6), 457-460.
6. Wing, D.M. (1995). Transcending alcoholic denial. Image: the Journal of Nursing Scholarship, 27(2), 121-126.

RECOMMENDED NANDA STAGING: 2.3

FATIGUE (NANDA Fatigue)

DEFINITION: An overwhelming sustained sense of exhaustion and decreased capacity for physical and mental work at usual level.[3,4]

SIGNS AND SYMPTOMS (Observed or Reported):
Drowsy [1,2]
Tired [2,4,6]
Listless [6,9]
Lack of energy/inability to maintain usual
  level of physical activity [1,2]
Irritable[8]
Increase in physical complaints [1]
Compromised concentration [1,3,9]
Compromised libido[3,9]
Unremitting and overwhelming lack of energy [9]
Perceived need for additional energy to finish
  required tasks [1,9]
Inability to restore energy even after sleep [1,9]
Increase in rest requirements [9]
Decreased performance [9]
Inability to maintain usual routine [9]
Disinterest in surroundings [9]
Feelings of guilt for not keeping up with
  responsibilities [9]

RELATED FACTORS:
Physiological:

Anemia [1]
Disease states [2,4,6,7]
Sleep deprivation [1,4,5,6,8]
Pregnancy [7]
Poor physical condition [8]
Malnutrition [1,4,6]
Increased physical exertion [8]

Psychological:
Stress [1,2,6,8]
Anxiety [4,5,7]
Depression [1,4,5,6,7]
Boring life style [1]

Situational: [4]
Negative life events
Occupation

Environmental:
Lights [2,5,8]
Noise [2,5]
Humidity [2,5,8]
Temperature [2,5,8]

REFERENCES:
1. Chun, L. (1997). The clinical validation of defining characteristics and related factors of fatigue in hemodialysis patients. In M.J. Rantz & P. LeMone. (Eds.), Classification of nursing diagnoses: Proceedings of the twelfth conference. (pp.89-96). Glendale, CA: CINAHL.
2. Hart, L.K., Freel, M., & Milde, F. (1990). Fatigue. Nursing Clinics of North America, 25(4), 967-976.
3. Johnson, M. & Maas, M. (1997). Nursing outcomes classification (NOC). St. Louis: The C.V. Mosby Company.
4. Lee, K.A., Lentz, M.J., Taylor, D.L., Mitchell, E.S., & Woods, N.F. (1994). Fatigue as a response to environmental demands in women's lives. Image: the Journal of Nursing Scholarship, 26(2), 149-154.
5. Potempa, K., Lopez, M., Reid, C., & Lawson, L. (1986). Chronic fatigue. Image: the Journal of Nursing Scholarship, 18(4), 165-169.
6. Robinson, K.D. & Posner, J.D. (1992). Patterns of self-care needs and interventions related to biological response modifier therapy: Fatigue as a model. Seminars in Oncology Nursing, 8(4 Suppl 1), 17-22.
7. Pugh, L.C. & Milligan, R.A. (1995). Patterns of fatigue during childbearing. Applied Nursing Research, 8(3), 140-46.
8. Stuifbergen, A.K. & Rogers, S. (1997). The experience of fatigue and strategies of self-care among persons with multiple sclerosis. Applied Nursing Research, 10(1), 2-10.
9. Tiesinga, L.J., Dassen, T.W.N., & Halfens, R.J.G. (1997). Validation of the nursing diagnosis fatigue among patients with chronic heart failure. In M.J. Rantz & P. LeMone (Eds). Classification of nursing diagnoses: Proceedings of the twelfth conference, North American Nursing Diagnosis Association. (pp.263-7). Glendale, CA: CINAHL.

RECOMMENDED NANDA STAGING: 2.3

FEAR (NANDA Fear)

DEFINITION: Response to perceived threat, real or imagined, caused by a consciously recognized and realistic danger.

SIGNS AND SYMPTOMS (Observed or Reported):

Self reported symptoms of feeling:
- Apprehension [1, 4, 5, 7]
- Increased tension [1, 5, 7]
- Decreased self assurance [4, 7]
- Impulsiveness [7]
- Excited [6]
- Scared [1, 3, 4, 5, 7]
- Jitteriness [1, 5, 7]
- Dread [1, 7]
- Alarm [1, 7]
- Terrified [7]
- Panic [4, 7]

Cognitive:
- Identifies object of fear [1,4,7]
- Diminished productivity [5]
- Diminished learning ability [5]
- Difficulty problem solving [5]

Psychological/Behavioral:
- Increased alertness [1,5,7]
- Avoidance or attack behaviors [1,7]
- Narrowed focus on "it" [1,4,5,7]

Physiological:
- Increased pulse [1,7]

Shunting of blood from skin to gastrointestinal tract, heart, central nervous system, and skeletal muscles [1,7]
- Anorexia [1, 7]
- Nausea [1, 7]
- Vomiting [1, 7]
- Diarrhea [1, 7]
- Muscle tightness [1, 7]
- Fatigue [1, 7]
- Increased respiratory rate and shortness of breath [1, 7]
- Pallor [1, 7]
- Increased perspiration [1, 7]
- Increased systolic BP [2,7]
- Pupil dilatation [1, 6]
- Dry mouth [2]

RELATED FACTORS:

Stimulus that is believed to be a threat [1,2]

Natural or innate origin e.g. sudden noise, height, pain, loss of physical support [1, 7]

Learned response e.g. conditioning, modeling from or identification with others [1, 7]

Separation from support system in a potentially threatening situation e.g. hospitalization, procedures [1, 7]

Unfamiliarity with environment experience(s) [1, 7]

Language barrier [1, 7]

Sensory impairment [1, 7]

Phobic stimulus [1]

Victimization [9]

REFERENCES:

1. Adams, P., Coler, M., Collins, J., Cottea, T., Delaney, C., Levin, R.F., Krainovich-Miller, B., Much, J. (1997). Anxiety/Fear. In M.J. Rantz & P. LeMone (Eds.), Classification of nursing diagnoses: Proceedings of the twelfth conference (pp.421-425). Pittsburgh, PA: NANDA.
2. Graham, L. E. & Conley, E. M. (1971). Evaluation of anxiety and fear in adult surgical patients. Nursing Research, 20(2), 113-122.
3. Jones, P. & Jakob, D. F. (1981). Nursing diagnosis: differentiating, fear and anxiety. Nursing Papers, 13(4), 20-9.
4. Taylor-Loughran, A. & O'Brien, M. et al (1989). Defining characteristics of the nursing diagnosis fear and anxiety: A validation study. Applied Nursing Research, 2(4).
5. Whitley, G.G. (1996). A multivariate approach for validation of anxiety and fear. Nursing Diagnosis, 7(3), 116-124.
6. Whitley, G.G. (1994). Expert validation and differentiation of the nursing diagnoses of anxiety and fear. Nursing Diagnosis, 5(4), 143-150.
7. Whitley, G.G. (1992). Concept analysis of fear. Nursing Diagnosis, 3(4), 155-161.

RECOMMENDED NANDA STAGING: 2.3

FEEDING DIFFICULTY (NANDA None)

DEFINITION: Problem with or inability to consume or retain adequate nutrients and fluids.

SIGNS AND SYMPTOMS (Observed or Reported):

Physiological:
Inadequate suck (infant) [1]
Inappropriate feeding reflexes for developmental age[1]
Hypersensitivity to oral stimulation[1]
Poor tongue control[1]
Swallowing dysfunction[1]
Gagging [2]
Vomiting/regurgitation during or after feedings [1]
Documented physiological compromise with feeding e.g. bradycardia, apnea, cyanosis [1]
Inability to self-feed [4] e.g. difficulty in handling food on plate, transporting food to mouth
Lack of hunger/satiety cues [1]

Behavioral:
Lack of cooperation [6]
Refusal to initiate compliance with instruction within five seconds [2]
Reluctant eater [2]
Highly selective eating preferences [2]
Consumes small amounts [2]
Passivity [6]
Excessive slowness [2]
Plays with food [7]
Requires excessive time to initiate and complete feedings [7]
Hold food in hand [2]
Not swallowing e.g. either unable, holds food in mouth, or allows food to drop out of mouth[2,5]
Refusal to eat e.g. turns head away, refuses to open mouth [2,5,7]
Refusal to self-feed [2]
Struggling or resisting during feeding [2]
Throws food [7]
Spitting [2,5,7]
Negative reaction to food or food source [1]

RELATED FACTORS:

Physiological:
Prematurity [1]
Developmental delay [1]
Neuromuscular impairment [1]
Dysfunctional sensory system [1]
Anatomical deformations
Oral-motor anatomical defects [2]
Swallowing problems [1]
Uncoordinated suck-swallow-breath cycles [7]
Maturational changes in anatomy and physiology[1]
Cognitive impairment (dementia) [4]
Persistent vomiting from gastroesophegeal reflux[2]
Respiratory problems e.g. aspiration, fatigue related to hypoxia [1]
Abdominal discomfort related to constipation [7]
Oral pain [7]
Physical factors of the wrist and hand e.g. limited range of motion, deformity, and/or decreased muscle strength [3]

Environmental/Psychosocial:
Past negative experiences associated with feeding/food [1]
Unrestrained access to food between meals [2]
Failure to have regular predictable mealtimes [2]
Mismanagement of food refusal episodes [2]
Negative comments about eating [2]

Client/Caregiver:
Negative interactions at mealtimes [2]
Dysfunctional parent-child interactions [7]
Emotionally entrapped in battle over food [2]
Coercive family processes [2]
Coercive power struggle [2]
Absence of effective cues or prompts [2]
Inappropriate social attention [2]
Negative prompts/reminders [2]
Ineffective feeding instruction [2]

REFERENCES:

1. Bottei, K. (1995). Feeding Dysfunction: A nursing diagnosis for infants who resist oral feeding. <u>Nursing Diagnosis,</u> 6(2), 80-88.
2. Sanders, M.R., Patel, R.K., KeGrice, B. & Sheperd, R.W. (1993). Children with persistent feeding difficulties: An observational analysis of the feeding interactions of problems and non-problem eaters. <u>Health Psychology,</u> 12(1), 64-73.
3. Wagner, M.B., Vignos, P.J., Carlozzi. C., & Hull, A.L. (1993). Assessment of hand function in Duchenne Muscular Dystrophy. <u>Archives of Physical Medicine & Rehabilitation,</u> 74(8), 801-804.

4. Watson, R. (1993). Measuring feeding difficulty in patients with dementia: Perspectives and problems. Journal of Advanced Nursing, 18(1), 25-31.

5. Watson, R. (1993). Measuring feeding difficulty in patients with dementia: Developing a scale. Journal of Advanced Nursing, 19(2), 257-263.

6. Watson, R. & Deary, I.J. (1994). Measuring feeding difficulty in patients with dementia: Multivariate analysis of feeding problems, nursing intervention and indicators of feeding difficulty. Journal of Advanced Nursing, 20(2), 283-287.

7. Zickler, C.F. & Dodge, N.N. (1994). Office management of the young child with cerebral palsy and difficulty in growing. Journal of Pediatric Health Care, 8(3), 111-120.

RECOMMENDED NANDA STAGING: 2.1

FEEDING SELF CARE DEFICIT (NANDA Self Care Deficit: Feeding)

DEFINITION: An impaired ability to perform or complete feeding activities.

SIGNS AND SYMPTOMS (Observed or Reported):
Inability to:
Prepare food for ingestion [10]
Open containers [10]
Handle utensils [10]
Get food onto utensil [10]
Pick up cup or glass [10]
Manipulate food in mouth [10]
Chew food [10]
Swallow food [10]
Complete a meal [10]
Bring food from receptacle to the mouth [3,5,8]
Ingest food in a socially acceptable
  manner [4,8]
Ingest food safely [4,8]
Ingest sufficient food [4,8]
Use assitive device [10]
Discomfort [1,5,6]

Suggested Functional Level Classification: [2]
0=Completely independent.
1=Requires use of equipment or device.
2=Requires help from another person for
  assistance, supervision, or teaching.
3=Requires help from another person and
  equipment device.
4=Dependant, does not participate in activity.

RELATED FACTORS:
Weakness/tiredness [4,6,7]
Pain [5,6]
Perceptual or cognitive impairment [5,6]
Neuromuscular impairment [5,6]
Musculoskeletal impairment [5,6]
Severe anxiety [5,6]
Environmental barriers [1,5,6]
Decreased/lack of motivation [8,9]

REFERENCES:
1. Baer, C.A., Delorey, M., & Fitzmaurice, J.B. (1984). A study to evaluate the validity of the rating system for self-care deficit. In Kim, M.J., McFarland, G.K., & McLane, A.M. (Eds.). Classification of nursing diagnoses: Proceedings of the fifth national conference. St. Louis, MO: C.V. Mosby Company.
2. Jones, E. (1974). Patient Classification for Long-Term Care: Users' Manual (Adapted from). HEW, Publication No. HRA-74-3107.
3. Levin, R.F., Krainovitch, B.C., Bahrenburg, E., & Mitchell, C.A. (1989). Diagnostic content validity of nursing diagnoses. Image- Journal of Nursing Scholarship, 21(1), 40-44.
4. Matteson, M.A. & McConnell, E.S. (1988). Gerontological nursing: Concepts and practice. Philadelphia, PA: W.B. Saunders Company.
5. McKeighen, R.J., Mehmert, P.A., & Dickel, C.A. (1990). Bathing/hygiene self-care deficit: Defining characteristics and related factors across age groups and diagnosis related groups in an acute care setting. Nursing Diagnosis, 1(4), 155-161.
6. McKeighen, R.J., Mehmert, P.A., & Dickel, C.A. (1991). Self-care deficit, bathing/hygiene: Defining characteristics and related factors utilized by staff nurses in an acute care setting. In Carroll-Johnson, R.M. (Ed.). Classification of nursing diagnoses: Proceedings of the ninth national conference. Philadelphia, PA: J.B. Lippincott Company.
7. Rhodes, V.A., Watson, P.M., & Hanson, B.M. (1988). Patients' descriptions of the influence of tiredness and weakness on self-care abilities. Cancer Nursing, 11(3), 186-194.
8. Smits, M.W. & Kee, C.C. (1992). Correlates of self-care among the independent elderly: Self-concept affects well-being. Journal of Gerontological Nursing, 18(9), 13-18.
9. Waters, K.R. (1994). Getting dressed in the early morning: Styles of staff/patient interaction on rehabilitation hospital wards for elderly people. Journal of Advanced Nursing, 19, 239-248.
10. Johnson, M. & Maas, M. (Eds.). (1997). Nursing outcomes classification (NOC). St. Louis: C.V.Mosby Company.

RECOMMENDED NANDA STAGING: 2.3

FLUID VOLUME DEFICIT (NANDA Fluid Volume Deficit)

DEFINITION: Isotonic loss of body fluids such that total fluid volume remains below normal (or expected) range for individual.

SIGNS AND SYMPTOMS (Observed or Reported):

Thirst [9,15,16]
Supine blood pressure normal [1]
Orthostatic hypotension [1,9,16]
Systolic blood pressure > 15 mmHg decrease
Heart rate > 15 beats per minute increase
Tachycardia [16]
Dizziness upon standing
Oliguria [9]
Concentrated urine [9,16]
Low urinary sodium [10]
Normal serum sodium [12]
Dry mouth [9]
Poor skin turgor [2,15,16]
Sudden weight loss (except in third spacing) [9]
Weakness [9,15,16]
Decreased venous filling [9]
Neck veins flat when fully reclined [1]
Elevated hematocrit [10,12,16]
Elevated blood urea nitrogen [10]
Lethargy [9]
Irritability in child [3,14]
Depressed fontenalle [3,16]

Absence of tears [3,16]
Hard stools [3,14]
Sticky mucous membranes [3]
Absence of saliva bubbles in babies
Diminished tearing [16]
Urine concentration normal if
   immature renal system [3]

RELATED FACTORS:

Vomiting [1,12,13]
Diarrhea [1,12,13]
Gastrointestinal fistulas,
   drainage, or obstruction. [1,13]
Third-spacing of fluid [9,12,13]
Burns [9,12,13]
Elevated environmental temperature
   or fever causing diaphoresis [4,5,6,7,13]
Diuretic therapy [8,9]
Fever [11]
Polyuria [1]
Inability to swallow [9]
Excessive laxative use [9]

REFERENCES:

1. Briggs, S.P., Sawaya, B.E. & Schnermann, J. (1990). Disorders of salt balance. In J. P. Kokko & R. L. Tannen (Eds.). Fluids and electrolytes, (2nd Ed.) (pp.70-138). Philadelphia: W.B. Saunders.
2. Dorrington, K.L. (1981) Skin turgor: Do we understand the clinical sign? Lancet, 1(8214), 264-266.
3. Driggers, D.A. (1982). Managing the dehydrated child. American Family Physician, 26(5), 189-194.
4. Eisenman, P.A. (1986). Hot weather, exercise, old age, and the kidneys. Geriatrics, 41(5), 108-10, 113-4.
5. Fish, P.D., Bennett, G.C. & Millard, P.H. (1985). Heatwave morbidity and mortality in old age. Age & Ageing, 14(4), 243-5.
6. Hart, G.R., Anderson, R.J., Crumpler, C.P., Shulkin, A., Reed, G. & Knochel, J. P. (1982). Epidemic classical heat stroke: Clinical characteristics and course of 28 patients. Medicine, 61, 189-197.
7. Irion G., Wailgum, T.P.D., Kendrick, Z.V. & Paolone, A.M. (1984.) The effect of age on the hemodynamic responses to thermal stress during stress. In V. J. Cristofalo, G. T. Baker, III, R. C. Adelman & J. Roberts (Eds.), Modern aging research, Vol 6. NY: Alan R. Liss
8. Madias, N.E. & Zelman, S.J. (1982) What are the metabolic complications of diuretic treatment? Geriatrics, 37(2), 93-96.
9. Metheny, N.M. (1996). Fluid and electrolyte balance: Nursing considerations. (3rd Ed.). Philadelphia: Lippincott.
10. Narins, R.G., Jones, E.R., Stom, M.C., Rudnick, M.R. & Bastl, C.P. (1982). Diagnostic strategies in disorders of fluid, electrolyte and acid-base homeostasis. American Journal of Medicine, (Mar), 72, 496-519.
11. Pals, J.K., Weinberg, A.D., Beal, L. F., Levesque, P.G., Cunningham, T.J. & Minaker, K.L. (1995). Clinical triggers for detection of fever and dehydration: Implications for long-term care nursing. Journal of Gerontological Nursing. 21(4), 13-19, 44-5.
12. Pestana, C. (1985). Fluids and electrolytes in the surgical patient, (3rd Ed.). Baltimore: Williams & Wilkins.

13. Reineck, H.J. & Stein, J.H. (1990). Disorders of sodium metabolism. In J.C.M. Chan & J.R. Gill, Jr. (Eds.). <u>Kidney electrolyte disorders,</u> (pp59-105). New York: Churchill-Livingstone.
14. Tejani, A., Dobias, B. & Mahadevan, R. (1981). Osmolar relationship in infantile dehydration. <u>American Journal of Diseases in Children, 135,</u> 1000-1005.
15. Delaney, C. & Mehmert, P. (1991). Utility of the Nursing Minimum Data Set in validation of computerized nursing diagnoses. In R.M. Carroll-Johnson (Ed.). <u>Classification of nursing diagnoses: Proceedings of the ninth conference,</u> (pp175-9). Philadelphia, PA: J.B. Lippincott.
16. Rios, H., Delaney, C., Kruckeberg, T. & Chung, Y. (1991). Validation of defining characteristics of four nursing diagnoses using a computerized database. <u>Journal of Professional Nursing, 7</u>(5), 293-299.

<u>**RECOMMENDED NANDA STAGING:**</u> 2.3

FLUID VOLUME EXCESS (NANDA Fluid Volume Excess)

DEFINITION: Equal gains of extracellular water and sodium.

SIGNS AND SYMPTOMS (Observed or Reported):

Intake exceeds output [7]
Normal serum sodium [3]
Weight gain over short period [3, 7]
Dependent edema [1,5, 7]
Pitting edema [1]
Distended neck veins when upright [1, 3]
Engorged neck veins [2]
Distended peripheral veins [3]
Slow emptying peripheral veins [3]
Bounding, full pulse [3]
Third heart sound (S3 gallop) [1]
Rales (crackles) [3,5, 7]
Dyspnea [5, 7]
Orthopnea [7]
Pleural effusion [3,7]
Hepatic congestion [1]
Hepatojugular reflux [1]

Ascites [3]
Decreased blood urea nitrogen [3]
Decreased hematocrit [3]
Central venous pressure > 11 centimeters of water [3, 8]
Bulging fontanel [6]
Polyuria with normal renal function [3]

RELATED FACTORS:

Renal failure [3, 4]
Congestive heart failure [3, 4]
Cirrhosis [3, 4]
Cushing's Syndrome [3]
Excess administration of sodium containing IV fluids [3]
Excess ingestion of sodium containing foods or medications [3]

REFERENCES:

1. Alpern, R.J., Saxton, C.R. & Seldin, D. W. (1990). Clinical interpretation of laboratory values. In J. P. Kokko & R. L. Tannen (Eds.).Fluids and electrolytes, (2nd Ed.). (pp.3-69). Philadelphia: W.B. Saunders.
2. Briggs, S.P., Sawaya, B.E. & Schnermann, J. (1990). Disorders of salt balance. In J. P. Kokko & R. L. Tannen (Eds.). Fluids and electrolytes, (2nd Ed.). (pp.70-138). Philadelphia: W.B. Saunders.
3. Metheny, N.M. (1996). Fluid and electrolyte balance: Nursing considerations. 3rd Ed. Philadelphia, PA: Lippincott.
4. Reineck, H.J. & Stein, J. H. (1990). Disorders of sodium metabolism. In J.C.M. Chan & J.R. Gill, Jr. (Eds.). Kidney electrolyte disorders, (pp.59-105). New York: Churchill-Livingstone.
5. Delaney, C. & Mehmert, P. (1991). Utility of the Nursing Minimum Data Set in validation of computerized nursing diagnoses. In R.M. Carroll-Johnson (Ed.). Classification of nursing diagnoses: Proceedings of the ninth conference. Philadelphia, PA: J.B. Lippincott.
6. Mott, S.R., James, S.R., & Sperhac, A.M. (1990). Nursing care of children and families. (2nd ed.). Redwood City, CA: Addison Wesley
7. Rios, H., Delaney, C., Kruckeberg, T., Chung, Y., & Mehmert P.A. (1991). Validation of defining characteristics of four nursing diagnoses using a computerized data base. Journal of Professional Nursing, 7(5), 293-299.

RECOMMENDED NANDA STAGING: 2.3

FUNCTIONAL URINARY INCONTINENCE (NANDA Functional Incontinence)

DEFINITION: Inability of usually continent persons to reach toilet in time to avoid unintentional loss of urine.[1]

SIGNS AND SYMPTOMS (Observed or Reported):
Accidents on way to toilet [5]
May only be incontinent in early a.m.[5]
Amount of time required to reach toilet
   exceeds length of time between sensing urge
   and uncontrolled voiding [4]
Senses need to void [4]
Able to completely empty bladder [3]

RELATED FACTORS:
Neuromuscular limitations [4,5]
Impaired vision [3,4]
Impaired cognition [3,4]
Psychological factors [3,4,5]
Environmental factors [3,54]
Weakened supporting pelvic structures [4]

REFERENCES:
1. Fantl, J.A., Newman, D.K., Colling, J., et al. (1996). Urinary incontinence in adults: Acute and chronic management. Clinical practice guidelines, No.2 1996 update. Department of Health and Human Services. Public Health Service, Agency for Health Care Policy and Research. AHCPR Publication No. 96-0682. Rockville, MD: U.S.
2. Gray, M. & Dougherty, M.C. (1987). Urinary incontinence: Pathophysiology and treatment. Journal of Enterostomal Therapy,14(4), 152-62
3. Penn, C. (Unpublished). Incontinence assessment: Examining the reliability of a structured assessment tool in guiding staff nurses through a focused assessment and accurate nursing diagnosis. Master's project, November, 1990. University of Iowa, Iowa City, IA.
4. Specht, J., Tunick, P., Maas, M., & Bulecheck, G. (1991). Urinary incontinence. In M. Maas, K. Buckwalter & M. Hardy (Eds.), Nursing diagnoses and interventions for the elderly (pp. 181-204). Redwood City, CA: Addison-Wesley.
5. Williams, M.E., & Pannill, F.C. (1982). Urinary incontinence in the elderly: Physiology, pathophysiology, diagnosis and treatment. Annals of Internal Medicine, 97(6), 895-907.

RECOMMENDED NANDA STAGING: 2.1

FUNCTIONAL URINARY INCONTINENCE RISK (NANDA None)

DEFINITION: Risk for involuntary loss of urine in a person who is usually continent which occurs when the person is unable to reach toilet in a timely manner.

RISK FACTORS:

Neuromuscular limitations:
 Gait/balance [3,4]
 Manual dexterity [2,3]
 Impaired transfer ability [3,4]
 Strength [3]
 Endurance [3]

Psychological factors:
 Attention seeking [2,3,4]
 Depression [2,3,4]
 Hostile/angry feelings [2,3,4]
 Lack of motivation [2,3,4]
 Reverse conditioning [2,3,4]

Environmental factors: [2,4]
 Placement in unfamiliar setting [2,4]
 Inconvenient toilet facilities [2,4]
 Lack of privacy [2,4]
 Physical restraint [2,4]
 Lack of caregiver assistance [2,4]

Physiological factors:
 Impaired vision [2,3]
 Impaired cognition/ sensation [1,2,3]
 Age related weakening of supporting pelvic
  structures [3]

REFERENCES:

1. Fantl, J.A., Newman, D.K., Colling, J. et al. (1996). Managing acute and chronic urinary incontinence clinical practice guidelines, quick reference guide for clinicians, 1996 update. Rockville, Maryland: AHCPR Publication 96-0686.
2. Penn, C. (Unpublished). Incontinence assessment: Examining the reliability of a structured assessment tool in guiding staff nurses through a focused assessment and accurate nursing diagnosis. Master's Project, November 1990. University of Iowa, Iowa City, IA.
3. Specht, J., Tunick, P, Maas, M. & Bulecheck, G. (1991). Urinary incontinence. In M. Maas, K. Buckwalter & M. Hardy (Eds.), Nursing diagnoses and interventions or the elderly, (pp. 181-204). Redwood City, CA: Addison-Wesley.
4. Williams, M.E. & Pannill, F.C. (1982). Urinary incontinence in the elderly: Physiology, pathophysiology, diagnoses and treatment. Annals of Internal Medicine, 97(6), 895-907.

RECOMMENDED NANDA STAGING: 2.1

GAS EXCHANGE IMPAIRMENT (NANDA Gas Exchange, Impaired)

DEFINITION: Excess or deficit in oxygenation and/or carbon dioxide elimination at the alveolar-capillary membrane.

SIGNS AND SYMPTOMS (Observed or Reported):
Abnormal arterial blood gases [1,2,3,5]
Hypercapnea [2,5]
Hypoxemia [1,3,5]
Cyanosis (neonates) [4,5,6]
Nasal flaring [4,5,6]
Dyspnea [5]
Restlessness [4,5]
Irritability [2,5]
Vision disturbances [5,6]
Somnolence [2,5,6]
Confusion [2,5,6]
Headache upon wakening [5]

RELATED FACTORS:
Alveolar-capillary membrane changes [1]
Ventilation/perfusion alterations [3]

REFERENCES:
1. Brukwitzki, G., Holmgren, C. & Maibusch, R. M. (1996). Validation of the defining characteristics of the nursing diagnosis ineffective airway clearance. Nursing Diagnosis, 7(2), 63-69.
2. Capuano, T.A., Hitchings, K.S. & Johnson, S. (1990). Respiratory nursing diagnoses: practicing nurses' selection of defining characteristics. Nursing Diagnosis, 1(4), 169-174.
3. Dossey, B.M., Guzzetta, C.E. & Kenner, C.V. (Eds.). (1990). Essentials of critical care nursing: Mind, body, and spirit. Philadelphia: J. B. Lippincott.
4. Hastings, B. (1989). Alterations in respiration. In C. Malloy & J. Hartshorn (Eds.). Acute care nursing in the home. New York: J. B. Lippincott.
5. NANDA. (1996). Nursing diagnoses: definitions & classification. Philadelphia, PA: NANDA.
6. Whaley, L.F. & Wong, D.L. (Eds.) (1991). Nursing care of infants and children. (4th Ed.). St. Louis: Mosby.

RECOMMENDED NANDA STAGING: 2.3

GROWTH ALTERATION (NANDA Altered Growth & Development)

DEFINITION: Growth above the 97th percentile or below the 3rd percentile for age, crossing two percentile channels; disproportionate growth pattern.

SIGNS AND SYMPTOMS (Observed or Reported):
Weight above 97th percentile or below the 3rd percentile the 1st two years of life [2,3,6,7]
Growth of less than 2 to 2.5 inches/year ages three to ten years [4,5]
Growth above or below three standard deviations from the mean [1,4,5,7]
Failure to maintain consistent pattern of growth [5,7,8,9]
Bone age greater or less than chronological age [1,3,6]
Delay or absence of puberty [2,4,6,7]
Precocious puberty [1,3,6]
Learning problems [1,4,5,7]
Behavioral difficulties [1,4,5,7,9]
Depression [5,9]
Reduced head circumference [10]
Reduced bone mass index [10]
Reduced mean body mass [10]

RELATED FACTORS:
Prenatal factors:
  Infection [2,5,8]
  Congenital / genetic disorders [1,2,3,4,5,7,8]
  Maternal nutrition [4,5,8]
  Multiple gestation [5,8]

Teratogen exposure [2,3,4,5,8]
Substance use/abuse [3,4,5,6,8]

Individual factors:
  Prematurity [3]
  Malnutrition [2,3,4,5,6,7,8]
  Organic and inorganic factors [2,5,6,8]
  Caregiver and/or individual maladaptive feeding behaviors [2,3,5,7,9]
  Anorexia [5,7]
  Insatiable appetite [7,9]
  Infection [1,2,3,7]
  Chronic illness [2,3,4,5,7,8]
  Substance abuse [1,5]

Caregiver factors:
  Abuse [3,5,7,8,9]
  Mental illness/mental retardation / severe learning disability [3,5,8]

Environmental Factors:
  Deprivation [7,8]
  Teratogen exposure [8]
  Lead poisoning [3,7]
  Poverty [3,7,8]
  Violence [3,7]

REFERENCES:
1. Connaughty, M.S. (1992). Accelerated growth in children. *Journal of Pediatric Health Care,* 6(5, Part 2), 316-324, 333-4.
2. Denniston, C.R. (1994). Assessing normal and abnormal patterns of growth. *Primary Care: Clinics in Office Practice,* 21(4), 637-654.
3. Frank, D.A., Needlman, R., & Silva, M. (1994). What to do when a child won't grow. *Patient Care,* 28(5), 107-110, 113, 117-120, 125-128, 135.
4. Giordano, B.P. (1992).The impact of genetic syndromes on children's growth. *Journal of Pediatric Health Care,* 6(5, Part 2), 309-315, 333-4.
5. Henry, J.J. (1992). Routine growth monitoring and assessment of growth disorders. *Journal of Pediatric Health Care,* 6(5, Part 2), 291-301, 333-4.
6. Lobo, M.L., Barnard, K.E., & Coombs, J.B. (1992). Failure to thrive: A parent-infant interaction perspective. *Journal of Pediatric Nursing: Nursing Care of Children & Families,* 7(4), 251-261.
7. Parker, S.H. (1992). The school nurse's role: early detection of growth disorders. *Journal of School Nursing,* 8(3), 30-32, 34, 36-38, 40-41.
8. Pinyerd, B.J. (1992). Assessment of infant growth. *Journal of Pediatric Health Care,* 6(5, Part 2), 302-308.
9. Stanhope, R., Wilks, Z., & Hamill, G. (1994). Psychosocial aspects of growth. Failure to grow: Lack of food or lack of love? *Professional Care of Mother & Child,* 4(8), 234-237.
10. Johnson, M., & Maas, M. (Eds). (1997) *Nursing outcomes classification.* St. Louis: Mosby

RECOMMENDED NANDA STAGING: 2.1

GROWTH ALTERATION RISK (NANDA None)

DEFINITION: At risk for growth above the 97th percentile or below the 3rd percentile for age, crossing two percentile channels; disproportionate growth pattern.

RISK FACTORS:

Prenatal factors:
Infection [2,5,8]
Congenital/genetic disorders [1,2,3,4,5,7,8]
Maternal nutrition [4,5,8]
Multiple gestation [5,8]
Teratogen exposure [2,3,4,5,8]
Substance use/abuse [3,4,5,6,8]

Individual factors:
Prematurity [3]
Malnutrition [2,3,4,5,6,7,8]
Caregiver and/or individual
maldaptive feeding behaviors [2,3,5,7,8]
Anorexia [5,7]
Insatiable appetite [7,9]
Infection [1,2,3,7]
Chronic illness [2,3,4,5,7,8]
Substance abuse [1,5]

Caregiver factors:
Abuse [3,5,7,8,9]
Mental illness/mental
retardation/severe learning disability [3,5,8]

Environmental Factors:
Deprivation [7,8]
Teratogen exposure [8]
Lead poisoning [3,7]
Poverty [3,7,8]
Violence [3,7]

REFERENCE:
1. Connaughty, M.S. (1992). Accelerated growth in children. Journal of Pediatric Health Care, 6(5, Part 2), 316-324, 333-4.
2. Denniston, C.R. (1994). Assessing normal and abnormal patterns of growth. Primary Care: Clinics in Office Practice, 21(4), 637-654.
3. Frank, D.A., Needlman, R., & Silva, M. (1994). What to do when a child won't grow. Patient Care, 28(5), 107-110, 113, 117-120. 125-128, 135.
4. Giordano, B.P. (1992).The impact of genetic syndromes on children's growth. Journal of Pediatric Health Care, 6(5, Part 2), 309-315, 333-4.
5. Henry, J.J. (1992). Routine growth monitoring and assessment of growth disorders. Journal of Pediatric Health Care, 6(5, Part 2), 291-301, 333-4.
6. Lobo, M.L., Barnard, K.E., & Coombs, J.B. (1992). Failure to thrive: A parent-infant interaction perspective. Journal of Pediatric Nursing: Nursing Care of Children & Families, 7(4), 251-261.
7. Parker, S.H. (1992). The school nurse's role: early detection of growth disorders. Journal of School Nursing, 8(3), 30-32, 34, 36-38, 40-41.
8. Pinyerd, B.J. (1992). Assessment of infant growth. Journal of Pediatric Health Care, 6(5, Part 2), 302-308.
9. Stanhope, R., Wilks, Z., & Hamill, G. (1994). Psychosocial aspects of growth. Failure to grow: Lack of food or lack of love? Professional Care of Mother & Child, 4(8), 234-237.

RECOMMENDED NANDA STAGING: 2.1

HEALTH ENHANCEMENT POTENTIAL (NANDA Health Seeking Behaviors (Specify))

DEFINITION: An individual, in stable health is actively seeking or passively receiving means to alter personal health habits and/or an environment in order to move toward a higher level of health. [1,2,3,4]

RISK FACTORS:

Expressed or observed desire to seek a higher level of wellness [2]

Expressed or observed desire for increased control of health practice [2]

Expression of concern about current environmental conditions on health status [2]

Stated or observed unfamiliarity with wellness community resources [2]

Demonstrated or observed lack of knowledge in health promotion behaviors [2]

Situational/maturational event precipitating concern re: current health status [1,5]

Legislation and/or workplace policies promoting safety and health behaviors [1]

REFERENCES:

1. NANDA (1994). Nursing diagnosis: Definitions & classification (p. 59). Philadelphia: NANDA.
2. Gettrust, K.V. & Barbec. P.D. (1992). Health seeking behaviors. In Nursing diagnosis in clinical practice: Guides for care planning (pp. 285-288). USA: Delmar Publishers.
3. Carpenito, L.J. (1992). Health seeking behaviors. In Nursing diagnosis: Application to clinical practice, (4th Ed). Philadelphia: Lippincott, 470-477.
4. Tripp, S. & Stachowiak, B. (1989). Nursing diagnosis: Health seeking behaviors (specify). In R.M. Carroll-Johnson (Ed.), Classification of nursing diagnosis: Proceeding of the eighth conference, (pp. 433-436). Philadelphia: Lippincott.
5. Ungemack, J.A. (1994). Patterns of personal health practice: men and women in the United States. American Journal of Preventative Medicine, 10(1), 38-44.

RECOMMENDED NANDA STAGING: 2.3

HOME MANAGEMENT DEFICIT (NANDA Impaired Home Maintenance Management)

DEFINITION: Inability or unwillingness to maintain a safe/personally satisfactory environment.

SIGNS AND SYMPTOMS (Observed or Reported):

Apparent unrepaired structural or utility defects or barriers [4]

Inadequate or contaminated water supply or sewage [4]

Smoke and/or fire hazards [4,5]

Inappropriate temperature or ventilation [4,5]

Lacking necessary equipment or aids [4,5,6]

Overcrowding of available space with lack of personal space [4]

Unwashed or unavailable cooking equipment, clothes, or linen [4,5,6]

Accumulated dirt, food/animal waste, garbage [5,6]

Offensive odors [4,5,6]

Presence of rodents and/or insects [4,5,6]

Repeated episodes of hygienic disorders, infestations, infections, and injuries [4,5]

Disorderly cluttered environment [3,6]

General household disrepair [3,6]

Express difficulty in maintaining home to their satisfaction [1,4,8]

Request assistance with home management maintenance/modification [3,4,5,6,7]

Inadequate furnishings [6]

Describe outstanding debts or financial crisis that impede maintenance [3,4,5,6]

RELATED FACTORS:

Lack of assistance or adaptation needed for home management/maintenance/modification [3,7]

Caregivers in exhausted, anxious, or depressed emotional state [2]

Lack knowledge [3,6]

Lack of motivation [3,6]

Negative responses to person needing assistance

Disease, injury or impairment in family member [3,4,5,6,7,8]

Change in family composition [2,4]

Insufficient family organization or planning [3,5,6]

Inadequate support systems [2,3,4,5,6,8]

Unfamiliarity with available resources [3,5,6]

Insufficient financial resources [3,5,6]

Inadequate community resources [4]

Inadequate dwelling and/or furnishings [4]

REFERENCES:

1. Artinian, N.T. & Duggan, C.H. (1995). Sex differences in patient recovery patterns after coronary artery bypass surgery. Heart & Lung: Journal of Critical Care, 24(6), 483-494.
2. Gjerdingen, D.K. & Chaloner, K. (1994). Mothers experience with household rules and social support during the first postpartum year. Women & Health, 21(4), 57-74.
3. Kim, M. & Moritz, D.A., (Eds) (1982). Classification of nursing diagnosis: Proceedings of the third and fourth national conferences, St. Louis: CV Mosby Company.
4. McFarland, G.K. & McFarland, E.A., (1989). Nursing Diagnosis and Intervention, St. Louis: CV Mosby Company.
5. NANDA (1994). Nursing diagnosis: Definitions & classification 1995-1996. North American Nursing Diagnosis Association: Philadelphia.
6. Randall, J. (1992). Home Maintenance Management Impaired. In K.V. Gettrust and P.D. Brabec, (Eds), Nursing diagnosis in clinical practice: Guides for care planning. Delmar Publishers, Inc.
7. Scmidt, M.F., Garvin, L.J., Heinemann, A.W., & Kelly, J.P., (1995). Gender-and-age related role changes following brain injury. Journal of Head Trauma Rehabilitation, 10(4), 14-27.
8. Sharpe, P.A., Clark, N.M., & Janz, N.K., (1991). Differences in the impact and management of heart disease between older women and men. Women & Health, 17(2), 25-43.

RECOMMENDED NANDA STAGING: 2.3

HOPE ALTERATION (NANDA Hopelessness)

DEFINITION: Decreased belief in anticipated future outcomes that are personally satisfying and life supporting.

SIGNS AND SYMPTOMS (Observed or Reported):

Passivity [9,4,13,16]
Lack of initiative [9,16]
Lack of involvement in care/passively allowing care [9]
Exhibits "giving up" behaviors [13]
Increased/decreased sleep [9]
Verbal cues (despondent content, "I can't," sighing) [9,1,2,15,16]
Shrugging in response to speaker [9]
Turning away from speaker [9]
Closing eyes [9]
Decreased positive affect [9,14]
Decreased appetite [9]
Decreased energy [10,11]
Decreased verbalization [9,11]
Decreased response to stimuli [9,16]
Decreased expressions of positive future orientation [4,15,16]
Decreased goal setting [4, 15]
Decreased expressions of inner peace [10,16]
Decreased optimism [4,14]
Questions self-worth [6]
Questions belief in self or expressions of self doubt [14,15]
Questions belief in others or doubts others [14,16]

Questions faith [12,15]
Questions meaning of life [14,15,16]
Questions reasons to live [5,8,16]
Questions will to live [13,16]

RELATED FACTORS:

Crisis situations (loss, life-threatening situations, hardships, change) [3,4,6,15]
Long-term stress [9]
Understanding of disease process [10]
Suffering [6]
Failing or deteriorating physiological condition [1, 3,9,10,12,16]
Prolonged activity restriction creating isolation [9,6]
Ineffective support systems [6,7,12]
Abandonment [9,6]
Personal attributes e.g. determination, courage, serenity [4,6]
Attainable aims/expectations [6,7]
Uplifting memories [6]
Ability to relive positive past experiences [6]
Spiritual awareness [6]
Spiritual base [6,12]
Interpersonal connectedness [4,6,7,16]
Lost belief in transcendent values/God [9,3,6]

REFERENCES:

1. Beck, A.T., Weissman, A., Lester, D. and Trexler, L. (1974). The measurement of pessimism: The hopelessness scale. Journal of Consulting and Clinical Psychology, 42(6), 861-865.
2. Bruss, C.R. (1988). Nursing diagnosis of hopelessness. Journal of Psychosocial Nursing and Mental Health Services, 26(3), 28-31, 38-9.
3. Farran, C.J., Salloway, J.C., & Clark, D.C. (1990). Measurement of hope in a community-based older population. Western Journal of Nursing Research, 12(1), 57-59.
4. Haase, J.E., et al. (1992). Simultaneous concept analysis of spiritual perspective, hope, acceptance and self-transcendence. Image: the Journal of Nursing Scholarship, 24(2), 141-147.
5. Hall, B.A. (1990). The struggle of the diagnosed terminally ill person to maintain hope. Nursing Science Quarterly, 3(4), 177-184.
6. Herth, K. (1990). Fostering hope in terminally-ill people. Journal of Advanced Nursing, 15(11), 1250-1259.
7. Herth, K. (1993). Hope in the family caregiver of terminally ill people. Journal of Advanced Nursing, 18(4), 538-548.
8. Hickey, S.S. (1986). Enabling hope. Cancer Nursing, 9(3), 133-137.
9. North American Nursing Diagnosis Association. (1994). Nursing diagnoses: Definitions and classification. Philadelphia: North American Nursing Diagnosis Association.
10. Owen, D.C. (1989). Nurses' perspectives on the meaning of hope in patients with cancer: A qualitative study. Oncology Nursing Forum, 16(1), 75-79.
11. Poncar, P.J. (1994). Inspiring hope in the oncology patient. Journal of Psychosocial Nursing and Mental Health Services, 32 (1), 33-38.
12. Raleigh, E.D. (1992). Sources of hope in chronic illness. Oncology Nursing Forum, 19(3), 443-448.

13. Smith, D.M. (1982). Guided imagination as an intervention in hopelessness. <u>Journal of Psychosocial Nursing & Mental Health Services.</u>, <u>20</u>(6), 29-32.
14. Steiger, N.J., and Lipson, J.G. (1985). Psychological and spiritual well-being. Chapter 10. In Steiger, N.J. and Lipson, J.G. <u>Self-care Nursing: Theory & Practice</u>. Bowie, Maryland: Brady Communications Company, Inc., 199-235.
15. Stephenson, C. (1991). The concept of hope revisited for nursing. <u>Journal of Advanced Nursing,</u> <u>16</u>(12), 1456-1461.
16. Wake, M.M. and Miller, J.F. (1992). Treating hopelessness: nursing strategies from six countries. <u>Clinical Nursing Research,</u> <u>1</u>(4), 347-365.

<u>**RECOMMENDED NANDA STAGING**</u>: 2.3

HOPE ALTERATION RISK (NANDA None)

DEFINITION: At risk for decreased belief in anticipated future outcomes that are personally satisfying and life supporting.

RISK FACTORS:

Low self-esteem
Blocks to self-love [46,13]
Negative future orientation [2]
Lack of optimism [9]
Suicidal behaviors [2,10]
Spiritual distress [5,6,12]
Suffering [4,5,14]
Failure of coping [8,11,12,13]
Poor relationships [14]
Physical deterioration/illness/stress [2,6,9,11,12,14,15]

Substance abuse [2,10]
Chronic and/or debilitating mental conditions e.g. depression, stress, anxiety [1,2,3,6,9,10,11]
Poorly controlled symptom management [6,7,8]
Lack of information [8,12]
War e.g. prisoner/concentration camp victim, isolation [4,6,7,8,13]
Natural disasters [5,6,13]
Losses [4,5,6,7,13]

REFERENCES:

1. Abraham, I.L., Neundorfer, M.M., and Currie, L.J. (1992). Effects of group interventions on cognition and depression in nursing home residents. Nursing Research, 41(4), 196-202.
2. Beck, A.T., Weissman, A., Lester, D. and Trexler, L. (1974). The measurement of pessimism: The hopelessness scale. Journal of Consulting and Clinical Psychology, 42(6), 861-865.
3. Drew, B.L. (1990). Differentiation of hopelessness, helplessness, and powerlessness using Erik Erikson's "Roots of Virtue". Archives of Psychiatric Nursing, 4(5), 332-337.
4. Farran, C.J., Salloway, J.C., and Clark, D.C. (1990). Measurement of hope in a community-based older population. Western Journal of Nursing Research, 12(1), 42-59.
5. Haase, J.E., et al. (1992). Simultaneous concept analysis of spiritual perspective, hope, acceptance and self-transcendence. Image: the Journal of Nursing Scholarship, 24(2), 141-147.
6. Herth, K. (1990). Fostering hope in terminally-ill people. Journal of Advanced Nursing, 15(11), 1250-1259.
7. Herth, K. (1993). Hope in the family caregiver of terminally ill people. Journal of Advanced Nursing, 18(4), 538-548.
8. Hickey, S.S. (1986). Enabling hope. Cancer Nursing, 9(3), 133-137.
9. Owen, D.C. (1989). Nurses' perspectives on the meaning of hope in patients with cancer: A qualitative study. Oncology Nursing Forum, 16(1), 75-79.
10. Page, R.M., Allen, O., Moore, L., and Hewitt, C. (1993). Co-occurrence of substance use and loneliness as a risk factor for adolescent hopelessness. Journal of School Health, 63(2), 104-108.
11. Poncar, P.J. (1994). Inspiring hope in the oncology patient. Journal of Psychosocial Nursing & Mental Health Services, 32(1) 33-38, 40-1.
12. Raleigh, E.D. (1992). Sources of hope in chronic illness. Oncology Nursing Forum, 19(3), 443-448.
13. Stephenson, C. (1991). The concept of hope revisited for nursing. Journal of Advanced Nursing, 16(12), 1456-1461.
14. Wake, M.M. and Miller, J.F. (1992). Treating hopelessness: nursing strategies from six countries. Clinical Nursing Research, 1(4), 347-365.
15. Yates, P. (1993). Towards a reconceptualization of hope for patients with a diagnosis of cancer. Journal of Advanced Nursing, 18(5), 701-706.

RECOMMENDED NANDA STAGING: 2.3

HOPE ENHANCEMENT POTENTIAL (NANDA None)

DEFINITION: Belief in anticipated future outcomes that are personally satisfying and life supporting.

SIGNS AND SYMPTOMS (Observed or Reported):

Expressions of:
 Faith[4,5,1,9]
 Reasons to live [3]
 Will to live[1]
 Meaning in life [2,11]
 Belief in self [7,9,10,11]
 Belief in others [7,9,10,11]
 Belief in treatments [3,9,10]
 Belief in physician successes [9,10]
 Positive future orientation [2,5,11]
 Inner peace [2,4,8]
 Optimism [2,7,8,10,11,13]

Demonstrates:
 Zest for life [3,8]
 Positive coping strategies [2,6,8,9,11]
 Goal setting [2,8,13]
 Exchanges, transforms, or moves energy to
  preserve hope e.g. setting goals that are smaller
  and more manageable [5,8]

RELATED FACTORS:

Interpersonal connectedness [2,4,5]
Spiritual base [4,9,12]
Personal attributes e.g. determination, courage,
 serenity [2,4,12]
Attainable aims/expectations [4,5]
Memories e.g. uplifting [4,12]
Ability to relive positive past activities e.g.
 meaningful vacations, significant events [4]
Spirit of lightheartedness [4]
Spiritual awareness [4]
Crisis situations e.g. loss, life-threatening situations,
 hardships, change [2,11]
Understanding of disease process [4]
Effective support system [5,9]
Value system [4,6,11]
Health status [1,9]

REFERENCES:

1. Farran, C.J., Salloway, J.C., and Clark, D.C. (1990). Measurement of hope in a community-based older population. Western Journal of Nursing Research, 12(1), 42-59.
2. Haase, J.E., et al. (1992). Simultaneous concept analysis of spiritual perspective, hope, acceptance and self-transcendence. Image: the Journal of Nursing Scholarship, 24(2), 141-147.
3. Hall, B. (1989). The struggle of the diagnosed terminally ill person to maintain hope. Nursing Science Quarterly, 3(4), 177-184.
4. Herth, K. (1990). Fostering hope in terminally-ill people. Journal of Advanced Nursing, 15(11), 1250-1259.
5. Herth, K. (1993). Hope in the family caregiver of terminally ill people. Journal of Advanced Nursing, 18(4), 538-548.
6. Hickey, S.S. (1986). Enabling hope. Cancer Nursing, 9(3), 133-137.
7. Hinds, P.S., Martin, J. and Vogel, R.J. (1987). Nursing strategies to influence adolescent hopefulness during oncologic illness. Journal of the Association of Pediatric Oncology Nurses, 4(1/2), 14-22.
8. Owen, D.C. (1989). Nurses' perspectives on the meaning of hope in patients with cancer: A qualitative study. Oncology Nursing Forum, 16(1), 75-79.
9. Raleigh, D.D.H. (1992). Sources of hope in chronic illness. Oncology Nursing Forum, 19(3),443-448.
10. Steiger, N.J., and Lipson, J.G. (1985). Psychological and spiritual well-being. Chapter 10. In Steiger, N.J. and Lipson, J.G. Self-care nursing: Theory & practice. Bowie, Maryland: Brady Communications Company, Inc., 199-235.
11. Stephenson, C. (1991). The concept of hope revisited for nursing. Journal of Advanced Nursing, 16(12), 1456-1461.
12. Wake, M.M. and Miller, J.F. (1992). Treating hopelessness: nursing strategies from six countries. Clinical Nursing Research, 1(4), 347-365.
13. Yates, P. (1993). Towards a reconceptualization of hope for patients with a diagnosis of cancer. Journal of Advanced Nursing, 18(5), 701-706.

RECOMMENDED NANDA STAGING: 2.3

HYPERCALCEMIA (NANDA None)

DEFINITION: An increase in the serum calcium concentration.

SIGNS AND SYMPTOMS (Observed or Reported):

Increased serum calcium levels [2]
Increased serum ionized calcium levels[2]
Arrhythmias [1,2]
Bradycardia[2]
Heart block[2]
EKG-shortening of QT interval[2,3]
   lengthened PR interval[1]
Increased sensitivity to digitalis[2]
Hypertension [1,2]
Anorexia [1,2,3]
Nausea[1,2,3]
Vomiting[1,2,3]
Constipation[2]
Polydipsia[3]
Polyuria[1,2,3]
Muscle weakness[1]
Decreased deep tendon reflexes [1]
Impaired concentration[1]
Decline in higher mental functioning2
Memory impairment[2]
Emotional instability[2]
Frank psychosis[2,3]
Confusion[1,2,3]
Lethargy [1,2]
Stupor[1]
Coma [1,2]
Sudden serum calcium >17 mg/dl[1]
Severe dehydration [1,2]
Azotemia [2]

Coma [1,3]
Chronic-pruritis [1]
Band keratopathy [1,3]
Soft tissue calcification [1,3]
Hypercalciuria[1,2]
Nephrolithiasis[1,3]
Joint pain[1]

RELATED FACTORS:

Primary hyperparathyroidism, e.g parathyroid
   adenoma, hyperplasia, or cancer[1,2,3]
Osteolytic extension with breast and lung
   cancer[1,2,3]
Multiple myeloma[1,3]
Disuse osteoporosis (prolonged
   immobilization)[1,2,3]
Sarcoidosis [3]
Tuberculosis [3]
Long-term lithium
   administration [1,2]
Theophylline [2]
Thiazide diuretics [1,2,3]
Large doses of vitamins A & D[1,2,3]
Excessive use of calcium containing
   antacids[2]
Hypophasphatemia [3]
Extracellular volume depletion [1,3]
Thyrotoxicosis [3]

REFERENCES:

1. Kainer, G., Chan, J.C.M. & Bell, N.H. (1990). Disorders of calcium metabolism. In J. C. M. Chan & J. R. Gill, Jr. (Eds.). Kidney electrolyte disorders, (pp. 171-221). New York: Churchill-Livingstone.
2. Metheny, N.M. (1996). Fluid and electrolyte balance: Nursing considerations. (3rd Ed.). Philadelphia: Lippincott.
3. Pak, C.Y.C. (1990). Calcium disorders: Hypercalcemia and hypocalcemia. In J. P. Kokko & R. L. Tannen (Eds.). Fluids and electrolytes, (2nd Ed.) (pp. 596-630). Philadelphia: W.B. Saunders.

RECOMMENDED NANDA STAGING: 2.1

HYPERKALEMIA (NANDA None)

DEFINITION: An increase in the serum potassium concentration.

SIGNS AND SYMPTOMS (Observed or Reported):
Increased serum potassium (K^+) [1,2]
Abnormal EKG:
  Peaking of T wave [1,2]
  Flattening of P wave [2]
  Prolonged PR interval [2,3]
  Widening QRS [1,2,3]
  Ventricular fibrillation [1,2]
Cardiac arrest [1]
Paresthesias-face, tongue, feet & hands [1]
Vague muscle weakness (> 8 mEq/L) [1,2]
Flaccid muscle paralysis [1]
Decreased deep tendon reflexes [2]
Nausea [1]
Intermittent intestinal colic or diarrhea [1]
Alert [2]

RELATED FACTORS:
Acidosis [1]
Respiratory acidosis [3]
Hyperglycemia-insulin deficiency [3]
Diabetic ketoacidosis [1]
Arginine HCl infusion [3]
Rapid IV infusion of potassium [1]
High oral intake of supplements [1]
Potassium-conserving diuretics [1]
Excessive use of salt substitutes [1]
Decreased glomerular filtration rate [1,2,3]
Oliguric renal failure [1]
Hypoaldosteronism [1,3]
Acute adrenal crisis [3]
Deficiency of adrenal steroids [1]
Malignant cell lysis after chemotherapy [1,3]
Tissue damage-crush injuries, burns [2,3]

REFERENCES:
1. Metheny, N.M. (1996). <u>Fluid and electrolyte balance: Nursing considerations</u>. (3rd Ed.). Philadelphia: Lippincott.
2. Pestana C. (1985). <u>Fluids and Electrolytes in the Surgical Patient</u>, (3rd Ed.). Baltimore: Williams & Wilkins.
3. Tanner, R.L. (1990). Potassium disorders. In J. P. Kokko & R. L. Tannen (Eds.). <u>Fluids and electrolytes</u>, (2nd Ed.). (pp.195-300). Philadelphia: W.B. Saunders.

RECOMMENDED NANDA STAGING: 2.1

HYPERMAGNESEMIA (NANDA None)

DEFINITION: An increase in the serum magnesium concentration.

SIGNS AND SYMPTOMS (Observed or Reported):

Increased serum magnesium (Mg^{2+}) [2,3]
Abnormal EKG:
   Shortening of QT interval[2,3]
   T wave abnormalities[2]
   Prolonged PR interval[2]
   Widening QRS [2]
Cardiac arrest [1,2]
Bradycardia[1,2]
Hypotension [1,2]
Facial flushing[2]
Sense of warmth[2]
Nausea [1,2]
Vomiting[1,2]
Muscle weakness[2]
Decreased deep tendon reflexes[1,2]

Loss of patellar reflex[2]
Respiratory paralysis [1,2,3]
Sedation [1,3]
Coma [1,2,3]

RELATED FACTORS:

Iatrogenic administration[1,2]
Renal failure[1,2]
Adrenal insufficiency[2]
Treatment for eclampsia or labor delay[2]
Hypocalcemia[2]
Use of magnesium containing antacids[2]
Use of magnesium containing laxatives[2]
Hemodialysis with high Mg^{2+} dialysate[2]
Increased gastrointestinal absorption[2]

REFERENCES:

1. De Castro, J.M. (1992). Age-related changes in natural spontaneous fluid ingestion and thirst in humans. <u>Journal of Gerontology,</u> <u>47</u>(5), 321-330.
2. Metheny, N.M. (1996). <u>Fluid and electrolyte balance: Nursing considerations</u>. (3rd Ed.). Philadelphia: Lippincott.
3. Pestana C. (1985). <u>Fluids and Electrolytes in the Surgical Patient,</u> (3rd Ed.). Baltimore: Williams & Wilkins.

RECOMMENDED NANDA STAGING: 2.1

HYPERNATREMIA (NANDA None)

DEFINITION: An increase in serum sodium concentration.

SIGNS AND SYMPTOMS (Observed or Reported):
Elevated serum sodium [9]
Elevated serum osmolality [9]
Thirst [2, 8, 9, 11]
Fever [9,11] with hyperpnea [2]
Tongue dry and swollen [3]
Dry, sticky mucous membrane [9]
Restlessness [3]
Weakness [11]
Hyperreflexia [11]
Muscle irritability [11]
Hypertonia [11]
Lethargy [11]
Disorientation [9,11]
Delusions [9]
Hallucinations [9]
Seizures [11]
Stupor [3]
Coma [9,11]
High pitched cry in infants [5]

RELATED FACTORS:
Water losses:
  Heat exhaustion [1, 7, 8, 12]
  Heat stroke [4, 12]
  Desert exposure [2, 13]
  Deprivation of water [12]
  Physically unable to obtain water
  Lack of thirst [5, 6, 12, 14]
  Insensible water loss with hyperventilation [12, 16]
  Excessive sweating [16]
  Watery diarrhea [12]
  Loop diuretics [11]
  Diabetes insipidus without fluid access [9,11]
  Hypertonic tube feedings without sufficient
    water [2, 11]

Sodium Gain:
  Hypertonic saline infusions [9,11]
  Large amount salt ingestion [9,11]
  Salt poisoning [11]
  Near drowning in sea water [11]
  Drinking sea water [2]
  Faulty hemo- or peritoneal dialysis [11]

REFERENCES:
1. Applegate, W.B., Runyan, J.W., Brasfield, L., Williams, M.L., Konigsberg, C. & Fouche, C. (1981). Analysis of the 1980 heat wave in Memphis. *Journal of the American Geriatric Society, 29*(8), 337-342.
2. Bartter, F.C. & Delea, C.S. (1990). Disorders of water metabolism. In J. C. M. Chan & J. R. Gill, Jr. (Eds.). *Kidney electrolyte disorders,* (pp.107-135). New York: Churchill-Livingstone.
3. Briggs, S.P., Sawaya, B.E. & Schnermann, J. (1990). Disorders of salt balance. In J. P. Kokko & R. L. Tannen (Eds.). *Fluids and electrolytes,* (2nd Ed.). (pp. 70-138). Philadelphia: W.B. Saunders.
4. Cronin, R.E. (1990). Magnesium disorders. In J. P. Kokko & R. L. Tannen (Eds.). *Fluids and electrolytes,* (2nd Ed.). (pp.631-645). Philadelphia: W.B. Saunders
5. Driggers, D.A. (1982). Managing the dehydrated child. *American Family Practice, 26*(5), 189-194.
6. Eisenman, P.A. (1986). Hot weather, exercise, old age, and the kidneys. *Geriatrics,* 41, 108-114.
7. Fish, P.D., Bennett, G.C.J., & Millard, P.H. (1985). Heatwave morbidity and mortality in old age. *Aging,* 14, 243-245.
8. Hughes-Davies, T.H. (1985). Thirst in the elderly. (Letter.) *New England Journal of Medicine, 312*(4), 247.
9. Metheny, N.M. (1996). *Fluid and electrolyte balance: Nursing considerations* (3rd Ed.). Philadelphia: Lippincott.
10. Phillips, P.A., Rolls, B.J., Ledingham, J. G., Forsling, M.L. Morton, J.J., Crowe, M.J. & Wollmer, L. (1984a). Reduced thirst after water deprivation in healthy elderly men. *New England Journal of Medicine, 311*(12), 753-759.
11. Sterns, R.H. & Spital, A. (1990). Disorders of water balance. In J. P. Kokko & R. L. Tannen (Eds.). *Fluids and electrolytes,* (2nd ed.) (pp. 139-194). Philadelphia: W.B. Saunders.

RECOMMENDED NANDA STAGING: 2.3

HYPERPHOSPHATEMIA (NANDA None)

DEFINITION: An increase in the serum phosphate concentration.

SIGNS AND SYMPTOMS (Observed or Reported):
Increased serum phophate[1]
Tingling around mouth, finger tips[1]
Muscle spasms[1]
Soft tissue calcification[1]
Hypocalcemia and its symptoms[1,2]

RELATED FACTORS:
Acute renal failure[1,2]
Large milk intake[1]
Excessive phosphate administration[1]
Excessive use of phosphasoda enemas[1]
Phosphate containing laxatives[2]
Excessive vitamin D intake[1]
Severe hemolytic anemia[2]
Chemotherhapy[1]

REFERENCES:
1. Metheny, N.M. (1996). Fluid and electrolyte balance: Nursing considerations. (3rd Ed.). Philadelphia: Lippincott.
2. Lau, K. (1990). Phosphate disorders. In J. P. Kokko & R. L. Tannen (Eds.). Fluids and electrolytes, (2nd Ed.) (pp.505-595). Philadelphia: W.B. Saunders.

RECOMMENDED NANDA STAGING: 2.1

HYPOCALCEMIA (NANDA None)

DEFINITION: A decrease in the serum calcium concentration.

SIGNS AND SYMPTOMS (Observed or Reported):
Decreased serum calcium [2]
Decreased ionized serum calcium [2]
Circumoral tingling, numbness [2]
Parethesias of hands, feet,[1] lips [2]
Chvostek's sign [2]
Trousseau's sign [2]
Muscle twitching [2]
Muscle cramping [2]
Carpopedal spasms [3]
Tetany [2]
Hyperactive reflexes [2]
Laryngeal spasms[1], stridor[3]
Irritability [3]
Anxiety [3]
Depression [3]
EKG with prolonged QT interval [3]
Bradycardia to ventricular tachycardia to asystole [2]
Hypotension [2]
Decreased response to digitalis [2]
Involuntary movements [1]
Epileptic seizures[3]
Convulsions [1,3]

RELATED FACTORS:
Alkalosis [2]
Infusions of citrated blood [2]
Hemodilution with normal saline [3]
Inadequate intake of calcium or vitamin D [1,2,3]
Poor exposure to sunlight[1]
Mithramycin therapy[3]
Chronic renal failure [1,3]
Intestinal malabsorption [1,2,3]
Liver disease[1]
Surgical hypoparathyroidism[1]
Primary hypoparathyroidism [1,3]
Hyperphosphatemia[2]
Phosphate therapy, [1,2]
Tumor induced osteomalacia[1]
Sepsis[2]
Magnesium deficiency [1,3]
Acute pancreatitis[1]
Anticonvulsants-phenytoin/phenobarbital [1,2]

REFERENCES:
1. Kainer, G., Chan, J.C.M. & Bell, N.H. (1990). Disorders of calcium metabolism. In J. C. M. Chan & J. R. Gill, Jr. (Eds.) Kidney electrolyte disorders, (pp.171-221). New York: Churchill-Livingstone.
2. Metheny, N.M. (1996). Fluid and electrolyte balance: Nursing considerations. (3rd Ed.). Philadelphia: Lippincott.
3. Pak, C.Y.C. (1990). Calcium disorders: Hypercalcemia and hypocalcemia. In J. P. Kokko & R. L. Tannen (Eds.). Fluids and electrolytes, (2nd Ed.). (pp.596-630). Philadelphia: W.B. Saunders.

RECOMMENDED NANDA STAGING: 2.1

HYPOKALEMIA (NANDA None)

DEFINITION: A decrease in the serum potassium concentration.

SIGNS AND SYMPTOMS (Observed or Reported):
Decreased serum potassium[1]
Abnormal EKG -arrhythmia: [1, 2, 3]
   ST segment depression
   Broad, flattened T waves
   Enlarge U wave
Cardiac arrest [1, 2, 3]
Heightened sensitivity to digitalis [1, 2]
Muscular weakness in legs [1, 2, 3]
Respiratory muscle weakness [1, 3]
Respiratory paralysis[1]
Prolonged gastric emptying[1]
Gaseous distention[1]
Constipation [3]
Paralytic ileus (adynamic) [1, 2, 3]
Dilute urine[1]
Polyuria[1, 3]
Nocturia[1]
Polydipsia [3]
Increased hydrogen excretion[1]
Myoglobinuria[1]
Rhabdomyolysis [1, 3]

RELATED FACTORS:
Decreased potassium intake [1, 3]
Alkalosis
Primary hyperaldosteronism
Secondary hyperaldosteronism[1]
High dose steroid administration[1]
Cushing syndrome[1]
Potassium-losing diuretics[1]
Medications: Amphotericin B, gentamicin,
   cisplatin, levodopa, & penicillin derivatives[1]
Osmotic diuresis[1]
Insulin hypersecretion[1]
Anorexia nervosa[1]
Alcoholism[1]

Extrarenal potassium losses:
   Vomiting[1, 3]
   Gastric suction[1, 3]
   Biliary drainage[1, 3]
   Diarrhea[1]
   Recent ileostomy[1]
   Villous adenomas[1]

REFERENCES:
1. Metheny, N.M. (1996). Fluid and electrolyte balance: Nursing considerations. (3rd Ed.). Philadelphia: Lippincott.
2. Pestana C. (1985). Fluids and Electrolytes in the Surgical Patient, (3rd Ed). Baltimore: Williams & Wilkins.
3. Tanner, R.L. (1990). Potassium disorders. In J. P. Kokko & R. L. Tannen (Eds.). Fluids and electrolytes, (2nd Ed.). (pp.195-300). Philadelphia: W.B. Saunders.

RECOMMENDED NANDA STAGING: 2.1

HYPOMAGNESEMIA (NANDA None)

DEFINITION: A decrease in the serum magnesium concentration.

SIGNS AND SYMPTOMS (Observed or Reported):

Decreased serum magnesium (Mg^{2+}) [2]

EKG changes: [2]
- Increased PR & QT intervals [1]
- Widened QRS complex
- ST segment depression
- T wave inversion [2]

Heightened cardiac sensitivity to digitalis [2,3]

Anorexia, nausea, vomiting [1]

Muscular weakness [1,2]

Muscle twitching [1,2]

Paresthesias [2]

Hyporeflexia [1]

Chvostek's sign [1,2]

Trousseau's sign [1,2]

Disorientation [2]

Ataxia [2]

Depression [2]

Psychosis [2]

Tremors [1,2]

Athetoid movements [2]

Tetany [2,3]

Generalized tonic/clonic seizures [1,2,3]

Focal seizures [2]

Small bowel resection or dysfunction [1,2]

Pancreatitis [1]

Malabsorption syndromes [1,2]

Laxative abuse [2]

Alcoholism [1,2]

Magnesium lack of intake [2]

Refeeding after starvation [2]

Protein calorie malnutrition [1]

Aminoglycoside, amphotericin B, cisplatin, and cyclosporin administration [1,2]

Loop diuretics [1,2]

Syndrome of Inappropriate Antidiuretic Hormone (SIADH) [2]

Osmotic diuresis [2]

Diabetic ketoacidosis [2]

Postoperative [2]

Renal impaired absorption of magnesium [2]

Insulin therapy [1,2]

Severe burn [2]

Sepsis [2]

Excessive Na^+ or Ca^{2+} urinary loss [2]

Hypothermia [2]

Extrarenal magnesium losses:
- Vomiting [1,2]
- Gastric suction [1,2]
- Fistular drainage [1,2]
- Diarrhea [1,2]

RELATED FACTORS:

Associated with hypokalemia, hypocalcemia, & hypophosphatemia [1,2]

REFERENCES:

1. De Castro, J.M. (1992). Age-related changes in natural spontaneous fluid ingestion and thirst in humans. Journal of Gerontology, 47(5), 321-330.
2. Metheny, N.M. (1996). Fluid and electrolyte balance: Nursing considerations, (3rd Ed.). Philadelphia: Lippincott.
3. Pestana C. (1985). Fluids and Electrolytes in the Surgical Patient, (3rd Ed.). Baltimore: Williams & Wilkins.

RECOMMENDED NANDA STAGING: 2.1

HYPONATREMIA (NANDA None)

DEFINITION: A decrease in serum sodium concentration.

SIGNS AND SYMPTOMS (Observed or Reported):

Decreased serum sodium[11]
Decreased serum osmolality[11]
Lethargy[4, 11]
Malaise[11]
Anorexia[11, 15]
Nausea[11]
Headache[5, 11]
Abdominal cramps[11]
Muscular twitching[11]
Dulling of sensorium[1, 2]
Disorientation[12]
Confusion[11]
Focal weakness[1, 3]
Hemiparesis[1, 2, 3, 6, 8,]
Ataxia[4]
Babinski's sign[1]
Convulsions[1, 2, 3, 11]
Decorticate posturing[1, 2]
Papilledema[11]
Coma[1, 2, 11]
Respiratory arrest[11]
Fingerprint edema[11]

Solute diuresis[13]
Hyperglycemia[10]
Mannitol administration[9]
Post-renal transplantation[9]
Low sodium tube feedings[14]
Adrenal insufficiency[11]
Addison's disease[13]
Adrenal cortical enzyme deficiencies[9, 13]
Chronic renal insufficiency[9, 13]
Salt losing nephropathies[13]
Heat exhaustion[11]

Water Gain: [dilutional]
  Excessive administration of water[11]
  Excessive administration of water with iso- or hypotonic tube feedings[11, 14]
  Vasopressin release under stress[7]
  Syndrome of Inappropriate Antidiuretic Hormone (SIADH) by drugs, tumors, pulmonary disorders, or head injury[5, 10, 11]
  Nephrotic syndrome[10]
  Decreased urine output[12]
  Postoperative menstruant women[6]
  Psychogenic polydipsia[10, 11]
  Labor induction with oxytocin[10]
  Tricyclic antidepressants[10,]

RELATED FACTORS:

Sodium Loss: [depletion]
  Gastrointestinal fluid losses[11]
  Diuretic therapy[2, 9, 11, 13]
  Theophylline[9, 11]
  Carbonic anhydrase inhibitors[9]
  Sodium restricted diets[9]
  Diuretic phase of acute renal failure[9, 13]
  Post-obstructive diuresis[9, 13]

Antineoplastic Drugs:[10, 11]
  Cyclophosphamide
  Vincristine

REFERENCES:

1. Arieff, A.l. & Witte, J.M. (1979) Death or permanent neurological disability despite correction of protracted hyponatremia. (Abstract.) Kidney International, 16, 955.
2. Ashouri, O.S. (1986) Severe diuretic-induced hyponatremia in the elderly. A series of eight patients. Archives of Internal Medicine, 146(7), 1355-1357.
3. Ayus, J. & Arieff, A. (1990). Symptomatic hyponatremia: Making the diagnosis rapidly. Journal of Critical Illness, 5(8), 846-856.
4. Ayus, J. Wheeler, J. & Arieff, A. (1992). Postoperative hyponatremic encephalopathy in menstruant women. Annuals of Internal Medicine, 117(11), 891-897.
5. Bartter, F.C. & Delea, C.S. (1990). Disorders of water metabolism. In J.C.M. Chan & J. R. Gill, Jr. (Eds.). Kidney electrolyte disorders, (pp.107-135). New York: Churchill-Livingstone.
6. Berkovic, S.F., Bladin, P.F. & Darby, D.G. (1984). Metabolic disorders presenting as stroke. Medical Journal of Australia, 140(7), 421-424.
7. Booker, J.A. (1984). Severe symptomatic hyponatremia in elderly outpatients: The role of thiazide therapy and stress. Journal of the American Geriatric Society, 32(2), 108-113.

8. Booker, J.A. & Crimmins, J. (1984) Hyponatremia or stroke? (Letter.) <u>Medical Journal of Australia,</u> <u>140</u>(13), 799-800.

9 Briggs, S.P., Sawaya, B.E. & Schnermann, J. (1990). Disorders of salt balance. In J. P. Kokko & R. L. Tannen (Eds.). <u>Fluids and electrolytes</u>, (2nd Ed.). (pp.70-138). Philadelphia: W.B. Saunders.

10. Kirch, D.G., Bigelow, L.B., Weinberger, D.R., Lawson, W.B. & Wyatt, R.J. (1985). Polydipsia and chronic hyponatremia in schizophrenic inpatients. <u>Journal of Psychiatry, 46</u>(5), 179-181.

11. Metheny, N.M. (1996). <u>Fluid and electrolyte balance: Nursing considerations</u>. (3rd Ed.). Philadelphia: Lippincott.

12. Pestana C. (1985). <u>Fluids and Electrolytes in the Surgical Patient</u>, (3rd Ed.). Baltimore: Williams & Wilkins.

13. Reineck, H.J. & Stein, J.H. (1990). Disorders of sodium metabolism. In J. C. M. Chan & J. R. Gill, Jr. (Eds.). <u>Kidney Electrolyte Disorders</u>, (pp.59-105). New York: Churchill-Livingstone.

14. Rudman, D., Racette, D., Rudman, I.W., Mattson, D.E. & Erve, P.R. (1986) Hyponatremia in tube-fed elderly men. <u>Journal of Chronic Disease, 39</u>,73-80.

15. Rymer, M.M. & Fishman, R.A. (1973). Protective adaptation of brain to water intoxication. <u>Archives of Neurology, 28</u>,49-54.

<u>RECOMMENDED NANDA STAGING</u>: 2.3

HYPOPHOSPHATEMIA (NANDA None)

DEFINITION: A decrease in the serum phosphate concentration.

SIGNS AND SYMPTOMS (Observed or Reported):
Decreased serum phosphate[1]
Hypotension[2]
Tachypnea[2]
Lethargy[2]
Apprehension[1]
Memory loss[2]
Confusion[1,2]
Delirium[1,2]
Coma[1]
Cardiac arrest [1,2]
Anorexia[2]
Nausea[2]
Malaise[2]
Paresthesias[1,2]
Myalgia[2]
Muscle weakness [1,2]
Muscle pain and tenderness[1]
Hyporelexia[2]
Ataxia[2]
Respiratory paralysis [1,2]
Seizures[1]

RELATED FACTORS:
Glucose administration[1]
Respiratory alkalosis[1]
Total parenteral nutrition without phosphorus supplement[1]
Hyperparathyroidism[2]
Poor intake[1]
Vomiting[1]
Vitamin D deficiency[1]
Malabsorption[1]
Recovery phase after burns[1]
Excess epinephrine release[1]
Nutritional recovery syndrome[1]
Phosphate-binding antacid use[1]
Diarrhea[1]
Renal tubular disorders[2]
Hyperparathyroidism[2]
Hypokalemia[1]
Hypocalcemia[1]
Hypomagnesemia[1]
Alcohol withdrawal [1,2]
Insulin administration[1]
Diabetic ketoacidosis[1,2]

REFERENCES:
1. Metheny, N.M. (1996). Fluid and electrolyte balance: Nursing considerations. (3rd Ed.). Philadelphia: Lippincott.
2. Lau, K. (1990). Phosphate disorders. In J. P. Kokko & R. L. Tannen (Eds.). Fluids and electrolytes, (2nd Ed.), (pp.505-595). Philadelphia: W.B. Saunders.

RECOMMENDED NANDA STAGING: 2.1

INSECURE PARENT-INFANT ATTACHMENT (NANDA Risk for Altered Parent/Infant/Child Attachment)

DEFINITION: Inadequate or unsatisfactory reciprocal interactions between parent and infant that result in lack of emotional/affectionate bond.

SIGNS AND SYMPTOMS (Observed or Reported):

Prenatal:
  Lack of recognition of pregnancy[3,5]
  Lack of talk about infant[3,5]
  Lack of visualization of infant[3,5]
  Lack of visualization of caring for infant[3]
  No name(s) selected for infant[3,5]

Maternal/Paternal:
  Negative perception of infant[5]
  Minimal verbal interaction with infant[2,8]
  Lack of tactile contact (touching & holding) with infant[8]
  Lack of eye to eye contact (en face position) with infant[5,8]
  Lack of desire for proximity to infant[1,5]
  Lack of affectionate tie[5,7]
  Lack of sensitivity to infant cues[5]
  Lack of attentiveness to infant[8]
  Lack of pleasure from interaction with infant[8]
  Lack of or inappropriate response to infant distress[5]
  Lack of attribution of family characteristics to infant[5]

Infant:
  Mistrust[5,7]
  Lack of eye contact with caregiver[8]
  Lack of verbal responsiveness to caregiver[8]
  Stiffens or cries when touched or held[8]
  Lack of pleasure during or after feeding[8]
  Abuse[5]
  Neglect[5]

RELATED FACTORS:

Maternal/Paternal:
  Stress during pregnancy[5,6]
  Medication used during labor and/or delivery[2]
  Low self esteem[6]
  Anxiety[2,6]
  Depression[6]
  Physical or mental illness[6]
  Lack of early contact with infant[2]
  Lack of rooming in with infant[2]
  Separation from infant[2]
  Inconsistent care and response to infant[7]
  Lack of social support[2]
  Lack of parental competence/parenting skills[6]
  Lack of knowledge about infant care[2]
  Lack of knowledge of infant's unique behavioral characteristics or cues[1,2]
  Lack of goodness of fit between parental expectations and infant behavior [4]

Paternal:
  No observation of feeding [2]

Infant:
  Physical illness[4]
  Developmental disability[4]
  Sensory impairment[4]
  Difficult temperament[2]
  Lack demonstration of cues[4]

REFERENCES:
1. Avant, K. (1979). Nursing diagnosis: Maternal attachment. <u>Advances in Nursing Science. 2</u>, 45-55.
2. Coffman, S. (1992). Parent and infant attachment: Review of nursing research 1981-1990. <u>Pediatric Nursing, 18</u>(4), 421-425.
3. Cranley, M.S. (1981). Development of a tool for the measurement of maternal attachment during pregnancy. <u>Nursing Research, 30</u>(5), 281-284.
4. Denehy, J.A. (1992). Interventions related to parent-infant attachment. <u>Nursing Clinics of North America, 27</u>(2), 425-443.
5. Gaffney, K.F. (1988). New directions in maternal attachment research. <u>Journal of Pediatric Health Care, 2</u>(4), 181-188.
6. Mercer, R.T., & Ferketich, S.L. (1990). Predictors of parental attachment during early parenthood. <u>Journal of Advanced Nursing. 15</u>(3), 268-280.
7. Pressler, J.L. (1990) Promoting attachment. In M.J. Craft & J.A. Denehy (Eds.). <u>Nursing Interventions for Infants and Children</u>, (pp. 4-17). Philadelphia, PA: W.B. Saunders.
8. Reiser, S.L. (1981). A tool to facilitate mother-infant attachment. <u>JOGNN: Journal of Obstetrical Gynecological Nursing, 10</u>(4), 294-297.

RECOMMENDED NANDA STAGING: 2.2

INSECURE PARENT-INFANT ATTACHMENT RISK (NANDA Risk for Altered Parent/Infant/Child Attachment)

DEFINITION: Risk for inadequate or unsatisfactory reciprocal interactions between parent and infant that result in lack of emotional/affectionate bond.

RISK FACTORS:

Maternal/Paternal:
Stress during pregnancy[5,6]
Medication used during labor and/or delivery[2]
Low self esteem[6]
Anxiety[2,6]
Depression[6]
Physical or mental illness[6]
Lack of early contact with infant[2]
Lack of rooming in with infant[2]
Separation from infant[2]
Inconsistent care and response to infant[7]
Lack of social support[2]
Lack of parental competence/parenting skills[6]
Lack of knowledge about infant care[2]

Lack of knowledge of infant's unique behavioral characteristics or cues[1,2]
Lack of goodness of fit between parental expectations and infant behavior[4]

Paternal:
No observation of feeding[2]

Infant:
Physical illness[4]
Developmental disability[4]
Sensory impairment[4]
Difficult temperament[2]
Lack demonstration of cues[4]

REFERENCES:

1. Avant, K. (1979). Nursing diagnosis: Maternal attachment. Advances in Nursing Science, 2, 45-55.
2. Coffman, S. (1992). Parent and infant attachment: Review of nursing research 1981-1990. Pediatric Nursing, 18(4), 421-425.
3. Cranley, M.S. (1981). Development of a tool for the measurement of maternal attachment during pregnancy. Nursing Research, 30(5), 281-284.
4. Denehy, J.A. (1992). Interventions related to parent-infant attachment. Nursing Clinics of North America, 27(2), 425-443.
5. Gaffney, K.F. (1988). New directions in maternal attachment research. Journal of Pediatric Health Care, 2(4), 181-188.
6. Mercer, R.T., & Ferketich, S.L. (1990). Predictors of parental attachment during early parenthood. Journal of Advanced Nursing, 15(3), 268-280.
7. Pressler, J.L. (1990) Promoting attachment. In M.J. Craft & J.A. Denehy (Eds.). Nursing interventions for infants and children, (pp. 4-17). Philadelphia, PA: W.B. Saunders.

RECOMMENDED NANDA STAGING: 2.2

LOW SELF-ESTEEM RISK (NANDA None)

DEFINITION: At risk for changes in self-perceptions of self-worth that may rise above or below basic level depending on various current life factors and may become long standing negative feelings.

RISK FACTORS:

Developmental changes [8]
Body image alterations [1,10]
Functional changes [2,8]
Loss of significant roles [5]
Significant early loss e.g. parent [6,9]
Social role changes e.g. decreased social interaction [9,11]
Long standing significant early relationship involving physical/emotional abuse, neglect, desertion [6,8,9]

Learned helplessness secondary to abuse, neglect, or abandonment e.g. children of alcoholics [3,6,7,9]
Unrealistic self-expectations [5,9]
Behavior inconsistent with values [5]
Life factors, e.g. recognition/rewards, failures/rejections [5]
Decreased power & control over environment [1]
Negative societal attitudes e.g. obesity [2]
Physical illness e.g. eating disorder [4]

REFERENCES:

1. Antaki, C. & Brewin, C. (Eds.). (1994) Attributions and psychological change. London: Academic Press.
2. Carpenito, L. (1997). Nursing diagnosis: application to clinical practice (self-esteem disturbance, chronic low self esteem, situational low self esteem). Philadelphia: J.B. Lippincott.
3. Coppersmith, S. (1967). The antecedents of self-esteem. San Francisco: W. H. Freeman.
4. Gibb, B., Kraynick, P., & Biebel, M. (1987). Validating a Nursing Diagnosis, Disturbance in Self-esteem: a comparison of Studies. In Classification of nursing diagnosis: Proceedings of the seventh conference A.McLane (Ed.). NANDA.
5. Gordon, M. (1986-87). Handbook of nursing diagnoses. New York, NY: McGraw-Hill.
6. Juhasz, A. (1989). Significant others and self-esteem: Methods for determining who and why. Adolescence, 24(95), 581-595.
7. Killeen M. R. (1988). Self-concept of children of alcoholics: Family influences... part 1. Journal of Child & Adolescent Psychiatric & Mental Health Nursing. 1(1), 25-30.
8. Norris, J. (1992). Nursing intervention for self-esteem disturbances. Nursing Diagnosis, 3(2), 48-53.
9. Norris, J. & Kunes-Connell. (1985). Self-esteem disturbance. Nursing Clinics of North America, 20, 745-761.
10. Norris, J. & Kunes-Connell, M. (1988). A multimodal approach to validation & refinement of an existing nursing diagnosis. Archives of Psychiatric Nursing, 2(2), 103-109.
11. Riffee, D. (1981). Self-esteem changes in hospitalized school-age children. Nursing Research, 30(2), 94-96.

RECOMMENDED NANDA STAGING: 2.3

ORAL SOFT TISSUE ALTERATION (NANDA Altered Oral Mucous Membrane)

DEFINITION: Disruption(s) of the lips and soft tissue of the oral cavity.

SIGNS AND SYMPTOMS (Observed or Reported):

Hyperemia ("beefy-red")[2]
Halitosis[2]
Edema (Gingival or mucosal)[5]
Bleeding[2,7]
Fissures, cheilitis[5]
Gingival hyperplasia[5]
Self report diminished/absent taste[2,6]
Self report bad taste[2]
Difficult speech (dysarthria)[2]
Self report difficulty eating/swallowing[2]
Purulent drainage or exudate[5]
Pain[2,7]
Macroplasia[5]
Coated tongue[2,5]
Smooth atrophic, sensitive tongue [2,5]
Geographic tongue[5]
Dryness (xerostomia)[2]
Mucosal denudation [2]
Ulceration[5,7]
White patches/plaques, spongy patches[5] or white curd-like exudate[2]
Vesicles, nodules or papules[5]
Gingival recession[2] - pockets deeper than four millimeters [4]
Gingival or mucosal pallor[5]
Enlarged tonsils beyond what is developmentally appropriate [2]
Presence of pathogens (per culture)[7]
Red or bluish masses, e.g. hemangioma[5]

RELATED FACTORS:

Pathology, e.g. cancer, infections, periodontal disease [2,5]
Loss of supportive structures[2]
Aging-related loss of connective, adipose or bone tissue[2]
Diminished hormone levels (women)[2]
Dehydration e.g. excessive fluid loss, e.g., sweating, vomiting [2]
Ineffective oral hygiene[1,2,4,5]
Mouth breathing [2]
Malnutrition/vitamin deficiency[2]
Decreased platelets[7]
Radiation therapy e.g. head/neck/mouth [2,7]
Chemotherapy[7]
Stress[2]
Depression[2]
Immunosuppression [2,6,7]
Immunocompromised[2,6,7]
Medication side effects[2]
Impaired salivation[2,6]
Barriers to oral self-care [6]
Barriers to professional care e.g., physical impairment[1,2,4,7]
Trauma [5]
Chemical, e.g. alcohol, tobacco, acidic foods, regular use of inhalers[2,4]
Mechanical e.g. poorly fitting dental prostheses, endotracheal or nasal gastric tubes, surgery, braces, biting/chewing [2, 5]
Cleft lip or palate[1,5]

REFERENCES:

1. Coulter, I.D., Marcus, M. & Atchison, K.A. (1994). Measuring oral health status: Theoretical and methodological challenges. Social Science and Medicine, 38(11), 1531-1541.
2. Eldredge, J.B. (1991). Altered oral mucous membrane. In M. Maas, K. Buckwalter and M. Hardy (Eds.). Nursing diagnoses for the elderly, (pp. 117-130). Fort Collins: Addison-Wesley.
3. Eilers, J., Berger A. & Peterson, M. (1988). Development, testing and application of the oral assessment guide. Oncology Nursing Forum, 15(3), 325-330.
4. Jette, A., Feldman, H. & Tennstedt, S. (1993). Tobacco use: A modifiable risk factor for dental disease among the elderly. American Journal of Public Health, 83(9), 1271-1276.
5. Kronmiller, J.E. (1987). Oral soft tissue abnormalities in children. Pediatric Nursing, 13(3), 161-165, 191.
6. Ofstehage, J. & Magilvy, K. (1986). Oral health and aging. Geriatric Nursing: American Journal of Care for the Aging, 7(5), 238-241.
7. Ransier, A., Epstein, J., Lunn, R. & Spinelli, J. (1995). A combined analysis of a toothbrush, foam brush and a chlorhexidine-soaked foam brush in maintaining oral hygiene. Cancer Nursing, 18(5), 393-396.

RECOMMENDED NANDA STAGING: 2.1

ORGANIZED INFANT BEHAVIOR ENHANCEMENT POTENTIAL
(NANDA None)

DEFINITION: Potential for enhanced physiological and neurobehavioral responses to the environment.

SIGNS AND SYMPTOMS (Observed or Reported):

Stability in Physiological/Autonomic System: [4]
 Baseline measures of:
   Heart rate
   Respiratory rate
   Color
   Oximeter saturation
   Feeding tolerance

Stability in Motor System: [3,4]
 Tone
 Movement: smooth synchronous, spontaneous
 Posture: flexion

Stability in State-Organization System: [2]
 Deep Sleep: near still; occasional
   suck/twitch; smooth regular breathing;
   arousal to intense stimuli
 Light Sleep: some activity; REM; eye
   flutter; closed lids; brief smile/cry/
   fussiness; irregular breathing pattern;
   more responsive to stimuli
 Drowsy: variable activity with mild startles;
   occasional eye opening/closing; heavy
   lidded; dull-glaze appearance; still face;
   irregular breathing pattern; delayed or
   changing response to stimuli
 Quiet-alert: minimal activity; eyes bright
   and wide; face bright/shiny/sparkling;
   regular breathing; attend/focus to most
   stimuli
 Active-alert: fussy/increased activity; open
   but less bright eyes; some facial
   brightness; irregular breathing; increasing
   sensitivity to stimuli
 Crying: increased motor activity, color
   change; closed or open eyes; grimaces;
   more irregular breathing pattern;
   increased response to unpleasant
   internal/external stimuli

Stability in Regulatory State: [4]
 Self-consolable: finger suck, hand-to-face;
   extremity anchoring; paying attention to
   voices/faces; position changes
 Alert for intake of surroundings

Stability in Attention-Interaction System: [3,4,7]
 Response to sensory stimulation e.g.
   alertness; habituation

RELATED FACTORS:

Prenatal: [8]
 Congenital/genetic disorders
 Teratogenic exposure

Postnatal: [4,8]
 Prematurity
 Malnutrition
 Feeding intolerance
 Oral/motor problems
 Invasive/painful procedure
 Pain

Individual Factors: [1,4,5,6,8]
 Gestational age
 Postconceptual age
 Immature neurological system
 Illness

Caregiver Factors: [5,6]
 Cue misreading
 Cue knowledge deficit
 Environmental stimulation contribution

Environmental Factors: [1,2,3,4,5,6,8,9]
 Sensory deprivation
 Sensory over stimulation
 Sensory inappropriateness
 Physical environment inappropriateness

REFERENCES:
1. Als, H., Lawhon, G., Duffy F.H., McAnulty G.B., Gibes-Grossman, R. & Bleckman, J.G. (1994). Individual developmental care for the very low birthweight premature infant. Journal of the American Medical Assn, 272(11), 853-858.
2. Blackburn, S. (1978). Sleep and awake states of the newborn. In KE Barnard et al. (Eds.). Early parent-infant relationships- Module 3- A staff development perinatal nursing care, (pp 17-21). The National Foundation: March of Dimes.

3. Blackburn, S. (1978). State-related behaviors and individual differences. In KE Barnard et al. (Eds.). <u>Early parent-infant relationships- Module 3- A staff development perinatal nursing care,</u> (pp. 22-32). The National Foundation: March of Dimes.

4. D'Apolito, K. (1991). What is an organized infant? <u>Neonatal Network, 10</u>(1), 23-33.

5. Lawhon, G. (1986). Management of stress in premature infants. In DJ Angeline, CM Whalen-Knapp & RM Gibes (Eds.). <u>Parental and neonatal nursing: A clinical handbook,</u> (pp. 30-31). Boston: Blackwell Scientific Publications.

6. Lawhon G. & Melzer A. (1988). Developmental care of the very low birthweight infant. <u>Journal of Pediatric and Neonatal Nursing, 2</u>(1), 56-65.

7. Lott J.W. (1989). Developmental care of the preterm infant. <u>Neonatal Network: Journal of Neonatal Nursing, 7</u>(4), 21-8.

8. National Association of Neonatal Nurses. (1993). <u>Infant developmental care guidelines</u>. Petaluma, CA: National Association of Neonatal Nurses.

9. Oehler, J. (1983). Sensory processing abilities of the preterm infant. <u>Journal of the California Perinatal Association, 3</u>(6), 55- 63.

<u>**RECOMMENDED NANDA STAGING:**</u> 2.1

OVERFLOW URINARY INCONTINENCE (NANDA None)

DEFINITION: Involuntary loss of urine that occurs when the reservoir capacity of the bladder is exceeded in the absence of detrusor muscle activity.

SIGNS AND SYMPTOMS (Observed or Reported):

Palpable and/or percussable bladder [7,8,10]
Suprapubic tenderness [1,10]
Post void residual [4,5,7,10]
Dribbling [1,2,4,5,8]
Leakage in small amounts throughout day and night [1,7,9]
Sense of incomplete emptying [2,5,7,8]
Lack of awareness of urine loss [5]
Urinary frequency with small amounts of urine [1,3,8]
Hesitancy [7,8]
Inability/difficulty passing a catheter [8]
Loss of urge sensation [10]
Retains ability to void but has infrequent voiding [3,10]
Diminished and/or interrupted urine flow [7,10]
Strains to void [7]

RELATED FACTORS:

Outlet obstruction:
  Prostatic hypertrophy [1,2,5,7,9,10]
  Urethral stricture (primary men) [1,2,7,9]
  Bladder neck contracture (primary men) [2,7,9]
  Fecal impaction [2,5]
  Pelvic or genital prolapse [1]
  Overcorrection of urethral detachment (primary women) [1]

Underactive detrusor due to myogenic or neurogenic factors: [1,2,5,6,10]
  Multiple sclerosis [2,9]
  Herpes zoster [2,9]
  Surgical trauma e.g. laminectomy, pelvic surgery [1,7,9]
  Peripheral neuropathy e.g. diabetes, alcoholism, pernicious anemia [1,7,9,10]
  Supra sacral spinal cord injuries [2]
  Impaired afferent sensation [2,10]
  Disruption of the motor innervation of the detrusor muscle [1,6]

Pharmacological: [1,2]
  Antispasmotics [2,4]
  Tri-cyclic antidepressants [2,4,6]
  Anti-Parkinson's [2,6]
  Antihistamines [2,4,6]
  Opiates [4,6]
  Antiarrymthics [6]
  Antidiahrreal [6]
  Spasms of external sphincter [6]
  Anxiety [6]
  Acute cystitis [6]

REFERENCES:

1. Fantl, J.A., Newman D.K., Colling, J., et al. (1996). Urinary incontinence in adults: Acute and chronic management. Clinical practice guidelines, No.2 1996 update. Department of Health and Human Services. Public Health Service, Agency for Health Care Policy and Research. AHCPR Publication No. 96-0682. Rockville, MD: U.S.
2. Gray, M. & Dougherty, M.C. (1987). Urinary incontinence – Pathophysiology and treatment. Journal of Enterostomal Therapy, 14(4), 152-62
3. National Institutes of Health. (1988). Urinary Incontinence in Adults. NIH Consensus Development Conference Statement. 7(5), 1-11. Bethesda, MD: U.S. Department of Health and Human Services.
4. Newman, D.K., Lynch, K., Smith, D.A. & Cell, P. (1991). Restoring urinary continence. AJN, (January), 28-36.
5. Palmer, M.H. (1990). Urinary incontinence. Nursing Clinics of North America, 25(4), 919-934.
6. Penn, C. (1990). Incontinence assessment: Examining the reliability of a structured assessment tool in guiding staff nurses through a focused assessment and accurate nursing diagnosis. University of Iowa, Iowa City, IA. [Unpublished Master's Project].
7. Resnick, N.M. & Yalla, S.V. (1985). Management of urinary incontinence in the elderly. The New England Journal of Medicine, 313(13), 800-805.

8. Specht, J., Tunick P., Maas, M. & Bulecheck, G. (1991). Urinary incontinence. In M. Maas, K. Buckwalter & M. Hardy (Eds.),. <u>Nursing diagnoses and interventions for the elderly,</u> (p. 181-204). Redwood City, CA: Addison-Wesley.

9. Wheatley, J. (1982). Bladder incontinence: Four types and their control. <u>Postgraduate Medicine, 7</u>(1), 75-81.

10. Willams, M.E. & Pannill, F.C. (1982). Urinary incontinence in the elders: Physiology, pathophysiology, diagnosis and treatment. <u>Annals of Internal Medicine, 97</u>, 895-907.

<u>**RECOMMENDED NANDA STAGING:**</u> 2.3

OVERFLOW URINARY INCONTINENCE RISK (NANDA None)

DEFINITION: Risk for involuntary loss of urine that occurs when the reservoir capacity of the bladder is exceeded in the absence of detrusor muscle activity.

RISK FACTORS:

Outlet obstruction:
Prostatic hypertrophy (primary men)[1,2,5,7,9,10]
Urethral stricture (primary men)[1,2,7, 9,]
Bladder neck contracture (primary men)[2,7,9]
Fecal impaction[2,5]
Pelvic or genital prolapse [1]
Overcorrection of urethra detachment (primary women) [1]

Underactive detrusor due to myogenic or neurogenic factors: [1,2, 5,6,10]
Multiple sclerosis[2,9]
Herpes zoster[2,9]
Surgical trauma e.g. laminectomy, pelvic surgery[1,7,9]
Peripheral neuropathy e.g. diabetes, alcoholism, pernicious anemia[1,7, 9,10]
Supra sacral spinal cord injuries[2]

Impaired afferent sensation[2,10]
Disruption of the motor innervation of the detrusor muscle[1,6]

Pharmacological: [1,2]
Antispasmodics [2,4]
Tri-cyclic antidepressants [2,4,6]
Anti-Parkinson's [2,6]
Antihistamines [2, 4,6]
Opiates[4,6]
Antiarrhythmics [6]
Antidiarrheal [6]

Spasms of external sphincter: [6]
Anxiety [6]
Acute cystitis [6]

REFERENCES:
1. Fantl, J.A., Newman D.K., Colling, J., et al. (1996). Urinary incontinence in adults: Acute and chronic management. Clinical practice guidelines, No.2 1996 update. Department of Health and Human Services. Public Health Service, Agency for Health Care Policy and Research. AHCPR Publication No. 96-0682. Rockville, MD: U.S.
2. Gray, M. & Dougherty, M.C. (1987). Urinary incontinence: Pathophysiology and treatment. Journal of Enterostomal Therapy, 14(4), 152-62
3. National Institutes of Health. (1988). Urinary Incontinence in Adults. NIH Consensus Development Conference Statement. 7(5). Bethesda, MD: U.S. Department of Health and Human Services.
4. Newman, D.K., Lynch, K. Smith, D.A. & Cell, P. (1991). Restoring urinary continence. AJN, 91(1), 28-36.
5. Palmer, M.H. (1990). Urinary incontinence. Nursing Clinics of North America, 25(4), 919-932.
6. Penn, C. (1990). Incontinence assessment: Examining the reliability of a structured assessment tool in guiding staff nurses through a focused assessment and accurate nursing diagnosis. University of Iowa, Iowa City, IA. [Unpublished Master's Project].
7. Resnick, N.M. & Yalla, S.V. (1983). Management of urinary incontinence in the elderly. The New England Journal of Medicine, 33(13), 800-805.
8. Specht, J., Tunick P., Maas, M. & Bulecheck, G. (1991). Urinary incontinence. In M. Maas, K. Buckwalter & M. Hardy (Eds.), Nursing diagnoses and interventions for the elderly, (pp. 181-204). Redwood City, CA: Addison-Wesley.
9. Wheatley, J. (1982). Bladder incontinence: Four types and their control. Postgraduate Medicine, 7(1), 75-81.
10. Willams, M.E. & Pannill, F.C. (1982). Urinary incontinence in the elders: Physiology, pathophysiology, diagnosis and treatment. Annals of Internal Medicine, 97, 895-907.

RECOMMENDED NANDA STAGING: 2.3

PARENTING INEFFECTIVENESS (NANDA Altered Parenting)

DEFINITION: Inability of the primary caretaker to create, maintain, or regain an environment which promotes the optimum growth and development of the child.[4]

SIGNS AND SYMPTOMS (Observed or Reported):
Parental:
  Insecure or lack of attachment to infant [2]
  Maternal-child interaction deficit [6]
  Little cuddling [6]
  Poor or inappropriate caretaking skills [6]
  Inconsistent care [4]
  Unsafe home environment [4]
  Poor parent-child interactions [6]
  High puntitiveness [4]
  Inconsistent behavior management [4]
  Inflexibility to meet needs of child, situation [5]
  Inappropriate visual, tactile, auditory stimulation [5]
  Negative statements about child [5]
  Rejection or hostility to child [6]
  Statements of inability to meet child's needs [6]
  Verbalization cannot control child [6]
  Verbalizations of role inadequacy, frustration [4]
  Inappropriate child care arrangements [1]
  Inadequate child health maintenance [6]
  Child abuse [1,2,4,6]
  Child neglect [1,6]

Infant or Child:
  Failure to thrive (FTT) [2,6]
  Lack of attachment [2,6]
  Lack of separation anxiety [2]
  Poor cognitive development [3]
  Poor academic performance [3]
  Poor social competence [2]
  Behavioral disorders [3]
  Frequent illnesses [5]
  Frequent accidents [5]
  Evidence of abuse [1,2,4,5]
  Runaway [5]

RELATED FACTORS:
Parental:
Social Factors:
  Single parent [4]
  Father of child not involved [6]
  Marital conflict, declining satisfaction [4,6]
  Lack of family cohesiveness [4]
  Poverty [4]
  Financial difficulties [4]
  Unemployment or job problems [4]
  Low socioeconomic class [4]

  Lack of resources [4]
  Lack of access to resources [4]
  Lack of transportation [3]
  History of being abused [4,6]
  History of being abusive [4]
  Legal difficulties [4]
  Lack of or poor parental role model [4]
  Poor home environment [4]
  Relocation [4]
  Change in family unit [4,7]
  Lack of value of parenthood [4]
  Social isolation [4]
  Lack of social support network [4,6]
  Stress [4]
  Role strain / overload [4,7]
  Maladaptive coping strategies [6]
  Poor problem-solving skills [1,4]
  Low self esteem [4]
  Inability to put child's needs before own [6]
  Unplanned or unwanted pregnancy [4]
  Inadequate child care arrangements [1]

Knowledge Factors:
  Unrealistic expectations of child [1,7]
  Lack of knowledge about child development [1,7]
  Lack of knowledge about parenting skills [3,7]
  Lack of knowledge about child health
    maintenance [6]
  Lack of cognitive readiness for parenthood [6]
  Low educational level / attainment [6]
  Low cognitive functioning [1]
  Poor communication skills [6]
  Inability to recognize and act on infant cues [2]
  Preference for physical punishment [1,6]

Physiological Factors:
  Lack of or late prenatal care [5]
  Young age - especially adolescent [3]
  High number or closely spaced of children [6]
  Multiple birth [4]
  Difficult labor and/or delivery [5]
  Separation from infant/child [5]
  History of substance abuse or dependence [3]
  History of mental illness [2]
  Depression [2]
  Physical illness [4]
  Disability [4]
  Sleep deprivation/disruption [7]

<u>Infant/Child</u>:
    Separation from parent at birth [5]
    Prolonged separation from parent [2]
    Premature birth [4]
    Illness [4]
    Handicapping condition or developmental delay [2]
    Difficult temperament [4]
    Lack of goodness of fit (temperament) with parental
        expectations [1]
    Attention Deficit Hyperactivity Disorder [3]
    Unplanned or unwanted child [4]
    Not gender desired [5]
    Multiple birth [4]
    Altered perceptual abilities [2]

<u>REFERENCES</u>:
1. Azar, S.T., Robinson, D.R., Hekimian, E. & Twentyman, C.T. (1984). Unrealistic expectations and problem-solving ability in maltreating and comparison mothers. <u>Journal of Consulting and Clinical Psychology, 52</u>(4), 687-691.
2. Call, J.D. (1984). Child abuse and neglect in infancy: Sources of hostility within the parent-infant dyad and disorders of attachment in infancy. <u>Child Abuse & Neglect, 8</u>(2), 185-202.
3. Denehy, J. (In press). Parenting Promotion. In M.J. Craft-Rosenberg & J.A. Denehy (Eds.) <u>Nursing interventions for childbearing and childrearing families</u>. Sage Publishing Co.
4. Garbarino, J. (1977). The human ecology of child maltreatment: A conceptual model for research. <u>Journal of Marriage and the Family, 39</u>, 721-735.
5. Hanrahan, K.M. (1994). <u>Altered parenting and high risk for altered parenting: validation and differentiation of the defining characteristics</u>. Unpublished master's thesis. The University of Iowa.
6. Nicoletti, A.M., Reitz, S.E. & Gordon, M. (1982). A descriptive study of the parenting diagnosis (1980). in M.J Kim, & D.A. Moritz, (Eds.). <u>Classification of nursing diagnoses: Proceedings of the third and fourth national conferences held in St. Louis, MO in 1978 and 1980</u>. New York: McGraw-Hill Book Company, 176-83.
7. Tiller, C.M. (1995). Fathers' parenting attitudes during a child's first year. <u>JOGNN: Journal of Obstetric, Gynecologic, & Neonatal Nursing, 24</u>(6), 508-514.

<u>RECOMMENDED NANDA STAGING</u>: 2.2

PARENTING INEFFECTIVENESS RISK (NANDA High Risk for Altered Parenting)

DEFINITION: Risk for inability of the primary caretaker to create, maintain, or regain an environment which promotes the optimum growth and development of the child.[4]

RISK FACTORS:

Parental:

Social Factors:
- Single parent [4]
- Father of child not involved [6]
- Marital conflict, declining satisfaction [4,6]
- Lack of family cohesiveness [4]
- Poverty [4]
- Financial difficulties [4]
- Unemployment or job problems [4]
- Low socioeconomic class [4]
- Lack of resources [4]
- Lack of access to resources [4]
- Lack of transportation [3]
- History of being abused [4,6]
- History of being abusive [4]
- Legal difficulties [3]
- Lack of or poor parental role model [4]
- Poor home environment [4]
- Relocation [4]
- Change in family unit [4,7]
- Lack of value of parenthood [4]
- Social isolation [4]
- Lack of social support network [4,6]
- Stress [4]
- Role strain / overload [4,7]
- Maladaptive coping strategies [6]
- Poor problem-solving skills [1,4]
- Low self-esteem [4]
- Inability to put child's needs before own [6]
- Unplanned or unwanted pregnancy [4]
- Inadequate child care arrangements [1]

Knowledge Factors:
- Unrealistic expectations of child [1,7]
- Lack of knowledge about child development [1,7]
- Lack of knowledge about parenting skills [4,7]
- Lack of knowledge about child health maintenance [6]

- Lack of cognitive readiness for parenthood [6]
- Low educational level / attainment [6]
- Low cognitive functioning [1]
- Poor communication skills [6]
- Inability to recognize and act on infant cues [2]
- Preference for physical punishment [1,6]

Physiological Factors:
- Lack of or late prenatal care [5]
- Young age - especially adolescent [3]
- High number or closely spaced of children [6]
- Multiple birth [4]
- Difficult labor and/or delivery [5]
- Separation from infant/child [5]
- History of substance abuse or dependence [3]
- History of mental illness [2]
- Depression [2]
- Physical illness [4]
- Disability [4]
- Sleep deprivation/disruption [7]

Infant/Child:
- Separation from parent at birth [5]
- Prolonged separation from parent [2]
- Premature birth [4]
- Illness [4]
- Handicapping condition or developmental delay [2]
- Difficult temperament [4]
- Lack of goodness of fit (temperament) with parental expectations [1]
- Attention Deficit Hyperactivity Disorder [3]
- Unplanned or unwanted child [4]
- Not gender desired [5]
- Multiple birth [4]
- Altered perceptual abilities [2]

REFERENCES:

1. Azar, S.T., Robinson, D.R., Hekimian, E. & Twentyman, C.T. (1984). Unrealistic expectations and problem-solving ability in maltreating and comparison mothers. Journal of Consulting and Clinical Psychology, 52(4), 687-691.
2. Call, J.D. (1984). Child abuse and neglect in infancy: Sources of hostility within the parent-infant dyad and disorders of attachment in infancy. Child Abuse & Neglect, 8, 187-202.
3. Denehy, J. (In press). Parenting Promotion. In M.J. Craft-Rosenberg & J.A. Denehy (Eds.) Nursing interventions for childbearing and childrearing families. Sage Publishing Co.

4. Garbarino, J. (1977). The human ecology of child maltreatment: A conceptual model for research. <u>Journal of Marriage and the Family, 39,</u> 721-735.

5. Hanrahan, K.M. (1994). <u>Altered parenting and high risk for altered parenting: validation and differentiation of the defining characteristics.</u> Unpublished master's thesis. The University of Iowa.

6. Nicoletti, A.M., Reitz, S.E. & Gordon, M. (1982). A descriptive study of the parenting diagnosis (1980). in M.J Kim, & D.A. Moritz, (Eds.). <u>Classification of nursing diagnoses: Proceedings of the third and fourth national conferences held in St. Louis, MO, in 1978 and 1980.</u> New York: McGraw-Hill Book, 176-83.

7. Tiller, C.M. (1995). Fathers' parenting attitudes during a child's first year. <u>JOGNN: Journal of Obstetric, Gynecologic, & Neonatal Nursing, 24</u>(6), 508-514.

<u>**RECOMMENDED NANDA STAGING**</u>: 2.2

PHYSICAL MOBILITY ALTERATION (NANDA Impaired Physical Mobility)

DEFINITION: A limitation in independent, purposeful physical movement of the body or of one or more extremities.

SIGNS AND SYMPTOMS (Observed or Reported):

Slowed movement[10, 17]

Decreased reaction time[14, 15]

Decreased muscle strength/mass[1,3,6,7,8,9,12,13,14,15,18]

Reluctance to initiate movement, e.g., fear, insufficient self-efficacy[7,9,12,16,17]

Postural instability during performance of routine ADL's[1,5,6,14, 15]

Difficulty turning [17]

Uncoordinated or jerky movements[3,7,8,9,12]

Limited range of motion[3, 6,7,8,9,12,13,14,15]

Limited ability to perform fine motor skills[4,5,16]

Limited ability to perform gross motor skills[2,5,6,8,10,16]

Gait changes, e.g. decreased walk speed, difficulty initiating gait, small steps, shuffles feet, exaggerated lateral postural sway [1,4,6,10,17]

Movement induced tremor[10]

Movement induced shortness of breath[5,17]

Engages in substitutions for movement, e.g. fixation on activity, increased attention to other's activity, controlling behavior, focus on pre-illness/disability activity [16]

Inability to purposefully move [9]

RELATED FACTORS:

Pain [5,7,8,12,17]

Discomfort [5,7,8,12,17]

Musculoskeletal impairment[1, 5,6,7,8,12]

Neuromuscular impairment[3, 6,7,8,12,17]

Sensoriperceptual impairment[3,8,12,14,16,17]

Cognitive impairment[7,8,12,16,17]

Limited cardiovascular endurance

Activity intolerance (cardiovascular condition)[3,5,16]

Joint stiffness/contractures[3]

Altered cellular metabolism[1,7]

Developmental delay[16]

Depressive mood states or anxiety[5, 7,8,17]

Sedentary life style/disuse/deconditioning[1,3,14,17,18]

Loss in integrity of bone structure[3]

Lack of physical or social environmental support[5,16]

Body mass index above 75th age appropriate percentile[5]

Selective or generalized malnutrition[1]

Prescribed movement restriction(s), e.g. physical or chemical restraints, bedrest prescription, use of mechanical equipment that restricts movement, therapeutic immobilization [1,7,8,9,12,13]

Lack of knowledge regarding value of physical activity[11]

Cultural beliefs regarding age-appropriate activity[17]

Medications[16]

REFERENCES:

1. Fiatarone, M.A, & Evans, J.E. (1993). The etiology and reversibility of muscle dysfunction in the aged. Journal of Gerontology, 48 (Special Issue), 77-83.

2. Fisher, N.M., Pendergast, D.R. & Calkins, E. (1991). Muscle rehabilitation in impaired elderly nursing home residents. Archives of Physical Medicine and Rehabilitation, 72(3), 181-185.

3. Graham, C. (1990). Exercise and aging: Implications for persons with diabetes. Diabetes Educator, 17(3), 189-195.

4. Jeffreys, M., Millard, J.B., Hyman, M. & Warren, M.D. (1969). A set of tests for measuring motor impairment in prevalence studies. Journal of Chronic Disease, 22(5), 303-319.

5. Jette, A.M., Branch, L. & Berlin, J. (1990). Musculoskeletal impairments and physical disablement among the aged. Journal of Gerontology, 45(6), M203-208.

6. Judge, J.O., Lindsey, C., Underwood, M. & Winsemius, D. (1993). Balance improvements in older women: Effects of exercise training. Physical Therapy, 73(4), 254-265.

7. Keenan, K. (1989). Clinical validation of the etiology and defining characteristics of the nursing diagnosis impaired mobility. In R. Carroll-Johnson (Ed.), Classification of nursing diagnoses: Proceedings of the eighth conference held in St. Louis, MO, March 1989 (pp. 291-295). Philadelphia: J. B. Lippincott.

8. Kraft, L.A., Maas, M. & Hardy, M.A. (1994). Diagnostic content validity of impaired physical mobility in the older adult. In R. Carroll-Johnson et al (Eds.), <u>Classification of nursing diagnoses: Proceedings of the tenth conference held on April 25-29, 1992 in San Diego, CA,</u> (pp. 197-199). Philadelphia: J. B. Lippincott.

9. Levin, R.F., Krainovitch, B.C., Bahrenburg, E., & Mitchell, C.A. (1989). Diagnostic content validity of nursing diagnoses. <u>Image: The Journal of Nursing Scholarship, 21</u>(1), 40-44.

10. Lueckenotte, A.G. (1996). <u>Gerontologic nursing.</u> St. Louis: Mosby-Year Book.

11. Maas, M. (1991). Impaired physical mobility. In M. Maas, K. Buckwalter & M. Hardy (Eds.), <u>Nursing diagnoses and interventions for the elderly,</u> (pp. 263-284). Redwood City, CA: Addison-Wesley.

12. Mehmert, P. & Delaney, C. (1991). Validating impaired physical mobility. <u>Nursing Diagnosis, 2</u>(4), 143-154.

13. Metzger, K.L. & Hiltunen, E.F. (1987). Diagnostic content validation of ten frequently reported nursing diagnoses. In A. McLane (Ed.), <u>Classification of nursing diagnoses: Proceedings of the seventh conference held in St. Louis MO, March 9-13,</u> (pp. 144-153). St. Louis: C. V. Mosby.

14. Mills, E.M. (1994). The effect of low-intensity aerobic exercise on muscle strength, flexibility and balance among sedentary elderly persons. <u>Nursing Research, 43</u>(4), 207-211.

15. Province, M.A., Hadley, E.C., Hornbrook, M.C., Lipsitz, L.A., Miller, J.P., Mulrow, C.D., Ory, M.G., Sattin, R.W., Tinetti, M.E. & Wolf, S.L. (1995). The effects of exercise on falls in elderly patients: a preplanned meta-analysis of the FIC SIT trials. <u>JAMA: Journal of the American Medical Association, 273</u>(17), 1341-1347.

16. Quellet, L.L. & Rush, K.L. (1992). A synthesis of selected literature on mobility: A basis for studying impaired mobility. <u>Nursing Diagnosis, 3</u>(2), 72-80.

17. Tinetti, M. (1986). Performance-oriented assessment of mobility problems in elderly patients. <u>Journal of the</u> American Geriatric Society, 34(2), 119-126.

18. Webster, J.A. (1988). Key to healthy aging: Exercise. <u>Journal of Gerontological Nursing, 14</u>(12), 8-15, 35-6.

<u>**RECOMMENDED NANDA STAGING:**</u> 2.3

POSITIVE SELF-ESTEEM (NANDA None)

DEFINITION: Relatively stable core sense of self-worth formed through consistently reflected appraisals of significant others. [4]

SIGNS AND SYMPTOMS (Observed or Reported):
Decreased need for social approval [6]
Comfortable with self disclosure [6]
Able to acknowledge and learn from short comings/failures [6]

RELATED FACTORS:
Unconditional self-acceptance [1]
Meaningful relationships [1]
Sense of personal power [1,2,4]
Sense of significance [1,2,4]
Virtue [1,2,4]
Competence [1,2,4]
Positive parenting [1]
Social support [2]

REFERENCES:
1. Coppersmith, S. (1967). The Antecedents of Self-esteem. San Francisco: W. H. Freeman.
2. Harter, S., Alexande, P., & Neimeyer, R. (1988). Long-term effects of incestuous child abuse in college women: Social adjustment, social cognition, and family characteristics. Journal of Consulting & Clinical Psychology, 56(1), 5-8.
3. Meisenhelder, J. (1985). Self-esteem: A closer look at clinical interventions. International Journal of Nursing Studies, 22(2), 127-135.
4. Norris, J. (1992). Nursing intervention for self-esteem disturbances. Nursing Diagnosis, 3(2), 48-53.
5. Norris, J. & Kunes-Connell, M. (1988). A Multimodal Approach to validation & refinement of an existing nursing diagnosis. Archives of Psychiatric Nursing, 2(2), 103-109.
6. Turkat, D. (1978). Defensiveness in self-esteem research. Psychological Record, 28, 129-135.

RECOMMENDED NANDA STAGING: 2.3

POST-TRAUMA SYNDROME (NANDA Post Trauma Response)

DEFINITION: A sustained maladaptive response to a traumatic overwhelming event.

SIGNS AND SYMPTOMS (Observed or Reported):

Intrusive dreams [5,6,9,10]
Nightmares [6,7,9]
Repression [1,2,8]
Aggression [2,3,5,7]
Detachment [1,7,9,10]
Psychogenic amnesia [1,4,6,9]
Hyper vigilance [6,9]
Substance abuse [5,6,9]
Compulsive behavior [6]
Avoidance [3,4,7,9]
Alienation [4,6,7,10]
Shame [3,6]
Guilt [1,2,3,6,7]
Grief [3,6,7,9]
Hopelessness [4,6,9]
Altered mood, sadness [3,6,7,9,10]
Depression [3,6,7,9,10]
Intrusive thoughts [1,3,5,6,9]
Denial [3,6,7,8]
Anxiety [2,3,4,5,6,7,8]
Horror [2,3,4,8,9]
Fear [3,6,7,9]
Anger/rage [3,6,9]
Irritability [6,7,9,10]
Difficulty in concentrating [1,6,7,9,10]
Numbing [1,3,4,10]
Flashbacks [4,5,6,9,10]

Exaggerated startle response [1,2,3,6,7,9]
Palpitations [6,7,8]
Panic attacks [3,6,8,9]
Gastric irritability [3,6]
Neurosensory irritability [3,6]
Headaches [1,3,8,9]
Enuresis (in children) [2]

RELATED FACTORS:

Natural disasters/man made disasters [2,4,6,9]
Witnessing mutilation, violent death, or other horrors [4]
Sudden destruction of one's home or community [6]
Events outside the range of usual human experience [6]
Tragic occurrence involving multiple deaths [4,7]
War [6]
Military combat [6,9]
Rape [3,4,5,9]
Serious threat or injury to one's self or loved ones [6,7]
Being held prisoner of war or criminal victimization (torture) [1]
Serious accidents [6]
Industrial and motor vehicle accidents [4]
Physical and/or psychological abuse [9]

REFERENCES:

1. Caldwell, M.F. (1992). Incidence of PTSD among staff victims of patient violence. H&CP: Hospital and Community Psychiatry, 43(8), 838-839.
2. Durkin, M.S., Khan, N. & Davidson, L.L. (1993). The effects of a natural disaster on child behavior: evidence for posttraumatic stress. American Journal of Public Health, 83(11), 1549-1553.
3. Kelley, S.J. (1990). Parental stress response to sexual abuse and ritualistic abuse of children in day-care centers. Nursing Research, 39(1), 25-29.
4. March, J.S. (1991). Posttraumatic stress in the emergency setting. Emergency Care Quarterly, 7(1), 74-81.
5. Mejo, S.L. (1990). Post-traumatic stress disorder: an overview of three etiological variables, and psychopharmacologic treatment. The Nurse Practitioner, 15(8), 41-45.
6. Moore, K. & Thompson, D. (1989). Posttraumatic stress disorder in the orthopedic patient. Orthopedic Nursing, 8(1), 11-18.
7. Norman, E.M., Getek, D.M. & Griffin, C.C. (1991). Post-traumatic stress disorder in an urban trauma population. Applied Nursing Research, 4(4), 171-176.
8. Ogilivie, B.C. (1987). Psychological aspects of rescue. Emergence Medical Services, 16(5), 34-44.
9. Shearer, R. & Davidhizar, R. (1995). Hidden scars: posttraumatic stress disorder. Nursingconnections, 8(1), 55-63
10. Spencer, M.L. (1995). Post-traumatic stress disorder and paralytic agents. Canadian Nurse, 91(5), 19-22.

RECOMMENDED NANDA STAGING: 2.3

POST-TRAUMA SYNDROME: RAPE (NANDA Rape-Trauma Syndrome)

DEFINITION: Sustained maladaptive response to a forced, violent sexual penetration against the victim's will and consent.

SIGNS AND SYMPTOMS (Observed or Reported):

Confusion [1, 2,6]
Disorganization [6, 7]
Anxiety [2, 3, 4, 5, 6, 8]
Agitation [2, 3, 5, 6]
Aggression [3,5]
Nightmares/sleep disturbance [2, 3, 5, 6, 8]
Dissociative disorders [1]
Shock [2, 5, 6, 8]
Anger [1, 2, 3, 4, 5, 6, 7, 8]
Revenge [1, 2, 7]
Shame [1, 2, 3,5, 6]
Guilt [1, 2, 5, 6, 7, 8]
Humiliation [1, 2, 5, 6, 7, 8]
Embarrassment [1, 3,7, 8]
Denial [4]
Change in relationships [3]
Self-blame [2, 6, 7,8]
Sexual dysfunction [1, 4]

Vulnerability [2, 4]
Mood swings [2, 6, 7]
Hyper-alertness [1, 7]
Helplessness [2, 4,6]
Powerlessness [4]
Inability to make decisions [1, 2, 4, 6]
Dependence [5, 6]
Depression [1, 3, 4,5, 6]
Fear [1, 4,5, 6, 8]
Phobias [3, 6]
Paranoia [6]
Loss of self-esteem [4, 6, 8]
Suicide attempts [1, 3]
Muscle tension/spasms [1, 4]
Physical trauma e.g. bruising, tissue irritation [4,7, 8]
Substance abuse [3]

RELATED FACTORS:
Rape

REFERENCES:

1. Caldwell, M.F. (1992). Incidence of PTSD among staff victims of patient violence. H&CP: Hospital and Community Psychiatry, 43(8), 838-839.
2. Durkin, M.S., Khan, N. & Davidson, L.L. (1993). The effects of a natural disaster on child behavior: evidence for posttraumatic stress. American Journal of Public Health, 83(11), 1549-1553.
3. March, J.S. (1991). Posttraumatic stress in the emergency setting. Emergency Care Quarterly, 7(1), 74-81.
4. Mejo, S.L. (1990). Post-traumatic stress disorder: an overview of three etiological variables, and psychopharmacologic treatment. The Nurse Practitioner, 15(8), 41-45.
5. Moore, K. & Thompson, D. (1989). Posttraumatic stress disorder in the orthopedic patient. Orthopedic Nursing, 8(1), 11-18.
6. Norman, E.M., Getek, D.M. & Griffin, C.C. (1991). Post-traumatic stress disorder in an urban trauma population. Applied Nursing Research, 4(4), 171-176.
7. Shearer, R. & Davidhizar, R. (1995). Hidden scars: posttraumatic stress disorder. Nursingconnections, 8(1), 55-63
8. Spencer, M.L. (1995). Post-traumatic stress disorder and paralytic agents. Canadian Nurse, 91(5), 19-22.

RECOMMENDED NANDA STAGING: 2.3

POST-TRAUMA SYNDROME RISK (NANDA None)

DEFINITION: A risk for sustained maladaptive response to a traumatic overwhelming event.

RISK FACTORS:
Non-supportive environment [4,7]
Inadequate social support [8]
Survivor's role in the event [4,7]
Exaggerated sense of responsibility [4,6]
Perception of event [4,5]
Duration of event [3,6]
Occupation e.g. police, fire, rescue, corrections,
  ER staff, mental health [1]
Displacement from home [2,7]
Diminished ego strength [1,4]

REFERENCES:
1. Caldwell, M.F. (1992). Incidence of PTSD among staff victims of patient violence. H&CP: Hospital and Community Psychiatry, 43(8), 838-839.
2. Durkin, M.S., Khan, N. & Davidson, L.L. (1993). The effects of a natural disaster on child behavior: evidence for posttraumatic stress. American Journal of Public Health, 83(11), 1549-1553.
3. March, J.S. (1991). Posttraumatic stress in the emergency setting. Emergency Care Quarterly, 7(1), 74-81.
4. Mejo, S.L. (1990). Post-traumatic stress disorder: an overview of three etiological variables, and psychopharmacologic treatment. The Nurse Practitioner, 15(8), 41-45.
5. Moore, K. & Thompson, D. (1989). Posttraumatic stress disorder in the orthopedic patient. Orthopedic Nursing, 8(1), 11-19.
7. Norman, E.M., Getek, D.M. & Griffin, C.C. (1991). Post-traumatic stress disorder in an urban trauma population. Applied Nursing Research, 4(4), 171-176.
8. Shearer, R. & Davidhizar, R. (1995). Hidden scars: posttraumatic stress disorder. Nursingconnections, 8(1), 55-63
9. Spencer, M.L. (1995). Post-traumatic stress disorder and paralytic agents. Canadian Nurse, 91(5), 19-22.

RECOMMENDED NANDA STAGING: 2.3

POWERLESSNESS (NANDA Powerlessness)

DEFINITION: Perceived lack of control over ones current situation and/or that ones own action will not significantly affect an outcome (influence others).

SIGNS AND SYMPTOMS (Observed or Reported):

Physical:
 Fatigue [10]
 Headache [10]
 Dizziness [10]
 Gasrointestinal complaints [10]
 Decreased appetite [6]
 Physical impairment e.g. inability to speak, use of limbs, etc. [7,8]

Verbal Expressions of:
 Lack of control over what is happening [3,4,5,6,7,8,9,10]
 Doubt that self-care measures can affect an outcome [5,6,7,8,9,10]
 Doubt regarding role performance [5,10]
 Uncertainty about fluctuating energy levels [5,8]
 Dissatisfaction/frustration over inability to perform previous tasks or activities [5,7,8,9,10,11]
 Giving up [6,10]
 Fatalism [6]

Emotional Response:
 Withdrawal [6,10]
 Undifferentiated anger [1,6,9]
 Pessimism/anxiety [1,6,10]
 Submissiveness/passivity [3,5,6,8,9]
 Depression [1,3,5,8,10,11]

Behavioral:
 Non-participation in self-care or decision-making [3,5,6,8,9,10,11]
 Does not seek information regarding self-care [3,5,6,8,9,11]
 Hesitant to set goals for future [5,6]
 Dependence on others for care that may result in anger/guilt/irritability [3,4,5,6,7,8,9,10]
 Restlessness/insomnia [10]

RELATED FACTORS:

Physiological:
 Chronic or acute illness (hospitalization, intubation, ventilator, suctioning) [1,3,4,5,6,10]
 Acute injury or progressive debilitating disease process e.g. spinal cord injury, multiple sclerosis [1,7,8,9]
 Aging e.g. atrophy of body, decreased self-esteem, decreased body image [6]
 Dying [9]

Psychosocial:
 Lack of knowledge of illness or healthcare system [3,4,6,9,10]
 Lifestyle of dependencies with inadequate coping patterns [3]
 Absence of integrality e.g. essence of power [2,6,11]

REFERENCES:

1. Boeing, M.H. & Mongera, C.O. (1989). Powerlessness in critical care patients. Dimensions of Critical Care Nursing. 8(5), 274-279.
2. Dzurec, L.C. (1994). Schizophrenic clients' experiences of power: using hermeneutic analysis. Image: The Journal of Nursing Scholarship. 26(2), 155-159.
3. Fuchs, J. (1987). Use of decisional control to combat powerlessness. Anna Journal, 14(1), 11-13, 56.
4. Lambert, V.A., & Lambert, C.E. (1981). Role theory and the concept of powerlessness. Journal of Psychosocial Nursing & Mental Health Services 19(9), 11-14.
5. Miller, J.F. (1984). Development and validation of a diagnostic label: powerlessness. In M.J. Kim et al, Classification of nursing diagnoses: Proceedings of the fifth national conference. 116-127.
6. Miller, J.F. & Oertel, C.B. (1983). Powerlessness in the elderly: Preventing hopelessness. In J.F. Miller, (Ed.), Coping with chronic illness: Overcoming powerlessness. Philadelphia, PA: F.A. Davis Co.
7. Richmond, T.S. & Metcalf, J. (1986). Psychosocial responses to spinal cord injury. Journal of Neuroscience Nursing. 18(4), 183-187.
8. Richmond, T.S., Metcalf, J., Daly, M. & Kish, J.R. (1992). Powerlessness in acute spinal cord injury patients: a descriptive study. Journal of Neuroscience Nursing. 24(3), 146-152.
9. Sheppard, K. Powerlessness: A nursing diagnosis. Dimensions in Oncology Nursing, 1(2), 17-20.
10. White, B.S. & Roberts, S.L. (1993). Powerlessness and the pulmonary alveolar edema patient. DCCN: Dimensions of Critical Care Nursing. 12(3), 127-137.
11. Zauszniewski, J.A. (1994). Nursing diagnosis and depressive illness. Nursing Diagnosis. 5(3), 106-114.

RECOMMENDED NANDA STAGING: 2.3

POWERLESSNESS RISK (NANDA None)

DEFINITION: Risk for perception of the lack of control over ones current situation and/or that ones own action will not significantly affect an outcome (influence others).

RISK FACTORS:

Physiological:
Chronic or acute illness e.g. hospitalization, intubation, ventilator, suctioning [1,3,4,5,6,10]
Acute injury or progressive debilitating disease process e.g. spinal cord injury, multiple sclerosis [1,7,8,9]
Aging e.g. atrophy of body, decreased self-esteem, decreased body image [6]
Dying [9]

Psychosocial:
Lack of knowledge of illness or healthcare system [3,4,6,9,10]
Lifestyle of dependencies with inadequate coping patterns [3]
Absence of integrality e.g. essence of power [2,6,11]

REFERENCES:

1. Boeing, M.H. & Mongera, C.O. (1989). Powerlessness in critical care patients. Dimensions of Critical Care Nursing. 8(5), 274-279.
2. Dzurec, L.C. (1994). Schizophrenic clients' experiences of power: using hermeneutic analysis. Image: The Journal of Nursing Scholarship. 26(2), 155-159.
3. Fuchs, J. (1987). Use of decisional control to combat powerlessness. Anna Journal, 14(1), 11-13, 56.
4. Lambert, V.A., & Lambert, C.E. (1981). Role theory and the concept of powerlessness. Journal of Psychosocial Nursing & Mental Health Services 19(9), 11-14.
5. Miller, J.F. (1984). Development and validation of a diagnostic label: powerlessness. In M.J. Kim et al, Classification of nursing diagnoses: Proceedings of the fifth national conference. 116-127.
6. Miller, J.F. & Oertel, C.B. (1983). Powerlessness in the elderly: Preventing hopelessness. In J.F. Miller, (Ed.), Coping with chronic illness: Overcoming powerlessness. Philadelphia, PA: F.A. Davis Co.
7. Richmond, T.S. & Metcalf, J. (1986). Psychosocial responses to spinal cord injury. Journal of Neuroscience Nursing. 18(4), 183-187.
8. Richmond, T.S., Metcalf, J., Daly, M. & Kish, J.R. (1992). Powerlessness in acute spinal cord injury patients: a descriptive study. Journal of Neuroscience Nursing. 24(3), 146-152.
9. Sheppard, K. Powerlessness: A nursing diagnosis. Dimensions in Oncology Nursing, 1(2), 17-20.
10. White, B.S. & Roberts, S.L. (1993). Powerlessness and the pulmonary alveolar edema patient. DCCN: Dimensions of Critical Care Nursing. 12(3), 127-137.
11. Zauszniewski, J.A. (1994). Nursing diagnosis and depressive illness. Nursing Diagnosis. 5(3), 106-114.

RECOMMENDED NANDA STAGING: 2.3

REFLEX URINARY INCONTINENCE (NANDA Reflex Incontinence)

DEFINITION: An involuntary loss of urine at somewhat predictable intervals when a specific bladder volume is reached.

SIGNS AND SYMPTOMS (Observed or Reported):

Predictable pattern of voiding [5,6]

Incomplete emptying with lesion above sacral micturition center [2,5]

Complete emptying with lesion above pontine micturition center [2]

No sensation of urge to void [2,4,5,6]

Unable to cognitively inhibit or initiate voiding [2,4,5,6]

No sensation of voiding [5,6]

No sensation of bladder fullness [5]

Sensation of urge without voluntary inhibition of bladder contraction [1,2]

Sensations associated with full bladder such as sweating, restlessness, and abdominal discomfort [3]

RELATED FACTORS:

Neurological impairment above level of sacral micturition center or pontine micturition center, e.g. myelomeningocele [2,4,5,6]

Tissue damage from [1]
  Radiation cystitis
  Inflammatory bladder conditions
  Radical pelvic surgery

REFERENCES:

1. Fantl, J.A., Neuman, D.K., Colling, J. et al (1996). Managing acute and chronic urinary incontinence. Clinical Practice Guideline, Quick Reference Guide. U.S. Department of Health and Human Services, Rockville, Maryland. AHCPR Pub. No. 96-0686.
2. Gray, M. & Dougherty, M.C. (1987). Urinary incontinence -- pathophysiology and treatment. Journal of Enterostomal Therapy, 14(4), 152-162.
3. Luckmann, J. & Sorenson, K.C. (1987). Medical-surgical nursing: A psychophysiologic approach. (Ed.). 3. Philadelphia: W.B. Saunders Co.
4. Palmer, M.H. (1993). Urinary incontinence. In V. Carrieri-Kohlman, A.M., Lindsey, & C. M. West. (Eds.). Pathophysiological Phenomena in Nursing (pp. 221-244). Philadelphia: W.B. Saunders Co.
5. Specht, J., Tunink, P., Maas, M. & Bulechek, G. (1991). Urinary incontinence. In M. Maas, K.C. Buckwalter, & M. Hardy (Eds.). Nursing Diagnosis and interventions for the elderly (p. 184). New York: Addison-Wesley.
6. Voith, A.M. (1986). A conceptual framework for nursing diagnoses: alterations in urinary elimination. Rehabilitation Nursing, 11(1), 18-21.

RECOMMENDED NANDA STAGING: 2.3

ROLE PERFORMANCE ALTERATION (NANDA Altered Role Performance)

DEFINITION: Patterns of behaviors and self-expression do not match the environmental context, norms, and expectations.

SIGNS AND SYMPTOMS (Observed or Reported):

Inadequate role competency and skills [1,3,4,5,6]
Inadequate adaptation to change/transition [4,6]
Altered role perceptions [3]
Inadequate confidence [4]
Inadequate motivation
Pessimistic [4]
Powerlessness [4]
Role ambivalence/denial [4]
Inadequate self-management
Inadequate coping [1,2]
Anxiety [3]
Role strain [2]
Role conflict [4]
Role confusion [1,3,4,5]
Role overload [2]
Uncertainty [3]
Role dissatisfaction [2]

RELATED FACTORS:

Knowledge Factors: [1,3,4,5,6]
   Lack of knowledge about role [1,3,4,5,6]
   Lack of knowledge about role skills [1,3,4,5,6]
   Lack of or inadequate role model [1,5]
   Lack of opportunity for role rehearsal [1,5]
   Role transition [1,3]
   Developmental transitions [1,3,4]
   Lack of role validation [1]
   Unrealistic role expectations [1,3]

Social Factors:
   Stress [2]
   Lack of rewards [2]
   Family conflict [2,3]
   Domestic violence [2]
   Job/schedule demands [2]
   Inadequate support system [1,2,4,5,6]
   Young age, developmental level [4,6]
   Poverty [4]
   Low social economic status [4]
   Lack of resources [1,2,4]
   Substance abuse [2]
   Inadequate/inappropriate linkage with health care
      system [3]

Physiological Factors:
   Physical illness [1]
   Pain [3]
   Fatigue [2]
   Body image alteration [2]
   Low self esteem [2,3]
   Mental Illness [1]
   Depression [2]
   Cognitive deficits [4]

REFERENCES:
1. Clarke, B.A. & Strauss, S.S. (1992). Nursing role supplementation for adolescent parents; prescriptive nursing practice. Journal of Pediatric Nursing, 7(5), 312-318.
2. McBride, A.B. (1988). Mental health effects of women's multiple roles. Image: The Journal of Nursing Scholarship, 20(1), 41-47.
3. Mercer, R.T. & Ferketich, S.L. (1994). Predictors of maternal role competence by risk status. Nursing Research, 43(1), 38-43.
4. Roosa, M.W., Fitzgerald, H.E. & Carlson, N.A. (1982). Teenage parenting and child development: a literature review. Infant Mental Health Journal. 3(1), 4-18
5. Rubin, R., (1967). Attainment of the maternal role. 2. Models and Referrants. Nursing Research, 16(4), 342-346.
6. Vukelich, C. & Kliman, D.S. (1985). Mature and teenage mothers' infant growth expectations and the use of child development information sources. Family Relations, 34, 189-196.

RECOMMENDED NANDA STAGING: 2.1

SECURE PARENT-INFANT ATTACHMENT (NANDA None)

DEFINITION: Reciprocal interactions between parent and infant that result in a satisfactory emotional/affectionate bond.

SIGNS AND SYMPTOMS (Observed or Reported):

Prenatal:
 Recognition of pregnancy [3,5]
 Talk about infant [3,5]
 Name(s) selected for infant [3,5]
 Visualization of infant [3,5]
 Visualize caring for infant [3]

Maternal/Paternal:
 Verbal interaction with infant [1,2]
 Talks to infant in soothing or playful manner [8]
 Tactile e.g. touching & holding contact with infant [1,2]
 Desire for proximity with infant [1,5]
 Protective of infant [7]
 Cradles infant close to body [8]
 Visual (en face position) eye contact with infant [1,5]
 Affectionate tie [1,5]
 Sensitivity to infant cues [5]
 Knowledge of unique aspects of infant's behavior and cues [1]
 Consistent care and response to infant [8]
 Appropriate response to infant distress [5]
 Attribution of family characteristics to infant [5]
 Positive perception of infant [5]
 Gratifying experiences with infant [6]
 Shows signs of pleasure during and after feeding [8]

Infant:
 Trust [5]
 Vocalizations or smiles in response to auditory stimulation from parent [8]
 Turns toward parent in response to touch, smell, sound [1]
 Curls up and cuddles in response to being held [8]
 Eye contact with parent [8]
 Responsiveness to care and attention [1,8]
 Shows signs of pleasure during and after feeding [8]
 Separation anxiety when separated from parent [1]

RELATED FACTORS:

Maternal/Paternal:
 Positive self esteem [6]
 Early contact with infant [2]
 Rooming in with infant [2]
 Consistent care and response to infant [7]
 Social support [2]
 Parenting skills and competence [6]
 Knowledge about infant care [2]
 Knowledge of infant's unique behavioral characteristics or cues [1,2]
 Goodness of fit between parental expectations and infant behavior [1]

Infant:
 Demonstration of cues [4]
 Responsive to parental care, verbalization [1,4]

REFERENCES:
1. Avant, K. (1979). Nursing diagnosis: Maternal attachment. ANS: Advances in Nursing Science, 2(1), 45-55.
2. Cranley, M.S. (1981). Development of a tool for the measurement of maternal attachment during pregnancy. Nursing Research, 30(5), 281-284.
3. Coffman, S. (1992). Parent and infant attachment: Review of nursing research 1981-1990. Pediatric Nursing, 18(4), 421-425.
4. Denehy, J.A. (1992). Interventions related to parent-infant attachment. Nursing Clinics of North America, 27(2), 425-43.
5. Gaffney, K.F. (1988). New directions in maternal attachment research. Journal of Pediatric Health Care, 2(4), 181-188.
6. Mercer, R.T., & Ferketich, S.L. (1990). Predictors of parental attachment during early parenthood. Journal of Advanced Nursing, 15(3), 268-280.
7. Pressler, J.L. (1990). Promoting attachment. In M.J. Craft & J.A. Denehy (Eds.). Nursing interventions for infants and children, (pp. 4-17). Philadelphia, PA: W.B. Saunders.
8. Reiser, S.L. (1981). A tool to facilitate mother-infant attachment. Journal of Obstetrical and Gynecological Nursing, 10(4), 294-297

RECOMMENDED NANDA STAGING: 2.2

SELF MUTILATION (NANDA None)

DEFINITION: Deliberate self-destructive behavior causing tissue damage with the intent of causing nonfatal injury to attain relief of tension.

SIGNS AND SYMPTOMS (Observed or Reported):
Picking at wounds [5]
Cuts/scratches on extremities or body usually covered by clothing [4]
Eraser burns [4,5]
Self-inflicted burns [5]
Self-inflicted tattoos [5]

RELATED FACTORS:
Adolescence [5]
Peers who self mutilate [5]
Isolation from peers
Perfectionism [5]
Substance abuse [5]
Eating disorders [5]
Sexual identify crisis [5]
Low or unstable self-esteem [5]
Low or unstable body image [5]
Labile behavior (mood swings) [5]
History of inability to plan solutions [3]
History of inability to see long-term consequences [3]
Uses manipulation to obtain nurturing relationship with others [5]

Chaotic/disturbed interpersonal relationships [5]
Feels threatened with actual or potential loss of significant relationship [5]
Loss of parent/parental relationship [5]
Experiences dissociation [5]
Experiences depersonalization [5]
Experiences mounting tension that is intolerable [5]
Experiences irresistible urge to cut/damage self [4,5]
Unable to express tension verbally [4,5]
Impulsivity [5]
Inadequate coping [5]
Needs quick reduction of stress [4,5]
Childhood illness or surgery [5]
Childhood sexual abuse [5]
Foster or group care [5]
Incarceration [5]
Violence between parental figures [5]
Family divorce [5]
Family alcoholism [5]
Family history of self destructive behaviors [5]
Character disorders [1]
Borderline personality disorders [1]

REFERENCES:
1. American Psychiatric Association. (1994). Diagnostic and statistical manual of mental disorders (4th ed.). Washington, DC: American Psychiatric Association.
2. Barstow, D.G. (1995). Self-injury and self-mutilation. Journal of Psychosocial Nursing & Mental Health Services, 33(2), 19-22, 38-39.
3. Haines, J., & Williams, C.L. (1997). Coping and problem solving of self-mutilators. Journal of Clinical Psychology, 53(2), 177-186.
4. Sebree, R., & Popkess-Vawter, S. (1991). Self-injury concept formation: Nursing diagnosis development. Perspectives in Psychiatric Care, 27(2), 27-35.
5. Walsh, B.W., & Rosen, P.M. (1988). Self-mutilation: Theory, research, and treatment. New York: Guilford Press.

RECOMMENDED NANDA STAGING: 2.3

SELF MUTILATION RISK (NANDA Risk for Self-Mutilation)

DEFINITION: Risk for deliberate self-destructive behavior causing tissue damage with the intent of causing injury, not death, to attain relief of tension.

RISK FACTORS:

Adolescence [5]

Peers who self mutilate [5]

Isolation from peers

Perfectionism [5]

Substance abuse [5]

Eating disorders [5]

Sexual identify crisis [5]

Low or unstable self esteem [5]

Low or unstable body image [5]

Labile behavior (mood swings) [5]

History of inability to plan solutions or see long-term consequences [3]

Uses manipulation to obtain nurturing relationship with others [5]

Chaotic/disturbed interpersonal relationships [5]

Feels threatened with actual or potential loss of significant relationship [5]

Loss of parent/parental relationship [5]

Experiences dissociation or depersonalization [5]

Experiences mounting tension that is intolerable [5]

Experiences irresistible urge to cut/damage self [5]

Unable to express tension verbally

Impulsivity [5]

Inadequate coping [5]

Needs quick reduction of stress

Childhood illness or surgery [5]

Childhood sexual abuse [5]

Foster or group care [5]

Incarceration [5]

Violence between parental figures [5]

Family divorce [5]

Family alcoholism [5]

Family history of self destructive behaviors [5]

Character disorders [1]

Borderline personality disorders [1]

REFERENCES:
1. American Psychiatric Association. (1994). Diagnostic and statistical manual of mental disorders (4th ed.). Washington, DC: American Psychiatric Association.
2. Barstow, D.G. (1995). Self-injury and self-mutilation. Journal of Psychosocial Nursing & Mental Health Services, 33(2), 19-22, 38-39.
3. Haines, J., & Williams, C.L. (1997). Coping and problem solving of self-mutilators. Journal of Clinical Psychology, 53(2), 177-186.
4. Sebree, R., & Popkess-Vawter, S. (1991). Self-injury concept formation: Nursing diagnosis development. Perspectives in Psychiatric Care, 27(2), 27-35.
5. Walsh, B.W., & Rosen, P.M. (1988). Self-mutilation: Theory, research, and treatment. New York: Guilford Press.

RECOMMENDED NANDA STAGING: 2.3

SITUATIONAL LOW SELF-ESTEEM (NANDA Situational Low Self-Esteem/ Self-Esteem Disturbance)

DEFINITION: Negative perceptions of self-worth that depend on current life factors.

SIGNS AND SYMPTOMS (Observed or Reported):

Sense of self-worth developed as a child [4]
Self negating verbalizations [2,5]
Indecisive [2,5]
Expressions of shame or guilt [2,5]
Evaluate self as unable to deal with situations or events [2,5]
Feelings of helplessness and uselessness [5]
Self neglect [2]
Social isolation [2]

RELATED FACTORS:

Developmental changes [3]
Body image alterations [1,5]
Functional impairment [2,3]
Loss of significant roles, objects e.g. relocation [2,3,5]
Social role changes, e.g. unemployment, divorce, hospitalization, relocation [2,3,6]
Life factors, e.g. recognition/rewards, failures/rejections [5]
Behavior inconsistent with values [5]

REFERENCES:

1. Antaki, C. & Brewin, C. (Eds.). (1994). Attributions and psychological change. London: Academic Press.
2. Carpenito, L. (1997). Nursing diagnosis: application to clinical. Philadelphia: J.B. Lippincott.
3. Norris, J. (1992). Nursing intervention for self-esteem disturbances. Nursing Diagnosis, 3(2), 48-53.
4. Norris, J. & Kunes-Connell. (1985). Self-esteem disturbance. Nursing Clinics of North America, 20, 745-761.
5. Norris, J. & Kunes-Connell, M. (1988). A multimodal approach to validation & refinement of an existing nursing diagnosis. Archives of Psychiatric Nursing, 2(2), 103-109.
6. Riffee, D. (1981). Self-esteem changes in hospitalized school-age children. Nursing Research, 30(2), 94-7.

RECOMMENDED NANDA STAGING: 2.3

SLEEP DEPRIVATION (NANDA None)

DEFINITION: Prolonged periods of time without sustained sleep (natural, periodic suspension of consciousness).

SIGNS AND SYMPTOMS (Observed or Reported):

Daytime drowsiness (sleepiness)[3,7,9,11]
Decreased ability to function [3,9,12]
Malaise [9,11]
Tiredness [11]
Lethargy [11]
Restlessness [11]
Irritability [11]
Heightened sensitivity to pain [11]
Listlessness [11]
Apathy [11]
Slowed reaction [11]
Inability to concentrate [11]
Perceptual disorders, e.g. disturbed body, sensation, delusions, feeling afloat [11]
Hallucinations [11]
Acute confusion [11]
Transient paranoia [11]
Agitated (combative) [11]
Anxious [11]
Mild, fleeting nystagmus [6]
Hand tremors [6]

Prolonged use of pharmacologic/dietary antisoporifics [3,9]
Aging-related sleep stage shifts [3]
Sustained circadian asynchrony [3,5,13]
Inadequate daytime activity [7,9,13]
Sustained (external) environmental stimulation [3,12]
Sustained unfamiliar/uncomfortable sleep environment [2,7]
Nonsleep inducing parenting practices [2,7]
Sleep disorders [3,12]
Sleep apnea [3]
Periodic limb movement, e.g., restless leg syndrome, nocturnal myoclonus [3]
Sundown syndrome [3]
Narcolepsy [3]
Idiopathic central nervous system hypersomnolence [3]
Sleep walking [3]
Sleep terror [3]
Sleep related enuresis [3]
Nightmares [3]

RELATED FACTORS:

Prolonged physical discomfort [2,3,7,12,13]
Prolonged psychological discomfort [3]
Sustained inadequate sleep hygiene [3,8,12]

Familial sleep paralysis [3]
Sleep-related painful erections [3]
Dementia [3]

REFERENCES:

1. Beyerman, K. (1987). Etiologies of sleep pattern disturbances in hospitalization patients. In A. McLane (Ed.). Classification of nursing diagnoses: Proceedings of the seventh conference (pp. 193-198). St. Louis: C.V. Mosby.
2. Chuman, M.A. (1988). Rhythmic alterations in consciousness: Sleep. In P. Mitchell, L. Hodges, M. Muwasives & C. Welleck (Eds.). AANN's Neuroscience Nursing: phenomena and practice (pp. 115-135). Norwalk, CT: Appleton & Lange.
3. Felton, G., Kruckeberg, T. & Moreno, E. (1992). Accommodation the biological clocks of shift workers. Management and Operations (June), 50-55.
4. Gordon, M. (1993). Manual of nursing diagnoses (pp. 219). St. Louis: C.V. Mosby.
5. Hammer, B. (1991). Sleep pattern disturbance. In M. Mass, K. Buckwalter & M. Hardy (Eds.). Nursing diagnoses and interventions for the elderly (pp. 317-326). Redwood City, CA: Addison-Wesley.
6. Jensen, D.P. & Herr, K.A. (1993). Sleeplessness. Nursing Clinics of North America, 28(2), 385-405.
7. Johnson, J.E. (1991). Progressive relaxation and the sleep of older noninstitutionalized women. Applied Nursing Research, 4(4), 165-170.
8. Kao Lo, C. & Kim, M.J. (1986). Construct validity of sleep pattern disturbance: A methodological approach. In M.E. Hurley, (Ed.). Classification of nursing diagnoses: Proceedings of the sixth conference. (pp. 197-206). St. Louis: C.V. Mosby.
9. Miceli, D. (1996). Sleep and activity. In A. Lueckenotte, (Ed.), Gerontologic nursing (pp. 224-243). St. Louis: C.V. Mosby.

10. Richardson, S. (1994). Sleep pattern disturbance and related factors in the critically ill. In R.M. Carroll-Johnson (Ed.). <u>Classification of nursing diagnoses: Proceedings of the tenth conference</u> (pp. 242). Philadelphia: J.B. Lippincott.

11. Rogers, A.E., Caruso, C.C. & Aldrich, M.S. (1993). Reliability of sleep diaries for assessment of sleep/wake patterns. <u>Nursing Research. 42</u>(6), 368-372.

12. Spenceley, S.M. (1993). Sleep inquiry: A look with fresh eyes. <u>Image: the Journal of Nursing Scholarship, 25</u>(3), 249-256.

13. Westfall, U. (1992). Nursing chronotherapeutics: A conceptual framework. <u>Image: the Journal of Nursing Scholarship, 24</u>(4), 307-312.

<u>**RECOMMENDED NANDA STAGING:**</u> 2.3

SLEEP PATTERN DISTURBANCE (NANDA Sleep Pattern Disturbance)

DEFINITION: Time limited disruption of sleep (natural, periodic suspension of consciousness) amount and quality.

SIGNS AND SYMPTOMS (Observed or Reported):
Less than age-normed total sleep time [7]
A feeling of not being well rested [7,10]
Dissatisfaction with sleep [7]
Decreased ability to function [7]
Increased proportion of Stage 1 sleep [16,17]

Decreased proportions of Stage 3 and 4 sleep: [16,17]
Hyporesponsiveness [17]
Excess sleepiness [17]
Decreased motivation [17]

Decreased proportion of REM sleep: [17]
REM rebound [17]
Hyperactivity [17]
Emotional lability [17]
Agitation and impulsivity [17]
Atypical polysomnographic features [3,15]

Sub-Categories of Sleep Pattern Disturbance:
Sleep Onset Insomnia (also referred to as
   "sleep latency" or sleep onset latency) [8,10]
Sleep onset greater than 30 minutes [4,13]
Self-reported difficulty falling asleep [6]
Sleep maintenance insomnia [7]
Three or more night time awakenings [4]
Prolonged awakenings [8,10,17]
Early AM insomnia [17,18]
Awakening earlier than desired awake time [7,10,17]
Self-induced impairment of normal pattern [19]

RELATED FACTORS:
Physical Discomfort/Pain: [2,7,12,13,17]
Nausea [13]
Fever [13]
Urinary urgency [2,7,13]
Position [12,17]
Wet [7,12]
Shortness of breath [7,13]
Stasis of secretions [7,9]
Oxygen desaturation [9]
Gastroesophageal reflux [3]

Psychological Discomfort:
Fear [9,13]
Anxiety [7,9,12,13]
Depression [7,9,12,13]
Grief [13]

Anticipation [13]
Separation from significant others [12,17]
Loneliness [7]
Loss of sleep partner, life change [12]
Thinking about home [2]
Boredom [2,7]
Fatigue [2,7]
Maldaptive conditioned wakefulness [3]
Ruminative presleep thoughts [3]
Preoccupation with trying to sleep [3]
Fear of insomnia [3]

Sleep Hygiene Factors: [3,8,14]
(Includes absence of sleep initiation
associations such as rocking, being held or
fed during nighttime awakening for infants)
Sustained use of antisleep agents, e.g.
   antisoporifics [3,9,14]
Pharmacological, e.g., xanthines, CNS
   stimulants [8,13]
Biochemical agents, e.g., catecholamines,
   neurotransmitters [8]
Dietary, e.g., caffeinated foods/beverages,
   alcohol [7,8]
Aging (developmentally) - related sleep shifts [3,9]
Delayed or advanced sleep phase syndrome [3]
Circadian asynchrony [3,5,12,16,18]
Body temperature [5,17]
Social schedule inconsistent with chronotype
   e.g. "morning" vs "evening person" [5]
Frequent travel across time zones [5]
Shift work [5,8]
Daylight/darkness exposure [13]
Frequently changing (or irregular) sleep-wake
   schedule [5,8]
Daytime activity pattern [7,9,18]
Periodic gender-related hormonal shifts, e.g.
   puberty, climacteric [3,8,15,16,17]
Childhood onset [3]
Temperament [8]

Environmental Factors: [13]
Excessive stimulation
Noise [2,7,9,10,13,17,18]
Noxious odors [17]
Lighting (continuous, less or more than
   desired) [2,7,17,18]
Physical restraint [12,17]
Other generated awakening [13]

Nurse (or other caregiver) for therapeutics,
  monitoring, lab tests [2,7,8,13,17]
Sleep partner (could be spouse, infant,
  child) [8,13,17]
Ambient temperature, humidity[7,18]
Unfamiliar (or change in) sleep (or bed)
  furnishings [2]
Unfamiliar sleep place [2,7,17]
Lack of sleep privacy/control [17]

Parental Factors:[8,16:]
  Mother's sleep-wake pattern [8]
  Parent-infant/interaction [8]
  Mother's emotional support [8]

REFERENCES:
1. Assousa, S.N. & Wilson, N.D. (1991). Validation of sleep pattern disturbance. In R.M. Carroll-Johnson (Ed.). Classification of nursing diagnoses: Proceedings of the ninth conference (pp. 242). Philadelphia: J.B. Lippincott.
2. Beyerman, K. (1987). Etiologies of sleep pattern disturbances in hospitalization patients. In A. McLane (Ed.). Classification of nursing diagnoses: Proceedings of the seventh conference (pp. 193-198). St. Louis: C.V. Mosby.
3. Chuman, M.A. (1988). Rhythmic alterations in consciousness: Sleep. In P. Mitchell, L. Hodges, M. Muwasives & C. Welleck (Eds.). AANN's neuroscience nursing: phenomena and practice (pp. 115-135). Norwalk, CT: Appleton & Lange.
4. Cohen, J., et al (1983). Sleep disturbance in the institutionalized aged. Journal of the American Geriatric Society, 31, 79-82.
5. Felton, G., Kruckeberg, T. & Moreno, E. (1992). Accommodation the biological clocks of shift workers. Management and Operations (June), 50-55.
6. Gordon, M. (1993). Manual of nursing diagnoses (pp. 219). St. Louis: C.V. Cosby.
7. Hammer, B. (1991). Sleep pattern disturbance. In M. Mass, K. Buckwalter & M. Hardy (Eds.). Nursing diagnoses and interventions for the elderly (pp. 317-326). Redwood City, CA: Addison-Wesley.
8. Jensen, D.P. & Herr, K.A. (1993). Sleeplessness. Nursing Clinics of North America, 28(2), 385-405.
9. Johnson, J.E. (1991). Progressive relaxation and the sleep of older noninstitutionalized women. Applied Nursing Research, 4(4), 165-170.
10. Johnson, S.E. (1989). Sleep pattern disturbance: Defining characteristics observable in practice. In R.M. Carroll-Johnson (Ed.). Classification of nursing diagnoses: Proceedings of the eighth conference (pp. 368-370). Philadelphia: J.B. Lippincott.
11. Kao Lo, C. & Kim, M.J.(1986). Construct validity of sleep pattern disturbance: A methodological approach. In M.E. Hurley, (Ed.). Classification of nursing diagnoses: Proceedings of the sixth conference. (pp. 197-206). St. Louis: C.V. Mosby.
12. Miceli, D. (1996). Sleep and activity. In A. Lueckenotte, (Ed.), Gerontologic Nursing (pp. 224-243). St. Louis: C.V. Mosby.
13. Richardson, S. (1994). Sleep pattern disturbance and related factors in the critically ill. In R.M. Carroll-Johnson (Ed.). Classification of nursing diagnoses: Proceedings of the tenth conference (pp. 218). Philadelphia: J.B. Lippincott.
14. Rodgers, A.E., Caruso, C.C. & Aldrich, M.S. (1993). Reliability of sleep diaries for assessment of sleep/wake patterns. Nursing Research. 42(6), 368-372.
15. Rossi, L., Fitzmaurice, J.B., Glynn, M.A. & Connors, K. (1987). Validation of the defining characteristics for sleep pattern disturbance. In A. McLane (Ed.). Classification of nursing diagnoses: Proceedings of the seventh conference (pp. 193-198). St. Louis: C.V. Cosby.
16. Shaver, J.L.F. & Giblin, E.C. (1989). Sleep. In J.J. Fitzpatrick, R.L. Taunton, & J.Q. Bencoliel (Eds.). Annual review of nursing research, (pp. 71-93). New York: Springer.

17. Spenceley, S.M. (1993). Sleep inquiry: A look with fresh eyes. Image: the Journal of Nursing Scholarship, 25(3), 249-256.
18. Westfall, U. (1992). Nursing chronotherapeutics: A conceptual framework. Image: the Journal of Nursing Scholarship, 24(4), 307-312.
19. Perez, V. & Coler, M. (1997). Sleep pattern disturbance: New defining characteristics and related factors are indicated. In M. Rantz & P. LeMone (Eds.) Classification of nursing diagnoses: Proceedings of the twelfth conference. Glendale, CA: CINAHL.

RECOMMENDED NANDA STAGING: 2.3

SPIRITUAL DISTRESS RISK (NANDA None)

DEFINITION: At risk for an altered sense of harmonious connectedness with all of life and the universe in which dimensions that transcend and empower the self may be disrupted.

RISK FACTORS: [6,12]
Energy-consuming anxiety [2,13]
Low self-esteem [1,2,4,13]
Mental illness, e.g. chronic depression [9,13]
Physical illness [2,10,13]
Blocks to self-love [1,2,7]
Poor relationships [2,5,9,12]
Physical or psychological stress [3,4,9,10,13]
Substance abuse [13]
Loss of loved one [10,13]
Natural disasters [13]
Situation losses [3,4,10,13]
Maturational losses [3,4,10,13]
Inability to forgive [1,9]

REFERENCES:
1. Burkhardt, M.A. (1989). Spirituality: An analysis of the concept. Holistic Nursing Practice, 3(3), 69-77.
2. Ellison, C.W. (1983). Spiritual well-being: Conceptualization and measurement. Journal of Psychology and Theology, 11(4), 330-339.
3. Emblen, J.D. (1992). Religion and spirituality defined according to current use in nursing literature. Journal of Professional Nursing, 8(1), 41-47.
4. Haase, J.E. et al., (1992). Simultaneous concept analysis of spiritual perspective, hope, acceptance and self transcendence. Image- The Journal of Nursing Scholarship, 24(2), 141-46.
5. Labun, E. (1988). Spiritual care: An element in nursing care planning. Journal of Advanced Nursing, 13(3), 314-320.
6. McHolm, F. (1991). A nursing diagnosis validation study: Defining characteristics of spiritual distress. In R.M. Carroll-Johnson (Ed.), Classification of nursing diagnoses: Proceedings of the ninth conference, Philadelphia: Lippincott, 112-119.
7. Moberg, D.O. (1984). Subjective measures of spiritual well-being. Review of Religious Research, 25(4), 351-364.
8. Paloutzian, R.F. and Ellison, C.W. (1982). Loneliness, spiritual well-being and the quality of life. In L.A. Peplau & D. Perlman (Eds.). Loneliness: A sourcebook of current theory, research and therapy, New York: Wiley Interscience, 224-237.
9. Reed, P.G. (1992). An emerging paradigm for the investigation of spirituality in nursing. Research in Nursing and Health, 15(5), 349-357.
10. Smucker, C. (1996). A phenomenological description of the experience of spiritual distress. Nursing Diagnosis, 7(2), 81-91.
11. Steiger, N.J. & Lipson, J.G. (1985). Psychological and spiritual well-being. In N.J. Steiger & J.G Lipson (Eds.). Self-care nursing: Theory and practice. Bowie, Maryland: Brady Communications Company, Inc., 208-235.
12. Weatherall, J. & Creason, N. (1987). Validation of the nursing diagnosis, spiritual distress. In A.M. McLane (Ed.), Classification of nursing diagnoses: Proceedings of the seventh conference, St. Louis: Mosby, 182-185.
13. Hill, L. & Smith, N. (1985). Self-Care nursing: Promotion of health. Englewood Cliffs, NJ: Prentice-Hall, Inc.

RECOMMENDED NANDA STAGING: 2.3

SPIRITUAL INTEGRITY ALTERATION (NANDA Spiritual Distress (Distress of the Human Spirit))

DEFINITION: Disrupted sense of harmonious connectedness with all of life and the universe in which dimensions that transcend and empower the self have been disrupted. [5]

SIGNS AND SYMPTOMS (Observed or Reported):

Expresses concern with meaning of life/death and/or belief systems [3,4,5,6,8,11,12,13]

Anger toward God [3,5,6,12]

Questions meaning of suffering [1,3,5]

Verbalizes inner conflict about beliefs [3,11]

Verbalizes concern about relationship with deity [6,12]

Questions meaning of own existence [10,12]

Unable to participate in usual religious practices [3,6]

Seeks spiritual assistance [6]

Questions moral/ethical implications of therapeutic regimen [3,4,6]

Displacement of anger toward religious representatives [6]

Description of nightmares/sleep disturbances [5,6]

Alteration in behavior/mood evidenced by anger, crying, withdrawal, preoccupation, anxiety, hostility, or apathy [6]

Altered transcendent relationships [1,3,5,12]

Perceived distress due to sudden disruption of life by some sudden or unexpected event/life transition/crisis [11,12]

Requests for assistance from "beyond" [12]

Experiences of spiritual pain, alienation anxiety, guilt, anger, loss, despair, regret [2,9,12]

RELATED FACTORS:

Separation from religious/cultural ties [6]

Challenged belief and value system, e.g., due to moral/ethical implications of therapy, due to intense suffering [1,3,5]

Psychological makeup which does not embrace spiritual capacity [4]

Traumatic experience [12]

Compromised upbringing [2,5]

Philosophy of life which does not include spiritual dimension [10]

Decreased integration of individual beliefs and values into daily life [3,6]

Inability to experience and express personal spirituality [6,9,10,12]

REFERENCES:

1. Burkhardt, M.A. (1989). Spirituality: An analysis of the concept. Holistic Nursing Practice, 3(3), 69-77.
2. Ellison, C.W. (1983). Spiritual well-being: Conceptualization and measurement. Journal of Psychology and Theology, 11(4), 330-339.
3. Emblen, J.D. (1992). Religion and spirituality defined according to current use in nursing literature. Journal of Professional Nursing, 8(1), 41-47.
4. Haase, J.E. et al., (1992). Simultaneous concept analysis of spiritual perspective, hope, acceptance and self-transcendence. Image: the Journal of Nursing Scholarship, 24(2), 141-147.
5. Hill, L. & Smith, N. (1985). Spirituality. In self-care nursing: Promotion of health, Englewood Cliffs, NJ: Prentice Hall, Inc.
6. Labun, E. (1988). Spiritual care: An element in nursing care planning. Journal of Advanced Nursing, 13(3), 314-320.
7. McHolm, F. (1991). A nursing diagnosis validation study: Defining characteristics of spiritual distress. In R.M. Carroll-Johnson (Ed.), Classification of nursing diagnoses: Proceedings of the ninth conference, Philadelphia: Lippincott, 112-119.
8. Moberg, D.O. (1984). Subjective measures of spiritual well-being. Review of Religious Research, 25, 4, 351-364.
9. O'Brien, M.E. (1982). The need for spiritual integrity. In H. Yura and M.B. Walsh (Eds.), Human Needs and the Nursing Process, Norwalk, Connecticut: Appleton-Century-Crofts.
10. Paloutzian, R.F. and Ellison, C.W. (1982). Loneliness, spiritual well-being and the quality of life. In L.A. Peplau, and D., Perlman, (Eds.) Loneliness: A source book of current theory, research and therapy, New York: Wiley Interscience, 224-237.

11. Reed, P.G. (1992). An emerging paradigm for the investigation of spirituality in nursing. <u>Research in Nursing & Health, 15</u>(5), 349-357.

12. Smucker, C. (1996). A phenomenological description of the experience of spiritual distress. <u>Nursing Diagnosis, 7</u>(2), 81-91.

13. Steiger, N.J. and Lipson, J.G. (1985). Psychological and spiritual well-being. In N.J. Steiger, and J.G. Lipson, (Eds). <u>Self-care nursing: Theory and practice</u>, (pp. 208-235). Bowie, Maryland: Brady Communications Company, Inc.,

14. Weatherall, J. & Creason, N. (1987). Validation of the nursing diagnosis, spiritual distress. In A.M. McLane (Ed.), <u>Classification of nursing diagnoses: Proceedings of the seventh conference</u>, St. Louis: Mosby, 182-185.

<u>**RECOMMENDED NANDA STAGING**</u>**:** 2.2

SPIRITUAL INTEGRITY ALTERATION RISK [9] (NANDA At Risk for Altered Spiritual Integrity)

DEFINITION: At risk for an altered sense of harmonious connectedness with all of life and the universe in which dimensions that transcend and empower the self may be disrupted.

RISK FACTORS: [8,14]

Energy-consuming anxiety [2,5]

Mental illness such as: chronic depression [5,11]

Physical illness [2,5,12]

Blocks to self-love [1,2,4,6,8,9,11]

Poor relationships e.g lack of shared values, communications [2,6,11,14]

Physical/ psychological stress [3,4,5,10,11,12]

Substance abuse [5]

Natural disasters [5]

Personal losses [3,4,5,12]

Situational losses [3,4,5,12]

Maturational losses [3,4,5,12]

REFERENCES:

1. Burkhardt, M.A. (1989). Spirituality: An analysis of the concept. Holistic Nursing Practice, 3(3), 69-77.
2. Ellison, C.W. (1983). Spiritual well-being: Conceptualization and measurement. Journal of Psychology and Theology, 11(4), 330-339.
3. Emblen, J.D. (1992). Religion and spirituality defined according to current use in nursing literature. Journal of Professional Nursing, 8(1), 41-47.
4. Haase, J.E. et al., (1992). Simultaneous concept analysis of spiritual perspective, hope, acceptance and self-transcendence. Image: the Journal of Nursing Scholarship, 24(2), 141-147.
5. Hill, L. & Smith, N. (1985). Self-care nursing: Promotion of health. Englewood Cliffs, NJ: Prentice-Hall, Inc.
6. Labun, E. (1988). Spiritual care: An element in nursing care planning. Journal of Advanced Nursing, 13(3), 314-320.
7. McHolm, F. (1991). A nursing diagnosis validation study: Defining characteristics of spiritual distress. In R.M. Carroll-Johnson (Ed.), Classification of nursing diagnoses: Proceedings of the ninth conference, Philadelphia: Lippincott, 112-119.
8. Moberg, D.O. (1984). Subjective measures of spiritual well-being. Review of Religious Research, 25(4), 351-364.
9. O'Brien, M.E. (1982). The need for spiritual integrity. In H. Yura & M.B. Walsh (Eds.), Human Needs and the Nursing Process, Norwalk, Connecticut: Appleton-Century-Crofts.
10. Paloutzian, R.F., & Ellison, C.W. (1982). Loneliness, spiritual well-being and the quality of life. In Peplau, L.A. & Perlman, D., (Eds.) Loneliness: A source book of current theory, research and therapy, New York: Wiley Interscience, 224-237.
11. Reed, P.G. (1992). An emerging paradigm for the investigation of spirituality in nursing. Research in Nursing and Health, 15(5), 349-357.
12. Smucker, C. (1996). A phenomenological description of the experience of spiritual distress. Nursing Diagnosis, 7(2), 81-91.
13. Steiger, N.J., & Lipson, J.G. (1985). Psychological and spiritual well-being. In N.J. Steiger, & J.G. Lipson, Self-care Nursing: Theory and Practice, (pp.208-235). Bowie, Maryland: Brady Communications Company, Inc.
14. Weatherall, J. & Creason, N. (1987). Validation of the nursing diagnosis, spiritual distress. In A.M. McLane (Ed.), Classification of nursing diagnoses: Proceedings of the seventh conference, St. Louis: Mosby, 182-185.

RECOMMENDED NANDA STAGING: 2.3

SPIRITUAL INTEGRITY ENHANCEMENT POTENTIAL (NANDA Potential for Enhanced Spiritual Well-Being)

DEFINITION: Heightened sense of harmonious connectedness with all of life and the universe through dimensions that transcend and empower the self.

SIGNS AND SYMPTOMS (Observed or Reported):

Expressions of :
Faith/Belief [4]
Hope (connectedness to possibilities
  and powers beyond the current situation) [5,8]
Meaning and purpose in life
  (connectedness with one's inner values and with
  a greater purpose in life) [1,4,5,8]
World view (outlook on life; cultural
  perspective) [9]
Peace/Serenity [4,8]
Love [5,8]
Forgiveness of self & others, e.g. avenue for
  facilitating connectedness by dissolving
  excessive guilt [5,8]

Behaviors:
Prays [5]
Participates in religious activities [5]
Church/spiritual rites and passages [5]
Reports mystical experiences [5]
Requests for and interactions with
  spiritual leaders [6]
Meditates [6]
Sings [6]
Displays creative energy [4]
Reads spiritual literature [6]

Provides service to others [6]

Patterns of Connectedness: [1,2,4,8]
  Intrapersonal (connectedness within oneself, inner
    values, greater purpose in life)
  Interpersonal (connectedness with others, e.g.)
  Transpersonal (connectedness to the unseen e.g.,
    a power/force greater than the self and ordinary
    resources, or God)
  Environmental (connectedness with all of life
    and nature; social and physical)

RELATED FACTORS: (as culturally appropriate)
Desire to transcend the realm of the material,
  capacity of transcendent values [2,3,9]
Wholesome self-concept [1,2]
Receptiveness to others, environment,
  universe, higher power [1,3]
Childhood experiences with family and friends [2,4]
Socialization experiences [2,4]
Supportive relationships with other people [2,4,7]
Realistic orientations toward loss and
  deprivation [2]
Satisfaction with life [4]
Level of spiritual maturity [1,2,3]
Crises/Opportunities [1]

REFERENCES:
1. Burkhardt, M.A. (1989). Spirituality: An analysis of the concept. Holistic Nursing Practice, 3(3), 69-77.
2. Ellison, C.W. (1983). Spiritual well-being: Conceptualization and measurement. Journal of Psychology and Theology, 11(4), 330-339.
3. Emblen, J.D. (1992). Religion and spirituality defined according to current use in nursing literature. Journal of Professional Nursing, 8(1), 41-47.
4. Haase, J.E. et al., (1992). Simultaneous concept analysis of spiritual perspective, hope, acceptance and self-transcendence. Image: the Journal of Nursing Scholarship, 24(2), 141-147.
5. Labun, E. (1988). Spiritual care: An element in nursing care planning. Journal of Advanced Nursing, 13(3), 314-320.
6. Moberg, D.O. (1984). Subjective measures of spiritual well-being. Review of Religious Research, 25(4), 351-364.
7. Paloutzian, R.F., & Ellison, C.W. (1982). Loneliness, spiritual well-being and the quality of life. In L.A. Peplau, & D. Perlman, (Eds.). Loneliness: A source book of current theory, research and therapy, (pp. 224-237). New York: Wiley Interscience
8. Reed, P.G. (1992). An emerging paradigm for the investigation of spirituality in nursing. Research in Nursing & Health, 15(5), 349-357.
9. Steiger, N.J., & Lipson, J.G. (1985). Psychological and spiritual well-being. In N.J. Steiger, & J.G. Lipson, Self-care nursing: Theory and practice, (pp. 208-235). Bowie, Maryland: Brady Communications Company, Inc.,

RECOMMENDED NANDA STAGING: 2.3

SWALLOWING IMPAIRMENT (NANDA Impaired Swallowing)

DEFINITION: Abnormal functioning of the swallowing mechanism associated with deficits in oral, pharyngeal, or esophageal structure or function.

SIGNS AND SYMPTOMS (Observed or Reported):

Oral Phase Impairment:
Food falls from mouth[1, 13]
Pooling in Lateral sulci[1, 11]
Sialorrhea or drooling[6, 8, 13]
Lack of tongue action to form bolus[1, 6, 11]
Lack of chewing [1, 10]
Premature entry of bolus[1, 11]
Inability to clear oral cavity[1, 11]
Abnormality in oral phase by swallow
    study [1, 4, 5, 7, 8, 10, 13, 14, 15]
Coughing, choking, gagging before a swallow [9, 11]
Incomplete lip closure[7, 9]
Food pushed out of mouth[1, 13]
Slow bolus formation[1, 13]
Piecemeal deglutition[1, 10]
Weak suck resulting in inefficient nippling[1, 11]
Long meals with little consumption[1, 11]
Nasal reflux[1, 2]

Pharyngeal Phase Impairment:
Delayed swallow[1, 10]
Gurgly voice quality[1, 6]
Choking, coughing or gagging[1, 6, 12]
Multiple swallows[1, 8]
Altered head positions[1, 10]
Effortful swallow[1]
Inadequate laryngeal elevation[1, 8]
Abnormality in pharyngeal phase by swallow
    study [1, 4, 5, 7, 8, 10, 13, 14, 15]
Recurrent pulmonary Infections[1, 11, 13]
Unexplained fevers[1]
Nasal reflux[1, 2]
Food refusal[1, 13]

Esophageal Phase Impairment:
Choking and or coughing with swallow [7, 8, 13]
Abnormality in esophageal phase by swallow
    study[1, 4, 5, 7, 8, 10, 13, 14, 15]
Regurgitation of gastric contents/wet burps[1, 7, 8, 13]
Vomiting[1, 7, 8, 13]
Heartburn or epigastric pain[1, 7, 13]

Complaints of "something stuck" [9, 13]
Unexplained irritability surrounding
    mealtime[1, 7, 11]
Hyperextension of head/arching during/after
    meals[1, 12]
Nighttime coughing/wakening[7, 13]
Odynophagia[1, 7, 13]
Vomitous on pillow [11, 13]
Repetitive swallowing/ruminating[1, 13]
Hematemesis[1, 12]
Acidic smelling breath[1, 7, 8, 13]
Bruxism [3]
Food refusal/volume limiting[1, 7, 8, 11]

RELATED FACTORS:

Neurologic Deficits:
Cerebral palsy [1, 4, 5, 13]
Premature infants [1, 8]
Traumatic head injury [1, 13]
Developmental delay[1, 8, 13]

Congenital and Anatomical Deficits:
Upper airway anomalies[1, 4, 5, 12, 13, 14, 14]
Oral cavity/oropharynx[1, 4, 5, 12, 13, 14, 15]
Laryngeal abnormalities[1, 4, 5, 12, 13, 14, 15]
Tracheal, laryngeal, esophageal defects[1, 5, 8, 13, 15]
Upper airway anomalies[1, 4, 5, 12, 13, 14, 15]
Nasal/nasopharyngeal cavity[1, 4, 5, 12, 13, 14, 54]
Gastroesophageal reflux disease[7, 11, 15]
Achalasia[7, 13, 15]
Acquired anatomical defects
External trauma[5, 13]
Internal trauma[5, 13]

Others:
Respiratory disorders[13, 15]
History of tube feeding[1, 14]
Failure to thrive/protein energy
    malnutrition[1, 8, 12, 13]
Behavioral feeding problems[1, 8, 13]
Conditions with significant hypotonia[1, 12, 13]
Cranial nerve involvement[1, 14]
Congenital heart disease[9, 15]
Self injurious behavior[2]

REFERENCES:
1. Arvedson, J. & Brodsky, L. (Eds.). (1993). Pediatric swallowing and feeding. San Diego: Singular Publishing Group, Inc.
2. Bosch, J., Van Dyke, C., Smith, S. & Poulton, S. (1997). Role of medical condition in the exacerbation of self-injurious behavior: An exploratory study. Mental Retardation, 35(2), 124-130.

3. Boyt, M.A. (1997). A refinement of the Nursing Diagnosis "Impaired swallowing". <u>Unpublished Master's Thesis</u>. University of Iowa. p. 57.

4. Christensen, J. (1989). Developmental approach to pediatric neurogenic dysphagia. <u>Dysphagia, 3</u>(3), 131-134.

5. Cohen, S. (1983). Difficulty with swallowing. In C. Bluestone & S. Stool (Eds.), <u>Pediatric otolaryngology</u>, (pp. 843-849). Philadelphia: W.B. Saunders.

6. Feinberg, M. (1997). The effects of medication on swallowing. In B. Sonies, <u>Dysphagia: A continuum of care,</u> (pp. 107-120). Gaithersburg, MD: Aspen.

7. Hendrix, T. R. (1993). Art and science of history taking in the patient with difficulty swallowing. <u>Dysphagia, 8</u>(2), 69-73.

8. Kramer, S. & Eicher, P. M. (1993). The evaluation of pediatric feeding abnormalities. <u>Dysphagia, 8</u>(3), 215-24.

9. Lespargot, A., Langevin, M., Muller, S. & Guillemont, S. (1993). Swallowing disturbances associated with drooling in cerebral-palsied children. <u>Developmental Medicine and Child Neurology, 35</u>(4), 298-304.

10. Logemann, J. (1983). <u>Evaluation and treatment of swallowing disorders</u>. Austin: Pro-Ed.

11. Morris, S., (1989) Development of oral-motor skills in the neurologically impaired child receiving non-oral feedings. <u>Dysphagia, 3</u>(3), 135-154.

12. Ramsay, M., Gisel, E. & Boutry, M. (1993). Non-organic failure to thrive: Growth failure secondary to feeding skills disorder. <u>Developmental Medicine and Child Neurology, 35</u>(4), 285-297.

13. Tuchman, D., & Walter, R. (Eds.). (1994). <u>Disorders of feeding and swallowing in infants and children</u>. San Diego: Singular Publishing Group, Inc.

14. Weiss, M. (1988). Dysphagia in infants and children. <u>Otolaryngologic Clinics of North America, 21</u>(4), 727-735.

15. Wolf, L. S., & Glass, R. P. (1992). <u>Feeding and swallowing disorders in infancy</u>. Tucson: Therapy Skill Builders.

<u>RECOMMENDED NANDA STAGING</u>: 2.1

TOILETING SELF CARE DEFICIT (NANDA Toileting Self Care Deficit)

DEFINITION: An impaired ability to perform or complete own toileting activities

SIGNS AND SYMPTOMS (Observed or Reported):

Inability to:
  Recognize & respond to full bladder [11]
  Recognize & respond to urge to have a bowel movement [11]
  Empty bowel or bladder [11]
  Go to toilet or commode [5,8,9]
  Sit on or rise from toilet or commode [5,8,9]
  Manipulate clothing [5,8,9]
  Carry out proper toilet hygiene e.g. wiping perineal area & washing hands [5,8,9,10]
  Flush toilet or commode [5,8,9]

Suggested Functional Level Classification: [4]
  0=Completely independent.
  1=Requires use of equipment or device.
  2=Requires help from another person for assistance, supervision, or teaching.
  3=Requires help from another person and equipment device.
  4=Dependant, does not participate in activity.

RELATED FACTORS:
Impaired transfer ability [9]
Impaired mobility status [4, 6,7,9]
Weakness/tiredness [6, 7,8]
Pain/discomfort [2, 6,7]
Perceptual or cognitive impairment [6,7]
Neuromuscular impairment [6, 7]
Musculoskeletal impairment [6, 7]
Severe anxiety [6, 7]
Environmental barriers [1, 6,7]
Decreased/lack of motivation [9]

REFERENCES:
1. Baer, C.A., Delorey, M. & Fitzmaurice, J.B. (1984). A study to evaluate the validity of the rating system for self-care deficit. In M.J. Kim., G.K. McFarland, & A.M. McLane, (Eds.). Classification of Nursing Diagnoses: Proceedings of the Fifth National Conference. St. Louis, MO: The C.V. Mosby Company.
2. Chang, B. (1994). Validity of concepts for selecting nursing diagnoses. Clinical Nursing Research, 3(3), 183-208.
3. Chang, B.L., Hirsch, M., Brazal-Villanueva, E. & Iverson, D.W. (1990). Self-care deficit with etiologies: Reliability of measurement. Nursing Diagnosis, 1(1), 31-36.
4. Jones, E. (1974). Patient Classification for Long-Term Care: Users' Manual (Adapted from). HEW, Publication No. HRA-74-3107.
5. Levin, R.f., Krainovitch, B.C., Bahrenburg, E., & Mitchell, C.A. (1989). Diagnostic content validity of nursing diagnoses. Image- Journal of Nursing Scholarship, 21(1), 40-44.
6. McKeighen, R.J., Mehmert, P.A. & Dickel, C.A. (1990). Bathing/hygiene self-care deficit: Defining characteristics and related factors across age groups and diagnosis related groups in an acute care setting. Nursing Diagnosis, 1(4), 155-161.
7. McKeighen, .R.J., Mehmert, P.A. & Dickel, C.A. (1991). Self-care deficit, bathing/hygiene: Defining characteristics and related factors utilized by staff nurses in an acute care setting. In Carroll-Johnson, R.M. (Ed.). Classification of nursing diagnoses: Proceedings of the ninth national conference. Philadelphia, PA: J.B. Lippincott Company.
8. Rhodes, V.A., Watson, P.M. & Hanson, B.M. (1988). Patients' descriptions of the influence of tiredness and weakness on self-care abilities. Cancer Nursing, 11(3), 186-194.
9. Smits, .W. & Kee, C.C. (1992). Correlates of self-care among the independent elderly: Self-concept affects well-being. Journal of Gerontological Nursing, 18(9), 13-18.
10. Waters, K.R. (1994). Getting dressed in the early morning: Styles of staff/patient interaction on rehabilitation hospital wards for elderly people. Journal of Advanced Nursing, 19, 239-248.
11. Johnson, M. & Maas, M. (Eds.). (1997). Nursing outcomes classification (NOC). St. Louis: The C.V.Mosby Company.

RECOMMENDED NANDA STAGING: 2.3

UNINTENTIONAL INJURY RISK: FALLS (NANDA Risk for Injury)

DEFINITION: Accentuated susceptibility to inadvertent falls that may cause physical harm and that can be prevented or controlled.

RISK FACTORS:

Demographic:
- History of falls [1,3,5,14]
- Under two years of age [6]
- Age 60 or over [2,3,7,9,10,11]
- Female (if elderly) [2,14]
- Unmarried [2]

Physiological:
- Presence of acute illness [12,13]
- Admission related to oncology or orthopedics [3]
- General pathological conditions with the majority being cardiac problems [10]
- Post-operative conditions [10]
- Visual difficulties [2,3]
- Hearing difficulties [2,13]
- Thin (Body Mass Index <21) [2]
- Weakness [3]
- Poor endurance [13]
- Poor back flexibility [13]
- Decreased lower extremity strength [12,13]
- Difficulty with gait [1,12,13]
- Mobility deficit [7]
- Arthritis [2]
- Osteoporosis/hip fracture [2]
- Drop of 20 mmHg or more in systolic blood pressure on standing [5,13]
- History of myocardial infarction or other cardiovascular disorders [9]
- History of diabetes mellitus [9]
- Sleeplessness [3]
- Faintness when turning or extending neck [13]
- Anemias [10]
- Vascular disease [2]

- Endoplasms [10]
- Temperature elevation [3]
- Urgency and/or incontinence [1,3]
- Diarrhea [3]

Cognitive:
- Mental status change [1,5,7,13,14]
- Dementia [5]

Environmental:
- Unfamiliar, dimly lit room [1]
- Confined to chair [1]
- Climbing over side rails [1]
- Ramps, curbcuts, and doorways were frequent settings for wheelchair tips/falls [8]
- No use of gate on stairs [15]
- No use of window gaurds [15]
- No protection on sharp corners in home [15]
- No anti-slip material in bath and/or shower [15]

Medications:
- Hypnotics or tranquilizers [10,12]
- Tricyclic antidepressants [11]
- Alcohol use [9]
- Antianxiety drugs [9]

Functional/Situational
- Difficulty with activities of daily living [1]
- Lack of parental supervision [6]
- Difficulty walking indoor [14]
- Cannot leave the institution without difficulty [14]

REFERENCES:

1. Berryman, E., Gaskin, D., Jones, A., Tolley, F., & MacMullen, J. (1989). Point by point: Predicting elders' falls. Geriatric Nursing: American Journal of Care for the Aging, 10(4), 199-201.
2. Dunn, J.E., Rudberg, M.A., Furner, S.E., & Cassel, C.K. (1992). Mortality, disability, and falls in older persons: The role of underlying disease and disability. American Journal of Public Health, 82(3), 395-400.
3. Hendrich, A.L. (1988). An effective unit-based fall prevention plan. Journal of Nursing Quality Assurance, 3(1), 28-36.
4. Henry, P.C., Hauber, R.P., & Rice, M. (1992). Factors associated with closed head injury in a pediatric population. Journal of Neuroscience Nursing, 24(6), 311-316.
5. Hernandez, M., & Miller, J. (1986). How to reduce falls. Geriatric Nursing: American Journal of Care for the Aging, 7(2), 97-102.
6. Hu, X., Wesson, D., & Kenney, B. (1993). Home injuries to children. Canadian Journal of Public Health,

84(3), 155-158.

7. Kilpack, V., Boehm, J., Smith, N., & Mudge, B. (1991). Using research-based interventions to decrease patient falls. Applied Nursing Research. 4(2), 50-56.

8. Kirby, R., Ackroyd-Stolarz, S.A., Brown, M.G., Kirkland, S.A., & MacLeod, D.A. (1994). Wheelchair-related accidents caused by trips and falls among noninstitutionalized users of manually propelled wheelchairs in Nova Scotia. American Journal of Physical Medicine & Rehabilitation, 73(5), 319-330.

9. Malmivaara, A., Heliovaara, M., Knekt, P., Reunanen, A., & Aromaa, A. (1993). Risk factors for injurious falls leading to hospitalization or death in a cohort of 19,500 adults. American Journal of Epidemiology, 138(6), 384-394.

10. Plati, C., Lanara, V., & Mantas, J. (1992). Risk factors responsible for patient's falls. Scandinavian Journal of Caring Sciences, 6(2), 113-118.

11. Poster, E.C., Pelletier, L.R., & Kay, K. (1991). A retrospective cohort study of falls in a psychiatric inpatient setting. H&CP: Hospital and Community Psychiatry, 42(7), 714-720.

12. Tinetti, M.E., Speechley, M., & Ginter, S.F. (1988). Risk factors for falls among elderly persons living in the community. The New England Journal of Medicine, 319(26), 1701-1707.

13. Tinetti, M.E., Williams, T.F., & Mayewski, R. (1986). Fall risk index for elderly patients based on number of chronic disabilities. The American Journal of Medicine, 80, 429-434.

14. Vellas, B., Cayla, F., Bocquet, H., dePemille, F., & Albarede, J.L. (1987). Prospective study of restriction of activity in old people after falls. Age and Aging Journal, 16(3), 189-193.

15. Wortel, E., & de Geus, G. (1993). Prevention of home related injuries of pre-school children: Safety measures taken by mothers. Health Education Research, 8(2), 217-231.

RECOMMENDED NANDA STAGING: 2.3

URINARY URGE INCONTINENCE RISK (NANDA None)

DEFINITION: Risk for involuntary loss of urine associated with a sudden, strong sensation or urinary urgency.

RISK FACTORS:
Detrusor muscle instability with impaired
   contractility [2,3]
Detrusor hyperreflexia from: [2,3]
   cystitis, urethritis, tumors, renal calculi, central
   nervous system disorders above pontine
   micturition center
Ineffective toileting habits[1]
Effects of pharmacologic agents[1], e.g.
   anticholinergics, beta adrenergics, alpha
   adrenergic blockers or agonists, calcium-channel
   blockers, diuretics, narcotics caffeine or alcohol
   intake[4]
Small bladder capacity [4]
Involuntary sphincter relaxation[2]

REFERENCES:

1. Engberg, D.I.H., McDowell, J. & Wilkerson, G. (1996). Urinary function. In A. G. Luekenotte. (Ed.). <u>Gerontological nursing</u> (pp. 693-726). St. Louis: C.V. Mosby.
2. Fantl, J.A., Newman D.K., Colling, J., et al. (1996). Urinary incontinence in adults: Acute and chronic management. <u>Clinical practice guidelines, No.2 1996 update</u>. Department of Health and Human Services. Public Health Service, Agency for Health Care Policy and Research. AHCPR Publication No. 96-0682. Rockville, MD: U.S.
3. Gray, M. & Dougherty, M. (1987). Urinary incontinence - pathophysiology and treatment. <u>Journal of Enterostomal Therapy, 14</u>(4), 152-62.
4. Specht, J., Tunink, P., Maas, M. & Bukecheck, B. (1991). Urinary incontinence. In M. Maas, K. Buckwalter & M. Hardy (Eds.). <u>Nursing diagnoses & interventions for the elderly</u>, Redwood City, CA: Addison-Wesley, 181-204.

RECOMMENDED NANDA STAGING: 2.3

Part III
Future Directions

The research plan outlined in Part I identifies remaining steps to be addressed. These include a) development of candidate labels, b) expert validation, and c) clinical validation. Further, future work must address classification/taxonomic structure.

Development of Candidate Labels

As discussed in Part I, development of candidate labels will continue. A database of candidate labels has been maintained throughout the refinement and development phases. Candidate diagnosis labels were identified in data collected in early research on diagnoses used and needed for critical care nursing and genetics nursing (Manuscript in process). Next, candidate diagnoses were identified through concept analysis methods used by the DWGs. These two methods have produced a large database of candidate diagnoses (approximately 400). The methodology for examination and analysis of this list of candidate diagnoses will be developed, piloted, and used for our next aim. It will include: (a) examination for conceptual redundancy; (b) comparison to existing lists of diagnoses, interventions, and outcomes using the Library of Medicine metathesaurus; c) prioritization of the candidate diagnoses for development; (d) use simultaneous concept analysis to differentiate those candidate diagnoses that may be conceptually close to existing labels; and (e) develop each prioritized label. Team members and satellite groups will using the same Concept Analysis Protocol adopted for all labels.

Eight (8) Satellite Diagnosis Work Groups (SDWG) have been organized through the efforts of nurses who are interested in developing new diagnosis concepts. These NDEC DWGs are external to the University of Iowa. Each group is developing diagnoses in areas of known gaps in the existing nomenclature. Their contributions will be added to the list of new diagnosis labels submitted by NDEC to NANDA.

The most distant SDWG is located in England, with June Clark as the chairperson. This SDWG is focusing on the development of diagnoses related to nausea, vomiting, post-natal depression, delayed surgical recovery, and diagnoses needed to care for people with diabetes. Another distant site is located in New Orleans, Louisiana, where Susan Burger-deRada is chairing a group whose interest is neurophysiological dimensions of massage therapy. A third site is Ann Arbor, Michigan, where Donna Algase is organizing and conducting concept analysis training for a group of nursing experts interested in the development of diagnoses on cognitive impairment. A fourth SDWG is centered in Steven's Point, Wisconsin, with T. Heather Herdmann as chair. The interest in this SDWG is neonatal diagnoses. A fifth SDWG, chaired by Petra Lamfers in Iowa, is developing diagnoses for Advanced Practice Nurses. A group in Missouri, chaired by Jane Bostrick, is developing diagnoses of health issues related to the elderly. Nutritional diagnoses are being refined and developed with the assistance of Mary Jane Oakland who is a Professor in Nutritional Science from Iowa State University in Ames, Iowa. Last, Jeffrey Fouche, Senior Business Analyst for Patient Care Documentation for Columbia/HCA Information Systems, is developing a list of potential candidate diagnoses through additions to the Diagnosis Dictionary component of their software.

Expert Validation

Expert validation is just beginning. Research instruments that can be administered electronically have been developed and piloted (methods and copies of the instruments to be used are available from the authors upon request). The results of the pilot tests indicate that the instruments were retrievable and could be easily read if the recipients downloaded the documents. However, because participants had a diversity of e-mail software and hardware, the ability to download was at times a barrier. Therefore, NDEC will use the NDEC website (http://www.nursing.uiowa.edu/ndec/) for discussion and expert validation. Nurses in nursing specialties will be invited to participate.

Particular attention is being given to nurse expert validation from the international community. NDEC has recently been given permission to use the World Wide Nursing Diagnosis Forum (htttp://www.cnh.nl/wwndf) for discussion and validation of nursing diagnoses. To date, the NDEC labels have been reviewed by Cecile Boisvert, RN, M.Sc.N., France. Specific care will focus on the use of gerunds and congruity with adoptions in non-U.S. countries.

Clinical Validation

Clinical validation will follow expert validation. Several methods exist for clinical testing. These methods include (a) matching diagnoses to clients; (b) content analysis of chart/client record; or (c) case reviews. The matching of diagnosis labels, signs and symptoms, and related factors to clients can be used across settings. Further, client records can be examined across a variety of health delivery settings to determine if the diagnoses capture the phenomena represented in the records. This examination will be structured through the used of validation criteria (examples may be obtained from the authors upon request). Last, case example discussion at unit/service meetings will be used as an opportunity to examine the extent to which the diagnoses to be validated capture and represent client phenomena seen in every care setting. Use of these manual methods will be dependent upon obtaining external fnding.

Clinical validation of diagnostic labels, signs/symptoms, and related factors/risk factors is being conducted using computerized nursing information systems. Two acute healthcare sites have been selected for the initial clinical validation. Site selection was based on a) the quality of the information system including capability of supporting a nursing data repository; b) the orientation and staff development related to use of information systems and standardized languages; and c) existing relationships with information system departments. The American Nurses Association Nursing Information and Data set Evaluation Center Standards and Guidelines (NIDSEC) (NIDSEC, 1997) were used to establish the quality of the nursing information systems and data sets. All refined labels are being incorporated into the nursing data set in each site.

The data collection procedure for electronic retrieval of the NMDS elements comprises four steps: 1) preparation for data collection in the clinical site; 2) collection of clinical data; 3) transfer of clinical data to the research data repository; and 4) establishing accuracy of the computerized data (see Table 5). Sensitivity scores will be computed for all signs/symptoms linked to each label and for all signs/symptoms linked to each label associated with each respective related factor.

Table 5

Establishing Accuracy of Computerized Data

a. Establish consistency checks/programmed requirements of specific logical relationships between certain data items to support some degree of data accuracy

b. Evaluate for coding errors

c. Calculate frequencies for all data elements to determine data quality

d. Review calculated frequencies of occurrence of all data elements with clinicians to verify consistency with in-house statistical reports

Classification/Taxonomic Issues

Organizing the NDEC labels into a classification is the next logical step in supporting clinical decision making and knowledge development. One of the major initial aims of the NDEC work was the inductive development of a classification system, after refinement and extension of the labels. Such study may prove to be redundant or not useful given recent initiatives within NANDA. A Proposed NANDA Taxonomy 2 was shared with the NANDA membership at the 1997 Conference. This Proposed Taxonomy 2 represented two major shifts, a shift away from using the "Human Response Patterns" and a shift toward adopting a multi-axial classification/taxonomy. Proposed axes included: acuity, unit of care, developmental state, potentiality, and descriptor. For purposes of experimentation and issue identification, the 96 labels included in Part II of this manuscript were incorporated into the Proposed Taxonomy II (See Table 6). Several questions related to label placement and multi-axial issues arose.

Label Placement

Over time, questions have arose as to the desirability and ability of nursing to maintain category exclusivity within classifications. This point addresses inheritance of characteristics from the higher order category. Several questions emerge on this issue. They include: a) Is it desirable that a label be categorized into one and only one category? B) If a label is categorized in two or more categories does this mean that greater specificity and conceptual clarity of the label are needed? C) Is the ability of a data repository to support knowledge discovery compromised by multiple placements of labels? D) If one assumes that the category conveys context, does the same label within two different categories symbolize the same concept/phenomenon? E) Can a category preserve philosophical/theoretical perspective? These questions can be illustrated through consideration of the placement of "Hope Alteration" and "Hope Alteration Risk." Depending upon theoretical origin, these labels could be categorized both within Domain 6, Class 1 Self-concept and Domain 10 Values -

Table 6

NDEC and NANDA Proposed Taxonomy 2

Domain 1	Health perception-Health management
Class 1	Health awareness
	Health Enhancement Potential
Class 2	Health management behaviors
	Development Alteration
	Development Alteration Risk
	Growth Alteration
	Growth Alteration Risk
	Health Management Deficit
Class 3	Health promotion behaviors
	Health Enhancement Potential
Domain 2	Nutrition - metabolism
Class 1	Ingestion
	Breastfeeding Difficulty
	Breastfeeding Effectiveness
	Dentition Alteration
	Eating Difficulty
	Eating Reluctance
	Feeding Difficulty
	Swallowing Impairment
Class 2	Digestion
Class 3	Absorption
Class 4	Metabolism
Class 5	Hydration
	Fluid Volume Deficit
	Fluid Volume Excess
Class 6	Integumentary system
	Oral Soft Tissue Alteration
Domain 3	Elimination
Class 1	Urinary
	Functional Urinary Incontinence Risk
	Overflow Urinary Incontinence
	Overflow Urinary Incontinence Risk
	Constant Urinary Incontinence
	Reflex Urinary Incontinece
	Urinary Urge Incontinence Risk

Table 6

NDEC and NANDA Proposed Taxonomy 2

Class 2	Bowel
	Constipation
	Constipation Risk
	Diarrhea
	Bowel Incontinence
Class 3	Skin
Class 4	Lung
Domain 4	Energy Maintenance
Class 1	Sleep-rest
	Fatigue
	Sleep Deprivation
	Sleep Pattern Disturbance
Class 2	Activity-exercise
	Physical Mobility Alteration
Class 3	Cardio-respiratory
	Airway Clearance Ineffectiveness
	Breathing Pattern Ineffectiveness
	Cardiac Output Alteration
	Gas Exchange Impairment
Class 4	Activities of daily living
	Bathing/Hygiene Self Care Deficit
	Dressing/Grooming Self Care Deficit
	Feeding Self Care Deficit
	Toileting Self Care Deficit
Class 5	Energy field
	Energy Field Disturbance
Domain 5	Cognitive - Perceptual
Class 1	Sensation - perception
Class 2	Cognition
Class 3	Communication
Domain 6	Self-perception - Self-concept

Table 6

NDEC and NANDA Proposed Taxonomy 2

Class 1	Self-concept
	Hope Alteration
	Hope Alteration Risk
	Hope Enhancement Potential
	Powerlessness
	Powerlessness Risk
Class 2	Self-esteem
	Chronic Low Self-esteem
	Defensive Self-esteem
	Low Self-esteem Risk
	Positive Self-esteem
	Situational Low Self-esteem
Class 3	Body-image
Domain 7	Role relationships
Class 1	Caregiving roles
	Caregiver Role Strain
Class 2	Family relationships
	Insecure Parent-infant Attachment
	Insecure Parent-infant Attachment Risk
	Family Process Alteration
	Family Process Alteration: Alcoholism
	Secure Parent-infant Attachment
	Parenting Ineffectiveness
	Parenting Ineffectiveness Risk
Class 3	Role performance
	Role Performance Alteration
Class 4	Social relationships
Domain 8	Sexuality - Reproduction
Class 1	Sexuality patterns
Class 2	Reproductive function
Domain 9	Coping - Stress tolerance
Class 1	Post-trauma responses
	Post-trauma Syndrome
	Post-trauma Syndrome Risk
	Post-trauma Syndrome: Rape

Table 6

Class 2	Coping processes
	Impaired Adjustment
	Community Coping Ineffectiveness
	Coping Ineffectiveness
	Family Coping Enhancement Potential
	Family Coping Ineffectiveness
	Family Coping Ineffectiveness Risk
	Fear
Class 3	Neuro-behavioral stress responses
	Decreased Intracranial Adaptive Capacity
	Decreased Intracranial Adaptive Capacity Risk
	Autonomic Dysreflexia
	Autonomic Dysreflexia Risk
	Organized Infant Behavior Enhancement Potential
	Disorganized Infant Behavior
	Disorganized Infant Behavior Risk
Domain 10	Values - Beliefs
Class 1	Spiritual values/beliefs
	Family Decisional Conflict
	Family Nonadherance
	Spiritual Integrity Alteration
	Spiritual Integrity Alteration Risk
	Spiritual Integrity Enhancement Potential
Class 2	Health values/beliefs
	Family Decisional Conflict
	Family Nonadherance
Class 3	Personal values/beliefs
	Family Decisional Conflict
	Family Nonadherance
Domain 11	Safety - Protection
Class 1	Infection
Class 2	Physical injury
	Unintentional Injury Risk: Falls

Table 6

NDEC and NANDA Proposed Taxonomy 2

Class 3	Violence
	Self Mutilation
	Self Mutilation Risk
Class 4	Environmental hazards
Domain 12	Comfort
Class 1	Pain
	Acute Pain
	Chronic Pain
Class 2	Nausea/vomiting
Class 3	Itching

Beliefs, Class 1 Spiritual values/beliefs. Further, consider "Family Decisional Conflict" as an illustration. Can this label most accurately be placed in Class 1 Spiritual values/beliefs, Class 2 Health values, or Class 3 Personal values/beliefs? Ten electrolyte imbalance labels have been developed by NDEC, e.g. Hypercalemia, hypocalemia. How are these labels categorized - Domain 2 Nutrition, Class 1 Ingestion, Class 2 Digestion, Class 3 Absorption, or Class 4 Metabolism? Does "Health Enhancement Potential" more appropriately fit within Domain 1, Class 1 Health Awareness or Class 3 Health Promotion?

Establishing a multi-axial classification supports greater granularity by increasing the combinatorial possibilities of labels and poses interesting questions. For example, if the axes of acuity, unit of care, developmental state, potentiality, and descriptor are adopted, is there a need for Domain 7, Class 2 "Family relationships"? Also, how is the community unit of care integrated into this taxonomy? Should Domain 11, Class 4 "Environmental violence" be renamed to "Environment"? Should the classes within Domain 11 be neutral vs unhealthy? Should a sixth axis be considered, an axis that captures the level of clinical validity and reliability of the label (certainty)? That is, should a sixth axis be used to specify the developmental stages of nursing diagnoses?

NDEC refinements have been based on the desirability and utility of greater granularity. Multi-axial classifications support this position. Frequently, nursing knowledge development conveyed in the literature supports the validity of specific signs/symptoms and/or related factors for specific axes combinations with a label. Consequently, specific NDEC labels have been specified for clinically logical dimensions of labels, for example, each NDEC concept has individual, family, community dimensions (unit of care), a health continuum dimension (actual, risk, health/potential for enhancement. Implementing the multi-axial classification must retain this specificity of nursing knowledge while promoting greater span of diagnoses. One might expect to see numerous placeholders for each logical combination of axes applied to each concept in such a multi-axial classification. This approach would preserve and support the state of nursing science in clinical decision making and clinical validation of signs/symptoms for each diagnostic label. Further, the identification of labels to be development would be enhanced.

Conclusion

As the familiar Carpenter lyrics go "We've Only Just Begun," even though the 25th NANDA Anniversary was just celebrated. The timing is right, the environment is rich, the professional energy is high leaving the questions: Can the timing, environment, and energy support continuing development of nursing diagnoses and a classification that will support nursing and patient/consumer visibility in the new millenium? Can this work support the interdisciplinary reality of the practice settings? Can international collaboration be enhanced? And can dialogues to strengthen the articulation of thesauri, classifications, and nomenclatures be more frequent and more productive?

Improving clinical outcomes is dependent upon the socialization and education of nurses as knowledge workers. How can the language/classification work address these needs? What strategies are needed to foster the integration of the classification work into curricula, to expand research agendas that capitalize on the newest knowledge discovery tools and nursing data repositories, and to implement these efforts into practice and clinical information systems? Language and classification work must address these needs.

The development of languages for diagnoses, interventions, and outcomes makes it necessary to consider several new and important questions. These questions included: A) Is it possible to maintain the integrity of any one nursing classification without intimate, intense deliberations with developers of other languages/classifications? B) Can NANDA/NDEC address diagnostic decisions involving signs/symptoms and related factors without consideration of NOC indicators? C) Can NANDA/NDEC and NOC support outcomes research without NIC interventions and activities? D) Are we prepared to enhance the mapping work between non-standardized and standardized vocabularies/languages/classifications? And E) Are we prepared, in mind and spirit, to support the umbrella work that must occur in nursing and within the interdisciplinary context to quantify and qualify what we do?

The collaborative agreement between NANDA and NDEC has stimulated dialogue on diagnosis concept development, refinement, and testing. It is the hope of the NDEC team that the outcome of this dialogue will be a nomenclature which captures client phenomena that is useful for the evaluation of care effectiveness and care costs.

References

American Nurses Association. (1995). *Nursing data systems: The emerging framework.* Washington, DC: Author.

Aydelotte, M.K., & Peterson, K.H. (1987). Keynote Address: nursing taxonomies — state of the art. In A. McLane (Ed.), *Classification of nursing diagnoses: Proceedings of the seventh conference* (pp. 1-16). St. Louis: Mosby.

Blewitt, K. K., & Jones, K. R. (1996). Using elements of the Nursing Minimum Data Set for determining outcomes. *Journal of*

Nursing Administration, 26(6), 48-56.

Carpenito, L. (1994). *Nursing diagnosis: Application to clinical practice.* Philadelphia: J.B. Lippincott.

Craft-Rosenberg, M., & Delaney, C. (1997) NANDA-NDEC Joint Venture Research Project. In M.J. Rantz, & P. LeMone, *Classification of nursing diagnoses: Proceedings of the twelfth conference.* Glendale, CA: CINAHL Information Systems.

Delaney, C., & Huber, D. (1996). *A Nursing Management Minimum Data Set (NMMDS): A report of an invitational conference.* Chicago, IL: American Organization of Nurse Executives.

Evans, D.A., Cimino, J. J., Hersh, W. R., Huff, S.M., & Bell, D.S. (1994). Toward a medical-concept representation language. *Journal of the American Medical Informatics Association, 1*(3), 207-217.

Fehring, R. (1986). Validation: Validating diagnostic labels. In R.M. Caroll-Johnson (Ed.), *Classification of nursing diagnoses.* St. Louis: The C.V. Mosby Company.

Fleishman, E.A. (1975). Toward a taxonomy of human performance. *American Psychologist, 30,* 1127-1149.

Gillenson, M. L. (1985). *Database: Step-by-step.* New York: John Wiley & Sons.

Gordon, M. (1994). *Nursing diagnosis: Process and application.* (3rd ed.) St. Louis: Mosby.

Hoskins, L. (1994). NANDA news. *Nursing Diagnosis, 5*(4), 141.

Iowa Interventions Project, J. McCloskey & G. Bulechek (Eds.) (1992). *Nursing interventions classification (NIC).* St. Louis: Mosby Year-Book.

Iowa Interventions Project, J. McCloskey & G. Bulechek (Eds.) (1996). *Nursing interventions classification (NIC)* (2nd ed.). St. Louis: Mosby Year-Book.

Iowa Interventions Project. (1995). Validation and coding of the NIC taxonomy. *Image, 27*(1), 43-49.

Iowa Outcomes Project, M. Johnson & Meridean Maas (Eds.). (1997). *Nursing outcomes classification (NOC).* St. Louis: Mosby Year-Book.

Jenny, J. (1994). *Advancing the science of nursing with nursing diagnosis.* Paper presented at the 11th conference of the North American Nursing Diagnosis Association, Nashville, TN.

Kerr, M., Hoskins, L.M, Fitzpatrick, J.J., Warren, J.J., Avant, K.C., Hurley, M., Lunney, M., Mills, W.C., & Rottkamp, B.C. (1993). Taxonomic validation: An overview. *Nursing Diagnosis, 41,* 6-14.

Kim, M.J. (1989). Nursing diagnosis. *Annual Review of Nursing Research, 7,* 117-142.

Kim, M.J., & Camilleri, D. (1994). Nursing diagnosis: is it essential for the nursing profession? In O.L. Strickland & D.J. Fishman (Eds.), *Issues in the 1990s.* Albany, NY: Delmar Publishing Inc

Loucopoulos, P., & Ziczi, R. (Eds) (1992). *Conceptual modeling, databases, and case: an integrated view of information systems development.* John Wiley & Sons, Inc.

Marek, K. (1989). Classification of outcome measures in nursing care. In *Classifications for describing nursing practice.* Kansas City, MO: American Nurses Association.

Martin, K., & Scheet, N. (1992). *The Omaha system: Applications for community health nursing.* Philadelphia: W.B. Saunders.

NIDSEC Committee (Zielstorff, R., Delaney, C., Marek, K., Kneedler, J., Marr, P., Averrill, C., Milholland, K. ANA staff).

(1997). *Nursing Information & Data Set Evaluation Center (NIDSEC): Standards and scoring guidelines*. Washington, DC: American Nurses Association.

North American Nursing Diagnosis Association. (1996). *Nursing diagnoses: Definitions and classification 1997-1998*. Philadelphia: Author.

Ozbolt, J., Fruchnight, J., & Hayden, J.H. (1994). Toward data standards for clinical nursing information. *J Am Med Info Assoc, 1*(2): 175-185.

Rodgers, B. L., & Knafl, K. A. (1993). *Concept development in nursing: Foundations, techniques, and applications*. Philadelphia: W. B. Saunders.

Saba, V., O'Hara, P., Zuckerman, A., Boondas, J., Levine, E., & Oatway, D. (1991). A nursing intervention taxonomy for home health care. *Nursing and Health Care, 12*, 296-9.

Smirvov, V. (1970). Levels and stages of knowledge. In Tavanec P. (Ed), *Problems in the logic of scientific knowledge*, Dordrecht, Holland: D. Reidel

Taylor, D. (1989). Interventions. In *Classifications for describing nursing practice*. Kansas City, MO: American Nurses Association

Waltz, C. F., Strickland, O., & Lenz, E. (1991). *Measurement in nursing research*. Philadelphia: F. A. Davis.

Warren, J. (1994). Nursing diagnosis taxonomy development: Overview and issues. In McCloskey, J. & Grace, H.(Eds.), *Current issues in nursing*, (4th ed.). St. Louis: The C.V. Mosby Company.

Warren, J. (1997). NANDA news. *Nursing Diagnosis, 8*(1), 5-6.

Nursing Diagnosis in Brazil: the Translation of NANDA's Taxonomy to Portuguese, Cultural Issues and Validation Process

Alba Lucia Botura Leite de Barros, RN, PhD

Jeanne Liliane Marlene Michel, RN, BS

Maria Miriam Lima da Nobrega, RN, MS

Telma Ribeiro Garcia, RN, DNS

The history of the translation of NANDA's Nursing Diagnoses Taxonomy started in 1986, in the state of Paraíba, when a small group began studies on the concept and the system of classification of diagnoses that was being developed in the United States. This was stimulated by Dr. Marga Coler, a teacher of the University of Connecticut, member of NANDA, that came to Brazil to develop a transcultural study focusing on nursing diagnoses related to crisis precipitants. The exchange of experiences contributed to the organization of a Group of Interest on Nursing Diagnoses, formed initially by professors of the Nursing Department of the Federal University of Paraíba. This group, using Gordon's Manual of Nursing Diagnoses (1985) and NANDA's Taxonomy I of 1986 (McLane 1987), started to discuss and to evaluate the possibility of the application of this taxonomy in the educational practice. With the growth of the group, and due to the lack of texts that presented the basic concepts and the taxonomy in Portuguese, emerged the idea of publishing a book presenting, in a didactic way, the contents necessary to the learning process and the application of nursing diagnoses.

In 1988, members of this group participated in the 8th NANDA Conference and made contact with the Taxonomy Committee, requesting and obtaining verbal authorization for translating the NANDA Taxonomy I to Brazilian Portuguese.

Thus, in 1990 the first book was published on nursing diagnoses in Brazil (Farias et al, 1990), which included the Revised Taxonomy I. During the process of writing that book, the first step was a free translation of the taxonomy, word by word, with no concern about the meaning of the terms. After that, the material was revised by a professor of the Department of Foreign Languages of the University, a specialist in English language, who advised the group in the translation of terms for which there were no corresponding ones in Portuguese. Next, the work was submitted to another professor, a specialist in Portuguese language, who compared the orig-

"

inal North American version with the translated one, unified and adapted the taxonomy to Brazilian Portuguese, and made the vernacular correction of all of the chapters of the book. Finally, since the authors had heard about another translation that had been done by a nurse from São Paulo, as part of her master's degree thesis (Maria, 1990), one of them met with this nurse and compared the two translations, thereby seeking consensus.

When the two translations became known, other versions began to appear, with some different translations for the diagnostic terms, thereby harming the standardization principle that characterizes the adoption of a taxonomy.

The First National Symposium on Nursing Diagnoses, in São Paulo, in 1991, pointed to the following difficulties: a) the lack of consensus in expressing the Human Response Patterns, which were sometimes translated as nouns, and other times as verbs, in either the gerund or in the infinitive form; b) differences in the translation of the meaning of some patterns; c) differences in the translation of diagnostic titles, defining characteristics, related factors and qualifiers suggested by NANDA; d) inadequacy of some defining characteristics that, in some cases, were not applicable to the Brazilian reality (Nobrega, 1991).

In order to discuss those difficulties, the Second National Symposium was organized in ParaÃba (1992). The theme was "Unifying nursing diagnoses in Brazil." Nurses from all over the country, who were working with nursing diagnoses, were divided in five groups, composed of experts in basic clinical areas. Each group was asked to compare some of the well-known translations and to propose a unified form for the translation of the diagnostic categories of a specific Human Response Pattern.

Thus, the translation of all the diagnoses of the NANDA Revised Taxonomy I, were discussed and revised. The results of this work were complied at the end of the Symposium, and sent to all the participants and to other nurses involved in the study of nursing diagnoses for evaluation. At the end of this process, a book was published that, although respecting the basic structure of NANDA's Taxonomy, included alterations in the gramatic form of the diagnostics components which had been translated to Portuguese and also some significant modifications in the structure of those diagnoses approved by NANDA for testing and clinical use (Nobrega and Garcia, 1994). This book has been widely used and referenced in the whole country.

After its publication, however, NANDA had approved and included twenty-six new diagnoses in the taxonomy. Consequently, there's a need to update. An attempt happened in the third National Symposium on Nursing Diagnoses, that happenned in Ceará, in 1996, when there were discussed proposals for the translation of the new diagnoses that were not yet included in the book, and alterations in those diagnoses already published. The result of this work has not yet published.

Cultural issues involved in the process of translation of nursing diagnoses taxonomy

It is necessary to consider that cultural differences have an important role in the process of adapting the taxonomy of nursing diagnoses to other countries. The North American reality is not the same as that of Brazil. There are predominantly North American cultural differences that differ from the characteristics of the Latin people. These determine distinct answers, behaviors and interpretations.

The translation process in Brazil, unifying

language with the help of many nurses from special interesting groups and from several regions of the country, permitted analysis of cultural issues.

The research that has been developed for the validation of diagnoses will contribute in the solution of the existing cultural differences.

Current situation of the use of nursing diagnoses in Brazil

The first reference to nursing diagnoses in Brazil occurred in the sixties, when Dr. Wanda de Aguiar Horta presented her thoughts on the subject, establishing the diagnosing as one of the phases of the nursing process. This author's influence was fundamental in the provision of systematic nursing care. The Brazilian literature continued to evidence resistance of nurses in the use of the diagnostic phase for many years after it was proposed by Horta.

The proposal of a taxonomy in the United States by the National Group for the Classification of Nursing Diagnoses (now, NANDA) brought a new impetus to the study and use of the diagnostic phase in Brazil, beginning in 1986, with the group of Paraíba.

Given the geographical dimensions and the socioeconomic and cultural differences among the several areas of our country, there is no uniformity in the provision of nursing care. Brazil has now 150 million inhabitants, and the nursing team is comprised of the following four categories:

> Nurses = 72,437
> Nursing Technicians = 65,411
> Nursing Auxiliaries = 296,863
> Nursing Aides = 144,903
> Total = 579,614

Such a distribution does not favor the use of the nursing process, and it sometimes ends in an undesirable nurse/patient relationship (Carvalho, 1996).

It is predictable that the technical-scientific progresses of the profession are more evident in areas where there is a strong nurse/patient relationship and also in areas linked to teaching and research. Thus, the study and application of nursing diagnoses had been accomplished by groups consolidated in the states of Paraíba, São Paulo, Paraná, Ceará, Minas Gerais and Rio Grande do Sul. These groups conduct study groups; scientific events (courses, congresses, seminars, conferences); continuing education activities; and launch research projects such as validation studies. These groups have been involved in translations and in the revision of the taxonomy.

In order to have an up-to-date evaluation of nursing diagnoses in our country, we conducted a brief survey of 17 institutions (16 universities and 1 hospital) that are using nursing diagnoses and publishing papers on the subject. From this survey we concluded that:

- 55% of those surveyed use nursing diagnoses in their practice (teaching or caring), as a phase of the nursing process;
- 95% of the respondents use the translated NANDA taxonomy (Farias, 1990; Nobrega and Garcia, 1994);
- 82% of the respondents believe that Brazilian nurses are motivated to use nursing diagnoses with a taxonomy. The major indicators of this motivation are:
  1) the potential of achieving professional autonomy;
  2) the possibility of developing more scientific work;

3) the frequent solicitation of courses about nursing diagnosis;

4) the increased participation in scientific events;

5) the increase of publications and presentations of papers on the subject;

6) the interest demonstrated by students of nursing schools;

- the difficulties related to the use of nursing diagnoses in daily practice are:

1) the nurses' lack of knowledge on the subject (86%);

2) the lack of institutional policies for using nursing diagnoses (86%);

3) insufficient number of nurses (68%);

4) erroneous concepts regarding nursing diagnosis (68%);

5) lack of relationship to the nursing process (50%);

6) deficit of bibliographical material in Portuguese (45%);

7) absence of diagnoses in practice situations (23%);

8) lack of linguistic consensus (23%);

9) inadequacy of some defining characteristics that, in some cases, are not applicable to our reality (27%);

10) differences in the translation (14%);

11) non insertion of the nursing process as obligatory content in the curricula (9%);

12) lack of the nurses' scientific knowledge, due to teaching deficiencies (9%).

- the translations of the diagnoses taxonomy were made with the following methods: free translation (50%); group consensus (50%);

technical revision of books already translated (17%);

- there are 8 institutions (47%) conducting validation studies on nursing diagnoses, using the methodologies of Fehring (87,5%); Gordon (25%); Hoskins (25%); comparison (25%); epidemiology (12.5%); multivariate analysis with logistic regression (12.5%); statistical methods of agreement between experts (12.5%).

From our findings, we conclude that nursing diagnoses have been increasingly studied and taught, as a phase of the nursing process, generally in undergraduate and graduate university courses. We believe that the fact that nursing diagnosis is utilized more in research and teaching than in nursing practice can be attributed to the natural course of evolution of nursing as science, because it is from research and the new nurses' formation that the practice gradually will be changed.

References

Carvalho, E. C. *The use of nursing diagnosis in Brazil. Presented at the session: International update – International nursing diagnosis.* In: 12th Biennial Conference – NANDA. Pittsburgh, April 14, 1996.

Farias, J. N. et al. *Diagnóstico de enfermagem: uma abordagem conceitual e prática.* João Pessoa: Santa Marta, 1990.

Gordon, M. *Manual of nursing diagnosis 1984-1985.* St. Louis: McGraw Hill, 1985.

Maria, V. L. R. *Preparo de enfermeiras para a utilização de diagnósticos de enfermagem: relato de experiência.* São Paulo: Escola de Enfermagem da USP, 1990. 130p. (Dissertação, Mestrado em Enfermagem

Fundamental).

Nobrega, M. M. L. Perspectiva da taxonomia dos diagnósticos de enfermagem: universalização dos termos. In: *Simposio Nacional Sobre Diagnosticos de Enfermagem, 1, 1991, São Paulo*. Anais. São Paulo: GIDE-SP/IDPC/EPM-Departamento de Enfermagem, 1991. P. 135-144.

Nobrega, M. M. L., & Garcia, T. R. (org.) *Uniformização da linguagem dos diagnósticos de enfermagem da NANDA: sistematização das propostas do II SNDE.* João Pessoa: União/CNRDE/GIDE-PB, 1994.

Nursing North American Diagnosis Association. *Taxonomy I revised 1990.*

NANDA's Language in Spain

Mercedes Ugalde Apalategui, R.N., C.N.S.

My dear colleagues, allow me first of all to thank NANDA for inviting me to take part in this International Panel and also the moderator, Mrs. Cécile Boisvert, an example to be followed for many European nurses for her teaching, her dynamism, her way of doing things and her constant support.

I would be delighted if, despite the language barrier, I could give you a general idea of the work we are doing in my country with the NANDA Nursing Diagnoses.

Introduction

Spain, as you know, is a country of the European Community, currently integrated in the building of the common European project along with fifteen other countries. The developments that have taken place over the last few years in Spanish nursing are parallel to those that have occurred in our society as a whole.

Our healthcare system in Spain, like that of all the other European countries, is Universal (for the whole population), public (the Health Ministry is responsible for organizing, managing and distributing resources) and free (paid for from the State budget). The economic resources are obtained from deductions from the salaries of the workers for the economic running of the Health and Pensions Systems. The National Health System has for several decades had a large network of hospitals and surgeries on a community level.

At the start of the eighties, there was a strong boost in the development of the Community Health System with the launch of an important reform, following the criteria of the WHO for "Health for all by 2000." This meant a parallel development in Community Nursing, which moved from a traditional role of doctors' helpers to a more professional one involving responsibilities for direct attention to the user, specific programs for the follow-up of chronic patients, healthcare education, etc., which has facilitated the implantation of nursing diagnoses in Spain. However, on the other hand, the greater technification of hospital treatment, the reduction in hospitals stays for patients and readjustments in management systems are hindering the use of nursing methodology and therefore of nursing diagnoses among the nurses working in hospital centers.

As I was saying, the Public Health System is the organizer and main contractor (there is not a long tradition of private practice among Spanish nursing staff). At the moment we are undergoing a political process of economic adjustment, which is calling into question what we call the "Welfare State." There is a tendency towards privatization, to a more medical-biological model centered on illness rather than on preventive aspects, and we are told that resources are in short supply, and people are starting to question certain forms of healthcare assistance and medical care.

This would mean a considerable step backwards in terms of the socio-sanitary achievements made and also for nurses, in that there would be fewer staff hired, workloads would increase and there would be greater job uncertainty. This would in the end translate into greater problems in the application of MOVE TOWARDS PROFESSIONALIZATION among Spanish nursing staff.

There are currently two identifiable trends. The first is a TECHNIFIED Nursing, the heir of the ATS (Technical Sanitary Aides), centered on the bio-medical model, with little professionalization and the consideration that it is unnecessary to use nursing language as such. The second is more PROFESSIONALIZED, centered on human needs, and the struggle to gain a specific own identity. Its practice is based on a nursing concept and tries to apply its work to the Nursing Process using NANDA diagnoses.

There are different types of professional organizations: The Medical Association (Colegio), which is the structure that groups together all nurses nationally and represents the Spanish nursing sector in the International Council of Nurses (ICN); membership of the Association is obligatory in order to practice. There are trade unions that defend our working interests in the different fields and, finally, there are scientific associations, whose interest is focused on the development of a given sector of nursing activity, such as community or geriatric nursing, teaching, the Internet and many more.

As regards nursing training, I consider it to be of a high level. From 1977 all Spanish nurses graduate from university with a middle grade academic title, a Diploma. That said, it is true that it is not possible to have access to the second or third level of university studies, degree courses or doctorates in nursing teaching and this is an important developmental problem. In the new Study Plan there is a subject called Fundamentals of Nursing in the first year, in which the theoretical fundamental of the nursing discipline are explained, as well as the Conceptual Frameworks (Models) and the Nursing Process (Methodology), and nursing diagnoses are used, and then worked on from different subjects. Over the last few years we have been able to see that the Taxonomy of NANDA is being used in most schools.

Development of Nursing Diagnosis in Spain

In the process of changes that we underwent in the eighties, most nurses gained type approval for our old qualification, to that of the new course of "University Diploma-holder in Nursing," through following a specific course. And it was on that course when we started to hear about the "Nursing Diagnoses." At that time, the publication of the Nursing magazine was also a key event, allowing us to see a first list of nursing diagnoses and articles on methodologically worked healthcare plans which also included nursing diagnoses.

From the beginning, one of the main problems we encountered in the dissemination and consolidation of the diagnoses was language translation. Some publications of mainly American authors translated the Process of Nursing Care by HEALTHCARE PROCESS. This created confusion as well as effectively hindering the clear recognition of the concept of Nursing Diagnoses, which had been translated as Healthcare Diagnoses. The also occured, for example, with the first texts to appear in Spanish by Yura and Walsh.

The Spanish Association of Nursing Teachers (AEED) had played a fundamental role in this entire process of change in the Spanish nursing sector. AEED is a teaching association of which I have been a member for more than ten years, gathering together teaching nurses, and has been the driving force behind many initiatives that have turned out to be fundamental for the development of nursing and diagnoses in our country. For example, in 1989, to mark the tenth anniversary of the founding of the Association, Linda J. Carpenito was invited to its annual Working Sessions, at which she gave a paper and led some workshops. This gave recognition to the work that we were doing in minority groups and meant the start of the expansion of the Nursing Diagnoses.

Following Carpenito's visit to Spain, the "Permanent Seminar for the Study of Nursing Diagnoses," led by her, and in which I took part, was set up in Barcelona. We worked for a year to reach a consensus on the translation of diagnostic labels. In the end that group ceased working.

Later, in the Association of Teaching Staff, a group was set up called GREDE (Group for the Study of Nursing Diagnoses), grouping together the members interested in the subject.

For our part, we saw the need to disseminate knowledge and the application of the diagnoses among the different healthcare nurses too. And, in order to accomplish this, a varied group of teaching nurses, managers and clinical specialists continues the work of translating and revising the Taxonomy of the NANDA, the results of which were published in 1995. At the same time, we take part in working sessions, congresses and other activities organized by the associations of nursing diagnoses of other countries, mainly in Europe, such as AFENDI, ACENDIO, and of course NANDA. We also established links with different Latin American nurses working with Nursing Diagnoses.

Setting of the AENTDE

I shall now explain to you the birth and brief history of the Spanish Association of Nomenclature, Taxonomy and Nursing Diagnoses (AENTDE).

At the beginning of 1995, on observing the importance that Nursing Classification Systems were acquiring internationally and growing increase in the use of Nursing Diagnoses, we saw the need to carry out some kind of activity that would provide an opportunity to get to know and put in touch with each other all nurses working with diagnoses in our country.

Three organizations were asked to take part. First of all, the academic authorities of the University of Barcelona, which gave us its unconditional support right from the start, and provided us with stimulation and help. Secondly, the Professional Association (Colegio) of Nurses of Barcelona, without whose initial financial support we should not even have been able to publicise the Symposium, and finally the healthcare authorities of the Hospital de Bellvitge, who were delighted to participate in the organization.

In this way we began to work on organizing the 1st International Symposium of Nursing Diagnoses "Towards a Common Language. Nursing Diagnoses?," held in Barcelona in May 1996. We were genuinely surprised by the response. Few of us suspected that close to 800 nurses would attend, from 15 countries, or that 100 scientific communications and posters would be presented. The figures themselves give us an idea of the great interest there was and the wisdom of our choice and appropriateness of holding the event.

At the same time, a founding group of four teachers from the School of Nursing of the University of Barcelona started to work on the creation of an Association, as we felt that it was necessary to provide the nurses working on Nursing Diagnoses around the country with a structure and an organization. We drew up the statutes and took all the bureaucratic steps necessary, and finally, in November 1995, AENTDE was registered as a professional nurses' non-profit-making Scientific Association with the following aims:

- To contribute to the development of a nursing terminology.
- To foster and promote a knowledge of the use of the Diagnoses and other own terminology among professional nursing staff.
- To work together with the national and international organizations to promote the exchange of research findings.

The official presentation took place in Barcelona at the 1st Symposium, where the participants were given the opportunity to become members of the Association. Over two days, about 300 of the participants joined and at the end of the Symposium a Constituent Assembly was held, at which the Management Board was elected, comprising 9 members from different areas of the country, representative of the nurses working in different ambits with Nursing Diagnoses, teaching, management, healthcare, universities, hospitals and community work.

At the first official act, unanimously approved by the Assembly of Members, Marjory Gordon, Cecile Boisvert and Jocelyn Mattewman were appointed Honorary Members in recognition of their work in favor of Nursing Diagnoses on the international level and in our country.

During the initial meetings, the Management Board drew up the working plan, which we have been developing over these last two years. We have created a four-monthly information bulletin "El Correo AENTDE," of which we have published five numbers to date, which is the medium through which we disseminate our news, opinions and new developments in the world of diagnoses. We also created some web pages with general information on the Association and the possibility to consult via e-mail.

One of the first activities that we carried out was the compilation of a survey for all the members, through which we have been able to discover the reality of the situation of the use of Nursing Diagnoses in Spain and see which topic aroused most interest. On the grounds of the results obtained, we are now working on the preparation of a working document defining the recommendation of the Association, the criteria to follow at the different levels of teaching of nursing diagnoses, and the lines of research that could be followed. This work will be presented officially in the Workshops to be carried out in the 2nd Valladolid '98 Symposium.

A documentary list is being created, which will allow acccess and consultation for all the professionals interested in having access to documentation on diagnoses, intervention and results.

As an extraordinary activity, in 1997 we held a Working Session with Marjory Gordon entitled "Nursing Diagnoses. Diagnostic Reasoning," which was attended by more than 600 nurses. And we are currently working on the organization of the 2nd International Symposium on Nursing Diagnoses to be held next month in Valladolid under the title "Nursing diagnoses as a means for professional development."

Future Developments

We can affirm that, despite its young age, the current situation of AENTDE is excellent. It is an organization that seems to have been developing considerably over the last two years — you only need to look at the results of the activities achieved — and we have found an outlet to a general unease by the nursing profession as a whole in our country.

There are currently about 400 members. The headquarters of the Association are at the School of Nursing of the University of Barcelona. We are organized around a central core, the Standing Board and five delegations in different areas of Spain. We are trying to consolidate and develop the regional delegations so that they can work in closer contact with the members in each area. We propose to draw up a "Directory of Working Groups" in order to facilitate contact between the different teams working on common subjects, such as groups of community nurses, protagonists in the use of nursing diagnoses, or groups working to establish standardized and computerized care plans in hospitals.

Therefore, it is a question of giving continuity and consolidating the projects that the Association had underway, propose lines of research and establish formal contacts with other national scientific associations, maintaining and consolidation international contacts, both on a European level, with ACENDIO and AFEDI, as with NANDA and specifically with Latin America, as we consider that, as we share a common language we have the possibility to work together in a particular way.

And finally, I would like to share a thought and a feeling with you. I have shared many hours of study and work on NANDA Diagnoses with other colleagues and we consider that we must recognize the importance and transcendence of the many, many hours given up freely by so many nurse in North America, whose names we sometimes do not even know, but whose efforts have made it possible to refine and develop a system of nursing classification. I think it is difficult to thank them enough for the contribution that they have made towards the development and consolidation of a system of scientific nursing throughout the world in this respect. I would like to transmit to NANDA, as the representative organization of this work, the gratitude of many colleagues for their effort and for having the generosity to share it.

References

Alfaro, R. (1966). *Aplicación del proceso de Enfermería. Guía práctica*. 3a ED. Mosby. Madrid.

American Psychiatric Association. (1995). *Manual diagnóstico y estadístico de los trastornos mentales (DSM-IV)*. Masson. Barcelona.

Campbell, C. (1987). *Tratado de Enfermería. Diagnósticos y Méthodos*. Doyma. Barcelona.

Carpenito, L. J. (1995). *Manual de diagnóstico de enfermería*. 5a Ed. Interamericana-McGraw-Hill. Madrid.

(1990). *Clasificaciones de la WONCA en atención primaria*. Masson. Barcelona.

Cuesta, A., Guirao, A., & Benavent, A. (1994). *Diagnóstico de Enfermería Adaptación al contexto español*. Diaz de Santos. Madrid.

Doenges, M. E., & Moorhouse, M. F. (1992). *Guía de bolsillo de Diagnósticos y Actuaciones de Enfermería*. Doyma. Barcelona.

Gordon, M. (1996). *Diagnóstico Enfermero*. Mosby/Doyma Libros. 3a Ed. Madrid.

Iyer, P. W., Tapich, B., & Bernocchi-Losey, D. (1997). *Proceso y diagnóstico de enfermería*. 3a Ed. Interamericana-McGraw-Hill. Madrid.

Lopez Martin, I. (1994). *Atención Domiciliaria. Diagnósticos de Enfermería*. Interamericana-McGraw-Hill. Madrid.

Luis, M. T. (1994). *Diagnósticos enfermeros*. 2a Ed. Mosby/Doyma Liros. Madrid. 1996.

Mi Ja K., McFarland, G. K., & McLane, A. M. (1994). *Guía clínica de Enfermería. Diagnóstico en Enfermería y plan de cuidados*. 5a Ed. Mosby. Madrid. (Traducción inadecuada).

North American Nursing Diagnosis Association (NANDA). (1997). *Diagnósticos Enfermeros de la NANDA. Definiciones y Clasificación 1997-1998*. Harcourt Brace. Madrid. (Traducción inadecuada).

Organización Mundial de la Salud. (1995). *Clasificación Estadistíca Internacional de Enfermedades y Problemas Relacionados con la Salud (CIE-10)*. Décima Revisión. Volumen 1. Publicación Científica No. 554. Organización Panamericana de la Salud. Washington.

Ugalde, M., & Rigol, A. (1995). *Diagnósticos de Enfermería. Taxonomía NANDA. Traducción, revisíon y comentarios*. Masson. Barcelona.

WEBwatch

Http://www.ub.es/aentde/welcome.htm
Asociación. Española de Nomenclatura, Taxonomía y Diagnósticos de Enfermería (AENTDE).

The Netherlands

Nico Oud, RN, Dip. N. Adm., MNSc

Firstly I would like to thank the organization and in particular Cécile Boisvert for the invitation to address you about the dissemination of NANDA's taxonomy in the Netherlands.

Background

The Netherlands has about 15.5 million inhabitants and on average they enjoy good health and a high life expectancy and low infant mortality. By 2010, the Central Bureau for Statistics (CBS) expects life expectancy to increase to 75.0 years for men and 81.5 years for women. However, the growing percentage of elderly people is one of the reasons why the demand for health care has been growing for some time, next to other factors like advanced treatment, improved medical appliances, modern standards of comfort, as well as the increasing lack of safety.

Health is human handy-work: by people for people and only sufficient personnel of sufficient quality will be able to supply health care that meets the demands of society. That's why labor-market policy is of great importance as within some years a shortage of personnel is being predicted again, especially for home-care. The number of working nurses and second-level nurses/caring personnel grew during the period 1990 -1995 with almost 17%; since then it is stabilizing. To cover health care there are about 370,000 nursing and caring personnel actively working in all kinds of intra-, semi- and extramural care settings.

With regard to the basic nursing education, the vocational and professional training courses for nurses and care providers have been subject to review and grouped together in a transparent and coherent new system since the implementation of it in August 1997. The new structure had to meet the demands made upon professional practitioners by the Individual Health Care Professions Act (Wet BIG) and the Decree on Educational Requirements in Nursing, which springs from it. The new qualification structure for nursing and care providing is now made up of four so-called 'qualification levels.' Each qualification level details the com-

"

petence (skills and knowledge) of a professional practitioner, based upon three criteria: responsibility, complexity and transfer. The competence of the professional practitioner increases per 'level: from mainly routine and standard procedural work at level 2 to the most complex activities at level 5. Qualification levels 2, 3, and 4 come under secondary vocational training while level 5 belongs to the higher professional educational level. The course leading to a qualification as a care helper (level 2) lasts for two year, the course to become a care worker (level 3) lasts for three years and the course leading to qualification as a (generic) nurse lasts for four years at both level 4 (Middle Vocational Training) and level 5 (Higher Professional Training), both leading to the official registered title of nurse.

To reach level 5, nurses must successfully complete a higher professional training course. They are capable of planning and providing nursing care according the nursing process. In addition level 5 nurses are able to :

- make a diagnosis and select appropriate activities and interventions, even in cases where no standards or procedural instructions are available, and set an example to fellow care providers in such cases;
- play an initiating and coordinating role in activities related to prevention, health education and provision of information;
- give consultations in every phase of the primary nursing process;
- fulfill an organizational function with regard to the content of care provided, such as determining the need for care, assignment of care seekers and coordinating the contribution of various disciplines to the care process;

- create conditions for improving the primary care process, with regard to aspects such as quality control.

With this mind it becomes clear that the developments of the NANDA and the NIC and the NOC becomes very important to those nurses, as well as the other international and national developments for this matter: the ICNP, ICIDH and the WWC/NRV classification of diagnostic terms for nursing.

For that purpose it was in 1995 that the first translations of the two books by Gordon were published in the Dutch language. The translation of most of the terms has been the result of a long way of weighing the pros and cons and numerous compromises. At that time the translators consulted Gordon several times about adjusting the terms to the Dutch language and nursing culture.

With regard to the translation of the NANDA labels and taxonomy it has been a matter of the work of a few nursing people, who were certainly not representative for the total nursing population. To their best knowing and abilities they have tried to translate according the spirit of the NANDA, and it was not always possible to translate directly from English to Dutch. That's why some of the labels can't also be translated backwards directly and differ from the original. But by reading and reading again the definitions some proper Dutch came forward and were discussed and decided upon. Other starting points during that time were briefness, specificity, comprehensibility, and simplicity. So brought specificity us to translation into more specific Dutch words for terms like alteration into 'tekort', 'verstoring', en 'stoornis', which sounded better the 'wijziging' of 'verandering'. And we were of the opinion that labels (nursing diagnoses) are also used for the communication between nurses and patients, and therefore the criteria of comprehensibility and simplicity.

Other examples are the difficult with translating "gerunds" like exchanging, communicating, relating, valuing, choosing, moving, perceiving, knowing and feeling. Therefore we had to choose for the option of the 'het' ('it') form before a verb, or just be the verb itself or by just a noun or description. Also, there are no direct Dutch equivalents for the terms impairment and disability, as we had noted much earlier for the translation of the ICIDH. So, we did follow most of the time the terms being used in that translation like: 'stoornis' and 'beperking' as being the most neutral and already used ones.

Since 1995 there is also now the handbook of Nursing Diagnoses, Interventions and Outcomes, in which next to translations of the main classifications also original Dutch work is being presented; a loose-leaf periodical which is being published 3 times per year with about 125 pages each time; and since 1997 also a newsletter, which is being published 4 times per year.

Next to this the publisher had also published the NANDA in a book form since 1997 and the new one just recently in 1998. In total about 1,500 copies are being sold.

All together it means that we opted for a very pragmatic and financially affordable way of dealing with the translation difficulties of the NANDA into the Dutch language. We therefore state always that the translation is a work-translation and we are open for any critique and suggestions. Till now only just a few did, so we hope we did a good job after all by providing our Dutch colleagues with the translation of this important work of the NANDA, in order to use it as proper as possible in the Dutch nursing language, but also with caution and with a critical view.

Thank you.
Nico Oud

Translation Issues and Recommendations from Japan

Shigemi Sato, PhD, RN

The NANDA labels translation have finally been standardized in Japan. I think this is a crucial step for Japanese nurses to have a common language and concepts.

Japan Society of Nursing Diagnosis

We have an active nursing diagnosis society called the Japan Society of Nursing Diagnosis (JSND), chaired by Dr. Mitsuko Matsuki, professor at Fukui Medical College. The JSND was established in 1995 as an outgrowth of the Japan Nursing Diagnosis Association which originally formed in 1991 (Matsuki, 1995). The JSND has increased its membership to approximately 1,500, issues a research journal twice a year, and holds an annual conference.

The Language Examination Committee

The JSND recognizes the importance of standardizing the NANDA labels translation, and therefore, the JSND has a language examination committee for this purpose. The language examination committee consists of seven members, all of whom have extensive knowledge about nursing diagnosis and are familiar with translation. The committee first published a proposed list of translation of NANDA diagnoses 1992-1993 in the Journal of JSND 1996. The second proposed translation was published next year based on the NANDA diagnoses 1995-1996. This latest translation is still in effect because the NANDA diagnoses 1997-1998 does not contain any new labels.

Standard Translation

Before the standard translation was published by the JSND, translators used their own words when translating American manuals and textbooks. For instance, for the translation of "Impaired Physical Mobility," one manual used "shintai undousei no shougai" while another manual used "shintai no kadousei no shougai." These differences may be subtle, but it was enough to make some Japanese nurses think that these are not the same diagnosis. The JSND translation 1997 was "shintai kadousei no shyougai" (Language Examination Committee, 1997). I have found that translators are more aware of the standard translation, and the JSND translation is now more often used in recent publications.

Need for Refinement

Although the importance of standard translation is being recognized, the list of current translation requires further refinement. Since many of the NANDA labels were translated word for word, some nurses think that translated labels sound somewhat awkward. Moreover, English expressions are used to describe several concepts without translating, such as parenting, sexuality pattern, coping, and noncompliance. Since these concepts are new in Japanese culture, it is difficult to find the matching Japanese words. However, people have expressed a concern for the numerous English expressions in Japanese. The aging population, which is increasing so rapidly and consuming health care resources, is not usually familiar with English expressions. I think that it is important for nurses to share nursing diagnoses with clients, but in order to do so, we have to discover or develop Japanese expressions which are understandable to the public.

Standard Translation of Definitions and Defining Characteristics

So, the translation of diagnosis labels is becoming uniform in Japan, but how about the definitions and defining characteristics? I think these should be also standardized, but it will surely require many more years. According to the JSND's meeting record, the language examination committee tried to translate the entire Nursing Diagnoses: Definitions & Classification 1997-1998. However, problems with publishing rights in Japan precluded JSND publishing it. The main reason seemed to be that NANDA sold the publishing rights to a Japanese publishing company instead of JSND. Unfortunately, the book did not become an official translation from JSND, but it was translated by people on the language examination committee, and it is available in Japanese.

Translating Defining Characteristics

Next, I would like to address the problems when translating the list of NANDA defining characteristics. Did any of you have problems with translating apprehension, distressed, worried, anxious in the diagnosis "Anxiety"? In Japanese, it is difficult to find different words for each of these, and so these words can be translated to a single Japanese word, "shinpai" or even "Anxiety." Is it really necessary to differentiate all these expressions? If so, I think NANDA has to develop some operational definitions. My point is that some of the current NANDA defining characteristics are too difficult or too ambiguous for translation.

Back-translation

I would like to share some of my experiences in translation. I have used the back-translation technique described by Brislin (1970) and translated 183 defining characteristics of 13 diagnoses for content validation. As you well know, back-translation is a technique to assure the equivalence of two instruments written in different languages for cross-cultural research. I hired two bilingual Japanese nurses as translators. One translator translated an instrument from English to Japanese, and another translator translated back from Japanese to English. Then an evaluator compared the similarity of two English versions: the original version and the back-translated version. When evaluating the similarity, emphasis was placed on meaning rather than exact wording.

Seventeen of 183 defining characteristics (or 9%) did not have equivalent meanings in the two English versions. Although most of the errors were due to translators' misunderstandings, I thought two errors were related more to the difficulty of the original English expressions. One was "foot shuffling" in Anxiety, and another was "shrugs in response to speaker" in Hopelessness. How will you translate these characteristics? Can you find more than one word in translation for these expressions? Three nursing diagnosis manuals by NANDA (1994), Gordon (1993) and Carpenito (1994) are available in Japanese, so I was able to compare these three manuals and the new translation from my translator.

Foot Shuffling?

For the translation of "foot shuffling," the NANDA (1994) translation was "ashi no kumi kae," the Gordon (1993) translation was "ashi no hiki tsure," and the translation from my translator was "binbo yusuri." According to an English to Japanese dictionary, all of these seemed to be acceptable, but which movement did NANDA mean originally? The differences may be subtle, but it provides different pictures to Japanese nurses. I had to clarify the meaning by discussion with an American expert on nursing diagnosis. After the discussion, the Japanese word "binbo yusuri," literally meaning "poor man's shake," was chosen for "foot shuffling."

Shrugs in Response to Speaker?

Again, there were three different translations for "shrugs in response to speaker" in Hopelessness. The NANDA (1994) translation was "kata wo sukumeru dousa." Gordon's (1993) was "kata wo subomete hannou." The Carpenito (1994) translation was "mukanshin wo shimesu." The translation from my translator was also "mukanshin wo shimesu."

Here again, according to the dictionary, any one of these expressions seemed to be OK, but which one did NANDA mean originally? The differences may be subtle, but it is enough to make some nurses think that these are not the same characteristics. I asked an expert to visually demonstrate "shrugs in response to speaker," and "gakkuri to kata wo otosu," literally meaning "drops shoulders with exhaling spirit," was chosen.

Recommendations

In summary, I would like to make two suggestions regarding the NANDA defining characteristics: one to the international members and another to NANDA. Dr. Coler (1994) recommended using culture-bound perceptions and interpretations instead of a word-for-word translation. I also think this is very important for the international members to consider. My Japanese translation of both "shrugs in response to speaker" and "foot shuffling" are, I would say, based on culture-bound interpretations. However, I was not able to use these interpretations without help from an American expert. So, my first recommendation is to discuss with American experts when translating difficult or ambiguous defining characteristics.

This idea led me to think of a suggestion for NANDA. Dr. Coler has also pointed out that the current list of the NANDA defining characteristics are difficult to translate to other languages because of the lack of a standard format for expressing characteristics or a linguistic protocol. I think this may be the time to review all defining characteristics for their translatability. By doing so, I believe some of the ambiguous or redundant defining characteristics can be eliminated from the current list.

References

Brislin, R.W. (1970). Back-translation for cross-cultural research. *Journal of Cross-Cultural Psychology, 1*(3), 185-216.

Carpenito, L.J. (1994). *Kango shindan handbook (T. Nakagi, Trans.) [Handbook of nursing diagnosis]*. Tokyo: Igaku Shoin. (Original work published 1993).

Coler, M.S. (1994). Achieving linguistic clarity: A model to aid translations. *Nursing Diagnosis, 5*(3), 102-105.

Gordon, M.S. (1993). *Kango shindan manual (S. Ito, J. Kusakari, K. Chikada, Y. Nojima, & M. Matsuki, Trans.) [Manual of nursing diagnosis]*. Tokyo: Health Publishing. (Original work published 1991).

Language Examination Committee. (1997). Kango shindan label no yakugo an (proposed translation of nursing diagnoses). *Nursing Diagnosis: Journal of Japan Society of Nursing Diagnoses, 2*(1), 91-95.

Matsuki, M. (1995). Japan: Nursing Diagnosis in Japan. In M.J. Rantz & P. LeMone (Eds.), *Classification of nursing diagnoses: Proceedings of the 11th conference* (pp. 313-316). Glendale, CA: CINAHL Information Systems.

North American Nursing Diagnosis Association (1994). *NANDA kango shindan: Teigi to bunrui 1992-1993 (M. Matsuki & T. Nakagi, Trans.) [NANDA nursing diagnoses: definitions and classification 1992-1993]*. Tokyo: Igaku Shoin. (Original work published 1992).

Association of Operating Room Nurses (AORN)

Aileen Killen

In contrast to our colleagues in AACN, The Association of Operating Room Nurses, Inc. (AORN) has embraced the concept of nursing diagnosis into the language of the Perioperative Data Set. Five expert perioperative nurses with interest and experience in nursing diagnosis were asked to form a subcommittee on Nursing Diagnosis of the AORN Data Elements Coordinating Committee (DECC).

The subcommittee was charged with identifying the current NANDA-approved nursing diagnoses that had relevance to perioperative nursing practice and to propose new diagnoses in areas of practice that were unique to the perioperative arena. At the initial meeting, the committee unanimously agreed that a survey consisting of all of the currently approved diagnoses would not only be cumbersome, but would potentially decrease the response rate as subjects were asked to respond to diagnoses that were foreign to their practice.

The subcommittee examined the literature to narrow down the list of nursing diagnoses to those with implications for the perioperative nurse. Current perioperative textbooks as well as five years worth of journal articles were reviewed. Journal articles included perioperative journals, general and specialty nursing journals, and journals from related fields such as psychology. Sixty diagnoses were identified and became the basis for a national survey.

The sample for the survey consisted, in part, of a convenience sample of the leaders of AORN and all members of the Educator/Clinical Nurse Specialty Assembly. Because AORN is an organization committed to individual members, a random sample of staff nurses was also included in the mailing. Respondents were asked to rate each potential nursing diagnosis as to the frequency with which it occurred in their practice and the priority with which the nurse must respond to the problem. A weighted score was computed for each nursing diagnosis using both the frequency and urgency scores.

Three categories of nursing diagnoses

were identified in the survey. The first category consisted of those nursing diagnoses which had both a frequency and a high priority score. Two diagnoses fell into this critical category. The second group consisted of nursing diagnoses with a high priority but a low frequency and the final group consisted of nursing diagnoses that had a low frequency and a low to moderate priority.

The highest weighted score was attributed to the nursing diagnosis *risk for perioperative positioning injury*. Interestingly, this diagnosis was submitted to NANDA by a member of the subcommittee as part of her master's thesis. We learned a lesson from this rating that perioperative nurses identify with specific language that they can easily relate to the work they do every day. This led us to address the second charge of submitting to NANDA new candidate diagnoses.

We began by suggesting revisions to some existing diagnoses that would include related factors and defining characteristics that would be applicable to perioperative nursing practice. Candidate nursing diagnoses such as latex allergy response, which has implications for both perioperative nurses as well as other groups of specialty nurses, were submitted to NANDA's Diagnosis Review Committee.

Although the work of the subcommittee has finished, the DECC of AORN continues to work with NANDA and the ANA to refine the Perioperative Data Set. Comments from the DRC regarding submissions will be reviewed by the current DECC and work will continue to refine proposed diagnostic categories.

American Association of Critical Care Nurses (AACN)

Kate Collopy

In order to respond to the question posed, AACN researched the use of nursing diagnosies in the organization. Both AACN leaders and members at large contributed to the positions presented. To summarize:

How is your specialty practice currently seeing the NANDA taxonomy incorporated into their standards of practice?

- Currently, nursing diagnosis taxonomy exits on our Outcome Standards for Care of the Critically Ill (1991). The current revision will not include the nursing diagnosis taxonomy but will probably mirror the ANA Standards of Nursing Care documents.
- The current Core Curriculum textbook includes key nursing diagnoses at the end of each disease or system section. The new edition will also incorporate the taxonomy in the same way.
- AACN's Practice Protocols do not include the taxonomy.
- The Certification Corporation exams use Bloom's taxonomy. Content areas of the exam reflect the nursing process. There are no plans to include the taxonomy in any new documents or resources.

If diagnoses are not used, why?

- Our members told us that NANDA taxonomy is useful in organization of work at the novice level and in education of care of complex patients, but have a decreased applicability in clinical practice. The taxonomy is too broad, generalized, and vague when describing a critically ill patient. The default is often to a systems language. Nursing diagnoses don't touch on the complexity and intertwining of problems and potential problems of complex patients.
- There are so many common or

standard problems for each patient, (i.e., psychosocial). Nursing diagnoses address norms and anticipated norms better than they address the changes and problems in an extremely dynamic environment.

- Some members have indicated that the use of nursing diagnoses is legally frightening. As stated by one nurse, "Some of my patients have 20 nursing diagnoses. If I spend the time to write each one and a care plan to address them, I wouldn't have time to provide care. So what should I do? List the top ten? Where am I legally if my patient dies from one of the ones that I didn't list?"
- NANDA taxonomy is considered restrictive and creates barriers for communication when dealing with a multi-disciplinary team. It inhibits communication and understanding across all disciplines.

Is the language of the current taxonomy useful to the specialty?

- The taxonomy helps the novice to organize and integrate the complexity of care, to assist in anticipatory planning and can serve as a guidepost for critical thinking. But critical care nurses find it bulky and unyielding in clinical practice, particularly for expert clinicians.

How do you see working with NANDA to improve the dissemination of nursing language while representing your specialty?

- Working with AACN's Synergy model, there is a potential to integrate the taxonomy in a meaningful way and describe nursing's unique contribution while being patient focused. The Synergy model describes the need for patient needs to drive nurse competency.
- Nursing diagnoses need to become more relevant to reality (i.e., health care systems, dynamic environments, decreased length of stay), and reflect that problems can change frequently in critical care: within shift, from RN to RN, as well as with resource availability, and emergencies.
- We are open to research in this area. For example, does skill level of the practitioner determine the ability to use the taxonomy (not just standardized nursing care plans for the problem, but driven by the specific need of the specific patient)? An alternate study could explore whether novice nurses use the taxonomy differently than experts.

The Association of Rehabilitation Nurses (ARN)

Ann McCourt

1. How is the specialty currently seeing the NANDA taxonomy incorporated into their standards of practice?

Before I discuss our involvement with nursing diagnosis, let me share with you some of the changes that have been occurring in rehabilitation nursing. There was a time when working in rehabilitation nursing meant you probably were working with patients who had sustained a spinal cord injury, a traumatic head injury or a stroke. Although we still care for these patients, the scope and location of our practice has considerably changed.

The aging population, increase in disability and chronic illness, the results of managed care and the transfer of general rehabilitation units from hospitals to extended care facilities have all had a significant impact on nursing. In the past few years we have broadened our scope of practice to include all patients with a multiplicity of problems, resulting form disability or chronic illness.

Regardless of the changes in the scope and setting of our practice we still have two major goals when caring for rehabilitation patients: to help patients to attain and maintain their optimal level of functioning and to cope and adapt to a change in lifestyle.

A. We do have both basic and advanced standards of practice, modeled after the ANA, which include nursing diagnosis. However, I think of equal importance is our basic certification exam in rehabilitation nursing. As many of you know, certification is very important to nurses in specialty practice, not just so they can wear the initials or receive higher pay, but it is increasingly becoming a requirement for employment. Ninety percent of the basic certification exam in rehabilitation nursing relates to Functional Health Patterns and nursing diagnosis. Therefore, it is highly unlikely that a nurse would pass the certification exam without a fundamental knowledge of NR-DX. As with many other specialties, by the year 2000, a bachelor of science degree in nursing will be required to take the certification exam. We also have an advanced certification exam. In order to take the advanced exam, a nurse must have passed the basic exam and have a master's or doctorate in nursing.

B. How do we know which diagnoses relate to rehabilitation nursing?

In the past few years our Rehabilitation Nursing Foundation has been involved in an extensive research project to determine the most important and frequently used diagnoses and the intervention and outcome linkages which go with them. Dr. Marjory Gordon was hired as our research consultant. The study involved four phases:

I.   The first survey was to identify the high frequency, high treatment priority nursing diagnoses. This is important for justifying the questions on the certification exam and for our basic core curriculum in rehabilitation nursing. There were no real surprises with the initial survey. Diagnoses included those relating to functional ability, elimination, roles and relationships, body image, coping, pressure ulcers, health management.

II. The second phase determined the defining characteristics of those diagnoses identified in the first survey. Important to assure accuracy in making the diagnoses.

III. and IV. Identified the outcome and intervention linkages for 21 diagnoses important to rehabilitation nursing.

Details of the study have been published in four separate articles in the *Journal of Rehabilitation Nursing Research*. The final arti-cle was published last year (1997).

The model that we used for our study, four phases and various methodologies, proved to be very effective in accomplishing our goal of determining our most important diagnoses and related interventions and outcomes. As a result of that study, two years ago the Foundation published clinical guidelines for the 21 nursing diagnoses important to rehabilitation nurses.

2. The publications of that booklet brings me to another question which we have been asked to address.

Is the language of the current taxonomy useful in to the specialty?
Yes and no, but essentially yes. The problem that we have with the current taxonomy is that many diagnostic labels are too broad to be clinically useful. One would never walk into a multidisciplinary rehabilitation team conference or write a case management report and state that the patient had a mobility problem, or was at risk for a skin impairment or had an altered thought process.

Impaired Mobility has been resolved, because the ARN Board of Directors authorized the practice committee to develop specific mobility diagnoses which would include Bed Mobility, Transfer, Ambulation (walking) and Locomotion (wheelchair mobility). They were submitted for the latest review process and were discussed Thursday. They have tentatively been approved by the NANDA board. Let me clarify, I am not implying that Impaired Mobility itself cannot be a useful diagnoses, but rather that its usefulness is limited with acute rehabilitation patients or those with complex mobility problems.

Pressure Ulcer and Attention/Concentration Deficit were also developed for our research study, but not for NANDA submission. We developed the attention/concentration deficit because it is frequently seen in patients with a traumatic head injury.

The lack of specific diagnoses for Impaired Skin Integrity is particularly dismaying for me because I worked on that diagnosis at the NANDA conference in 1978. We realized that there were multiple nursing diagnoses under this category. In fact, we got involved with pressure ulcers, burns, rashes, wounds, etc. All we have at the moment is a label for pressure ulcers. How are we going to resolve this?

Perhaps by having nurses from several specialties work in Impaired Skin Integrity. Consider the skin problems diagnosed and treated by the specialties represented on this panel. (Wounds, pressure ulcers, burns, etc.)

3. How does the specialty see working with NANDA to improve the disseminations of nursing language while representing the specialty?

To me, this is an interesting and difficult question. We could continue to use nursing diagnoses in the many ways that have been mentioned:

- Adhere to our standards of practice which include nursing diagnoses
- Include nursing diagnosis in the certification process
- Include nursing diagnoses in documentation formats: nursing care plans – either written or computerized, nursing minimum data sets, managed care reports
- Continue to include nursing diagnoses is in our publications.

In addition to disseminating information, we could also:

- further refine existing diagnoses or develop new ones which relate to our specialty; and
- really think broadly and creatively and consider developing cross-specialty diagnosis-specific, clinical practice guidelines. Perhaps have several specialty organizations working together on the same diagnosis. The expected outcomes might be the same but the etiologies and interventions would be different. Example: Pain. On this panel we have nurses working with patients who might have post-operative pain, pain from terminal cancer, chest pain, or pain related to acute muscle spasm.

There is much that could be done, providing we have the interest, the leadership, the commitment, the knowledge and clarification of roles.

Oncology Nursing Society (ONS): The Use of Nursing Diagnoses in Oncology Nursing Practice

Rose Mary Carroll-Johnson, MN, RN

The Oncology Nursing Society (ONS) is a national professional organization of more than 62,000 registered nurses working in the field of oncology. Members represent a variety of professional positions and practice settings. We have two journals, an active researcher group, and a large group of advanced practice nurses. When discussing the use of nursing diagnoses in oncology nursing one must consider nursing diagnoses in practice (i.e., by nurses caring for patients at the "bedside") and the way in which nursing diagnosis is reflected in the specialty's literature and research.

ONS has incorporated nursing diagnosis for some time into its standards (ANA & ONS, 1996) and its practice guidelines (McNally, Somerville, Miaskowski, & Rostad, 1991). In practice settings, the use of nursing diagnoses is driven largely by institutional requirements and the extent to which nursing diagnoses are incorporated into computerized nursing systems. Time to do thoughtful assessment and care planning is limited. Particular gaps in the use of nursing diagnosis in practice may involve less available time, lack of comfort applying nursing diagnoses in alternate or ambulatory care settings, and the increased use of unlicensed assistive personnel. Based on the level of knowledge of most professional oncology nurses about nursing diagnosis, the problems of use seem to have more to do with these logistics rather than a lack of acceptance.

The one area where we see nursing diagnoses used consistently is in our literature. Journal articles and book chapters regularly employ nursing diagnoses to characterize the nursing care necessitated by cancer and its treatments. In addition, certain key nursing diagnoses – pain, fatigue, ineffective coping, to name only a few – are primary areas of focus in our research efforts.

Clinical Practice

Many nursing diagnoses are fundamental to the cancer experience (See Table 1). Assessment and intervention in many of these areas becomes as basic and automatic to oncology nurses as the taking of vital signs. Our researchers have provided a substantial base of information in regard to these

Table 1

High Frequency Nursing Diagnoses in Oncology Nursing Practice

Anxiety

Body image disturbance

Pain, Chronic pain

Grieving

Fatigue

Ineffective individual coping

Risk for infection/altered protective mechanisms

Knowledge deficit

Altered nutrition: less than body requirements

Altered oral mucous membrane

Altered sexuality patterns

diagnoses and many of these diagnoses are evident in our list of oncology nursing research priorities (Stetz, Haberman, Holcombe, & Jones, 1995), which is updated every few years (See Table 2).

Table 2

1994 Oncology Nursing Research Priorities

1. Pain
2. Prevention (Health Seeking Behaviors)
3. Quality of life
4. Risk reduction/Screening (Health Seeking Behaviors)
5. Ethical issues
6. Neutropenia/immunosuppresion (altered protective mechanisms)
7. Patient education (Knowledge deficit)
8. Stress, coping, adaptation (Ineffective individual coping)
9. Detection
10. Cost containment

#12: Fatigue, #19: Nausea, #20: Stomatitis

In addition to those diagnoses used regularly, certain diagnoses, though not frequently seen in care plans, are an important part of our practice, dialogue, and research (See Table 3).

Table 3

Oncology Nursing High Interest Areas

Caregiver role strain
Decisional conflict
Diarrhea
Health Seeking Behaviors
Spiritual distress
Powerlessness

Oncology nurses can and will contribute to the concept development of these diagnoses, as well as to identification of the associated interventions and outcomes.

Caregiver role strain: Family issues in general are an important focus for oncology nurses who view the family as the unit of care. Oncology nurse researchers are looking at physical aspects, psychological challenges, and financial burden in this area.

Decisional conflict: This has been a longstanding area of interest in regard to treatment choices. It is even more critical now as we deal with end-of-life care, assisted suicide, and the burgeoning field of genetic testing and prevention.

Health seeking behaviors: Increasing interest in cancer prevention and alternative and complementary therapies gives new meaning to this diagnosis.

Spiritual distress: ONS has a special interest group devoted to the area of spiritual care and a number of research studies have examined aspects of spirituality in the patient with cancer.

Powerlessness: Cancer is a unique context in which to evaluate this nursing diagnosis especially in regard to genetic research.

Issues in the Use of Nursing Diagnoses

Oncology nurses struggle with a number of issues in regard to use of nursing diagnosis. These issues are by no means unique to oncology nursing but bear highlighting. A difficulty staying current with NANDA work and low dissemination of changes in and additions to the nursing diagnosis taxonomy, as well as the work of the Nursing Intervention Classification (NIC) and Nursing Outcomes Classification (NOC) teams, inhibits their use. The widespread use of automated information systems can however drive some of these changes, as well as facilitate familiarity and use.

Reducing the complexity of the language used in the taxonomy and allowing use of alternate language in some situations (e.g., when no diagnosis seems appropriate to describe the nursing problem) will facilitate acceptance. Nursing can learn from the translation efforts of our international colleagues in this regard.

Lastly, changes in advanced practice nursing must be monitored for their effects on the use of nursing language. The clinical nurse specialists, our clinical mentors and teachers of nursing models and nursing diagnosis, are disappearing while the numbers of nurse practitioners, who are more likely to use a medical model and medical vocabulary, are increasing (Carlson-Catalano, 1998). The impact of these practice changes on nursing's efforts to foster the use of a nursing taxonomy for diagnosis, intervention, and outcomes must be monitored.

What Lies Ahead

NANDA, in conjunction with NIC and NOC project teams, needs to expand efforts to collaborate with specialty organizations to identify and develop specialty-specific or high incidence diagnoses/syndromes. In turn, the specialty organizations need to consider devoting time and resources to an effort to track the use of these taxonomies and contribute to the research efforts to more accurately define and elucidate specialty-specific diagnoses, interventions, and outcomes.

Journal editors and specialty organization research directors would seem to be particularly important contacts to establish and maintain. Journal editors can facilitate use of the taxonomies in published material and disseminate information and continually update their readers. Research directors can build strategic alliances to share methodologies, carry out multisite studies, and forward pertinent results.

Conclusion

Oncology nurses face barriers to widespread use of nursing diagnosis, NIC, and NOC just like most nurses. Specialty organizations, however, have much to contribute to the efforts to develop these classifications, as well as to disseminate information about and facilitate their use. Formal collaboration among NANDA, the NIC and NOC research teams, and specialty nursing organizations should be pursued aggressively.

References

American Nurses Association & Oncology Nursing Society. (1996). *Statement on the scope and standards of oncology nursing practice.* Washington, DC: American Nurses Publishing.

Carlson-Catalano, J. (1998). Nurse practitioners' use of nursing diagnoses. *Nursing Diagnosis, 9*(2), 39-40.

McNally, J., Somerville, E., Miaskowski, C., & Rostad, M. (Eds.) (1991). *Oncology Nursing Society guidelines for oncology nursing practice.* Philadelphia, PA: Saunders.

Stetz, K., Haberman, M., Holcombe, J., & Jones, L. (1995). 1994 Oncology Nursing Society research priorities survey. *Oncology Nursing Forum, 22,* 785-789.

An International Perspective on Nursing Diagnosis Development

June Clarke, RN, PhD

My first visit to a NANDA conference — to Pittsburgh in 1996 — opened a new window on my nursing world. It marked the beginning of a sabbatical which enabled me to spend some time in the USA and several countries of Europe, finding out how nurses in different countries were developing and using standardized languages and clinical information systems to describe nursing practice. This paper describes my intellectual wanderings, but more significantly the "wonderings" for each new thing I saw and heard raised new questions, and what I saw and heard in one place interacted with what I saw and heard in other places. Each time, I came back to a core conclusion – that the concept of nursing diagnosis was central. But the question which puzzled me was, "Why is it so different in different countries? What is so different about nursing in one country from nursing in another that makes the concept of nursing diagnosis in one country central to the way nurses see their work, while in another country the very word produces apoplexy?"

Many things are explained by history. The history of nursing diagnosis in the USA has been well documented, and this week we have had the opportunity to treasure its pearls. But I would pick out as especially significant two features: the first is the role played by the American Nurses Association; in particular, the incorporation of the concept of nursing diagnosis into its Standards for Nursing Practice in 1974, and its position statement Nursing: A Social Policy Statement, in 1980; the second is the American health care system, in particular its systems for reimbursement and accreditation. These two factors, which seem to me to have been important drivers of developments in the USA, are simply not part of the experience of European countries.

In Europe the first formal initiative of which I am aware came from the Dutch nurses, and as the participation in this conference shows, they are still ahead of the rest of Europe. After attending the 10th NANDA conference in San Diego in 1992, some Dutch nurses, including Nico Oud who has been honored at this conference for his achievements, organized the first Dutch conference on nursing diagnosis under the title NANDA: Line of Action for the Netherlands?

The conference was also attended by nurses from other countries, specifically from Denmark, where the Danish Institute of Health and Nursing Research had been the co-ordinating organization between 1976 and 1985 for the WHO project "People's Need for Nursing Care". This multinational study, in which 11 European countries participated, used as its conceptual framework the nursing process, an idea which was at that time still new to Europe. The development, interpretation and use of the nursing process in different countries emerges as another key issue, to which I will return later.

So a year later, in November 1993, the first European conference on nursing diagnosis was held in Copenhagen. That conference was my first real exposure to the developments in nursing diagnosis that were going on in the various countries of Europe, and it identified another issue to which I shall return: that of the 300 or so nurses from 19 countries who attended, only two (myself and one other) came from the UK.

From the conference emerged the idea of developing a pan-European association for nurses who were interested in this field. A steering group was established with a brief for two tasks: to organize another European conference in two years time, and to put together proposals for establishing such an association. Two years later, the second European conference, held in Brussels in 1995, saw the launch of ACENDIO — the Association for Common European Nursing Diagnoses, Interventions and Outcomes. Randi Mortensen was elected the first President, with me as Secretary, and last

year I was elected President. The third European conference, which became the first ACENDIO conference, was held in 1997 in Amsterdam, and the next one, the second ACENDIO conference, will be held in Italy, in March 1999.

The birth and development of ACENDIO in the mid-1990s is remarkably like the birth and development of NANDA in the 1970's – including all the difficulties. We have the additional difficulties of language: our first Board of Directors consisted of eight people from eight different countries with eight different languages. This brings problems of organizational management and costs, but it is also an important source of our richness. The translation and cross-cultural validation of nursing diagnosis is part of our mission, albeit one that we haven't been able to do much about as yet. There is another difference too: you will notice that our title includes interventions and outcomes not just diagnoses. ACENDIO is a child of its time, and the world into which we were born is driven by political and financial imperatives that focus on interventions and outcomes in health care, more than by the needs of our own science as expressed in nursing diagnosis. Advocates of nursing diagnosis have always argued that the purpose of identifying the diagnosis is to enable the selection and prescription of the appropriate intervention; in most countries, however, people want to know what nurses do because they want to know what it costs, and they do not yet understand that nursing interventions cannot be explained without reference to nursing diagnoses.

Meanwhile, other forces and events in Europe quite outside the field of nursing have been interacting with and influencing these developments. The European Union, which began as an economic institution designed to develop a Common Market, has become a political institution whose agenda is concerned with standardization (or more euphemistically, har-monization) of everything from the content of sausages to a common currency. Standardization activities include health informatics. So Europe has a committee called CEN/TC251 which is exactly like the USA's ANSI. It has four work-groups covering information models, data security, safety and quality, technology for interoperability, and terminology and knowledge bases.

The European Union is also a major source of funding for research and development, which is especially important since, unlike the USA, Europe does not have the big foundations such as Kellogg for grants, nor (at least in the UK) tax breaks for individuals who make donations. But EU funding reflects the original purposes of the EU which you will remember were economic, so eligibility depends on making consortia with commercial organisations, and requires the applicants to be able to match any funding awarded.

One of the funding programmes is for medical informatics, and since the mid-1980s nurses in several European countries have been trying to break into this funding programme. The first to be successful were Gunnar Neilson and Randi Mortensen from Denmark, who in 1991 put up a project called ID-ENTITY (Informatics and Diagnoses — European Nursing Terminology as a Basis for Information Technology). The bid was not successful, but the EU Commission awarded a smaller grant for what is known as a Concerted Action — that is, money to enable participants in an enterprise to develop the kind of networks and consortium that is likely to be more successful in a bid next time.

This Concerted Action project became known as the TELENURSING project, and its specific purpose was to find out the "state of the art" in respect of the computerization of nursing documentation in Europe. Fifteen countries participated in two meetings and a questionnaire study. As a research project, it was poor, but it demonstrated that all over Europe nurses were documenting their practice; they were using the nursing process and a very, very few were using nursing diagnosis. As a political activity it was a huge step forward, for it led to a successful bid in the next funding round for what became the TELENURSE project.

Meanwhile, the ICNP project, which had begun in 1990, was also developing. Norma Lang and I were the first two consultants; then, when we learned of the work going on in Denmark, we invited Randi Mortenson, who brought with her Gunnar Neilson who became our first technical adviser, soon to be joined by Margie Murphy, Madeline Wake and Amy Coenen, and together we became the Development Team for the Alpha version. You have already heard a great deal in the last few days about the ICNP project. The link between ICNP and TELENURSE is that TELENURSE needed ICNP to achieve its purpose of developing the electronic patient record and ICN saw a golden opportunity to develop and test its emerging product.

The Journey: USA

So I began my journey at Pittsburgh in April 1996. The conference itself was rather like the "immersion courses" which language students do. I had the opportunity to meet and ask questions of the "pearls" of the nursing diagnosis movement; my learning curve was almost vertical. Next I spent a wonderful month at the

University of Iowa where I was immersed in the NIC, NOC and NDEC projects, joining in the work groups and visiting clinical sites to find out how things worked out in practice. Then I went to Washington where as well as seeing more systems in use, I learned about the Unified Medical Language System, and had the privilege of attending, as observer, a meeting of the ANA Steering Committee on Databases. I want publicly to thank all those who made my visit such a wonderfully enriching experience.

A Whistle-Stop Tour of Europe

While I was in Iowa, I returned briefly to Europe — to Spain, where, along with Marjorie Gordon, I spoke at the first Spanish conference on nursing diagnosis, which was attended by over 800 nurses. The NANDA taxononomy has been translated into Spanish, and, under the leadership of Mercedes Ugalde, Spain now has its own nursing diagnosis association.

Developments in France grew from the experience of French-speaking Canada. The NANDA taxonomy has been translated into French, there is a large and active Francophone nursing diagnosis association (AFEDE), and nursing diagnosis is taught as a compulsory component of the basic nursing curriculum.

In Germany there is still a long struggle ahead to establish nursing as a profession, and nursing education generally is still at quite a low level, but interest in nursing diagnosis is developing fast. Hanneke van Maanen, who is Professor of Nursing at Bremmen, and Theo Dassen, who has recently been appointed Professor of Nursing at Berlin, are among the founder members of ACENDIO. Significantly, both are Dutch.

In Italy a new law has recently moved nursing education into universities. A major problem is the shortage of doctorally prepared nurses. Renzo Zanotti, a founder member and Board member of ACENDIO and (at this time) Italy's only doctorally prepared nurse, has been teaching and translating books about nursing diagnosis for several years.

Developments in Eastern Europe are just beginning but are moving fast. Slovenia was represented at the First European Conference on Nursing Diagnosis in Copenhagen in 1993; Maijda Slaimer-Japeli is a founder member of ACENDIO, and a paper from Slovenia is included in this week's conference.

In Switzerland, where I went primarily to touch base with the International Council of Nurses, whose headquarters is of course in Geneva, I arrived just at the time when a new federal law on health statistics was creating a wonderful opportunity for Swiss nurses to establish a position and a language for nursing in the newly developing minimum data set.

Europe: The Grand Tour

These countries have been part of my intellectual and e-mail travels, but my sabbatical in Europe focused on the Nordic countries, Belgium and Netherlands.

The Nordic Countries

The Medical Informatics Europe conference (MIE96) which was held that year in Copenhagen provided a golden opportunity to find out what was happening in Denmark, Norway, Sweden, Finland and Iceland. There was lots of exciting work both in nursing language and in nursing informatics generally. In Iceland, Asta Thoroddsen was testing the emerging ICNP in a clinical setting. In Denmark, in addition to the work of the Danish Institute of Health and Nursing Research, the

National Board of Health is developing classifications for both nursing diagnoses and nursing interventions. In Sweden, where Margreta Ehnfors and Anna Erenberg have been developing the VIPs system, there has been a nursing diagnosis interest group since 1998. In both Sweden and Finland the national nurses associations have established specific projects to work on the ICNP.

Belgium

I went to Belgium to talk with Walter Sermeus, the nurse member of the team who developed the Belgian Nursing Minimum Data Set, and George Evers, who is working on nursing diagnosis within the framework of Orem's model of nursing. Both are professors at the Catholic University of Leuven. Belgium has had a mandatory NMDS and a system for collecting hospital data through a twice-yearly census since 1985, but surprisingly, I found (other than Evers' work) little interest in nursing diagnosis.

Netherlands

Of all the countries I visited, Netherlands was by far the most active in the field of nursing diagnosis. In addition to all the people I had met at NANDA and other conferences, I learned of the work of several agencies such as the National Centre for the Nursing and Caring Professions (LCVV) and WCC, which was the government agency responsible for developing classification and information system for all the healthcare professions, and is the WHO Collaborating Centre for the International Classification of Impairments Disabilities and Handicaps. I saw clinical information systems being developed or in use in several hospitals, including the university hospitals at Groningen and Leiden, and at Vught (the oldest psychiatric hospital in the Netherlands), and the paper based but nevertheless very effective system used by the community nursing service in Breda. I talked with nurses in the universities like Theo Dassen and his team of researchers at Groningen who were doing wonderfully careful work on the validation of several nursing diagnoses; Harry van der Bruggen and Maike Groen who are working on the definition of nursing outcomes at the University of Limberg in Maastricht, and many others.

Questions and Issues

I did not get a lot of sleep, but as I sat on trains and in airports (lots of them), questions kept bubbling up in my mind:

- What can explain the similarities and differences I have found? I can understand why USA might be different from Europe, but why is Belgium so different from the Netherlands when they are so close and speak the same language?
- What drives the development in those countries where there is such a lot going on, that is missing in neighbouring countries who have never heard of nursing diagnosis?
- And why is the UK so far behind?

Driving Forces

First of all the driving forces. A major driving force in all countries is the development of computerized information services for management and financial purposes. One reason for the USA's headstart has been the imperatives of the reimbursement and accreditation system which, until the market-oriented healthcare reforms of the early 1990s, European countries did not have. But there have also been other forces. I mentioned the development of nationally mandated minimum data sets in Belgium and Switzerland; and in Sweden tremendous impetus was given by the 1986 Patient Record Act, which makes it compulsory for nurses to record their care alongside that of the physician, and the subsequent govenment guidance which identifies diagnosis as part of nursing care. In the Netherlands, the concept of nursing science is important. In France, nursing diagnosis is included in the national nursing curriculum.

The UK has had none of these imperatives — no reimbursement or accreditation systems, no legal requirements for nursing documentation, no concept of nursing science, nothing in the curriculum, and a huge emotional barrier to the word diagnosis. The new driver in the UK is a massive development of information technology and the UK government's new emphasis on information systems for the National Health Service. My worry is that because nursing is so unprepared, there is a risk that what nursing cannot do for itself will be done by others. The risk is that we will repeat the early mistakes which US nurses have worked so hard to overcome – of minimum data sets which do not include nursing, patient information systems based on a medical model, and perpetuation of our invisibility.

National Nursing Associations

The second significant factor is the role and influence of nursing associations, especially the national nursing association in each country. In the USA the contribution of the American Nurses Association has been enormous. I earlier pointed to the significance of the incorporation of nursing diagnosis into the ANA Standards for Nursing Practice, but I am also impressed by the political commitment reflected in resolutions of the ANA House of Delegates, the many ANA publications, and especially the work of the Steering Committee on Databases. The politics of the ANA systems for approving nursing languages for inclusion in the NLM Unified Medical Language System, and most recently for systems vendors (NIDSEC), has been quite brilliant. One of the products of my sabbatical was a report to the Royal College of Nursing of the UK entitled "Information is Power" — How the American Nurses Association Manages Nursing Information.

The Nursing Process

The third factor which emerges is the use and interpretation of the nursing process. I was fascinated by an article by Pesut and Herman in *Nursing Outlook* earlier this year called "OPT: Transformation of Nursing Process for Contemporary Practice." What fascinated me was not so much the model which they were proposing, but their analysis of its precursors — three generations of the nursing process. The first generation (1950-1970) used a four-step linear model of assessment, planning, intervention and evaluation to identify patient problems and procedures to deal with the problems. Because this first generation model focused on the nursing needs of people with particular medical conditions, its orientation remained within the medical model.

Once nurses began to think more about the independent domain of nursing, they say, a new approach to thinking and reasoning — a second-generation nursing process — emerged. Its midwife, as identified by Pesut and Herman, was the 1973 ANA publication on Standards of Nursing Practice, which established a five–step nursing process, which specifically identified nursing diagnosis as a fifth step between assessment and planning. This period (1970-1990) used the work of Gordon and others on diagnostic reasoning, information processing models, decision-making theory. Pesut and Herman describe this as a "significant transformation" and so it is.

Then as the 1980s moved into the 1990s, they say, attention shifted from problems and diagnoses to specification and measurement of outcomes. Significant for this third generation, for which Pesut and Herman propose their new model, are the terminologies and classification systems for nursing diagnoses, intervention and outcomes which provide a clinical language for clinical reasoning and require new models and approaches.

The nursing process started to cross the Atlantic during the mid-1970s and gradually became consolidated in nursing curricula (if not in nursing practice) in the 1980s — by which time the US, according to Pesut and Herman, was already moving into the second generation. The key is that the UK, and probably most of the rest of Europe, for a variety of reasons which there is not time to discuss now, remains stuck in the time warp of the first generation — the four-step nursing process which does not include nursing diagnosis.

Nursing Education

The fourth significant factor is nursing education. I have often suggested that if, in what has been called "the battle of the nurses, " Florence Nightingale had lost and Ethel Bedford Fenwick had won, nursing education in the UK and probably the rest of Europe would be very different from what we have today. The UK and most of the rest of Europe still has what I call the Nightingale vocational training model rather than the Bedford Fenwick university model.

The European Union Advisory Committee on Training in Nursing which sets the standards for the basic education which regulates the free movement of nurses in Europe, has recently been trying to shift nursing education in Europe to the level of university education which is advocated by ICN, WHO, the Council of Europe and most of the rest of the world. The Nordic countries, the Netherlands and Spain are more or less there; in the UK the profession is at best lukewarm, and the ACTN representatives for Germany and Austria are actively resisting.

The achievement of university preparation for nursing is important for 3 reasons:

1. because, as Virginia Henderson once pointed out, nurses can practice only to the level to which they have been prepared;

2. because in the multidisciplinary activity of health care, I believe that nurses will never be perceived as equal members of the team, or achieve status and influence equal to their potential contribution, while their education (and therefore their ability to articulate and argue their case) is so much less than that of the other members of the team;

3. and thirdly, and most significantly for the present issue, because a proper university education is based on habits of thinking and ways of developing and using knowledge which support the cognitive processes of clinical decision making and knowledge–based practice, and that includes of course nursing diagnosis.

Two Ways of Conceptualizing Nursing

And that brings me to my final issue, which I think underpins all the rest. It is how nurses conceptualize the nature of nursing practice. This factor is linked with education, because it is through the processes of basic education, and most significantly through socialization into the profession, that each nurse's personal concept of nursing is formed.

There are two ways of conceptualizing nursing. In the UK nursing is doing. Our values are reflected in our language. In the UK we value "hands-on care"; our formal educational aspiration is a "knowledgeable doer." We advocate research-based practice as a means of justifying what we do. We teach tasks. I do not know of any basic nursing curriculum in the UK which includes courses on clinical decision making or diagnostic reasoning. The result is that when nurses continue their education after their personal concept of nursing and their ways of practising are established, they may learn about nursing theory and research methods, even about nursing diagnosis, but when the chips are down and time is short, what matters is to get on with the doing.

The second way conceptualizes the core of nursing practice not as doing, but as deciding what to do, why, when and how – that is, clinical decision making based on reasoning. This way does not devalue the doing, but it recognizes the importance of cognitive as well as technical skills. When nursing is seen in this way, things like theory, the literature, cognitive skills, clinical reasoning are not unaffordable extras – they are the basic tools needed to do the job.

Conclusion

So I have wandered and wondered and learnt a lot. I am passionate about the need to identify and articulate those phenomena which are nursing's special concern and the focus of nursing intervention, and I am excited about the work that is going on everywhere, and the work I am beginning to do myself. I have a lot to learn. Thank you for giving me the opportunity to be part of such a wonderful learning community.

References

Gordon, M. (1994). *Nursing diagnosis: Process and application.* St Louis: Mosby-Year Book.

American Nurses Association. (1974). *Standards for nursing practice.* Kansas City: ANA.

American Nurses Association. (1980). *Nursing: A social policy statement.* Kansas City: ANA.

Ashworth P. et al. (1987). *People's need for nursing care: A European study.* Copenhagen: WHO.

Neilsen, G., & Mortensen, R. (1994). *Telenursing: Documentation of the nursing process in hospitals by computers in Europe.* Copenhagen: Danish Institute for Health and Nursing Research.

International Council of Nurses. (1997). *The international classification for nursing practice: A unifying framework. The alpha version.* Geneva: ICN.

Apalategu, M. U., & Cuadra, A. R. (1995). *Diagnosticos de enfermeria: Taxonomia NANDA.* Barcelona: Masson S.A.

Brender J., Christensen J., Schepper J., & McNair, P. (Eds) (1996). *Medical informatics. Europe 96.* Amsterdam: 1OS Press.

Thoroddsen, A. (1997). ICNP from a clinical nursing point of view. In Mortensen, R. *ICNP in Europe: TELENURSE.* Amsterdam: 1OS Press.

Sermeus, W., & Delesie, L. (1994). The registration of nursing minimum data set in Belgium: Six years of experience. In S.J. Grobe & E.S. Pleuter-Wenting (Eds), *Nursing information: An international overview for nursing in a technological era*. Amsterdam: Elseview.

Pesut D.J., & Herman, J. (1998). OPT: Transformation of nursing process for contemporary practice. *Nursing Outlook, 46,* 29-36.

McGann, S. (1992). *The battle of the nurses*. London: Scutari Press.

UKCC. (1986). *Project 2000: A new preparation for practice*. London: UKCC.

Nursing Interventions Classification (NIC) — Current Status and New Directions

Joanne C. McCloskey, PhD, RN
Gloria M. Bulechek, PhD, RN

This paper is based upon two presentations, one at the NANDA, NIC and NOC conference in St. Charles, IL, in November 1997 and one at the NANDA conference in St. Louis in April 1998. The paper is submitted for inclusion in the *NANDA Proceedings of the Thirteenth National Conference* and to the *On-line Journal of Nursing Informatics*.

Introduction

The ongoing work at the University of Iowa to name and classify nursing interventions is 11 years old. The impetus for the work on interventions partially evolved from the NANDA work – once a nurse makes a diagnosis, there is an obligation to do something about it. Prior to the development of the Nursing Interventions Classification, the profession of nursing had no language with which to communicate the interventions that nurses perform. In the past decade, the development of this language and its implementation in practice and education has evolved rapidly. The purpose of this paper is to overview NIC and then to discuss some current work and related issues.

Overview of NIC

The Nursing Interventions Classification (NIC) (McCloskey & Bulechek, 1996) names and describes interventions that nurses perform. An intervention is defined as "any treatment, based upon clinical judgment and knowledge, that a nurse performs to enhance patient/client outcomes" (p. xvii). NIC is useful for clinical documentation, communication of care across settings, aggregation of data across systems and settings, effectiveness research, productivity measurement, competency evaluation, reimbursement, and curriculum design. Each of the 433 interventions in the classification is composed of a naming label, a definition, and a list of activities that describe what a nurse does to carry out the intervention. The label and definition are the standardized language and cannot be changed unless through a formal review process; the activities can be modified somewhat to meet

Table 1

2540 Cerebral Edema Management

DEFINITION: Limitation of secondary cerebral injury resulting from swelling of brain tissue

ACTIVITIES:
Assess for confusion, changes in mentation, complaints of dizziness, syncope
Establish means of communication: ask yes or no questions; provide magic slate, paper and pencil, picture board, flashcards, vocaid device
Monitor neurologic status closely and compare to baseline
Monitor CSF drainage characteristics: color, clarity, consistency
Record CSF drainage
Decrease stimuli in patient's environment
Give sedation as needed
Note patient's change in response to stimuli
Monitor respiratory status: rate, rhythm, depth of respirations; PaO2, PCO2, pH, bicarbonate
Allow ICP to return to baseline between nursing activities
Screen conversation within patient's hearing
Administer anticonvulsants as appropriate
Avoid neck flexion, or extreme hip/knee flexion
Avoid Valsalva maneuvers
Administer stool softeners
Hyperventilate patient
Position with head of bed up 300 or greater
Avoid use of PEEP
Analyze ICP waveform
Plan nursing care to provide rest periods
Monitor patients ICP and neurologic response to care activities
Administer paralyzing agent
Encourage family/significant other to talk to patient
Restrict fluids
Avoid hypotonic IV fluids
Adjust ventilator settings to keep PaCO2 at prescribed level
Limit suction passes to less than 15 seconds

Monitor for CSF rhinorrhea/otorrhea
Monitor lab values: serum and urine osmolality, sodium, potassium
Monitor volume pressure indices
Perform passive range of motion
Monitor CVP
Monitor ICP and CPP
Monitor PAWP and PAP
Monitor P and BP
Monitor intake and output
Drain CSF according to standing orders
Hyperventilate prior to suctioning
Maintain normothermia
Administer loop active or osmotic diuretics
Implement seizure precautions
Titrate barbiturate to achieve suppression or burst-suppression of EEG as ordered

BACKGROUND READINGS:

Ackerman, L.L. (1992). Interventions related to neurological care. In G.M. Bulechek & J.C. McCloskey (Eds.), Symposium on nursing interventions. *Nursing Clinics of North America, 27*(2), 325-346.

Alpers, R., & Hertig, V.L. (1990). Cerebral edema management. In M.J. Craft &
J.A. Denehy (Eds.), *Nursing interventions for infants and children* (pp. 345-354). Philadelphia: W.B. Saunders.

American Nurses' Association Council in Medical-Surgical Nursing Practice & American Association of Neuroscience Nurses (1985). *Neuroscience nursing practice: Process and outcome for selected diagnoses.* Kansas City, MO: ANA.

Cammermeyer, M., & Appledorn, C. (Eds.). (1990). *Core curriculum for neuroscience nursing* (3rd ed.) (pp. ldl-ldl 1). Chicago: American Association of Neuroscience Nurses.

Hickey, J.V. (1992). *The clinical practice of neurological and neurosurgical nursing* (3rd ed.). Philadelphia: J.B. Lippincott.

Johanson, B.C., Wells, S.J., Hoffmeister, D., & Dungca, C.U. (1988). *Standards for critical care* (3rd ed.). St. Louis: Mosby-Year Book.

Mitchell, P.H., & Ackerman, L.L. (1992). Secondary brain injury reduction. In G.M. Bulechek & J.C. McCloskey (Eds.), *Nursing interventions: Essential nursing treatments* (2nd ed.) (pp. 558-573). Philadelphia: W.B. Saunders.

Source: McCloskey, J.C. & Bulechek, G. M. (Eds.) Nursing Interventions Classification (NIC), 2nd ed. St. Louis: Mosby Year Book.

the needs of the situation and to provide for individualized care planning. Each intervention also has a short list of background readings that supports the intervention and a unique four letter code. See one example in Table 1.

The classification includes all treatments that nurses perform, from the most basic (e.g., Body Mechanics Promotion – facilitating the use of posture and movement in daily activities to prevent fatigue and musculoskeletal strain or injury) to those that are highly complex and specialized (e.g., Anesthesia Administration – preparation for and administration of anesthetic agents and monitoring of patient responsiveness during administration and Electronic Fetal Monitoring: Intrapartum – electronic evaluation of fetal heart rate response to uterine contractions during intrapartal care). NIC interventions include both the physiological (e.g., Acid-Base Management – promotion of acid-base balance and prevention of complications resulting from acid-base imbalance) and the psychosocial (e.g.,

Anxiety Reduction – minimizing apprehension, dread, foreboding, or uneasiness related to an unidentified source of anticipated danger). There are interventions for illness treatment (e.g., Hyperglycemia Management – preventing and treating above normal blood glucose levels), injury prevention (e.g., Fall Prevention – instituting special precautions with patient at risk for injury from failing), and health promotion (e.g., Exercise Promotion – facilitation of regular physical exercise to maintain or advance to a higher level of fitness and health). Interventions are for individuals or for families (e.g., Family Integrity Promotion – promotion of family cohesion and unity). Indirect care interventions (e.g., Emergency Cart Checking – systematic review of the contents of an emergency cart at established time intervals) and interventions for communities (e.g., Environmental Management: Community – monitoring and influencing of the physical, social, cultural, economic, and political conditions that affect the health of groups and communities) are also included.

The interventions are coded in a three-level taxonomic structure easy for clinicians to use. At the top, most abstract level, of the taxonomy are six domains: Physiological: Basic, Physiological: Complex, Behavioral, Safety, Family, and Health System. At the second level are 27 classes organized within the domains. At the third level are the interventions themselves, grouped according to class and domain. All domains, classes, and interventions have definitions. Some (not many) interventions are located in more than one class, but each has a unique code (see Table 1 – unique code number for Cerebral Edema Management is 2540) which identifies the primary class and is not used for any other intervention.

NIC can be used in all settings (from acute care intensive care units, to home care, to hospice, to primary care) and specialties (from critical care to ambulatory care and long term care). While the entire classification describes the domain of nursing, some of the interventions in the classification are also done by other providers. NIC can be used by other non-physician providers to describe their treatments.

The classification is continually updated with an ongoing process for feedback and review. In the back of the NIC book, there are instructions for how users can submit suggestions for modifications to existing interventions or propose a new intervention. These submissions are then put through a two-level review process, first by selected experts in the area and then by the entire research team. Interventions which need further work are sent back to the author for revision. All contributors whose changes are included in the next edition are acknowledged in the book. The next edition of the classification will be published in fall of 1999 with a 2000 copyright and new editions of the classification are planned for every four years. Work between editions and other relevant publications that enhance the use of the classification are available from the Center for Nursing Classification at The University of Iowa, Iowa City, IA.

Several tools are available that assist in the implementation of the Classification. Included in the NIC book are two tools that assist with selecting an intervention: the taxonomic structure and linkage lists with all NANDA diagnoses. In addition, available from the Center for Nursing Classification, there is an implementation manual, an anthology of past publications, linkages with Omaha health problems, a listing of interventions core to 39 clinical specialties, a thesaurus of synonyms and related terms, and linkages with NOC outcomes. A 40-minute video that is useful for implementation in practice and education has been produced by the National League for Nursing and is available for the Center for Nursing Classification. The Center also maintains a listserv for users and a listing of users by state and country.

NIC is recognized by the American Nurses Association (ANA) and is included as one data set that will meet the uniform guidelines for information system vendors in the ANA's Nursing information and Data Set Evaluation Center (NIDSEC). NIC is included in the National Library of Medicine's Metathesaurus for a Unified Medical Language. Both the Cumulative Index to Nursing and Allied Health Literature (CINAHL) and SilverPlatter have added NIC to their nursing indexes. NIC is included in the Joint Commission on Accreditation for Health Care Organization's (JCAHO) as one nursing classification system that can be used to meet the standard on uniform data. Many health care agencies are adopting NIC for use in standards, care plans, competency evaluation, and nursing information systems; nursing education programs are using NIC to structure curriculum and identify competencies of graduating nurses; authors of major texts are using NIC to discuss nursing treatments; and researchers are using NIC to study the effectiveness of nursing care. Licenses are granted by Mosby Year Book for commercial or institutional use. Licensing fees are determined by the number of users per site and are renewable every two years. Interest in NIC has been demonstrated in several other countries, notably Canada, Denmark, England, France, Iceland, Japan, Korea, Spain, Switzerland, and The Netherlands.

New Directions and Issues

At every stage of major projects there is ongoing work and related issues to be resolved. In this section, we address some of these.

Development of Community Interventions: While the second edition of NIC does include some interventions that can be used with communities (aggregates), this area is still incomplete. Several of the interventions in the classification, including Environmental Management: Community, Environmental Management: Worker Safely, Health Education, Health Screening, Immunization/Vaccination Administration, Risk Identification, and Smoking Cessation, will be used by community health nurses when working with both individuals and groups. However, more interventions aimed at whole populations or communities still need to be developed. Several of the suggestions for interventions on the current "Under Consideration List" which have been submitted by reviewers and users of NIC are community interventions, e.g., Community Advocacy, Community Mobilization, Community Resource Development, Disaster Preparedness, Epidemic Prevention, Environmental Management: Adequate Housing, Environmental Protection: Air Pollution, Environmental Protection: Waste Disposal, Environmental Protection: Water Pollution, and Program Development. This area of intervention is especially important in Third World countries where nursing action is often aimed at the entire community. It is also an area of growing importance in the US as health care becomes more prevention and community focused. According to Deal (1994), "as the devastating impact of public health problems such as AIDS, infant mortality, adolescent pregnancy, child abuse, and domestic violence become more evident nationwide, a clear need exists for effective population-based health programs... it is imperative that community health nurses define their services and provide evidence supporting the effectiveness of interventions they offer." (p. 315). The American Nurses Association Division on Community Health Nursing (1980) defines community health nursing as a synthesis of nursing practice and public health practice applied to promoting and preserving the health of populations, with the dominant responsibility to the population as a whole. A population is a collection of individuals who have one or more personal (e.g., gender, age) or environmental (e.g. country, worksite) characteristics in common (Stanhope & Lancaster, 1966). We have tentatively defined a community health intervention as follows: A community (or public health) intervention is targeted to promote and preserve the health of populations. Community interventions emphasize health promotion, health maintenance, and disease prevention of populations and include strategies to address the social and political climate in which the population resides. We hope that in the third edition of NIC we will include many more interventions for the community.

Ongoing Refinement of Existing Interventions and Development of Other New Interventions: In addition to paying special attention to the area of community we are continuing to refine existing interventions and to develop other interventions as user feedback indicates. As the Classification is becoming better known and used, we are receiving increasing amounts of feedback. Sometimes when new interventions are developed, existing related interventions need some modification and this is done as part of the review and revision process. Some of the new interventions that have been developed and will be in the third edition of

NIC include: Abuse Protection: Domestic Partner, Anaphylaxis Management, Breast Examination, Case Management, Circulatory Care: Arterial Insufficiency, Circulatory Care: Venous Insufficiency, Community Disaster Preparedness, Cost Containment, Developmental Care, Forgiveness Facilitation, Reminiscence Therapy, Religious Ritual Enhancement, Staff Development, and Triage: Emergency Center.

Need for Effectiveness Research: The essential effectiveness question is "what works best for which patients"? Nursing effectiveness research (also called outcomes research), is about studying the effects of nursing interventions. In the future, when nurses systematically document their care with standardized languages (NANDA, NIC, NOC), databases concerning nursing practice information generated from care delivered will become available. Questions concerning which interventions work best for which patients at what cost can readily be studied from the existing sources of data. The progress of nursing science should move more quickly when existing data can be used rather than each researcher having to collect new data each time a research question or hypothesis is proposed. With the help of these databases, we will be able to determine which nursing interventions work best for a given population. We will address research questions such as the following:

1. What intervention works best for the achievement of a specific outcome?
2. What interventions are typically used together?
3. What interventions are typically used in certain areas or specialties?

In order to answer the above questions, we need to collect information about the patient, the providers, and the care environment. We have suggested elsewhere (Iowa Intervention Project, 1997a) that data about the following variables should be collected to confidently answer the previous three questions: the patient's identity number (to allow linking of information), age, sex, race/ethnicity (these three to provide some demographic information), episode admission or encounter date, discharge or termination date, disposition (where the patient went after discharge), and outcomes (both expected and achieved); the physician's diagnoses and interventions; the nurse's diagnoses and interventions, including the specific medications administered (in order to control for the medications' effects in relationship to other nursing interventions); and the work unit's type, staff mix, average patient acuity, and work load (also necessary as controls). Each of these variables needs a standardized definition and measure. (See the chapter by the Iowa Intervention Project, 1997a for the definitions and measures of 24 variables proposed for the basis of a nursing database.)

Our work with the identification and measurement of variables necessary for the conduction of effectiveness research demonstrates that the profession still needs to grapple with several issues related to the collection of standardized data. For example, the collection and coding of medications in easily retrievable form is not yet available in most facilities. While nursing effectiveness research can be done without the knowledge of medications, many of the outcomes that are achieved by nurses are also influenced by certain drugs and so the control for medication effect is desirable. Also, at the present time there is also no unique number that identifies the primary nurse. Consequently, it is not currently possible to attribute clinical interventions or outcomes to particular nurses based upon documentation data. Additionally, health care facilities do not yet collect the unit data in a standardized way. Despite the remaining challenges, we have made enormous progress in our ability to engage in effectiveness research. With the development of standardized language that can be used for documentation of actual clinical practice, we can now add effectiveness methods to our ability to study the impact of our interventions.

Determination of Average Time for Each Intervention: Hand in hand with knowing what works in practice is knowing the cost of what works. Administrators' top concern these days is keeping health care costs affordable (at an acceptable level of quality). As managed care continues to grow, health care and nursing administrators need to be able to know and articulate the cost of nursing care in order to be able to contract for services. The treatment or intervention can be considered the "product" of nursing care and therefore provides an acceptable and explainable item for billing. (That is, the intervention is not everything that nurses do but is a reasonable proxy; other services can be included in the overhead charge or as an add on charge). The steps to determining the costs of nursing interventions can be listed as follows:

- Identify the interventions delivered to the patient.
- Affix a price per intervention taking into account the level of provider and time spent delivering the intervention, as well as supplies and equipment required.
- Determine an overhead or indirect care charge (allocate evenly to all patients) and be able to provide justification.

- Determine the cost of delivering care per patient (direct care interventions plus overhead).
- Determine the charge per patient or use the information to contract for nursing services (Iowa Intervention Project, 1997b).

The first step in determining nursing cost is to identify the interventions that will be delivered to the patient (or patient population). This step is now possible with the use of NIC. The next step of affixing a price per intervention hinges on knowing who needs to deliver the intervention and, on average, how much time it takes. While each agency/managed care group needs to determine these issues for their own practice, some overall guidelines would assist in this process. It is not, in our opinion, desirable to conduct time in motiontwork sampling studies for all of the interventions included in NIC. These methods take a good deal of time, are resource intensive and have other problems related to sample size, timing of data collection periods, and the potential influence of the observer on the study subjects (Scherubel & Minnick, 1994). Estimates of time to perform interventions by nurses who do the interventions has been shown to be an accurate and efficient method to determine time values (Albrecht, 1987; McCloskey, Bulechek, Moorhead, & Daly, 1996). While we think it desirable to obtain time estimates for each intervention, at the present time, we do not have plans to conduct this research. While it is a desirable goal, we do not have the resources to do the research without additional funding. *Funding for Ongoing Work*: As indicated, funding to continue this work is an ongoing concern. We have been fortunate to have received seven years of funding (two R01 grants) from the National Institute of Nursing Research (NINR). We did submit a third grant which was approved but not with a high enough priority score to obtain continued funding. We revised and resubmitted this but the results were similar — the reviewers' comments indicated that while the work was very important, the expectation was that we should now be able to move to the stage of effectiveness research (use of data from information systems using NIC). While many health care institutions are beginning to use NIC and NOC, the implementation takes many years before useful data can be generated. In addition, most institutions do not systematically collect the other variables addressed in the previous section on effectiveness research. In fact, a recent survey of health care executives (Serb, 1998) revealed that only 2 percent of 1,700 respondents indicated that they have a fully operational electronic patient record system. Many health care systems still cannot electronically keep track of patients with no common coding for the same patient. We are, in our opinion, still years away from having good data for effectiveness research in nursing.

We feel that the ongoing refinement and maintenance of NIC is an important contribution to the profession but resources are an ongoing concern. We are fortunate that the College of Nursing is supporting one staff person for three years to assist the investigators of NIC and NOC in the Center for Nursing Classification. The Center was proposed by the investigators three years ago as a structure to keep the work ongoing when grant funding was no longer available. The Center is located in the College of Nursing and provides working and meeting space for staff and investigators. The purposes of the Center are to: a) facilitate the continued development of the Nursing Interventions Classification and the

Nursing Outcomes Classification to reflect current nursing practice, b) conduct the review processes and procedures for updating the Classifications, c) publish, sell, and otherwise disseminate materials related to the Classifications, d) provide office support to assist faculty investigators to write grants and obtain funding, and e) offer opportunities for student research assistants' and fellows' education and research experience. In order to have some permanent support for the Center, we are working to raise an endowment. Our goal is to raise $1 million and we need to reach this goal in the next three years when our College support will end. To date we have raised $190,000. We would very much appreciate your donation — without your support, the continued upkeep of these classifications is at risk. Gifts and pledges to the Center for Nursing Classification Endowment Fund should be sent to the University of Iowa Foundation, Iowa City, Iowa. All gifts qualify as charitable contributions. *Copyright and Licensing:* NIC is published and copyrighted by Mosby Year Book in St. Louis and they process requests for permissions to use the Classification. We have been asked on several occasions why we decided to allow a publisher to have copyright rather than retain this. There are several reasons. When we first began working on the classification we had little idea of the magnitude of the work or its current widespread use. We were looking for a way to get the work in print and disseminated quickly. As academics, we were familiar with the book publishing world and after some very serious review of alternative mechanisms and talks with other publishers, we selected Mosby as the publisher. Publication with Mosby has several advantages. First, they have the resources and the contacts to produce a book, to market it, and to sell it. (We produce and distribute related products from the Center but we

do not have the staff or the expertise to do this on a larger scale.) In addition, Mosby has the legal staff and resources to process requests for permissions and protect the copyright. This is especially important with standardized language where alteration of terms will impede the goal of communication among nurses across specialties and between delivery sites. We continue to have a good relationship with Mosby which involves frequent and active participation in permissions requests. We view our relationship as a partnership.

We want to address some of the facts about copyright and licensing as it is our experience that the nursing community has little knowledge in this area. Copyright does not restrict fair use. According to guidelines by the American Library Association (1977), fair use allows materials to be copied if: 1) the portion copied is selective and sparing in comparison to the whole work; 2) they are not used repeatedly; 3) no more than one copy is made for each person; 4) the source and copyright notice is included on each copy; and 5) persons are not assessed a fee for the copy beyond the actual cost of reproduction. The determination of the amount that can be copied under fair use policies has to do with the effect of the copying on sales of the original material. The American Library Association says that no more than 10% of a work should be copied.

When someone puts NIC on an information system that will be used by multiple users, copyright is violated (one book is now being "copied" for use by hundreds of nurses) and so a licensing agreement is needed. Also, when someone uses large amounts of NIC in a book or software product which is then sold and makes money for that individual then a permissions fee is necessary. Schools of nursing and health care agencies that want to use NIC in their own organizations and have no intention of selling a resulting product are free to do so. Fair use policies exist however. For example, NIC should not be Xeroxed and used in syllabi semester after semester — the NIC book should be one of those adopted for use. Similarly, health care agencies need to purchase a reasonable number of books (say, one per unit) rather than Xerox and put the interventions in some procedure manual.

Requests for use of NIC should be sent to the permissions department of Mosby (see the front of the NIC book for the address). Many requests for permission to use do not violate copyright and permission is given with no fee. Fees for use in a book depend on the amount of material used. Fees for use in information systems depend upon the number of users and averages about $5.00 per user for two years. There is a $2500 flat fee for incorporating NIC into a vendor's database and then a sublicense fee for each sublicense undertaken based on the number of users. The fees are very reasonable and a substantial portion of the fees which are returned to the authors are being reinvested into the endowment fund to be used in the future for further development and refinement of NIC.

Multiple classifications: One additional issue that is of some concern at this crucial stage of dissemination and need for adoption in practice is the confusion that multiple classifications create. The American Nurses Association has recognized five classifications: NANDA nursing diagnoses, Nursing Interventions Classification (NIC), Nursing Outcomes Classification (NOC), the Home Health Care classification (Saba, 1992), and the Omaha system (Martin & Scheet, 1992, Visiting Nurse Association of Omaha, 1986). In addition there are writings and publications about other "classifications" such as the State Board of Nursing's nomenclature developed for their computerized licensure test, Grobe's (1992) lexicon, and Osbolt's database (Osbolt, Fruchtnight, & Hayden, 1994). The International Classification of Nursing Practice (ICNP) (International Council of Nurse, 1996) being produced and disseminated by the International Council of Nurses in collaboration with Randi Mortinson and Gunar Neilson of Denmark also contains different emerging classifications. Some nursing specialty organizations such as the Association of Operating Room nurses are also developing languages for their own specialty. While the profession may be too large for one language, there is still a need to communicate with a common language. The National Library of Medicine which has incorporated the five ANA-recognized languages is working to map relationships between these languages but, to date, that work is unavailable to most nurses and has not been evaluated or clinically tested. We believe that the profession is best served by the continued use and development of NANDA, NIC and NOC, which are comprehensive across setting and specialty and each of which has an ongoing research effort to continue development of the classification. Linkages based on expert opinion have been established between NANDA and NIC, NANDA and NOC, and NIC and NOC and linkages among all three classifications are in development. Currently each of these classifications has its own taxonomic structure. Another future task is to determine if one taxonomic structure can accommodate all three classifications. While this is highly desirable from a user perspective, it may not be possible from a theoretical perspective.

Conclusion

The work to develop a comprehensive classification of nursing interventions began in 1987 with the formation of a small group of interested individuals at the University of Iowa. The work continues today with the assistance of a large research team and users around the country and in other countries who provide feedback and suggestions for refinement. As the work matures and the use grows, new issues emerge. The challenges with limited funding are enormous but we continue to be gratified by the overwhelming interest.

References

Albrecht, C.A. (1987). Hours of direct nursing care: Assessing baseline data for an automated system. *Computers in Nursing, 5*(2), 46-49.

American Library Association. (1977). *Librarian's copyright kit*. Washington, DC: Author.

American Nurses Association. (1980). *A conceptual model of community health nursing practice*. Kansas City, MO: The Association.

Deal, L.W. (1994). The effectiveness of community health nursing interventions: A literature review. *Public Health Nursing, 11*(5), 315-323.

Grobe, S. J. (1992). Nursing intervention lexicon and taxonomy. In K.C. Lun, P. DeGoulet, T.E. Piemme, & 0. Rienhoff (Eds.). *Medinfo 92* (pp. 981-986). New York: B. V. Elsevier Science Publishing co.

Iowa Intervention Project. (1997a) Defining nursing's effectiveness: Diagnoses, interventions, and outcomes. In M. Rantz & P. LeMone (Eds.), *Classification of nursing diagnoses: Proceedings of the twelfth conference*. Glendale, CA: CINAHL Information Systems, 293-303.)

Iowa Intervention Project. (1997b). Proposal to bring nursing into the information age. *Image, 29*(3), 275-281.

International Council of Nurses (1996). *The International classification for nursing practice: A unifying framework*. Geneva, Switzerland: ICN.

Johnson, M. & Maas, M. (1997). *Nursing outcomes classification (NOC)*. St. Louis: Mosby Year Book.

Martin KS., & Scheet N. J. (1992). *The Omaha System: Applications for community health nursing*. Philadelphia: WB Saunders.

McCloskey, J.C. & Bulechek, G.M. (Eds.) (1996) *Nursing interventions classification (NIC)*. (2nd ed.). St Louis: Mosby Year Book.

McCloskey, J.C., Bulechek, G.M., Moorhead, S., & Daly, J. (1996). Nurses' use and delegation of indirect care interventions, *Nursing Economic$, 14*(1), 10-17.

Osbolt, J.G., Fruchtnight, J.N., & Hayden, JR. (1994). Toward data standards for clinical nursing information. *Journal of the American Medical Informatics Association 1*(2), 175-185.

Saba V.K. (1992). The classification of home health care nursing: diagnoses and interventions. *Caring Magazine, 11*(3), 50-57.

Scherubel, J.C. & Minnick, A.F. (1994). Implementation of work sampling methodology. *Nursing Research, 43*(2), 120-123.

Serb, C. (1998). Techtravails. *Hospitals and Health Networks, 72*(8), 39-40.

Stanhope, M., & Lancaster, J. (1996). *Community health nursing: Promoting the health of aggregates, families and individuals*, (4th ed). St. Louis: Mosby Year Book.

Visiting Nurse Association of Omaha (1986). *Client management information system for community health nursing agencies* (Pub. No. HRP-0907023) US Washington, DC: US Government Print Office.

Overview of the Nursing Outcomes Classification (NOC)

Marion Johnson, PhD, RN

This paper overviews the Nursing Outcomes Classification (NOC) and identifies some of the issues related to the use of NOC. Work on the classification began in August, 1991 when a research team was formed to develop a taxonomy of patient outcomes sensitive to nursing interventions. The research team currently consists of three Co-Pls, 17 investigators, over 20 clinicians, and a number of master's and doctoral students. Funding for the research was provided by Sigma Theta Tau International and the Institute of Nursing Research. Purposes of the research were to:

- Identify, label, validate and classify patient outcomes influenced by nursing,
- Evaluate the validity and usefulness of the outcomes in field tests, and
- Define and test measurement procedures.

The first two purposes of the research have been completed and validation of the measures is underway in the second phase of the research.

Description of NOC

The Nursing Outcomes Classification, containing 190 outcomes listed alphabetically, was published by Mosby in 1997 (Iowa Outcomes Project, 1997). Since publication, an additional 28 outcomes and the taxonomy have been developed. For this work, an outcome is stated as a variable concept representing a patient or family caregiver state, behavior, or perception that is measurable along a continuum and responsive to nursing interventions. Stating the outcomes as variable concepts, rather than as goals, allows for the identification of positive or negative changes or no change in a patient's status. Each NOC outcome has a definition, a list of indicators that are useful in evaluation of patient status, a measurement scale, and a short list of references used in development of the outcome as illustrated in Figure 1. Sixteen 5-point Likert scales have been developed for use with the out-

Figure 1. Example of NOC Outcome

Knowledge: Treatment Regimen - Extent of understanding and skills conveyed about a specific treatment regimen					
Knowledge: Treatment Regimen: (Specify disease)	**Never** **1**	**Slightly** **2**	**Moderately** **3**	**Substantially** **4**	**Extensively** **5** **NA**
Indicators:	**Never**	**Slightly**	**Moderately**	**Substantially**	**Extensively** **NA**
Describes prescribed diet	1	2	3	4	5 NA
Describes prescribed medication	1	2	3	4	5 NA
Describes prescribed activity	1	2	3	4	5 NA
Describes prescribed exercise	1	2	3	4	5 NA
Describes prescribed procedures	1	2	3	4	5 NA
Describes rationale for treatment regimen	1	2	3	4	5 NA
Describes self-care responsibilities for ongoing treatment	1	2	3	4	5 NA
Describes self-care responsibilities for emergency situations	1	2	3	4	5 NA
Describes expected effects of treatment	1	2	3	4	5 NA
Demonstrates self-monitoring techniques	1	2	3	4	5 NA
Other ________________ (Specify)	1	2	3	4	5 NA

Used with permission of Mosby-Year Book from Iowa Outcomes Project. M. Johnson & M. Maas (Eds.). (1997) Nursing Outcomes Classification (NOC). St. Louis: Mosby, p. 197

comes to measure patient status in relation to the outcome. The scale for Knowledge: Treatment Regimen in Figure I uses a measurement scale from none to extensive. Examples of other scales are: 1 = extremely compromised to 5 = not compromised and 1 = never demonstrated to 5 = consistently demonstrated. All of the scales are developed so that 1 is the least desirable patient state and 5 is the most desirable patient state. One of the 16 scales is used with each outcome to measure patient status for both the outcome and the indicators. For example, in the outcome Knowledge: Treatment Regimen, 1 = none or no knowledge and represents the least desirable state while 5 = extensive knowledge and represents the most desirable state. It is important to recognize that a 5 rating on the scale may not be achieved by all patients. For example, an aphasic patient may never achieve a 5 on communication ability, but improvement may be measured, for example if they move from a 1 to a 3 on the scale.

Outcomes in the current classification are developed for use at the individual level and relate to the patient or family caregiver. Outcomes applicable to other social units, such as families and communities, are being developed. The term "patient" is used for conciseness, but refers to any individual receiving nursing care in any setting, for example a nursing home or the patient's home. Outcomes for caregivers are those that apply to any individual who cares for or acts on behalf of the patient, such as a family member, significant other, or personal friend. Caregiver does not apply to professional caregivers paid to provide care. Examples of outcomes for caregivers are Caregiver Emotional Health and Caregiver Performance: Direct Care.

The outcomes were developed at varied levels within a middle range of abstraction. Thus, some are more general with broader scope than others. For example, Self-Care: Activities of Daily Living (ADL) is defined as the "ability to perform the most basic physical tasks and personal care activities" and has ten indicators that include: eating, dressing, toileting, bathing. If required, more specific outcomes for each of the dimensions of self-care are available. For example, Self-Care:

Eating is defined as the "ability to prepare and ingest food" and the indicators include: handles utensils, picks up cup or glass, chews food.

Description of the Taxonomy
The outcomes are organized in 24 categories referred to as classes. The classes are grouped in the following six broad domains: Functional Health, Physiologic Health, Psychosocial Health, Health Knowledge & Behavior, Perceived Health, and Family Health. Consistent terminology and format were used in the development of domain and class labels and definitions. Each class and domain has a definition that facilitates placement of newly developed outcomes within a particular class. The classes with the number of outcomes in each class for the domain Functional Health are: Energy Maintenance, 4; Growth & Development, 22; Mobility, 11; Self-Care, 11; and Sensory Function, 5.

Each of the domains reflects a dimension of personal or family health and classes represent components of the health dimension. Although NOC is the most inclusive classification of patient and caregiver outcomes currently available to evaluate nursing interventions, it will continually evolve and become more complete. Additional classes may be identified if new outcomes cannot be subsumed in the existing classes and additional domains and classes may be required as outcomes characterizing family and community units are developed.

Each element of the taxonomy has been coded for application in computerized clinical information systems. The code for each outcome places it within a particular class and consequently also within a domain. For example, Figure 2 illustrates the coding for the outcome Comfort Level and one of the indicators, reported physical

Figure 2.

Coding for Outcome Comfort Level	
CODE	**DIMENSION**
Domain 5	Perceived Health
Class V	Sympton Status
Outcome 2100	Comfort Level
Indicator 01	Reported Physical Well-Being
Scale i	None to Extensive
Rating 1 to 5	Individual Patient Status
5V210001i3	Complete code for a patient evaluated at a 3 on the outcome Comfort Level

well-being. It is important to note that the scale as well as the patient state is also coded.

Issues Related to NOC

Although comprehensive, a number of developmental issues should be considered. Outcomes continue to be identified and developed. Examples of outcomes developed since publication of the book include: Fetal Status: Antepartum; Knowledge: Infant Care; Sensory Function: Hearing; and Risk Control: Cancer. Family outcomes, such as Family Integrity, Family Communication, Family Safety, and Family Cohesiveness are being developed and work on community outcomes is underway. Outcomes must also be linked with diagnoses and interventions. The outcomes in NOC have been linked to NANDA diagnoses and NIC interventions and these linkages are being used to develop links between NANDA, NIC, and NOC. The outcomes are also being linked to the Resident Assessment Protocols (RAPS) used in long-term care and the Omaha system used in community nursing.

The need for nursing-sensitive outcomes continues to be a topic of debate with the move to develop collaborative outcomes. While collaborative outcomes are important as measures of health care system and organization effects, they do not provide any one discipline with the knowledge necessary to evaluate that discipline's interventions. Nursing-sensitive outcomes are necessary for the evaluation of nursing practices, nursing interventions, and system and organizational changes that impact the practice of nursing. They are also needed if nursing is to be a collaborative partner in the identification of interdisciplinary outcomes.

The use of measures rather than goals requires a shift in thinking related to the evaluation of nursing care. While the measurement of patient status in relation to selected outcomes allows for the evaluation of change or lack of change following nursing interventions, it may require a more detailed evaluation of patient status when determining the outcome level. The use of NOC, however, does not eliminate setting goals. The outcomes can be converted to goal statements by determining the desired point on the measurement scale for an individual patient or for a specified patient population.

Although selected outcomes have been piloted in three field sites (two hospitals and one nursing home) with favorable results, further evaluation of the outcomes in clinical practice is necessary. The second phase of the research to evaluate the reliability, validity, and sensitivity of the measurement scales is beginning. During this phase of the research, an attempt will be made to isolate risk adjustment factors for the more common nursing-sensitive outcomes. The identification of personal characteristics that contribute to outcome achievement is an important factor when evaluating outcome attainment across organizations and health care systems.

The outcomes use of the outcomes in practice settings and computerized information systems will provide additional information for the evaluation of NOC. Data generated from these sources can be used to determine the frequency with which each outcome is selected, the nursing diagnoses and interventions associated with each outcome, and characteristics of the patient populations for which specific outcomes are selected.

The use of standardized outcome measures, such as NOC, offers nursing the opportunity to assume accountability for the effects of nursing interventions on the health of individual patients and patient populations it serves. The ability to quantify the effects of the care nurses provide is essential for describing the value of nurses to consumers and other providers.

References

Johnson, M., & Maas, M. (Eds.) (1997). *Iowa Outcomes Project: Nursing outcomes classification (NOC)*. St. Louis: Mosby.

A Message from the Incoming President

Dorothy A. Jones, EdD, RN, C, FAAN

It is with a great sense of responsibility that I accept the honor of serving as the fifth president of the North American Nursing Diagnosis Association (NANDA). As the association journeys toward the year 2000 and beyond, I am grateful to Judy Warren for her leadership as NANDA president during the past two years. In addition, I would like to acknowledge the significant accomplishments of the NANDA Board of Directors and Committee Chairs. Because of their hard work, the association is well positioned to meet the challenges of the next millennium. The current stability of NANDA will enable continued development, utilization, and refinement of nursing diagnosis worldwide.

During our recent 25th anniversary celebration, conference participants had an opportunity to observe firsthand the many contributions NANDA has made to revolutionize nursing education, practice, and research. In retrospect, it was clear that many of the outstanding nursing leaders of the past three decades have contributed a great deal to NANDA, clarifying our message and guiding the developments in nursing diagnosis. Nurses in clinical practice – as well as the nurse theorists, researchers, administrators, and educators – have all partnered in the advancement of nursing diagnosis and helped trnasform professional nursing forever.

During a summer meeting (1997), the NANDA board members accepted an offer to archive NANDA's historical documents at the Burns Library on the Boston College campus. In honor of this occasion, Dr. Barbara Munro, Dean of the Boston College School of Nursing, described the library's historical holdings and personally invited nurses from around the world to visit the library through the website or in person. This achievement enables NANDA to preserve its contributions to nursing language development over the past 25 years. In addition, the site will offer students of nursing diagnosis a chance to study the concept and the language of nursing as it continues to emerge.

As a collective whole, NANDA has promoted the naming and classifying of human responses experienced by individuals and groups across the health spectrum. This contribution has given voice to patient phenomena of concern and nursing practice. Over time, the work of NANDA has attracted the attention of nurses globally. It is incredible that the work of a relatively small cohort of nurses across North America has so dramatically shaped nursing as a discipline internationally. While we celebrate NANDA's many remarkable contributions, we must also recognize that in a rapidly changing and complex healthcare delivery system, the human experience of individuals and groups continues to emerge. As a result, the work of NANDA remains unfinished.

During the presidential address at the conclusion of the 13th NANDA conference, I outlined a strategic plan that will be used by the Board to move NANDA into the next century. The major purpose of this plan reflects NANDA's commitment to increasing the visibility of nursing's contributions to patient care by continuing to develop, refine, and classify phenomena of concern to nursing.

To accomplish this vision, I identified seven goals: 1) fostering the inclusion of NANDA's taxonomy into standardized language systems and data bases; 2) developing a collaborative relationship between NANDA and specialty organizations; 3) promoting the use of nursing diagnosis in educational curricula and clinical practice; 4) maintaining the NANDA archives to preserve the association's history; 5) promoting the dissemination of NANDA's work internationally; 6) expanding NANDA's membership and financial base; and 7) promoting the development and clinical testing and validation of nursing diagnosis.

The NANDA Board is ready to embark on an evolving journey that is challenging and exciting. The committees and members have been energized by the 13th conference and the 25th anniversary celebration of the association. It is my hope that NANDA members and nurses everywhere come together and continue the work begun by Kristine Gebbie and Mary Ann Lavin at the first Invitational Conference. Through these efforts the developments and classification of nursing diagnoses can be expanded, and NANDA can continue tis contribution to the shaping of nursing practice and structuring nursing knowledge.

Paper Presentations

Validation of the Nursing Diagnosis *Ineffective Breastfeeding*

Ana Cristina Freitas de Vilhena Abrão, MNSC
Maria Gaby Rivero de Gutierrez, DNSC

The present study is part of a larger project concerning the identification and validation of the accepted nursing diagnoses related to maternal breastfeeding in order to improve the nursing care provided to the woman during her reproductive cycle. According to the WHO/UNICEF (1989), "maternal breastfeeding represents an irreplaceable mode of supplying the infant with the ideal type of food likely to improve its healthy development and growth in addition to favorably influence either the mother's and infant's biological and emotional status." However, the breastfeeding practice is a most complex endeavor as a consequence of the biological, psychological, social, and cultural aspects involved. (Caetano, 1992).

The breastfeeding act is related to a number of factors which influence its successful results. Giugliani (1994) suggested that strategies concerning breastfeeding promotion should be flexible enough to fit the target population and its culture, habits, beliefs, and socioeconomic status, as well as other characteristics. Thus, the development of human resources for a program directed towards the stimulation of maternal breastfeeding and the assistance provided to the woman who desires to breastfeed or is breastfeeding are essential strategies to be used for this program's successful outcome. (WHO/UNICEF, 1989).

Within this context, the nurse has a most significant and conclusive role in identifying the needs, problems, or the nursing diagnoses related to maternal breastfeeding and implementing the necessary actions to have them solved, as well as evaluating the results achieved by the mother-infant dyad.

This way, we decided to select the following nursing diagnoses: *effective breastfeeding*, *ineffective breastfeeding*, and *interrupted breastfeeding*; however, greater emphasis was placed in identifying the defining characteristics and factors related to the *ineffective breastfeeding* diagnosis.

OBJECTIVES
- Identify the occurrence of *ineffective*

Table 1.

Distribution of women by age

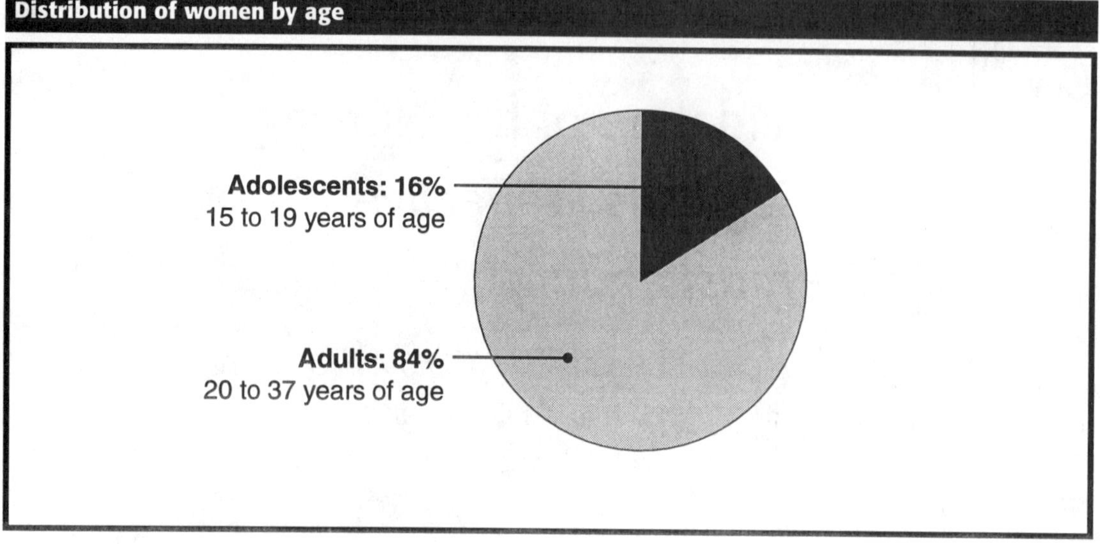

breastfeeding among an adult and adolescent puerperal women population.

- Describe the defining characteristics and factors related to the *ineffective breastfeeding* diagnosis and compare them with those proposed by the North American Nursing Diagnosis Association (NANDA 1997-1998).

METHODS

This analitical descriptive study was carried out in a Public Maternity Hospital and within a Nursing Care Ambulatory setting, located in the city of São Paulo, Brazil, from March to April, 1997.

The subjects included 100 puerperal women and infants in stages ranging from 12 hours to 60 days post-partum. Two nursing teachers from the Obstetrical Nursing Department of "Universidade Federal de São Paulo" collected related data by means of an interview with the mother followed by the dyad's thorough physical examination.

The instrument used for data collection was separated into two parts: the first one included the establishment of a nursing consultation protocol supported by NANDA's human response patterns. The second part included a directing chart showing either characteristics or factors related to the maternal breastfeeding diagnoses. The factors and characteristics identified by the authors were also included in that list.

RESULTS

First, data related to some characteristics shown by the studied population will be presented; followed by the frequency of the selected diagnostic occurrences in adult and adolescent puerperal women.

Tables 1 and 2 show that most of the studied population included adult puerperal women (84%) with low educational level (80% grammar school); these findings show the need for an adequate selection of materials and teaching methods in

Table 2.

Distribution of women according to educational level

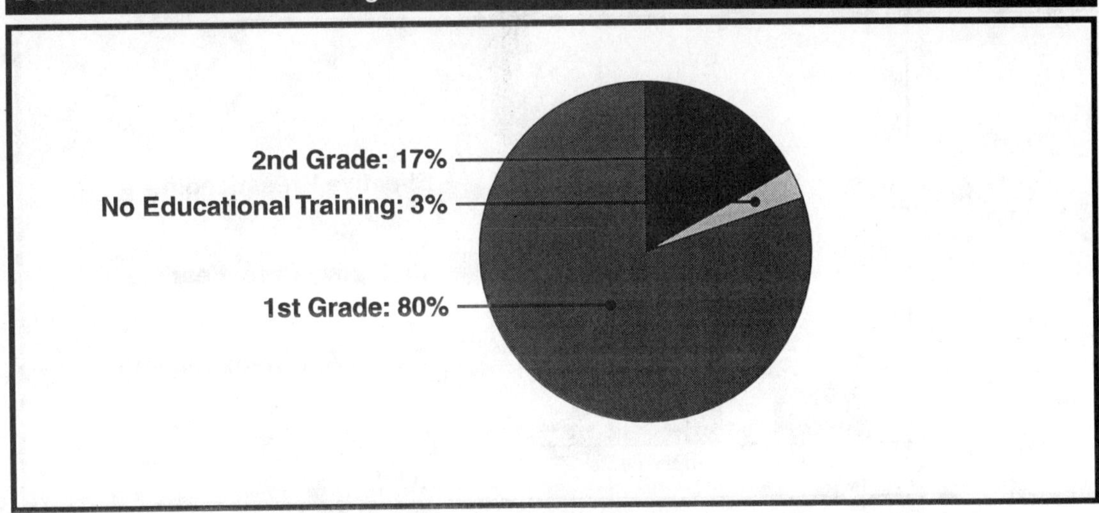

Table 3.

Distribution of women according to parity

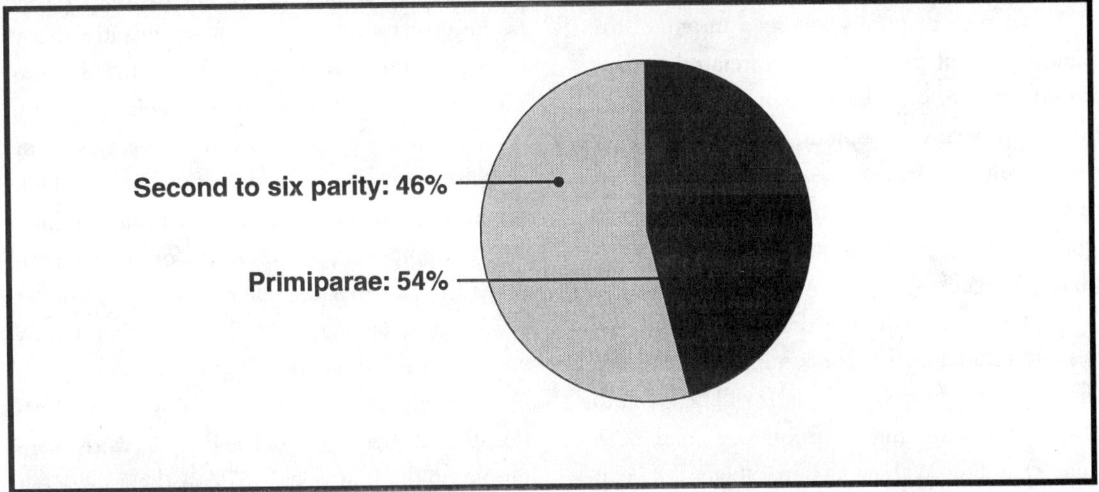

maternal breastfeeding promotion.

Table 3 shows that as to parity, more than half of the subjects were primiparae and the remaining were between the second and sixth parity. This finding is significant for nursing since it may influence the breastfeeding practice.

As to the studied nursing diagnoses shown in Table 4, it could be verified that 51% of the women showed an effective situation of breastfeeding; eight of them were still adolescents and 43% were adults, thus pointing to a positive situation. The diagnosis of *ineffective breastfeeding* was evidenced in 43% of the investigated women; 7% of them were adolescents and 36%

Table 4.

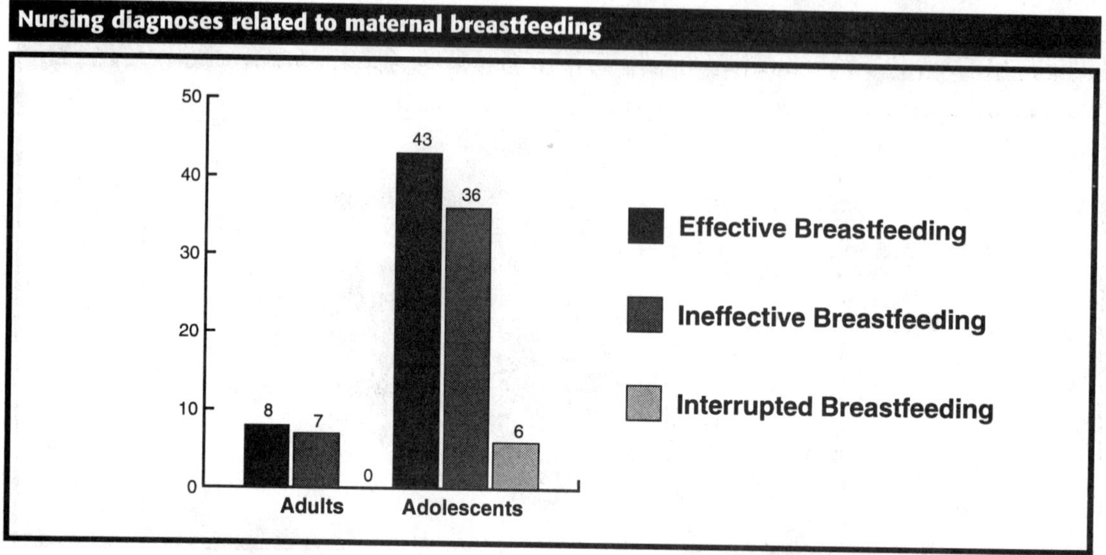

adults; only 6% of all the adult women presented the interrupted breastfeeding diagnosis.

No such diagnosis was seen in any of the adolescents but this fact may be related to their attendance period which occurred during the first 72 hours of hospitalization time. These results suggest similar percentages of occurrence between adult women and adolescents when related to *effective* and *ineffective breastfeeding* diagnoses.

When analyzing the defining characteristics and related factors concerning the diagnosis *effective breastfeeding*, emphasis will be given to those presenting higher frequency than 80% (major) and those showing percentages between 50 and 79% (minor). Defining characteristics identified as lower than 50% will not be approached in the present discussion.

Concerning the major defining characteristics related to the *ineffective breastfeeding* diagnosis, only the defining characteristic unsatisfactory breastfeeding process was identified in the total sampling of investigated women (Table 5). This fact may be due to the assumption that every woman presenting with *ineffective breastfeeding* is found to be in an unsatisfactory breastfeeding situation. Also, consideration must be given to the fact that this characteristic is very generic since it fails to show any sign or symptom, or else, any indicative factor which might explain that ineffective breastfeeding. Another important issue to be discussed concerns the fact that this characteristic was never observed as isolated but always concomitantly with other defining characteristics.

The minor identified defining characteristics, that is, between 50% and 79%, were "sore nipples in the first week" (57% of the adolescent mothers) and "nonsustained suckling at the breast" (57.1% in adolescents' infants). These occurrences may be related to the lacking experience in breastfeeding practice since most of those mothers were primiparae. Applebaum (1970), Vinha (1987), Vinha et al. (1987) suggested that the presence of sore nipples was likely to impair maternal breastfeeding.

Table 5

Defining characteristics identified in *"ineffective breastfeeding diagnosis"*

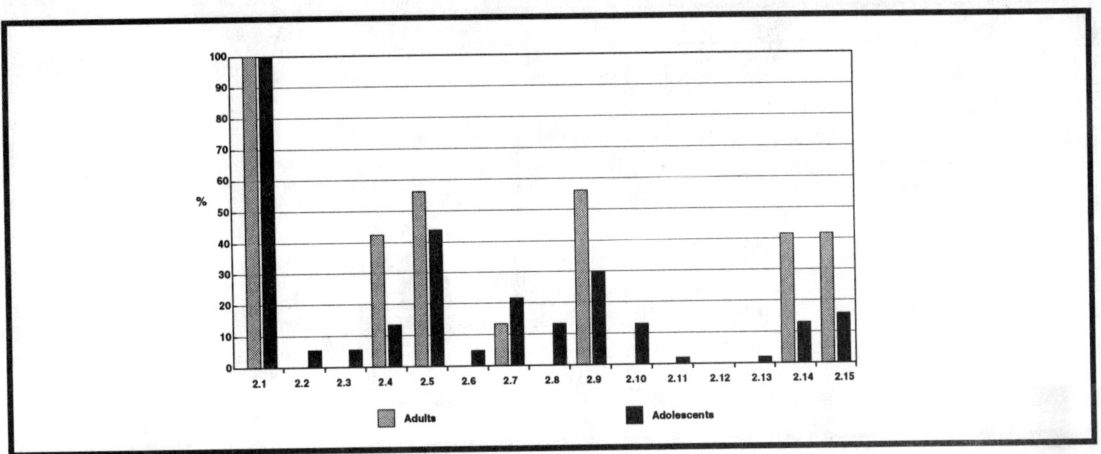

Legend:

2.1 = insatisfactory breastfeeding process

2.2 = actual or perceived inadequate milk supply

2.3 = no observable signs of oxytocin release

2.4 = insufficient emptying of each breast per feeding

2.5 = persistence of sore nipples in the first week of breastfeeding

2.6 = persistence of sore nipples beyond the first week of breastfeeding

2.7 = infant inability to attach to maternal breast correctly

2.8 = observable signs of inadequate infant intake

2.9 = nonsustained suckling at the breast

2.10 = insufficient opportunity for suckling at the breast

2.11 = infant exhibiting fussiness and crying within the first hour after breastfeeding

2.12 = unresponsive to other comfort measures

2.13 = infant arching and crying at the breast

2.14 = resisting latching on

2.15 = pain at breastfeeding

Table 6

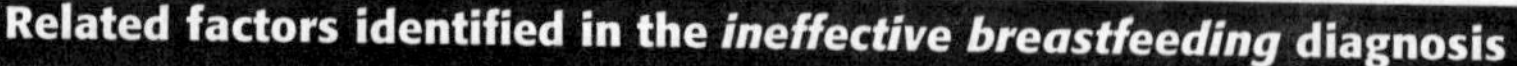

Related factors identified in the *ineffective breastfeeding* diagnosis

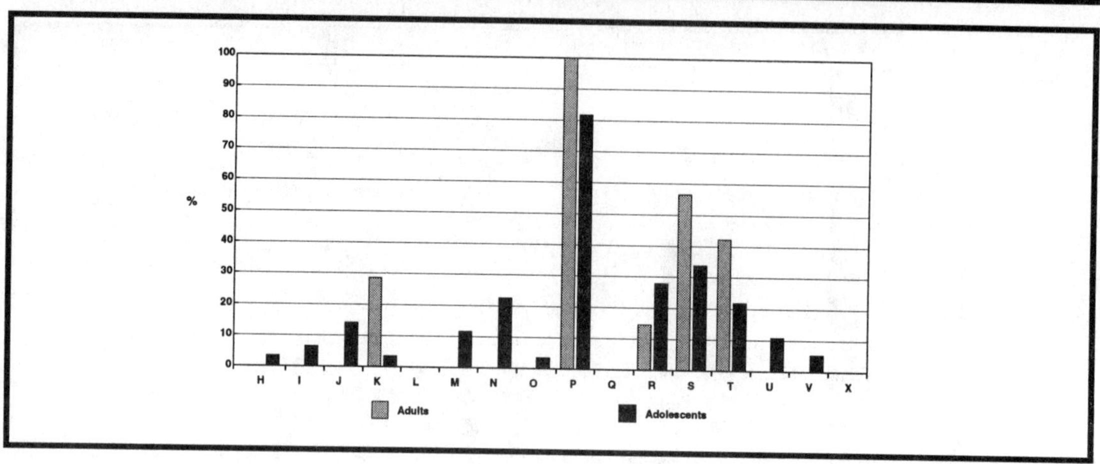

Label:

H = prematurity

I = infant anomaly

J = deficient suckling reflex

K = maternal breast anomaly

L = previous breast surgery

M = history of previous breastfeeding failure

N = supplemental feedings with artificial nipple

O = lacking support from partner/family

P = knowledge deficit

Q = maternal breastfeeding interruption

R = anxiety or maternal ambivalence

S = incorrect attaching or latching to maternal nipple

T = excessive suckling time

U = previous trauma in healing process

V = excessive use of pacifier

X = improper technique when withdrawing infant from breast

As to "nonsustained suckling at the breast," studies carried out by the La Leche League International (1982), Pontes and Sá (1987) and Savage (1990), concluded that the low frequency and short duration of mammary suckling have a direct influence in the prolactin levels, and as a consequence, in milk production.

Regarding the major related factors concerning the *ineffective breastfeeding* diagnosis (Table 6), a knowledge deficit was seen in 100% of the investigated adolescents and in 83% of the adult women. Problems resulting from lacking orientation on maternal breastfeeding are very well known.

Gulik (1982) and Nobrega et al. (1983) express the opinion that the mother's previous and faulty knowlege regarding the maternal breastfeeding process may lead to low milk production and ejection. Morse and Harrison (1987) and also Hill and Humenick (1989) stated that a knowledgeable mother is likely to perform successful breastfeeding and also emphasize the importance of support provided by partner, family, friends, and healthcare providers during this stage.

The benefits resulting from the orientation provided and the mothers' follow-up during the breastfeeding process were validated in a study carried out by Abrao (1991), in which most of the assisted puerperal women showed lower incidence of breast engorgement and mamillary traumas when compared to women who had not received that type of orientation. Another factor related to the *ineffective breastfeeding* diagnosis but not included in NANDA's official classification listings was identified by the present authors as "incorrect mamillary-areolar latching" and observed in 57.1% of the breastfed infants, all of them adolescent mothers' newborns. Authors like Woolridge (1986),

Escott (1989), Richard and Alade (1992), stated that infants' correct mouth-nipple position at breastfeeding is essential for successfful breastfeeding since it provides adequate suckling.

Cadwell (1981), Gulick (1982), Vinha (1987), and King (1991) related the inadequate latching and suckling with the presence of hypogalactia and mamillary traumas.

The findings shown by the present study support the inference that the *ineffective breastfeeding* diagnosis and the defining characteristics and related factors concerning this same diagnosis identified in this study, show powerful bonds with the mothers' inexperience in the breastfeeding process. Thus, the need for the nurse's educational intervention is essential for this process to achieve its maximum success.

When comparing the defining characteristics and related factors of the *ineffective breastfeeding* diagnosis identified in this study and NANDA's proposals, it is possible to verify that only some of them could be validated in practice. It must be emphasized that this study is still in its preliminary stage but its continuity is going through a developmental stage carried out by one of the authors.

Also, it should be stressed that the utilization of a structured instrument for providing the puerperal woman with a nursing consultation based in the human response patterns was of great value because it created the means for obstetrical nurses to improve their practice and as a consequence benefit the women assisted by those nursing healthcare providers.

References

Abrao, A.C.F.V. *Aleitamento materno: efeito de um programa educativo para o auto cuidado com as mamas na incidencia de ingurgitamento mamario e traumas mamilares*. Sao Paulo, 1993.125 p. Dissertacao (Mestrado) – Departamento de Enfermagem da Escola Paulista de Medicina.

Applebaum, R.M. *Tecnicas modernas para o exito da amamentacao*. Trad. de Maria Teresa Maldonado. Liga do leite materno do Brasil. RJ, 1970. 31p. (publicacao avulsa).

Cadwell, K. Improving nipple graspability of success at breastfeeding. *Journal of Obstetric, Ginecologic, and Neonatal Nursing*, n.10, p. 277-79, 1981.

Caetano, L.C. *Aleitamento materno-fatores que contribuem para a sua pratica*. Sao Paulo, 1992. 156p. Dissertacao (Mestrado) – Departamento de Enfermagem da Escola Paulista de Medicina.

Escott, R. Posicionamento, pega e transferencia de leite. Trad. Tereza S. Toma, *Breastfeeding Review*, May, 1989.

Giugliani, E.R.J. Amamentacao: como e porque promover. *J. Pediatr.* (RJ), v.70, n.3, p.138-147, 1994.

Gulick, E.E. Informational correlates of successful breastfeeding. *American Journal of Maternal-Child Nursing*, n.7, p.370-75, 1982.

Hill, P., & Humenick, S. Insufficient milk supply. *Image*, n.21, p.145-48, 1989.

King, S.F. *Como ajudar as maes a amamentar*. Trad. de Zuleika Thomson e Orides Navarro Gordan. Londrina, 1991.

La Leche League International. *Como aumentar a quantidade de leite materno*. Franklin Park, Illinois, n.85, 1982. (Folheto informativo).

Morse, J., & Harrison, M. Social coersion for weaning. *Journal of Nurse Midwifery*, n.32, p.204-210, 1987.

NANDA. *Nursing diagnoses*. Philadelphia, 1997/1998.

Nobrega, S. et al. A erva doce e seu efeito galactogeno-um estudo experimental. *Rev. Bras. Enf.* (RS), v.36, p.163-177, 1983.

Organizacao Mundial da Saude/Fundo das Nacoes Unidas Para a Infancia. Promocao, protecao e apoio em aleitamento materno. Genebra, 1989.

Pontes, A.G., & Sa, M.F.S. Efeito da succao mamilar sobre os niveis plasmaticos de prolactina em puerperas normais. *Rev. Bras. Ginecol. Obstetr.*, v.5, n.9, p.116-19, 1987.

Righard, L. & Alade, M.O. Sucking technique and its effect on success of breastfeeding. *Birth*, v.19, n.4, p.185-89, 1992.

Savage, F. Breastfeeding in the 1990s. *National Medical Journal of India*, v.3, n.4, p.155-59, 1990.

Vinha, V.H.P. *Amamentacao materna-incentivos e cuidados*. Sao Paulo, Sarvier, 1987.

Vinha, V.H.P. et al. Trauma mamilar-uma proposta de tratamento. *Femina*, v.15, n.5, p.370-78, 1987.

Woolridge, M.W. The anatomy of infant sucking. *Midwifery*, v.2, p.164-71, 1986.

Comparison of Use of Nursing Language in Documentation of Rehabilitation Nursing

Jean M. Arnold, EdD, RNC

Partial Funding by Rutgers University College of Nursing Office of Research

Health care charting systems have focused on documentation of care for an individual patient, but not as a basis for aggregate data collection. Nursing classification systems using standardized nursing language provide a means for developing common documentation systems. The Twelfth Conference of the North American Nursing Diagnosis Association (NANDA) (1996) informed participants that there were several methodologies to support this endeavor. These methodologies include (1) the design of computer-based databases that capture patient outcomes sensitive to the effects of nursing care; (2) a formal research relationship with the University of Iowa School of Nursing to conduct a study entitled Nursing Diagnosis Extension Classification; (3) collaboration with the American Nurse Association's Steering Committee on Databases Supporting Nursing Clinical Practice; and (4) collaboration with accepted classification systems including Home Health Care Classification, the Omaha VNA system and the Nursing Outcome Classification (Warren, 1997, p. 75).

The NANDA Classification system, the first step toward the development of standardized language in nursing, began over 20 years ago. The other classification systems — Home Health Care Classification, The Omaha VNA system, Nursing Intervention Classification (NIC) and Nursing Outcome Classification (NOC) — were developed as parallel efforts within the last 10 years. The American Nurses Association has recognized these classification systems and supports their use in the development of nursing information systems (Lang, 1995).

Purposes
- To compare the use of nursing language in documentation of rehabilitation nursing practice at two research sites.
- To develop a coding structure for a custom relational database using standardized nursing language.

Definitions
- Length of stay was the time period from the

client's admission to rehabilitation unit to time of discharge.

- Documentation was the notes written by nurses on their client records.
- The problem component of 32 NANDA diagnoses identified by expert panels in previous research (Arnold, 1994) were used to begin identification of those used in rehabilitation nursing practice. These diagnoses will be referred to as U-Diagnose™ problems in this paper.
- Outcome description was a specific description of desired outcome related to each of the selected NANDA problems. Outcome category was one selected from Nursing Outcomes Classification (Johnson & Maas, 1997).

Methods

Major questions addressed in this report were the client demographics, client length of stay on the rehabilitation unit, nursing diagnosis frequency, and identification of outcomes related to nursing diagnoses used in the rehabilitation setting and their relationship to standardized nursing language. There were two time periods for data collection: day 14 and at discharge.

A bridge was built between narrative nursing documentation and a custom relational entitled the U-Diagnose™ Rehabilitation Database. This bridge was the author's revised Gerontological Nursing U-Diagnose™ Instrument (GNUDI). The development of the reliability and validity of the original GNUDI with an expert panel was described in previous research (Arnold, 1997). The instrument consisted of three sections: Part I: Demographic Data, Part II: Listing of Gerontological Nursing Diagnoses and Part III: Checklist of Selected Nursing Diagnoses with Outcomes and Interventions.

Demographic variables included the client's initials, identification number, age, marital status, and sex. Admission date, discharge date and discharge prognosis was also included in this section. Part II was used to identify the diagnoses documented for the given subject. In Part III, the researcher checked off the diagnoses, actions and outcome descriptions documented in the narrative charting by the nurses in this study.

The U-Diagnose™ problems were identified by using a conversion sheet, which listed Resident Assessment Protocols (RAPs), based on gerontological minimum data set assessment for nursing home residents and care screening. Two master's-prepared gerontological nursing specialists active in practice at the research sites validated the conversion sheets. U-Diagnose™ problems were also identified from examination of the nursing care plans. Another nurse researcher supports this procedure for problem identification. "Nursing knowledge processing in each nurse's head is more extensive that the information within the 18 RAPs" (Rantz, 1994). In Part II, the actions and outcomes transposed to the GNUDI were based on the nurses' narrative nursing care plans, notes and discharge plans. The same data collection procedures were used at both research sites. The time frame for data collection was about 20 weeks at each research site. Diagnoses, interventions and outcomes were added to the GNUDI during the data collection periods.

Human Subjects Procedures

The researcher received approval from the two health agency review panels as well as an educational institution review board. Each nurse signed a consent form allowing the researcher to examine her documentation. The identity of

Table 1

Frequency of the Top Ten U-Diagnose™ Problems in Agency A and Agency B

Agency A	Agency B
Impaired physical mobility	Impaired physical mobility
Impaired skin integrity	Altered nutrition, less than
Altered nutrition, less than	Risk for injury
Diversion activity deficit	Hygiene self-care deficit
Ineffective individual coping	Pain
Altered tissue perfusion	Dressing/grooming self-care deficit
Pain	Impaired skin integrity
Risk for infection	Sensory perceptual alterations
Risk for injury	Feeding self care deficit
Constipation	Impaired home main management

each client record was protected by the assignment of a research number in place of the health agency identification number.

The next phase of the research was to code the GNUDI to facilitate the development of the U-Diagnose™ Rehabilitation Database. The U-Diagnose Problems™ selected were coded using five of the six domains within the NIC. Those five domains used were Physiological: Basic, Physiological: Complex, Behavioral, Health System and Safety (McCloskey & Bulechek, 1996). The GNUDI outcome descriptions were labeled using the NOC outcome category (Johnson & Maas, 1997).

Sample

The subjects included 31 client records at Agency A and 38 client records at Agency B. An agency representative selected the client records by using a list of random numbers provided by the researcher. Each client record was examined for approximately 90 minutes at two designated data collection times periods: day 14 of the subject's hospitalization and upon their discharge.

Results

The gender distribution of the Agency A sample was 58% female (18) and 42% male (13). For this sample, 87% (27) were white and 13% (4) were black. The ages ranged from 61 to 94. The gender distribution of the Agency B sample was 84% (32) female and 16% (6) male. For this sample, 97% (37) were white and 3% (1) black. The ages ranged from 57 to 93.

The average length of stay for clients at Agency A was 34 days with a range of 7 to 87 days. Prior to this study the agency representative estimated that the average length of stay was 28 days. The mean length of stay at Agency B was 25 days, ranging from 14 days to 68 days.

Table 1 illustrates the top 10 nursing diagnoses that occurred in samples from Agencies A and B. The diagnosis of impaired physical mobility had the highest occurrence in both samples. The five diagnoses that were common to both samples were impaired physical mobility, impaired skin integrity, altered nutrition: less than body requirements, pain, and risk for injury. These findings were supported by findings from a random sample of members of the

Table 2

Five Common Diagnoses in Agency A and B: Linkages between U-Diagnose™ Problems, NOC Outcomes and NIC Domains

U-Diagnose™ Problem	NOC Outcome	NIC Domain
Impaired physical mobility	Mobility level	Physiological: Basic
Impaired skin integrity	Tissue integrity: skin	Physiological: Complex
Altered Nutrition: less	Nutritional status	Physiological: Basic
Risk for injury	Safety status: falls	Safety
Pain	Comfort level	Physiological: Basic

American Rehabilitation Nurses, who identified 21 diagnoses through a mail survey (Rehabilitation Nursing Foundation, 1995). The five common diagnoses described above were among the 21 rehabilitation-nursing diagnoses. In this study, 15 different diagnoses were included in the top 10 across the two samples. Five additional nursing diagnoses were included in the 21 described by the rehabilitation nurses. These include ineffective individual coping, colonic constipation, self-care deficit: hygiene, self-care deficit: dressing and grooming, and self-care deficit: feeding. Four of these 15 diagnoses were not included in the 21 rehabilitation nursing diagnoses. These diagnoses included diversional activity deficit and altered peripheral tissue perfusion documented by nurses in Agency A and sensory perceptual alterations and impaired home maintenance management documented in Agency B.

Nine diagnoses listed in Table 1 were also among the frequently used nursing diagnoses used in nursing care plans in a long-term care setting (Daly, Maas, & Buckwalter, 1995, Fielding, Beaton, Baier, Rallis, Ryan & Siripornsawan, 1997). These include impaired physical mobility, risk for injury, self-care deficit: hygiene, pain, impaired skin integrity, ineffective individual coping, self-care deficit: dress-

ing/grooming, sensory perceptual alterations and self-care deficit: feeding. The common finding of similar diagnoses across research studies indicates that nursing science is identifying diagnoses for specific populations. Table 2 lists the five common diagnoses identified in the documentation of patient care at both Agencies A & B with their linkages to the NOC outcomes (Johnson and Maas (1997) and the NIC domains (McCloskey and Bulechek, 1996). The researcher readily selected the corresponding outcomes and interventions domain from these classification listings. Table 2 indicates the logical relationship among the three nursing classification systems. It also demonstrates how it is possible to develop coding structures that can be used in the development of nursing information systems.

Table 3 illustrates how the NANDA problem impaired physical mobility can be used to illustrate how the GNUDI outcome description compares with NOC language. The GNUDI outcome is a descriptive phrase whereas the NOC outcome is a noun. Although the language structure differs, the descriptions have similar meaning.

There were six additional nursing diagnoses identified in this research through the use of the GNUDI at Agency A and Agency B.

Table 3

Comparison between GNUDI Outcome Description and NOC Outcome Category

GNUDI Outcome Description	NOC Category
Free of contractures	Muscle function
Ambulate with walker	Ambulate with wheelchair
Move joints ROM	Joint movement: active
Receive ROM	Joint movement: passive
Maintain body positioning	Body positioning

Table 4

Linkages between U-Diagnose™ Problems, NIC Domain and NOC

Diagnosis	NIC Domain	NOC
Colonic constipation	Physiologic Basic	Bowel Elimination
Fluid volume deficit	Physiologic Complex	Fluid balance
Ineffective coping	Behavioral	Coping
Impaired home maint	Health System	Role performance
Risk for injury	Safety	Safety behavior

Thirty of the U-Diagnose™ problems were used at Agency A with two new diagnoses. The additional diagnoses included self-care deficit: hygiene and cerebral tissue perfusion, altered. Thirty-nine nursing diagnoses were used at Agency B. The diagnoses that surfaced at Agency B were self-care deficit: feeding, self-care deficit: dressing/grooming, bowel incontinence, body-image disturbance, impaired verbal communication, peripheral tissue perfusion, and violence.

Table 4 illustrates the relationships between diagnoses documented in Agency A and B. Five of the six NIC domains were used. Only the family domain was not used because it was not applicable to the older adult client. The outcomes were selected arbitrarily by the researcher to represent the diagnosis in order to develop a coding structure for the relational database. The dilemma with using NOC is that more than one outcome can be used to represent a given diagnosis.

Conclusions

- The GNUDI instrument was a bridge between narrative charting and a custom relational database.
- The NANDA, NIC and NOC classification systems can be used to interrelate nursing diagnoses, interventions and outcomes.

- Coding structures for relational databases can be constructed using the NANDA, NIC and NOC classification systems. There were common diagnoses identified in Agencies A and B.
- The examination of documentation of rehabilitation nursing practice using the nursing elements of diagnosis, interventions and outcomes at an atomic level provided the opportunity to convert the data to standardized language.

Implications

The use of standardized nursing language and computerization of nursing documentation will lead to further identification of what we know and do.

References

Arnold, J.M. (1997). A gerontological nursing instrument for coding nursing U-Diagnose™ diagnoses, interventions and outcomes. In M. J. Rantz and P. LeMone (Eds.), *Classification of nursing diagnoses: Proceedings of the twelfth conference* (pp.222-227). Glendale, CA: CINAHL

Arnold J. M. (1995). Validation of nursing diagnoses across six gerontological U-Diagnose™ case studies. In M. J. Rantz and P. LeMone (Eds.), *Classification of nursing diagnoses: Proceedings of the eleventh conference* (p. 239). Glendale, CA: CINAHL.

Daly, J. M., Maas, M., & Buckwater, K. (1995). Use of standardized nursing diagnoses and interventions in long-term care. *Journal of Gerontological Nursing, 21*(8), 29-36.

Fielding, J. Beaton, S, Baier, L., Rallis, D. Ryan, R. M., & Sirpornsawan, D. Nursing diagnoses and related outcome objectives for long-term care facilities. In M. J. Rantz and P. LeMone (Eds). *Classification of nursing diagnoses: Proceedings of the eleventh conference* (pp. 182-188). Glendale, CA: CINAHL

Johnson, M., & Maas, M. (Eds.) (1997). *Nursing outcomes classification: Iowa outcomes project*: St. Louis: Mosby

Lang, N. M. (Ed.). (1995). *An Emerging framework: Data system advances for clinical nursing practice*. Washington, DC: American Nurses Association.

McCloskey, J., & Bulechek, G. (1996). *Nursing interventions classification (NIC)*. (2nd ed.). St. Louis: Mosby.

Rantz, M. J. (1994). Development of a nursing-diagnosis based integrated computerized documentation and care planning system for long-term care. In S. J. Grobe & E. S. P. Pluyter-Wennting (Eds.) *Nursing informatics: An International overview for nursing in a technological era: Proceedings of the fifth IMIA* (pp. 372-382). Amsterdam: Elsevier.

Rehabilitation Nursing Foundation. (1995). *21 Rehabilitation Nursing Diagnoses: A Guide to interventions and outcomes*. Glenview, IL.

Warren, J. J. (1997). Nursing diagnosis: The keystone to a unified nursing language. In M. J. Rantz and P. LeMone (Eds.) *Classification of nursing diagnoses: Proceedings of the twelfth conference:* (pp. 73-76). Glendale, CA: CINAHL

Perioperative Data Elements: The Contribution of a Specialty to Nursing Language

Suzanne C. Beyea, RN, CS, PhD
Aileen R. Killen, RN, PhD, CNOR
Donna Watson, RN, MSN, CNOR
Association of Operating Room Nurses, Denver, Colorado

The Association of Operating Room Nurses (AORN) is a professional specialty organization of 43,000 nurses committed to providing cost-effective, quality perioperative nursing care. Since 1993, members of this organization have been involved in activities to define, describe, define, and establish a database that represents perioperative nursing practice. This work has been spearheaded by the Data Elements Coordinating Committee (DECC) of the AORN and has resulted in a Perioperative Nursing Data Set (PNDS).

At its inception, the four main goals of the Data Elements Coordinating Committee were to: 1) develop a methodology to identify data elements; 2) develop and compile definitions; 3) implement and evaluate the data element framework; and 4) disseminate information. The DECC also recognized the need for standardized languages for computerized records and validation of outcomes effectiveness. Committee members were committed to the premise that for perioperative nursing to be vis-

ible to administrators, financial officers, and health care policy makers uniform computerized records of perioperative nurse/patient activities must be accessible. The motto of the group was, "If we cannot name it, we cannot control it, finance it, teach it, research it, or put it into public policy" (Lang, 1989, p 71).

Data elements are defined as the smallest unit of information that has meaning, such as a raw fact or observation. Each data element is a discrete entry that is described without and does not require further interpretation or information. The DECC seeks to identify the data elements in the perioperative record that define and describe nursing activities that contribute to patient outcomes. Individual entries in the patient record are the data elements and when combined, they serve as a perioperative database.

Patient-specific information in the record contributes information to the data set. The DECC members proposed that nursing diagnoses, interventions, outcomes, and structure elements are the foundation of a perioperative

"

nursing data set. When multiple, individual data sets are combined, a perioperative nursing data set is formed. DECC members project that such a perioperative nursing data set will assist perioperative nurses to document, examine, and evaluate the quality and effectiveness of the care they provide.

Nursing Diagnosis

The DECC created three subcommittees representing the areas of diagnosis, intervention, and outcome to examine perioperative nursing practice. The primary objective of the DECC Subcommittee on Nursing Diagnoses was to identify those clinical judgments that are integral to perioperative nursing practice. Using a consensus process, DECC subcommittee members developed an operational definition of nursing diagnosis for operating room nurses: "Nursing Diagnosis is a concise clinical judgment label of a perioperative patient problem formulated for the purpose of directing nursing actions intended to achieve the expected outcomes" (Killen, Kleinbeck, Golar, Schuchardt, & Uebele, 1997, p. 102).

Following that effort, subcommittee members conducted a systematic review of the literature, including the *AORN Journal*, other nursing journals, current perioperative textbooks, and related psychology, sociology, education, and physical therapy references. From this review of the literature, it was determined that more than 100 nursing diagnoses were mentioned at least once in the literature. Based on the context and frequency of each diagnosis in the literature, the DECC Diagnoses Subcommittee members identified 60 diagnoses that were related to perioperative nursing practice.

The previously established definition for nursing diagnoses and the identified 60 periop-

erative nursing diagnoses were the basis of a survey instrument designed to establish the validity of the labels. Survey participants were asked to rank the frequency that each nursing diagnosis occurred on a daily basis in their practice. The ranking used a one to five scale, ranking items from "never" to "almost all of the time." Respondents were also asked to rank how often the diagnosis occurred and the priority they assigned to that specific patient problem on a scale one to five. The highest priority was assigned to conditions requiring immediate attention such as a life-threatening situation. The lowest priority was assigned to conditions that never required a perioperative nurse's attention (Kleinbeck, 1996; Killen et al.,1997).

The survey was mailed to one thousand AORN members, AORN board members, national committee leaders, and educator and clinical specialist specialty assembly group members consisting of a convenience sample (n=550) and a random sample of staff nurse members who were staff nurses (n=450). There were 239 surveys returned for a response rate of 24%. The average age of respondents was similar to the average age of the AORN membership at large. Most respondents were certified operating room nurses and were involved in the provision of patient care. Twenty-two percent (n = 53) of respondents reported that they provided direct patient care for 100% of the time. Clinical specialists were the largest group of respondents (34%; n = 81) of the sample.

Based on the responses to the frequency and priority question on the survey, a weighted mean score was calculated for each diagnosis. These scores were then used to rank order the nursing diagnoses. Diagnoses that were scored as high frequency, high urgency, or high priority were categorized as "critical" to patient outcomes. From this analysis, the nursing diagnoses "risk of perioperative position injury" and "risk of infection" emerged as the only two diagnoses that were of the highest concern to perioperative nurses.

The second tier of this ranking procedure categorized low frequency, high priority diagnoses as "primary." DECC committee members identified a total of 24 diagnoses in this subset. Examples include pain, neurovascular dysfunction, risk of aspiration, risk of injury, hypothermia, and impaired gas exchange. When most of these diagnoses occur in the perioperative arena, they pose a physical threat to the surgical patient and can result in an unwanted patient outcome.

The final tier of this classification process identified "secondary diagnoses." These 34 diagnoses do not occur very often, do not require immediate attention, and have a moderate priority. Examples include impaired verbal communication, acute confusion, sensory perception alterations, and decision conflict. Most of these human responses are not observed during the intraoperative phase, but are phenomena of concern to nurses caring for patients during the pre- and post-operative phases of the surgical experience.

Based on respondents' feedback, the extensive literature review, and the combined expertise of the DECC committee members, a number of proposed perioperative nursing diagnoses were identified. Some of the recommended new labels included "risk for latex allergy response," " risk of malignant hypothermia," and "delayed surgical recovery." A number of revisions and additions to existing NANDA nursing diagnostic categories were also suggested. The intent of this effort is to make existing nursing diagnostic language more reflective of the needs of the perioperative patient by identifying signs and symptoms and related factors that are observed in the perioperative arena. These recommendations have been forwarded to NANDA's Diagnosis Review Committee.

Interventions

The DECC Subcommittee on Nursing Interventions was charged with identifying and validating perioperative nursing interventions. Once again, by using a consensus process and reviewing pre-exiting AORN documents related to patient outcomes, standards of care, and competencies, the subcommittee members initially identified 115 criteria as nursing interventions. Following an extensive review of the literature and consultation with practice experts, the list contained 145 interventions.

The committee decided to survey members in an effort to validate the interventions. The "Nursing Intervention(s)/Treatment(s)/ Patient Outcome(s) Survey" was developed to determine if the identified interventions reflected the contributions of perioperative nurses to surgical patient outcomes. Participants were asked to link the interventions to six outcomes and answer two open-ended questions: 1) What nursing actions are not listed?, and 2) What patient outcomes are not listed? Respondents agreed that nursing actions could be linked to outcomes and that this validation process must occur with expert perioperative nurses.

The survey was mailed in July 1994 to a panel of 210 perioperative nursing experts. One hundred forty-five (69%) of the surveys were returned. Based on the responses of the survey, the subcommittee revised the nursing action statements, resulting in a document that consisted of 91 interventions and six outcome standards. The survey was then revised and mailed in

January 1995, to the original panel plus 22 additional members (n=232). The second survey asked respondents to indicate whether or not nursing actions contributed to patient outcomes and whether or not statements required additional revision. Response choices included: 1) the nursing action is not relevant, 2) the statement needs major revision, 3) the nursing action is relevant, but needs minor revision, and 4) the nursing action is very relevant and is clearly stated.

One hundred fifty-eight (68%) of panel members responded during this round of the survey process. Analysis of the survey results led to the development of the first version of the "Perioperative Nursing Data Elements: Interventions (PNDS:1.0)." The identified interventions were deemed to be: 1) applicable across all perioperative settings; 2) focused on patient care; and 3) amenable to future computerized coding. The subcommittee further refined the PNDS: 1.0 and version two is the current working document. Currently, several interventions are being considered for incorporation into version three.

Outcomes

AORN developed and published the first standards for perioperative nursing care in 1983. This document was intended to reflect the standards of care a patient can expect to receive during surgical, diagnostic, or therapeutic interventions. In 1991, these standards were renamed "Patient Outcomes: Standards of Perioperative Care." The DECC Outcomes Subcommittee first convened in 1995, and its initial charge was to review and revise this document. This recommendation was the result of the earlier survey related to interventions and outcomes. The goal of this subcommittee was to develop outcomes that reflected collaborative, interdisciplinary efforts as well as independent nursing activities.

Patient outcomes were defined as observable, measurable, physiological, and psychological responses to perioperative nursing interventions. These outcomes, interpretive statements, and accompanying criteria served as a framework for measuring and documenting patient outcomes. The outcomes reflected the nurse's scope of responsibility in all phases of the perioperative period and were guided by ethical, legal, and moral principles. Examples of outcome statements include: 1) The patient is free of signs and symptoms of physical injury; and 2) the patient is free from signs and symptoms of infections.

Following an extensive literature and research review, the outcome statements were reviewed and revised through the consensus process. Next, a decision to survey members was made. A survey was developed and mailed to a stratified, randomized sample of 1030 AORN members. Participants were asked to rate each outcome statement and criterion for their usefulness in practice, teaching, research, and policy development. Participants were also asked to answer yes or no to three statements/questions: 1) the intent of this statement is clear to me; 2) the interpretative statement and criterion support the outcome statement; and 3) do you currently document information about this outcome?

Although the response rate was only 17%, the subcommittee believed that the respondents adequately represented the current stratification of the membership at large. If there was agreement at the 80% level or greater, an outcome was judged valid. All items for which there was 69% to 79% agreement were reviewed and/or revised by the expert committee utilizing the comments of survey participants. Any item with less than 69% was deleted from the proposed list. This process resulted in the current list of 28 nurse-sensitive perioperative outcomes.

Future Directions

Major efforts continue from the organizational perspective to refine this perioperative nursing data set, disseminate information to members at large, and create a national perioperative data base. In our current health care environment, we must have an organized approach to collect, organize, classify, and capture clinical nursing data to communicate nursing practice. The PNDS is a specialty nursing language that will provide for a systematic method of collecting the basic elements of perioperative nursing care. This data will allow nurses to predict cost, determine necessary resources, and validate perioperative nursing practice.

References

Killen, A.R., Kleinbeck, S.V.M., Golar, K., Schuchardt, J.T., & Uebele, J. (1997). The prevalence of perioperative nurse clinical judgments. *AORN Journal, 65*(1), 101-108.

Kleinbeck, S.V.M. (1996). In search of perioperative nursing data elements. *AORN Journal, 63*(3), 926-931.

Lang, N.M., Galliher, J.M., & Hirsch, I.L. (1989). Challenges to the profession. In *Classification Systems for Describing Nursing Practice.* Washington, DC: American Nurses Association.

Nursing Interventions in School Settings

Roberta Cavendish PhD, RN, CPN

Margaret Lunney PhD, RN, CS

Barbara Kraynyak-Luise, EdD, RN

Kathryn Richardson, MS, RN

Background

Nurses in school settings across the country are working to meet the diverse healthcare needs of school children (Igoe, 1995). School environments offer prime opportunities for nurses to assist children and families with health promotion and health protection (Adams, 1995). With the complexity of such services and the high number of students under the care of school nurses (e.g., 250 to many thousands), computerization of health records will be necessary for documentation of nursing services (Gardner, 1991), comparison of data across populations of school children, and integration of the services provided in schools with the services provided in other settings. To achieve computerization, nursing classification systems such as the Nursing Interventions Classification (NIC) contain standardized terms to support the comparison of data across populations and the communication of nurses with each other, the health care system, and consumers. It is important to describe the number and types of NIC interventions likely to be used in school nursing to support the efficiency and effectiveness of computerized school health records. The NIC was developed through research (Iowa Intervention Project, 1996) and consists of 433 standardized terms for interventions that nurses perform. Each intervention has a definition, a list of activities, and a bibliography. The interventions are nurse-initiated, e.g., patient education, and physician-initiated, e.g., medicine administration.

Purposes

The purposes of this national survey were to: (1) determine which NIC interventions are used in school settings for all populations; (2) describe the frequency of NIC interventions that are used by nurses who work with three age groups of children and children with special needs; (3) identify interventions that are not included in the NIC but should be developed for school nurses.

Methods

The study was conducted using survey research

Table 1

High Frequency Intervention

Intervention	n	m
Documentation	505	4.69
First Aid	502	4.69
Medication Management	513	4.56
Infection Control	503	4.35
Health Screening	504	4.18
Health Education	505	4.16
Telephone Consultation	505	4.12
Heat/Cold Application	511	4.10
Presence	504	4.05
Emotional Support	499	4.02
Infection Protection	501	3.88
Health Care Information Exchange	506	3.78
Pain Management	511	3.72
Learning Facilitation	501	3.72

methods (Babbie, 1990), and the NIC Use Survey. This instrument includes the names of each intervention, definitions and a five-point likert scale (1= not at all; 2= about once a year; 3= about once a month; 4= about once a week; 5= everyday). The NIC questionnaire and a demographic data form were mailed to a stratified random sample of members of the National Association of School Nurses (N=1200). Of these 75 were ineligible (N=1125). The 515 usable responses from 49 states is a 46% response rate. Standard survey protocols as described by Babbie (1990) were followed, e. g., two rounds of reminder postcards were sent to facilitate a high response rate. Completion and return of the research instrument provided evidence of consent. Confidentiality was maintained. Data cleaning was done to verify accuracy of the data. Data were analyzed using descriptive statistics. Percents, Chi square was used to examine the association of demographic characteristics such as grade level of children to frequencies of nursing interventions. The analyses were conducted with SPSS 6.1, Windows 97.

Findings

High frequency interventions used in all school settings were identified. Selected interventions with means ranging from 3.72 to 4.69 are included in Table 1. Only three NIC interventions were not used by any subjects (Autotransfusion, Infection Control: Intraoperative, Phlebotomy: Blood Unit Acquisition); 267 interventions were not used on average by most subjects (m = 1.0 - 1.99); 103 interventions were used on average from once a year to once a month (m = 2.0 - 2.99); 48 interventions were used on average from once a month to once a week (m = 3.0 - 3.99); 12 interventions were used on average from once a week to every day (m = 4.0 - 4.69).

A number of NIC interventions were associated with grade level of children (p <.05). Teaching sexuality, substance abuse, and anger control were interventions significantly associated with the nursing care of the intermediate school population. Family Planning and Smoking Cessation Assistance were interventions significantly associated with the nursing care of high school population. Attachment Promotion and Music Therapy interventions were significantly associated with the the nursing care of children with special needs. Other significant NIC interventions in this population were in the domain of Activity and Exercise Management, and Elimination Management.

Conclusions and Implications

The implications of the findings are that specific NIC interventions are used by nurses in school settings. Core interventions identified can be used for computerization of the health records of school children, and further development of the NIC. There is significant evidence for adoption of the Nursing Intervention Classification by school nurses. These data support services for the health promotion, disease protection and injury management of the nation's children (Lunney, 1996; Pender, 1996). The results of this study will be submitted for publication to the Journal of School Nursing.

This study was partially funded by the Professional Staff Congress of the City University of New York.

References

Adams, R.M. (1995). *School nurse survival guide.* New Jersey: Prentice Hall.

Babbie. E. (1990). *Survey research methods* (2nd ed.). California: Wadsworth Publishing Company.

Gardner, E. (May, 1991). Computerize all patient records by 2001. *Modern Healthcare, 21*(19), 4.

Igoe, J.B. (1995). School health: Designing the policy environment through understanding. *Nursing Policy Forum, 1*(3), 13-36.

Iowa Intervention Project-McCloskey, J. C., Bulchek, G.M. (Eds.). (1996). *Nursing Interventions Classification (NIC)* (2nd ed.). St. Louis: Mosby-Year Book.

Lunney, M. (1996). The significance of nursing classification systems to school nursing. *Journal of School Nursing, 12*(2),16-18.

Pender, N. (1996). *Health promotion in nursing practice,* (3rd ed.). Norwalk, CT: Appleton & Lange.

Documentation of Nurse Practitioner Practice: Challenges and Opportunities

Susan K. Chase, EdD, RNCS, FNP
Jean D'Meza Leuner, PhD, RN

Nurse practitioner practice developed over the last 30 years as a way of responding to a physician shortage and as a means of providing health care to underserved populations. Manpower levels for all health care providers have been in a state of change and recent pressure by the federal government to decrease economic support for specialty physician training has again changed the shape of advanced practice nursing. As advanced practice developed, nurse practitioners have argued that their contributions are unique from physician practice (Roberts, 1996). The challenge of identifying unique contributions that nurse practitioners make and of having those contributions recognized and reimbursed remains. One essential piece in recognition is recording. This requires that nurse practitioner contributions be documented in a retrievable way.

Documentation of nursing practice in general and nurse practitioner practice in particular serves several functions. Some of these functions have been outlined in a 1997 publication by the Iowa Intervention Project. They include to:

- communicate to facilitate care coordination,
- determine a baseline,
- record nursing orders,
- illustrate how general plans or guidelines have been individualized,
- protect oneself from malpractice,
- provide evidence necessary for billing for services,
- provide retrievable data to show care effectiveness, and
- show compliance with accreditation guidelines.

All these purposes have direct application to nurse practitioner practice settings. Documentation of nurse practitioner activities and effectiveness is required for full recognition of nurse practitioner contributions to health care.

Documentation of activities is also required for reimbursement of services by third party payers. Reimbursable documentation requires that an International Classification of

"

Disease (ICD-9) code be designated and that data be provided that justifies the level of care that is being billed. Evaluation and management (E&M) Services codes are listed among Current Procedural Terminology (CPT) codes and vary according to the complexity of the visit. Health care providers are reimbursed for their decision making, for consultation and for preventative health examinations. A routine visit for an established patient might be classified as 99213, and must include an expanded problem focused history, and expanded problem focused examination, decision making of low complexity, counseling and coordination of care, and at least 15 minutes of face time, not counting documentation. Documentation that does not supply enough data to support the level of billing can be denied by the third party payer. Not documenting adequately and not documenting all the skills provided to a patient results in lost revenue for a practice (Buppert, 1998).

Documentation of nurse practitioner practice has been problematic. Nurse practitioners' (NP) practice includes elements of nursing as well as medical diagnosis and treatment. Nurse practitioners function in environments in which nursing diagnosis concepts are relatively unknown. The time pressure for scheduling office visits and the effort to streamline documentation may have implications for nurses practicing in collaborative settings. Encounter forms that are invented to document the most frequent patient problems and care provider activities structure data collection, problem identification and planning in such a way as to limit the documentation of individualization of nurse practitioner activities. How nurse practitioner respond to these challenges is generally unknown.

A study was conceived to address the ways in which nurse practitioners conceptualize and document their practice. Specific research questions included:

1. Do nurse practitioners report using a different data base, problem conceptualization or interventions as compared with physicians?
2. How do nurse practitioners report the activities of their practice, including data base, problem conceptualization, interventions, and patient outcomes?
3. Do nurse practitioners who report unique patient outcomes differ in how they report their practice?
4. What are the barriers to recording unique data, diagnoses, interventions and outcomes?

Methods

A researcher-designed open ended questionnaire was mailed to a national random sample of 400 NP's with a response rate of 49% (n=197). Verbal responses were analyzed for content. Quantitative responses were subjected to descriptive and bivariate analysis.

Results

Responses were obtained from subjects in 37 states. The states with the largest number of responses were Florida (23), Massachusetts (19), California (18), New York (16), and Texas (10). The sample was predominantly female (96%), most worked full time (74%), and the majority were master's prepared (73%). See Table 1 for details on demographic data. The nurse practitioners in the sample had a mean of 10.6 years experience in a mean of 2.71 settings. These were nurse practitioners who were experienced and were qualified to speak to our research questions.

The largest number of respondents were

Table 1

Sample Description:		
Gender	n	percent
male	8	4
female	186	96
Employment Status		
full time	135	74
part time	37	20
not working	12	6
Educational Preparation		
BS	102	54
MS	139	73
PhD	10	5
Years as NP	Range 0-26	Mean 10.53
Number of Settings	Range 0-13	Mean 2.7
Years at Present Setting	Range 0-28	Mean 5.95

Family Nurse Practitioners, followed by Adult, Women's Health, Pediatric, and Gerontologic. Those who described their practice as "other" included hospital based practice and anesthesia. See Table 2 for a description of the types of practice reported by respondents.

Table 2

Type of Practice		
Type of Practice	n	percent
Family	74	39
Adult	50	50
Women's	26	26
Pediatric	24	24
Gerontologic	3	2
Other	15	8

The respondents practiced in a variety of settings. Table 3 provides information about the practice settings. The largest number worked in private group practice settings. Others worked in public clinics or health centers, acute care settings, and Health Maintenance Organizations (HMO's), with some in school health settings or nurse managed clinics.

Table 3

Practice Settings		
Type of Setting	n	percent
Private Practice	64	32
Public Clinic	28	14
Acute Care	22	11
HMO	14	7
School Health	14	7
Nurse Managed Clinic	8	4

Findings

1. Do NP's report using a different data base, problem conceptualization, or interventions as compared with physicians?

Just under half of the nurse practitioners in our sample reported that their assessment differed from that of the physician. Chi square analysis revealed that for those who reported that their assessment was unique, there was a statistically significant difference in documenting their assessment differently, defining the patient problems differently, in carrying out interventions that were not coded on encounter forms, and that the outcomes for their care was different from the outcomes for physician care. Some of the responses to the item describing their assessment data base included, "It's more wellness oriented," "We look at the situation differently, more holistically." Some reported using "more of a holistic approach, more of the impact of health and illness on the individual." NP assessment more comprehensive and time consuming.

Table 4

Unique Assessment Data Base

47% stated NP assessment differs from MD. If said yes,

document assessment differently	p= .000
define problems differently	p= .000
carry out interventions not coded	p= .000
outcomes for NP care differ	p= .000

Findings

1. How do NP's report the activities of their practice including interventions, and patient outcomes?

Although we could say that approximately half of our sample are practicing with a nursing model we also note that all nursing interventions used are not recorded. Some respondents shared, "There is so much that goes on in a visit that it's virtually impossible to record it all. I am especially thinking of a physical exam visit because with adolescents, even younger kids, behavioral issues, psychosocial problems" do not get recorded. Specific interventions that are described as part of nurse practitioner include both psychosocial and psychomotor skills. Examples are suturing, counseling, active listening, and contraception-related procedures. One nurse responded, "I consider much of what I do a nursing intervention, for example, teaching health promotion activities, anticipatory guidance."

2. Do NP's who report unique patient outcomes differ in how they report their practice?

In response to the survey tool, 37% of respondents stated that patient outcomes to nurse practitioner care differ from that of physicians. In the open-ended portion of the questionnaire, respondents listed outcomes to their care that were unique from physician practice.

Unique outcomes to NP care include:
- increased patient satisfaction
- increased understanding of illness and medications
- patients more involved in decision making
- better compliance with regimen
- patient self management
- decreased anxiety

For those respondents who stated that their outcomes to care differed from physician practice, Chi square analysis shows they are more likely to answer that nursing assessment differs from MD assessment (p=.000) and that nursing defines problems differently (p= .005). Those NP's reporting unique outcomes were more also likely to have used a different data base (p<.000) and to have define their problems differently (p=.005).

Related to documentation issues, for those NP's reporting unique outcomes for NP care, Chi square analysis shows they are more likely to answer that nursing assessment is documented differently (p= .027), some nursing assessment issues are not recorded in the patient record (p=.038), and nursing interventions are implemented that are not recorded (p= .039). It is possible that nurses functioning from a nursing model may be more aware than nurses who do not see their unique contribution to recognize difficulties with documentation.

3. What are the barriers to recording unique data, diagnoses, interventions and outcomes?

Our survey shows that only 49% of the NPs report that outcomes to nursing interventions are recorded. One person responded, "Outcomes are not linked directly to nursing. The practice is collaborative." Another reported "after counseling on spousal abuse, encouraging restraining orders, then I document if spouse is in or out of home." Another reported, "wound care outcomes are wound healing, preventing an impending mastitis."

Although it is possible to conceive of nursing outcomes, problems with documentation remain. Only 15% of nurse practitioner respondents report using nursing diagnosis terminology. Problems with nursing diagnosis terminology described by nurse practitioners include the problems that other disciplines are not familiar with the terminology and that encounter forms lack check boxes for nonmedical concepts. "There are no ICD-9 codes or if there are, it becomes very cumbersome and doubles work for data input people." A criticism of nursing diagnosis terminology is that it is too wordy and not specific enough to direct intervention. One person noted that they call the medical issues what they are, and nursing diagnoses may be helpful for some psychosocial issues.

Several respondents noted that their nurse practitioner education programs trained them to use medical terminology. One person noted, "I think problems are problems, whether you think they come under the domain of medicine or nursing, they are the patients'." How is it that nurse practitioner programs are educating their students?

Discussion

Our survey has shown that nurse practitioner assessment can differ from physician assessment, that if assessment is different from physician assessment, unique problems can be defined, and unique outcomes achieved. Furthermore, we have shown that unique contributions of nurse practitioners are not always documented. This challenge must be addressed. Nurse practitioner programs must examine what they are teaching as the proper data base for a nursing assessment. If popular physical assessment texts are used as the guide for nursing assessment, then we are missing functional assessment and many lifestyle factors. Functional health pattern data can be considered part of the subjective health data. Patient problems frequently include family, coping, and functional issues. These problems need to be carried on patient problem lists even in interdisciplinary practices. Projecting outcomes for patients is part of the new focus on "Disease Management." Nursing needs to record outcomes to their participation in patient management. If interdisciplinary providers need education about nursing terminology, then we have a responsibility to educate them through interdisciplinary journals and conferences.

Documentation systems must be expanded to include the contributions of nurse practitioner care. Nurse practitioners provide effective care using a data base and problem conceptualization that may be different from that of either RN's or physicians. Research into effectiveness of care using and documenting a nursing model must be conducted. Interventions by NPs will only be reimbursable if they are recorded and if nurses advocate strongly to have their unique contributions recognized.

References

Buppert, C. (1998). Reimbursement for nurse practitioner services. Nurse Practitioner: *The American Journal of Primary Health Care, 23*(1), 67, 70, 72-74, 76, 81.

Iowa Intervention Project (1997). State of the science: Proposal to bring nursing into the information age. Image: *The Journal of Nursing Scholarship, 29,* 275-281.

Roberts, S.J. (1996). Breaking the cycle of oppression: Lessons for nurse practitioners? *Journal of the American Academy of Nurse Practitioners, 8,* 209-214.

Documentation of Nursing in Structured Multi-Disciplinary Practice Setting

Joyce M. Dungan, RN, MSN, EdD
Donna Jean Gardner, MSN, CNS

This paper presents a method of documentation to reflect practice based on the conceptual Model of Dynamic Integration (DMDI) (Dungan, 1997) using Gordon's Functional Health Patterns (Gordon, 1994) as the framework for assessment. Dynamic Integration supports holistic, autonomous and collaborative practice of nursing. The model supports linkage of clinical judgment to nursing modalities of care that promote functional integrity and self responsibility. It has been applied in a number of nursing protocols over the past decade in a variety of practice settings (Lamm, Dungan, & Hiromoto, 1991; Kumasaka & Dungan, 1993; Mynchenberg & Dungan, 1995, Sciarini & Dungan, 1996; Georgesen & Dungan, 1996, Dungan, Brown & Ramsey, 1996; Nishio, 1997).

The DMDI is comprised of concepts and constructs that are well documented in nursing literature. It is an interaction model consistent with the Reciprocal Interaction World View described by Fawcett (1995). This model views humans as having three dimensions, body, mind and spirit, in a relationship of dynamic integration and in open communication with an ever changing environment. Integration between the three dimensions allows for optimum functioning and is experienced as health. Any human dimension that is not functioning properly disrupts the whole for the client and all others within the intimate environment. The model must be considered across three axes in each nursing situation. The first axis represents the Client focus of the therapeutic relationship which may be an individual, family or larger aggregate of society. The next axis is Development which must be assessed to set the standards of function that may be expected of the client. The third axis is the Wellness/Illness Scale that will determine the nature of the intervention that is appropriate in each nursing situation.

Broken lines signify open communication between the three dimensions and with the environment which includes significant relationships. Cultural beliefs, values and practices form the context of nursing interactions and are of

"

Figure 1

Conceptual Framework of Dynamic Integration Practice Model

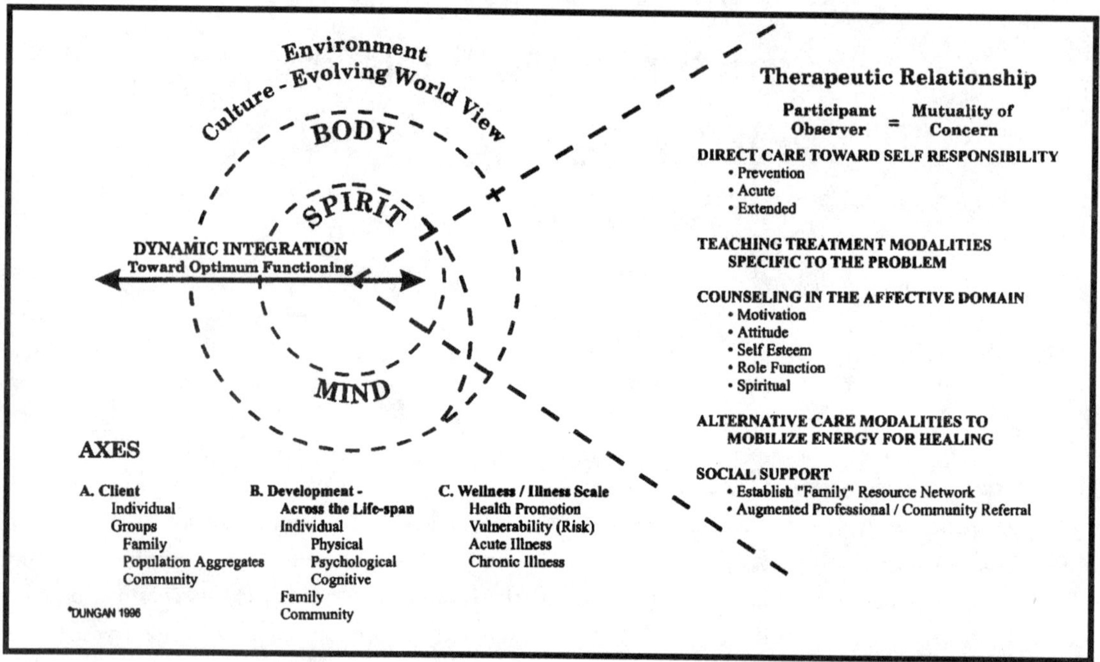

utmost importance in developing the therapeutic relationship through which nursing process is possible (Figure 1).

Energy (life force) is exchanged across all three dimensions and is shared. Any condition that demands energy (illness/life transition) from one dimension may deplete energy from another. Also, energy generated from one dimension may be shared across all three. Appropriate nursing intervention, especially in the context of complimentary healing strategies, may increase energy for re-integration. Spiritual resources may be recruited to heal the body. Cognitive reappraisal strategies may be employed to help clients view situations as challenges rather than threats (Lazarus & Folkman, 1984) and engage in self responsibility. The outcome of dynamic integration may actually yield a higher level of functional development.

Establishment and maintenance of a therapeutic relationship in support of the patient toward independent functioning is an essential element of the model's management strategy. Nursing interaction is represented by an interactive wedge that may touch all three dimensions of the client tofacilitate reintegration. Modalities of care are based upon a caring relationship built on trust and mutual respect between client and

Table 1

Dynamic Integration Model Approach to Transition

NURSING MODALITIES OF CARE

DIRECT CARE – This phase embraces (1) health promoting care as well as disease prevention protocols, (2) the relatively short term care or management of care in acute situation and (3) extended care in chronicity and aging.

TEACHING – (Cognitive Domain) Abount specific health care needs identified related to situation. Should be initiated during the direct care phase. Teach what client needs to know to become independent.

COUNSELING – (Affective Domain)

1. Cognitive Reappraisal
   Threat to Challenge
2. Role Change – Family Negotiation
   - Illness Role
   - Health Seeking Role
   - Care Giver Role
   - Co-Dependency Issues
3. Energy Management – Finite Energy For All Dimensions
4. Self-Concept (Sexuality and Body Image)
5. Reframing World View
   Accommodate cultural beliefs to necessities of life-style change to manage vulnerability
6. Validation Therapy
7. Grieving Losses
8. Strengths and Effective Coping Skills

COMPLIMENTARY HEALING MODALITIES (Spiritual Domain)

1. Spiritual Counseling
2. Meaning of Experience
3. Realistic Hope
4. Therapeutic Touch
5. Music Therapy

SOCIAL SUPPORT

1. Family Resources –Teaching the family skills & attitudes about maintenance, reintegration and return to relative independence.
2. Teach Appropriate Assertiveness and Use of Family

AUGMENTED SOCIAL SUPPORT

1. Short Term Professional Care During Transition
2. Intermittent Professional Care
3. Case Management
4. Community Resources for Client and Care Giver – Referral
5. Teaching Appropriate Assertive To Use Augment Services

nurse. This concept has its roots in the work of Peplau (1952) and is achieved through use of presence, caring, unconditional positive regard, active listening and consensual validation. The current works of Montgomery (1991) and Swanson (1991, 1993) describe a caring relationship that gives nurses permission to coach clients through difficult situations.

Healing must come from within but may be influenced by nursing interventions that function to increase energy available to clients for integration of body, mind and spirit. Key to integration and re-integration are strategies of direct care, teaching/learning, counseling, complimentary healing modalities and social support geared toward clients' affected dimension (Table 1). Practical information is used to increase the power of decision making and give as much control as possible to clients. Teaching is targeted to specific knowledge needed to cope with effects of transition, disease and/or treatment. Appropriate counseling is provided to engage mind and spirit to maintain or restore integration. Social support is a nursing intervention used during transition to incorporate healing into daily demands.

Social support is typified by reciprocal interpersonal relationships that enhance security, mutual respect and positive feelings (Jennings, 1987). Within the context of health care, the term is often reserved for family members. Norbeck (1988) recognized that a sparse social matrix necessitated surrogate social support. The Dungan model acknowledges need for augmented social support from professionals, paraprofessionals and/or peer-help groups for variable lengths of time. Judicious assessment of the amount and type of augmented support to return families to relatively independent functioning is an important feature of the model.

In the spring of 1994, the Nursing Directorate of Naval Medical Center, Portsmouth, Virginia adopted the Dungan Model of Dynamic Integration as the theoretical framework to guide practice and advance the concepts of nursing. In Navy nursing, staff are representative of a wide variety of educational levels and backgrounds. Adopting a conceptual framework was a way to unify nursing practice by bringing different perspectives into focus and giving direction to practice.

Key factors leading to the selection of the DMDI were its new, flexible framework using terminology that is commonly used in nursing and it's congruence with the nursing process. In preparation for an upcoming JCAHO inspection in the fall of 1994, a critical appraisal of the documentation process was conducted and ideas were generated regarding integration of the conceptual framework.

Assessment/Diagnosis

To begin the process of revamping the documentation, outcome goals were identified from a review of the literature. Specifically, information included in the chart must be legally sound and provide current, complete, and concise description of patient status. There should be minimal replication of information. The caring process must be reflected in the documentation along with observations, treatments and patient responses to medical and nursing care. Another goal was that the documented information would be complementary and communication among disciplines would be enhanced. Finally, information in the chart could be retrieved for audit and/or research (Lampe, 1994).

In an attempt to improve the quality of documentation, a core group of Clinical Nurse Specialists (CNSs) was formed to develop a comprehensive patient care data base consistent with the Dungan Model of Dynamic Integration. Facilitation of interdisciplinary collaboration was a key objective. Greater accessibility to data collected by all members of the health care team would establish a comprehensive baseline against which problems, needs and concerns could be identified and outcomes compared. A review of the literature seeking such a collaborative tool provided no examples.

The CNS group shifted the focus from a single tool to consider a unified process to gather complimentary information and enhance collaborative practice. From a nursing perspective, the format needed to be structured enough to minimize variation from one unit to the next, yet adaptable enough to allow for age specific and problem focused differences. The nursing input (History Part 4) also needed to expand data collected by physicians in the health history, review of systems and physical assessment findings (History Parts 1, 2, & 3 respectively). Another factor considered was the transferability to an electronic system planned for the near future.

Gordon's Functional Health Patterns (Gordon, 1994) were selected to provide the structure for the data base through which the tenants of the DMDI could be applied. This framework for assessment is familiar to many nursing staff because of its wide acceptance by the nursing community. Questions were generated from concepts presented in the Dungan Model and supported by the nursing literature (Dungan, 1997; Fuller & Schaller-Ayers, 1994; Lampe, 1994). The goal was to stimulate critical thinking and promote development of simultaneous processing.

Utilizing a consistent format, data collection tools were developed specifically for adult, pediatric, perinatal and neonatal populations.

These tools are designed to be completed by the patient/significant other whenever possible to encourage involvement and promote self-responsibility. For each Functional Health Pattern, screening questions are grouped into clusters to help identify associated diagnoses and facilitate further investigation. Related diagnoses are listed to link clinical judgments with observed data. Learning Resource Guides were generated to address factors related to developmental phenomena characteristic of neonatal, pediatric, adolescent and geriatric clients. To enhance the multi-disciplinary perspective, this form, History 4 follows the Physician History 3 in the chart to provide a complete "picture" of the patient.

After History 4 is completed by the patient/significant other, the RN is responsible for reviewing data with patient and clarifying any uncertainties. Using participant/observer interaction, therapeutic relationship is begun, additional information is gathered, diagnoses are confirmed and mutuality of understanding is explored. During this transaction short term goals are set. Through a review of specific questions, data about cultural beliefs that may influence health decisions are identified. The nature of the Functional Health Patterns facilitates assessment of functional integrity in relationship to an ideal of optimal function for each situation. Information about availability of appropriate social support is gathered during the assessment phase and the impact of the diagnoses on support systems is addressed.

Planning/Implementation

From the assessment phase, a prioritized problem list is generated. In keeping with the goal of multi-disciplinary collaboration, an integrated problem list has been developed on which all

History Part 4

Functional Health Patterns – Adult

1. Health Perception/Management
Client Section

Identified Problems/Focus

What brings you in for medical care? _______________________

❏ No problem

What do you expect to happen during this visit? _______________________

❏ Altered health maintenance

Previous hospitalizations/surgeries/major illness/chronic medical problems? _______________________

❏ Non-adherence

____

❏ Knowledge deficit

How is your general health? ❏ Good ❏ Fair ❏ Poor

❏ Allergies

Date of last: (FEMALE)   (MALE)

❏ Other:

Breast exam ______   Menstrual period ______   Prostate exam ______

Comments:

Mammogram ______   Pap smear ______   Testicular exam ______

Do you use tobacco? ❏ No ❏ Yes Type ______ How long? ______ How much? ______

Do you drink alcohol? ❏ No ❏ Yes How much? ______ How often? ______

Do you use other substances? ❏ No ❏ Yes Describe: _______________________

Are any of these of concern for you? _______________________

Any allergies to meds, foods, dyes, tape? ❏ No ❏ Yes Describe: _______________________

❏ Medications

____

Meds you are currently taking: _______________________

Do you have a: Yes   No   Need/Want information

  Living Will   ❏   ❏   ❏

  Advance Directive   ❏   ❏   ❏

  Medical Power of Attorney   ❏   ❏   ❏

If yes, where are these documents located? _______________________

Height __________   Weight __________

2. Nutritional/Metabolic

❏ No problem

Do you have a skin condition? ❏ No ❏ Yes Describe: _______________________

❏ Nutrition Consult

Do you have a special diet? ❏ No ❏ Yes Describe: _______________________

❏ Altered fluid volume status

Any major changes in your weight, appetite or thirst over the last year? ❏ No ❏ Yes

❏ Impaired skin integrity

Describe: _______________________

❏ Knowledge deficit

Any difficulty with eating, swallowing or indigestion? ❏ No ❏ Yes Describe: _______________________

❏ Other:

Comments:

Do you have dentures? ❏ No ❏ Yes: ❏ partial ❏ lower ❏ upper

3. Elimination

❏ No problem

Any changes or difficulties with urinary elimination? ❏ No ❏ Yes Describe: _______________________

❏ Altered urinary elimination

❏ Altered bowel elimination

Any changes or difficulties with your bowel habits (e.g., diarrhea, constipation, hemorrhoids, or

❏ Other:

bleeding): ❏ No ❏ Yes Describe: _______________________

Comments:

Do you use laxatives or other aids for regularity? ❏ No ❏ Yes Describe: _______________________

4. Activity/Exercise

❏ No problem

Do you have enough energy for your desired/required activities? ❏ No ❏ Yes Explain: ______

❏ Activity intolerance

❏ Self care deficit

Please rate your ability to do the following:

❏ Impaired physical mobility

	Independent	Need Assist	Unable	Explain
Walking	❏	❏	❏	_______
Bath/Shower	❏	❏	❏	_______
Dressing	❏	❏	❏	_______
Eating	❏	❏	❏	_______
Using toilet	❏	❏	❏	_______
Moving from bed/chair	❏	❏	❏	_______

❏ Fall risk

❏ Other:

Comments:

Check if you use or need any of the following:

❏ crutches   ❏ walker   ❏ wheelchair   ❏ cane   ❏ artificial limb

❏ elevated toilet   ❏ other: _______________________

Have you fallen recently? ❏ No ❏ Yes

Addressograph

(Adapted from Lampe, 1994)

History Part 4

Functional Health Patterns – Adult

5. Cognitive/Perceptual

What is the highest level of education you completed? ______________________

Any recent changes in memory? ☐ No ☐ Yes Describe:______________________

____

Any difficulty with hearing and/or vision? ☐ No ☐ Yes Describe:____________

Do you use hearing aids/glasses/contacts? ☐ No ☐ Yes Type:______________

Do you regularly experience pain or discomfort? ☐ No ☐ Yes Describe:________

____

Place a mark (X) on the scale below that reflects how much pain you feel now:

0 ——— 1 ——— 2 ——— 3 ——— 4 ——— 5 ——— 6 ——— 7 ——— 8 ——— 9 ——— 10

No sensation of pain   As much pain as could possibly be

What do you do to relieve pain? ______________________

Identified Problems/Focus

☐ No problem
☐ Pain
☐ Chronic pain
☐ Sensory perceptual alteration
☐ Altered thought process
☐ Teaching protocol modification
☐ Other:
Comments:

6. Sleep/Rest

Do you have any difficulty sleeping? ☐ No ☐ Yes Describe:______________

Is there anything you do or use to help you sleep? ☐ No ☐ Yes Describe: ______________

____

☐ No problem
☐ Sleep pattern disturbance
☐ Other:
Comment:

7. Self-perception/concept

Has your illness/condition caused changes in the things you can do? ☐ No ☐ Yes
Describe:______________________

Has it caused changes in the way you feel about yourself? ☐ No ☐ Yes
Describe:______________________

Do you have any questions about your illness or your hospital stay? ______________

____

☐ No problem
☐ Body image disturbance
☐ Self-esteem disturbance
☐ Knowledge deficit
☐ Other:
Comments:

8. Roles/Relationships

Who will care for you after discharge? ______________________

Any family/work difficulties as a result of your illness/condition? ☐ No ☐ Yes
Describe:______________________

Do others depend on you? ☐ No ☐ Yes How are they managing? ______________

____

Does anyone come to your home to help you? (e.g., visiting nurse, housekeeper) ☐ No ☐ Yes

Who and how often? ______________________

(For dependents) If your sponsor is active duty, is he/she deployed? ☐ No ☐ Yes

☐ No problem
☐ Altered role performance
☐ Social isolation
☐ Discharge Planner assistance needed
☐ Other:
Comments:

9. Reproductive/Sexuality

Some people have a concern that their condition may effect their intimacy/relationship(s).

Is this a concern for you? ☐ No ☐ Yes Explain:______________________

Method of contraception or protection: ☐ N/A ______________________

☐ No problem
☐ Knowledge deficit
☐ Other:
Comments:

10. Coping/Stress

Do you feel afraid or depressed by your illness? ☐ No ☐ Yes Describe:________

Other than this hospitalization, have there been any big changes in your life in the last year
or so? ☐ No ☐ Yes Describe:______________________

When you have problems or stress in your life, how do you generally handle it? ______________

Place a mark (X) on the line below that reflects how you feel now:

●——————●——————●——————●——————●——————●——————●——————●

No sensation of anxiety   As much anxiety as could possibly be

☐ No problem
☐ Ineffective coping
☐ Anxiety
☐ Fear
☐ Depression
☐ Other:
Comments:

11. Values/Beliefs/Spiritual Resources

Do you have any important spiritual and/or cultural practices and concerns?______________

Would you like to see the Chaplain? ☐ No ☐ Yes Religious Preference: ______________

☐ No problem
☐ Spiritual distress
☐ Other:
Comments:

______________________________   ______________________________
Patient's/Significant Other's Signature   Date/Time   RN Signature   Date/Time

disciplines may identify problems. The process facilitates communication and minimizes fragmentation of the patient status. Several areas within the hospital have been using collaborative treatment plans for some time and have demonstrated effectiveness of an integrated approach.

Expected Outcomes (EO) for each problem are discussed with the patient/significant other(s) and listed to identify goals, plan interventions and give focus to discharge planning for care team members. The four components of EO include: an observable behavior of the patient, established measurement criteria, condition under which behavior should occur (i.e., with a walker, assisted by one staff, independently) and the time frame in which the behavior should occur (i.e., by discharge, within 24 hours, by a specific date).

There has been significant resistance from both physicians and nurses to the Collaborative Problem List and the efficacy of this component of the process is still being tested. Support of this tool from a nursing perspective would replace the lengthy "care plan" format with a more individualized problem focused format.

The Patient Profile is the tool used to communicate the plan of care to nursing staff from one shift to the next. The Direct Care needs of the patient are traditionally reflected as specific physician orders and nursing initiated orders (NIO). Nursing orders include standard interventions related to care as well as complimentary interventions such as Healing Touch, Music Therapy, Massage, and Relaxation Techniques.

In support of transition from illness toward wellness and optimal functioning, augmented professional/community referrals are initiated by the Registered Nurse (RN). Several speciality departments accept Nurse Initiated Consults and further contribute to the multi-disciplinary plan of care. These include Dietary, Infection Control, Ostomy/Skin Care, Family Advocacy, Chaplain, Social Work, Psychiatric Liaison, CNS, Asthma Clinic and Discharge Planning.

As part of the process, the problems on the Collaborative Problem List are included on the Patient Profile for use during report and to plan continuity of care for the next shift. Night nurses, during chart verification, update the Collaborative Problem List and Profile. At report, the status of each problem is reviewed and plans of care for the next shift are discussed. These discussions stimulate critical thinking and provide relevant information to reflect patient progress toward meeting EO's.

Implementation/Evaluation

Implementation of the plan of care and patient response are reflected in the documentation. For our purpose, a variety of flowsheets have been developed over time to meet the needs of different patient populations. To give consistency to the charting process and enhance data communication and retrieval, a Focus Charting® format (Lampe, 1994) has been adopted. This format supports problem identification and tracking, reflects specific interventions, allows for application of Complimentary Care Modalities, and includes an evaluation of patient response to care. This directly links the Collaborative Problem List, Expected Outcomes, and the Nursing Process as well as meets JCAHO requirements.

A Learning Resource Guide or Programmed Self-Instruction has been developed to educate nursing staff in use of Focus Charting. Two categories of Focus Notes have been identified. The first is documented on the Activities of Daily Living (ADL) Flowsheets to reflect patient variance in response to interventions. The use of a focus statement minimizes non-essential charting. The second category of Focus Notes is recorded in multi-disciplinary Progress Notes to update the status of current problems in chronological order every 24 hours and to reflect new problems identified.

Assessment of teaching and counseling needs is an ongoing process determined by information gathered through the therapeutic relationship. Two components have been identified to support a unified multi-disciplinary approach. The first is the incidental or spontaneous teaching/counseling that is less structured and often occurs at the point of need expressed by the patient. Topics that may be covered using this approach are related to information about medication, safety measures, wound care, mobility assistance and others arising out of specific patient encounters and in response to patient inquiries. This teaching is documented on a form titled "Patient Teaching Record." This form is maintained at the bedside or in the front of the chart to facilitate multi-disciplinary documentation of incidental teaching.

The second component of patient education focuses on high risk/high volume populations and provides structured teaching for specific topics: Diabetes, Asthma, Newborn Care etc. A standardized template has been titled "Patient Education Flowsheet" and specific topic outlines are being developed at each unit level for these. The emphasis is on multi-disciplinary patient and family teaching based on Standards of Care for specific conditions. This education flowsheets supports Clinical Pathways and facilitates communication of educational needs from inpatient to outpatient settings. A copy of this form is given to the patient as well as to the clinic staff to document what has been taught and learned and what information needs reinforcement.

The final element in our documentation process is the Trans-disciplinary Discharge Form, designed by physicians to provide for continuity of care. This form has streamlined the discharge process by facilitating documentation of the inter-disciplinary plan of care during the inpatient episode and allowing for easy relay of data for outpatient follow-up. It also links with the Patient Education Flowsheets to minimize duplication of effort.

To provide staff training about the changes in the documentation process, each unit identified an Implementation Member to conduct in-service teaching sessions and serve as a resource for the current staff. New staff members are introduced to the Dungan Model of Dynamic Integration and the documentation process during orientation. In addition, Focus Charting videos and workbooks are available within each area of the hospital and clinics for clarification of information and to answer questions about the charting format.

In the near future Portsmouth Naval Medical Center plans to institute a system of electronic documentation. The entire care process outlined in this article was designed for easy transition. It is hoped that the flexibility of our system of Dynamic Integration (Dungan, 1997) will allow us to easily establish standardized templates that can be adapted to population specific needs while maintaining a consistent structure of Functional Health Patterns (Gordon, 1994). Staff familiarity is important to ease the transition to electronic documentation and will help move from a hard copy system to a paper-less process.

References

Dungan, J. (1997) Dungan model of dynamic integration, *Nursing Diagnosis,* 8(1), 17-28.

Dungan, J., Brown, A., & Ramsey, M. (1996). Health maintenance forthe independent frail older adult: Can it improve physical and mental well being? *Journal of Advanced Nursing, 23,* 1185-1193.

Fawcett, J. (1995) *Analysis and evaluation of conceptual models of nursing* (3rd ed.). Philadelphia: Davis.

Fuller, J., & Schaller-Ayers, J. (1994). *Health assessment: A nursing approach,*(2nd Ed.), Philadelphia: Lippincott

Georgesen, J., & Dungan, J. (1996). Managing spiritual distress in patients with advanced cancer pain. *Cancer Nursing, 19*(5), 376-383.

Gordon, M. (1994), *Nursing diagnosis, process and application*, (3rd Ed.), St. Louis: Mosby.

Jennings, C. (1987). Social support: A way to a climate of caring. *Nursing Administration Quarterly, 11*(4), 63-70.

Kumasaka, L., & Dungan, J. (1993). Nursing strategy for initial emotional response to cancer diagnosis. *Cancer Nursing 16*(4), 296-303.

Lamm, B., Dungan, J., & Hiromoto, B. (1991). Long-term lifestyle management. *Clinical Nurse Specialist 5*(4), 182-188.

Lampe, S. (1994). *Focus charting: Documentation for patient-centered care*, (6th Ed.), Minneapolis: Creative Nursing Management, Inc.

Lazarus, R., & Folkman, S. (1984). *Stress, appraisal and coping*. New York: Springer.

Montgomery, C. (1991). The care-giving relationship: Paradoxical and transcendent aspects. *The Journal of Transpersonal Psychology 23*(2), 91-104.

Mynchenberg, T., & Dungan, J. (1995). A relaxation protocol to reduce patient anxiety. *Dimensions of Critical Care Nursing 14*(2), 78-85.

Nishio, K. (1997). A family affected by mitochondrial encephalomyopathy: A nursing protocol. *Clinical Nurse Specialist 11*(5): 195-201.

Norbeck, J. (1988). Social support. *Annual Review of Nursing Research, 6,* 85-109.

Peplau, H. (1952, 1988). *Interpersonal relations in nursing*. New York: Macmillan.

Sciarini, P., & Dungan, J. (1996). A holistic protocol for management of fluid volume excess in hemodialysis patients. *American Nephrology Nurses' Association Journal, 23,* 299-305.

Swanson, K. (1991). Empirical development of a middle range theory of caring. *Nursing Research, 40,* 161-166.

Swanson, K. (1993). Nursing as informed caring for the well-being of others. *Image, 25*(4), 352-357.

Patient Involvement in Nursing Diagnosis Research

Kathryn Van Dyke Hayes, DNSc, RN, C

As nursing diagnosis research moves into the next millennium, a deliberate analysis of the specific patient roles in nursing diagnosis research is warranted. Numerous nursing diagnosis research studies have included patient subjects. An analysis of the specific patient roles in nursing diagnosis research has not previously been explicated. The purpose of this paper is threefold: (a) to critically review the literature on patient participation in nursing diagnosis research, (b) to discuss the results of a descriptive study in which persons with spinal cord injury rated the importance of risk factors for disuse syndrome, and (c) to propose implications for future nursing diagnosis research.

Review of Patient Participation in Nursing Diagnosis Research

Several research studies involving patient subjects were identified via the Cumulative Index for Nursing and Allied Health Literature (CINAHL), previous editions of the North American Nursing Diagnosis Association's (NANDA) proceedings, and the comprehensive bibliography developed by the NANDA Research Committee (Dougherty, Jankin, Lunney, & Whitley, 1993). For the purpose of this review, patient subjects were defined as any subject in a nursing diagnosis research study except nurses or nursing students. This review includes both research studies of NANDA accepted nursing diagnoses and nonaccepted nursing diagnoses.

The literature review does not include research studies whose only sampling methods incorporated record reviews including computerized records, nurse subjects, nursing student subjects, secondary analyses of data, or case control methods. Qualitative case studies were included, however, nonresearch articles with case studies or scenarios fabricated for illustration of a nursing diagnosis were not reviewed.

The literature review revealed a number of issues. For example, a few titles had solely published as abstracts in NANDA proceedings; these abstracts lacked clarity regarding the exact role of the patient subjects in the study. The lack of clarity or specific details in the abstracts made categorization of studies difficult. Retrieval of each actual study, when available, was needed to determine the inclusion of patient subjects. This resulted in a labor intensive process for one writer. At times, clear and specific information regarding the patient subjects' roles was still lacking in full length articles. Several studies had multiple purposes and may be classified in more than one category. In a few studies, patient involvement was minimal or tangential to the study's primary purpose, however, these studies were reviewed in order to construct comprehensive and detailed categories.

The discussion and presentation of studies is not intended to be all inclusive. Studies cited are used as illustrations for each category of patient involvement in nursing diagnosis research. Future plans include publication of a comprehensive list of nursing diagnosis research studies with patient subjects.

After an extensive review of the literature, 148 studies were located that included patient subjects. The research studies spanned nearly two decades: a time period from 1979 to 1997. Patient involvement in nursing diagnosis research can be categorized as follows: concept clarification, elucidation of the etiology of a disorder, instrument testing, clinical diagnostic validation, and miscellaneous roles. The miscellaneous roles category was created for a variety of studies that were fewer in number and are grouped for convenience.

Concept Clarification

Concept clarification refers to patient subjects who provided descriptions, personal perspectives, analyses, or judgments about a particular concept or phenomena. Fifteen research studies were located in this category. Concepts or phenomena studied include Sick Role Conflict (Kubsch & Wichowski, 1992), Powerlessness (Shaw, 1987), and the perception of being disrobed (de Arajo Silveira, Coler, & da Nobrega, 1997). An example includes a phenomenological approach used by Smucker (1995) to describe the phenomena of spiritual distress in 10 adults. Analysis of in-depth interview data revealed the experience of spiritual distress occurred over time in two phases (Smucker). Fowler (1997) described the experience of Impaired Verbal Communication during short-term oral intubation in 10 previously intubated patients subjects. Using a semistructured interview approach, patient subjects reported feelings of pain, discomfort, fear, and frustration throughout intubation (Fowler).

Semistructured and structured interview guides were used as the principal data collection method. Occasionally, observation (de Arajo Silveira et al., 1997) or participant observation (Downey, 1995) was used to capture patient subject behavior and/or supplement interview data.

Elucidation of the Etiology of Certain Disorders

Ten studies were located involving patient subjects who elucidated the etiologies of certain disorders. Specifically, this category consists of studies that obtain the patient's perspective on factors, causes, or reasons for the etiology of certain disorders. McLane, McShane, and Sleifert (1984) conducted interviews to assess factors indicative of Alteration in Bowel Elimination: Constipation in 20 subjects aged 50 and older. A study was conducted to examine the sleep problems of 141 hospitalized women (Cox & Halfens, 1995). Analysis of interview data revealed the most frequently reported sleep problems involved difficulty falling asleep and frequent awakenings.

The majority of research studies utilized small convenience samples; however, some studies had convenience samples of 100 or more subjects (Beyerman, 1987; Cox & Halfens, 1995). Convenience samples were usually obtained from one site, but McLane and McShane (1986) used several sites to obtain 300 subjects for a survey. Patient subjects ranged in age from adolescents to retirees. Data collection methods consisted of semi-structured or structured interviews (Beyerman, 1987; Cox & Halfens, 1995; Rossi, Fitzmaurice, Glynn, & Connors, 1987). Due to multiple purposes, some studies utilized multiple data collection methods, such as interview and observations (Norris & Kunes-Connell, 1987; Norris & Kunes-Connell, 1989) or interview and standardized instrument (Norris & Kunes-Connell, 1985). Both standardized instruments as well as researcher designed instruments were used. Documentation of reliabilty and validity information for data collection instruments wall standardized instruments was inconsistent.

Instrument Testing

Patient subjects have been utilized to test instruments and establish reliability and validity indices. Twenty research studies were located that included patient subjects for the testing of instruments, including NANDA accepted nursing diagnoses and other nursing diagnoses. For example, investigator designed instruments for risk of homicide (Campbell, 1986), boredom and confusion (Savitz & Friedman, 1981), Mixed Incontinence (Woodtli, 1995), and Self Care Deficit (Chang, Hirsch, Brazal-Villanueva, & Iverson, 1990) have been tested using patient subjects. Savitz and Friedman (1981) estab-

lished the reliability and validity of an interview schedule for diagnosing individuals as being in a bored, confused, or adaptive state of mind. In two phases, Chang et al. (1990) examined the reliability of an assessment guide for the diagnostic label, Self Care Deficit. Using the modified standardized instrument, clinical nurse specialists assessed 30 in-patients and formulated the diagnostic label, its etiologies, and contributing factors (Chang et al.). Other studies developed and tested instruments completed by the patient subjects themselves. Thirty elderly women in a pilot study completed the Stress and Urge Incontinence Instrument (SUII) to determine its reliability and validity (Sidani & Woodtli, 1994).

The majority of research studies including patient subjects for instrument testing used convenience or purposive sampling methods. Overall, samples sizes tended to be small (< 30). Most studies used a sample from a singular site or setting probably due to the lack of extensive resources needed for conducting multisite, multisample investigations (Maas, Hardy, & Craft, 1990). Research instruments tested included interview guides, questionnaires, observational checklists, and assessment guides.

Clinical Diagnostic Validation

Clinical diagnostic validation (CDV) is the largest category of patient involvement in nursing diagnosis research. Ninety research studies were located with patient subjects that clinically validated defining characteristics, etiologies, or related factors of nursing diagnoses. In order to establish a database for the validation of nursing diagnoses, patient subjects were interviewed, responded to questionnaires and/or other instruments, were observed, or gave had health assessment data collected by nurses.

In 21 of the 90 studies, patient subjects were assessed by nurse subjects for the presence of specific nursing diagnoses for a particular patient population. Nursing diagnoses have been identified for several patient populations, including patients with the medical diagnosis of multiple sclerosis (Gould, 1983), the chronically ill (Hoskins, McFarlane, Rubenfeld, Walsh, & Schreier, 1986), seriously ill psychiatric patients (Holmes et al., 1995), and adults with insulin-dependent diabetes mellitus (Beaulieu, 1989).

A total of 69 out of the 90 studies included patient subjects for CDV. Few nursing diagnoses were studied more than once. For example, more than one CDV study with patient participation was located for powerlessness (Mullins, 1994; Richmond, Metcalf, Daly, & Kish, 1992; Shaw, 1987), urge incontinence (Gaffney & Zirker, 1994; Woodtli & Yocum, 1994), and fatigue (Chung, 1997; Tiesinga, Dassen, & Halfens, 1997). Both NANDA accepted nursing diagnoses and nonaccepted diagnoses were studied.

CDV studies had similar limitations as the studies in previous categories. Primarily, small sample size and solitary site studies with minimal integration of qualitative and quantitative methods were located. Frequently, documentation of psychometric qualities of data collection instruments is incomplete. A rare CDV study, such as Whitley's (1997) clinical validation study of anxiety and fear, included both patient subjects and nurse subjects.

Miscellaneous Roles

The miscellaneous category consists of a variety of less common patient roles in nursing diagnosis research. These thirteen studies are grouped together for convenience. Miscellaneous patient involvement includes roles in formulating nursing diagnoses, methodology development, identification and/or rating of risk factors or defining characteristics for a nursing diagnosis, and identification of nursing diagnoses by patient subjects.

Each miscellaneous role will be illustrated with an example. In a study to systematically formulate and develop a nursing diagnosis, Avant (1979) observed 15 primigravidas and their infants to demonstrate the nursing diagnosis maternal attachment. Several studies have included patient subjects for methodology development, such as Bayesian methods (Magnan, 1995) and investigator designed strategies for validating nursing diagnoses (da Cruz, 1995; Swehla, 1988). Hayes (1994) interviewed 35 persons with spinal cord injuries to determine the importance of risk factors for disuse syndrome from their perspective. This study will be discussed in detail in the next section. Whitley and Tousman (1996) conducted a study to reduce the defining characteristics for the nursing diagnoses Anxiety and Fear. Sixty-nine hospitalized psychiatric and medical-surgical patients rated a list of defining characteristics for how closely they represented their own anxious state (Whitley & Tousman). A singular study was located in which 231 postpartum women completed questionnaires and identified nine nursing diagnoses of concern 72 hours after birth (Triboti, Lyons, Blackburn, Stein, & Winters, 1988).

Descriptive Study Involving Patients with Spinal Cord Injury

Purpose

A descriptive survey was designed to identify the importance of risk factors for disuse syndrome from the perspective of persons with spinal cord injuries. This survey was part of a larger study designed to validate the nursing diagnosis Risk for Disuse Syndrome (Hayes, 1994).

Rationale

Patients are a valuable resource for the identification and refinement of defining characteristics or risk factors for nursing diagnoses. Fehring (1994) has proposed the patient-focused clinical diagnostic validity (CDV) model in which individuals with a particular nursing diagnosis, if psychological or behavioral in nature, are asked to rate defining characteristics. It seems short-sighted to fail to obtain patient input when it comes to nursing diagnoses, such as Risk for Disuse Syndrome, that are primarily physiological in nature. This failure to obtain patient input is especially contradictory to current trends in the provision of health care in which patient input is solicited and essential to the development of the plan of care. Furthermore, patient's lived experiences provide a wealth of information not available from any other source.

Sample

The average spinal cord injured subject fit the following profile: (a) a 37.4 year old male; (b) a high school graduate; (c) sustained a complete, cervical spinal cord injury due to a motor vehicle accident 10.51 years ago; (d) received surgical treatment as a result of the injury; and (e) had attended the outpatient follow-up clinic for 6.5 years.

Instrumentation/Procedure

Using a structured interview format, a total of 35 persons with spinal cord injury were interviewed to determine the importance of risk factors from their point of view. A researcher-designed instrument, the Persons with Spinal Cord Injury: Structured Interview Guide (PSCI: SIG) consisting of 13 demographic data questions, 48 questions on risk factors, and one open-ended question on medications, was developed. Risk factors were stated in general terms or layman's language. First, patient subjects were asked whether they had experienced the risk factor. If the patient subject had experienced the risk factor, the investigator asked the subject to rate how important the risk factor was to the development of the complications of immobility using a 3-point Likert scale with not important (1), somewhat important (2), and very important (3). Expert reviewers suggested the term complications of immobility be used in place of disuse syndrome, because patient subjects would be more familiar with that term. If the patient subject had not experienced the particular risk factor, the investigator moved to the next question on the PSCI:SIG. Completion of the PSCI:SIG took an average of 45 minutes.

Protection of Human Subjects

All subjects with spinal cord injuries voluntarily agreed to participate and were interviewed at the outpatient follow-up clinic at a large rehabilitation hospital in the Mid-Atlantic region of the United States. The research proposal was approved by the Institutional Review Board at a large rehabilitation hospital.

Study Results

As shown in Table 1, ten risk factors were experienced by all patient subjects and were rated by the majority of subjects as very important. One item, cultural/ethnic background, was rated by 35 patient subjects, but it did not achieve a majority in any of the three response categories. Two more items, paralysis rated by 24 patient subjects and lack of knowledge to relieve or control a painful condition rated by 22 patient subjects, achieved a rating as very important by a

Table 1

Items on the PSCI: SIG Rated by More Than Half of the Patient Subjects

Item/Question	n^a	Not Important %	Somewhat Important %	Very Important %
Weakened/Run Down Condition	35	2.9	8.6	88.6
Overall Nutritional Condition	35	2.9	14.3	82.9
Type/Amount of Fluid	35	5.7	11.4	82.9
Lack of Motor Control	35	0.0	20.0	80.0
Loss of Sensation	35	2.9	20.0	77.1
Type/Amount of Exercise	35	0.0	25.7	74.3
Kind of Food Eaten	35	5.7	25.7	68.6
Pain	35	2.9	34.3	62.9
Feeling Fatigued/Tired	35	2.9	40.0	57.1
Medications	35	2.9	40.0	57.1
Cultural/Ethnic Background	35	40.0	45.7	14.3
History of a Fall	31	16.1	32.3	51.6
Acute Pain	26	19.2	42.3	38.5
Paralysis	24	0.0	25.0	75.0
Impaired Balance	24	4.1	29.2	66.6
Bed Rest/Enforced Rest	24	0.0	41.7	58.3
Recent Admission to Health Care Institution	24	20.8	37.5	41.7
Lack of Knowledge to Relieve/Control Painful Condition	22	0.0	13.6	86.4
Severe Pain	22	4.5	27.3	68.2
Powerlessness	22	4.5	40.9	54.5
Chronic Pain	22	9.1	36.4	54.5
Fluid Retention/Edema	22	13.6	59.1	27.3
Major Surgery	20	25.0	10.0	65.0
Fear of Falling	19	0.0	31.6	68.4
Contractures	19	10.5	31.6	57.9
Treatments That Limit Movement/Activity	19	15.8	47.4	36.8
Paraplegia	18	0.0	27.8	72.2
Hopelessness	18	5.6	22.2	72.2
Splints	18	33.3	22.2	44.4

n^a = number of patient subjects who rated the item.

majority of subjects (≥18). A total of 12 risk factors out of 48 were rated as very important to the development of complications of immobility by the majority (≥18) of the persons with spinal cord injuries.

Although not rated by a majority of patients, 13 additional risk factors achieved the highest percentage of responses in the very important category as shown on Table 1. Three items, acute pain, fluid retention, and treatments that limit movement/activity were rated by less than the majority as somewhat important by the highest percentage of subjects.

The responses to an additional 19 items rated by 1 to 17 patient subjects are shown in Table 2. Although not a majority (≥18), 16 additional items achieved the highest percent of responses in the very important category. Diabetes/high blood sugar, obesity/extreme overweight, and amputation were rated as very

Table 2

Items on the PSCI: SIG Rated by More Than Half of the Patient Subjects

Item/Question	n^a	Not Important %	Somewhat Important %	Very Important %
Quadriplegia	17	0.0	5.8	94.1
Underweight	17	17.6	29.4	52.9
Treatment with Immobilization Device	16	18.8	18.8	62.5
Fractured Bone	16	0.0	25.0	75.0
Depression	14	7.2	0.0	92.9
Inability to Cope/ Adapt	12	0.0	33.3	66.6
Illness Affecting Breathing	11	9.0	0.0	90.9
Illnesses of Joints/ Arthritis	11	18.2	18.2	63.6
Recent Weight Loss	11	18.2	18.2	36.6
Ventilator/Breathing Machine	10	20.0	0.0	80.0
Illnesses Affecting the Heart	7	14.3	28.6	57.1
Severe Phobia/Fear	7	0.0	14.3	85.7
Osteoporosis	5	0.0	80.0	20.0
Poor/Decreased Eyesight	5	60.0	20.0	20.0
Obesity/Extreme Overweight	4	0.0	0.0	100.0
Diabetes/High Blood Sugar	3	0.0	0.0	100.0
Low Blood Sugar	3	33.3	0.0	66.6
Fracture Treatment With External Stabilization Devices	2	50.0	0.0	50.0
Amputation of Arm or Leg	1	0.0	0.0	100.0

n^a = number of patient subjects who rated the item.

important by 100% of the patient subjects who experienced these risk factors. Diabetes was rated by three subjects, obesity by four subjects, and amputation by one subject, respectively.

Of the three remaining items, 80% of the patient subjects who experienced osteoporosis (n = 5) rated this item as somewhat important. Poor/decreased eyesight was rated by three out of five patient subjects as not important (60%). Fracture treatment with external stabilization devices was rated equally as not important (50%0 and very important (50%) by two subjects.

Two open-ended questions at the end of the PSCI:SIG provided patient subjects with the opportunity to make suggestions for risk factors and spontaneous comments in their own words. The majority of patient subjects (87%) suggested risk factors. A total of 52 suggested risk factors were summarized into four categories: (a) psychiatric-mental health factors, (b) environmental factors, (c) social support factors, and (d) miscellaneous factors (e.g., financial constraints, smoking). A total of 15 (42.8%) of patient subjects made general comments on a range of one to six topics. General comments made by patient subjects were grouped into six categories: (a) environmental issues, (b) spinal cord injury prevention issues, (c) community resources, (d) psychological/coping issues, (e) public education issues, and (f) miscellaneous issues.

Discussion of Study Results

Patient involvement in the validation of nursing diagnoses that are primarily physiological in nature has been limited. An examination of the results on the PSCI:SIG reveals patient subjects rated nearly all the risk factors, especially those they personally experienced, as important or very important. Patient subjects suggested additional risk factors that were not on the PSCI:SIG (e.g., substance abuse, smoking, denial). Suggested risk factors were primarily in the psychiatric-mental health factor category. Insight into the patient subjects' lived experiences of coping with immobility and spinal cord injury were apparent in their responses to open-ended questions. It is evident that patient subjects can add to the body of knowledge of risk factors for Risk for Disuse Syndrome, but caution is necessary in the interpretation of results. Future research to correlate patient's and nurse's perceptions of risk factors for disuse syndrome across multiple settings may assist in increasing confidence in the content validity of this nursing diagnosis (Schroeder, 1991).

Twenty-nine additional risk factors were rated as very important by less than a majority of patient subjects. For example, diabetes/high blood sugar, obesity/extreme overweight, and amputation were experienced and rated by small numbers of subjects. Yet, 100% of the patient subjects who experienced these risk factors rated them as very important to the development of complications of immobility. Future research using a larger sample of patient subjects might consider the relative importance of these items.

The length of time post spinal cord injury or duration of immobility or inactivity may impact on the patient's perception of risk factors. In this study, 85.7% of patient subjects had been injured for at least three years; 62.8% had been injured for at least six years. Patient subjects with spinal cord injuries who were immobilized for shorter periods of time may rate risk factors in a different manner. Risk factors may also vary among patient subjects of different ages (younger or older) and medical diagnoses. Consideration of these issues is needed in future studies on the nursing diagnosis of Risk for Disuse Syndrome.

Implications for Future Nursing Diagnosis Research

After a review of the specific patient roles in nursing diagnosis research, implications for future patient involvement in nursing diagnosis research include: (a) conducting multiple site and multiple, diverse sample studies (Mass, Hardy, & Craft, 1990); (b) establishing acceptable reliability and validity indices for data collection instruments; (c) refining instruments for specific and general patient populations (Tiesinga et al., 1997); (d) increasing the integration of qualitative and quantitative methods (Kim, 1991); (e) comparing patient subject and nurse subject perceptions of the same phenomena across multiple settings (Schroeder, 1991); and (f) replicating existing nursing diagnosis research involving patient subjects.

Summary

Nurse researchers have included patient subjects in a variety of nursing diagnosis research studies. Further patient input in nursing diagnosis research is essential to validate nursing diagnoses that are meaningful and useful in clinical practice. Future strategies to strengthen nursing diagnosis research include placing more emphasis on determining the effectiveness and sensitivity of patient data for the validation of specific nursing diagnoses.

References

Avant, K. (1979). Nursing diagnosis: Maternal attachment. *Advances in Nursing Science, 1*, 45-55.

Beaulieu, J.A. (1989). Nursing diagnoses co-occurring in adults with insulin-dependent diabetes mellitus. In R.M. Carroll-Johnson (Ed.), *Classification of nursing diagnoses: Proceedings of the eighth conference, North American Nursing Diagnosis Association* (pp. 199-205). Philadelphia: Lippincott.

Beyerman, K. (1987). Etiologies of sleep pattern disturbance in hospitalized patients. In A.M. McLane (Ed.), *Classification of nursing diagnoses: Proceedings of the seventh conference, North American Nursing Diagnosis Association* (pp. 193-198). St. Louis: Mosby.

Campbell, J.C. (1986). Nursing assessment for risk of homicide with battered women. *Advances in Nursing Science, 8*(4), 36-51.

Chang, B., Hirsch, M., Brazal-Villanueva, E., & Iverson, D.W.R. (1990). Self-care deficit with etiologies: Reliability of measurement. *Nursing Diagnosis, 1*, 31-36.

Chung, L. (1997). The clinical validation of defining characteristics and related factors of fatigue in hemodialysis patients. In M.J. Rantz & P. LeMone (Eds.), *Classification of nursing diagnoses: Proceedings of the twelfth conference, North American Nursing Diagnosis Association* (pp. 89-96).

Cox, K., & Halfens, R. (1995). Sleep pattern disturbance: A nursing diagnosis. In M. J. Rantz & P. LeMone (Eds.), *Classification of nursing diagnoses: Proceedings of the eleventh conference, North American Nursing Diagnosis Association* (pp. 180-181). Glendale, CA: CINAHL Information Systems.

da Cruz, I.C.F. (1995). Nursing diagnoses: Strategy for formulation and validation. In M.J. Rantz & P. LeMone (Eds.), *Classification of nursing diagnoses: Proceedings of the eleventh conference, North American Nursing Diagnosis*

Association (pp. 238). Glendale, CA: CINAHL Information Systems.

de Arajo Silveira, M.D.F., Coler, M.S., & da Nobrea, M.M.L. (1997). Assessment of the perception of being disrobed in Brazilian ICU patients: Evolution of a nursing diagnosis. In M.J. Rantz & P. LeMone (Eds.), *Classification of nursing diagnoses: Proceedings of the twelfth conference, North American Nursing Diagnosis Association* (pp. 406-410). Glendale, CA: CINAHL Information Systems.

Dougherty, C. M., Jankin, J. K., Lunney, M. L., & Whitley, G. G. (1993). Conceptual and research-based validation of nursing diagnoses: 1950 to 1993. *Nursing Diagnosis, 4,* 156-165.

Downey, T. A. (1995). Illuminating the defining characteristics of the nursing diagnosis of fear: An application to transient-developmental fear in children. In M.J. Rantz & P. LeMone (Eds.), *Classification of nursing diagnoses: Proceedings of the eleventh conference, North American Nursing Diagnosis Association* (pp. 265). Glendale, CA: CINAHL Information Systems.

Fehring, R. J. (1994). The Fehring model. In R.M. Carroll-Johnson & M. Paquette (Eds.), *Classification of nursing diagnoses: Proceedings of the tenth conference, North American Nursing Diagnosis Association* (pp. 55-62). Philadelphia: Lippincott.

Fowler, S. B. (1997). Impaired verbal communication during short-term oral intubation. *Nursing Diagnosis, 8,* 93-98.

Gaffney, J., & Zirker, W. S. (1994). Empirical validation of urge incontinence in a sample of elderly women. In R.M. Carroll-Johnson (Ed.), *Classification of nursing diagnoses:*

Proceedings of the tenth conference, North American Nursing Diagnosis Association (pp. 186-187). Philadelphia: Lippincott.

Gould, M. T. (1983). Nursing diagnoses concurrent with multiple sclerosis. *Journal of Neurosurgical Nursing, 15,* 339-345.

Hayes, K. V. (1994). *Diagnostic content validation and operational definitions of risk factors for the nursing diagnosis high risk for disuse syndrome,* The Catholic University of America [Order No. 95117721]. Ann Arbor, MI: University Microfilms.

Holmes, H., Covington, K., Evans, T., Smith, N., Kennedy, B., & Williams, C. (1995). Correlates of nursing diagnoses among seriously ill psychiatric patients. In M.J. Rantz & P. LeMone (Eds.), *Classification of nursing diagnoses: Proceedings of the eleventh conference, North American Nursing Diagnosis Association* (pp. 270-271). Glendale, CA: CINAHL Information Systems.

Hoskins, L.M., McFarlane, E.A., Rubenfeld, M.G., Walsh, M.B., & Schreier, A.M. (1986). Nursing diagnosis in the chronically ill: Methodology for clinical validation. *Advances in Nursing Science, 8*(3), 80-89.

Kim, M.J. (1991). Integrated methods for nursing diagnosis research. In R. M. Carroll-Johnson (Ed.), *Classification of nursing diagnoses: Proceedings of the ninth conference, North American Nursing Diagnosis Association* (pp. 201-206). Philadelphia: Lippincott.

Kubsch, S.M., & Wichowski, H.C. (1992). Identification and validation of a new nursing diagnosis: Sick role conflict. *Nursing Diagnosis, 4,* 141-147.

Maas, M.L., Hardy, M.A., & Craft, M. (1990).

Some methodologic considerations in nursing diagnosis research. *Nursing Diagnosis, 1,* 24-30.

Magnan, M.A. (1995). A Bayesian methodological approach to validation of a nursing diagnosis: Activity intolerance. In M. J. Rantz & P. LeMone (Eds.), *Classification of nursing diagnoses: Proceedings of the eleventh conference, North American Nursing Diagnosis Association* (pp. 97-111). Glendale, CA: CINAHL Information Systems.

McLane, A.M., & McShane, R.E. (1986). Empirical validation of defining characteristics of constipation: A study of bowel elimination practices of healthy adults. In M.E. Hurley (Ed.), *Classification of nursing diagnoses: Proceedings of the sixth conference, North American Nursing Diagnosis Association* (pp. 448-455). St. Louis: Mosby.

McLane, A.M., McShane, R.E., & Sleifert, M. (1984). Constipation: Conceptual categories of diagnostic indicators. In M.J. Kim, G.K. McFarland, & A.M. McLane (Eds.), *Classification of nursing diagnoses: Proceedings of the fifth national conference* (pp. 174-179). St. Louis: Mosby.

Mullins, D.L. (1994). Powerlessness: Concept analysis and validation of the defining characteristics. In R.M. Carroll-Johnson & M. Paquette (Eds.), *Classification of nursing diagnoses: Proceedings of the tenth conference, North American Nursing Diagnosis Association* (pp. 208-210). Philadelphia: Lippincott.

Norris, J., & Kunes-Connell, M. (1985). Self-esteem disturbance. *Nursing Clinics of North America, 20,* 745-761.

Norris, J., & Kunes-Connell, M. (1987). Self-esteem disturbance: A clinical validation study. In A.M. McLane (Ed.), *Classification of nursing diagnoses: Proceedings of the seventh conference, North American Nursing Diagnosis Association* (pp. 121-128). St. Louis: Mosby.

Norris, J., & Kunes-Connell, M. (1989). Nursing diagnoses: Chronic low self esteem, situational low self esteem, defensive coping. In R.M. Carroll-Johnson (Ed.), *Classification of nursing diagnoses: Proceedings of the eighth conference, North American Nursing Diagnosis Association* (pp. 437-442). Philadelphia: Lippincott.

Richmond, T.S., Metcalf, J., Daly, M., & Kish, J.R. (1992). Powerlessness in acute spinal cord injury patients: A descriptive study. *Journal of Neuroscience Nursing, 24,* 146-152.

Rossi, L., Fitzmaurice, J.B., Glynn, M.A., & Connors, K. (1987). Validation of the defining characteristics for sleep pattern disturbance. In A.M. Lane (Ed.), *Classification of nursing diagnoses: Proceedings of the seventh conference, North American Nursing Diagnosis Association* (pp. 279). St. Louis: Mosby.

Savitz, J., & Friedman, M.I. (1981). Diagnosing boredom and confusion. *Nursing Research, 30,* 16-20.

Schroeder, M.A. (1991). Quantitative methods for nursing diagnosis research. In R.M. Carroll-Johnson (Ed.), *Classification of nursing diagnoses: Proceedings of the ninth conference, North American Nursing Diagnosis Association* (pp. 192-200). Philadelphia: Lippincott.

Shaw, R.J. (1987). Powerlessness in a nursing home population. In A.M. McLane (Ed.), *Classification of nursing diagnoses:*

Proceedings of the seventh conference, North American Nursing Diagnosis Association (pp. 189-192). St. Louis: Mosby.

Sidani, S., & Woodtli, M.A. (1994). Testing and validation of an instrument to assess the defining characteristics of stress and urge incontinence. In R.M. Carroll-Johnson & M. Paquette (Eds.), *Classification of nursing diagnoses: Proceedings of the tenth conference, North American Nursing Diagnosis Association* (pp. 179-181). Philadelphia: Lippincott.

Smucker, C. (1995). A phenomenological description of the experience of spiritual distress. In M.J. Rantz & P. LeMone (Eds.), *Classification of nursing diagnoses: Proceedings of the eleventh conference, North American Nursing Diagnosis Association* (pp. 136-149). Glendale, CA: CINAHL Information Systems.

Swelha, M. A. (1988). Nursing diagnosis as a standard: Methodology for identifying and validating diagnoses in an ambulatory care setting. *Nursing Administration Quarterly, 12*(2), 16-23.

Tiesinga, L.J., Dassen, T.W.N., & Halfens, R.J.G. (1997). Validation of the nursing diagnosis fatigue among patients with chronic heart failure. In M.J. Rantz & P. LeMone (Eds.), *Classification of nursing diagnoses: Proceedings of the twelfth conference, North American Nursing*

Diagnosis Association (pp. 263-267). Glendale, CA: CINAHL Information Systems.

Triboti, S., Lyons, N., Blackburn, S., Stein, M., & Withers, J. (1988). Nursing diagnoses for the postpartum woman. *Journal of Obstetrical, Gynecological, and Neonatal Nursing, 17,* 410-416.

Whitley, G. G., & Tousman, S. A. (1996). A multivariate approach for validation of anxiety and fear. *Nursing Diagnosis, 7,* 116-124.

Whitley, G.G. (1997). A comparison of two methods of clinical validation of nursing diagnosis. In M.J. Rantz & P. LeMone (Eds.), *Classification of nursing diagnoses: Proceedings of the twelfth conference, North American Nursing Diagnosis Association* (pp. 103-110). Glendale, CA: CINAHL Information Systems.

Woodtli, A. (1995). Mixed incontinence: A new nursing diagnosis. *Nursing Diagnosis, 6,* 135-142.

Woodtli, M.A., & Yocum, K. (1994). Urge incontinence: Identification and clinical validation of defining characteristics. In R.M. Carroll-Johnson & M. Paquette (Eds.), *Classification of nursing diagnoses: Proceedings of the tenth conference, North American Nursing Diagnosis Association* (pp. 182-185). Philadelphia: Lippincott.

An Evaluation of the Impact of Nursing Diagnosis at Chelsea & Westminster Hospital, London, UK (abstract)

Dickon Weir-Hughes, MA, RN

Chelsea & Westminster Hospital, London, is the only hospital in the UK with a formal research-funded program for the implementation of nursing diagnosis, specifically the NANDA taxonomy. As a result the project has had a high profile. The challenges of implementing nursing diagnosis in the UK have been explored by a number of authors, including Weir-Hughes (1996) and Lister (1997). The implementation program, which is linked to the development of an electronic patient record, is on target to be completed in 1998.

The purpose of this paper is to describe the impact of nursing diagnosis at Chelsea & Westminster Hospital, using a case study approach. The paper builds on previously presented work which described the implementation strategy and the pilot project. Ways in which nursing diagnosis has helped nurses to care for patents more effectively and to promote and communicate the caring role of nursing in an increasingly technical world are discussed. The benefits of nursing diagnosis in role clarification and the positively changes perceptions of nurses and physicians are explored. The views of service users are also discussed. The implementation of nursing diagnosis has prompted a number of very positive interrelated developments, such as the introduction of an assessment tool based on Gordon's Functional Health Patterns. The rationale for such developments are explored. The benefits of using the NANDA taxonomy and networking with NANDA members are highlighted. In response to the positive globalism of nursing ways in which a UK hospital could contribute to the development of nursing diagnosis internationally are suggested and explored. In summary, this paper outlines the impact of an exciting process of organizational development which we would like to share and celebrate with colleagues.

Nursing Diagnoses and Defining Characteristics at 24 and 72 hours Post-Surgery with General Anesthesia: Preliminary Results

Dorothy A. Jones, EdD, RNC, FAAN
Jane Flanagan, RNC, MSN
Amanda Coakley, RNC, PhD(c)

The refinement of surgical interventions, increased consumer demands for quality care and health care restructuring have continued to expand outpatient surgeries on a daily basis. From 1991-1992, ambulatory surgery increased 4.1% while inpatient surgery decreased 2.9% (OR Manager, March 1992). Reforms in health care delivery continue to decrease hospital stays in an effort to reduce health care costs. Within this climate of change, the professional nurse continues to be the core person responsible for the comprehensive management and monitoring of patients' responses to the surgical experience.

Within the current environment of change in North America, individuals having surgery in ambulatory care settings are discharged to home several hours after surgery. Despite this emerging trend, there has been little research conducted to study patients' response to the experience. Additionally, with the rapid increase in the number and complexity of same day surgeries, concern has been raised as to the relevance of data found in earlier studies to adequately describe the current experience (Hackbarth, Haas, Kavanaugh & Vlasses, 1995).

Purpose of the Study
The American Organization of Operating Room Nurses (AORN) support the belief that "comprehensive care should be provided for all patients during the surgical experience" (Abbott & Rodriquez, 1989, p. 338). However, describing how this occurs, particularly with discharge on the same day as the surgery, requires further study (Leske, 1993). Findings from a previous investigation (Jones, Coakley, Dauphinee & Fernsebner, 1996), studying responses of six women having same day surgery for breast biopsies with local anesthesia reported patients had many concerns, questions and reactions to the same day surgical (SDS) experience following hospital discharge. This work promoted the important role nurses play in positively affecting the care outcome related to comfort management and patient satisfaction during the experience.

The preliminary findings of this study and

Table 1

Operational Definitions Study Variables

Perioperative experience – defined by the Association of Operating Room Nurses as "the commencing with the decision for surgical intervention and ending with a follow-up home/clinic evaluation. This period includes the preoperative, intraoperative and post operative phase." (AORN, 1995, p. 1:3-1)

Same day surgery – defined as the same day surgery where the entire perioperative experience occurs on an outpatient basis and within a period of less than 24 hours.

General Anesthesia – refers only to admission of a general anesthetic by a licensed anesthesiologist that results in an unconscious state.

Postoperative follow-up – refers to the period of 24 and 72 hours following discharge from the hospital as measured by The 24 and 72 Hour Post Operative and Follow-Up Telephone Interview Schedule. Patients responses (diagnoses) were recorded on appropriate forms.

Nursing Diagnosis – is a category name within a classification system of the North American Nursing Diagnosis Association derived form clinical judgement.

Defining Characteristics – is defined as information which influences the decision (Gordon, 1994).

the literature support the need to investigate the effect of SDS experiences with general anesthesia and care outcomes in the home environment (Kleinbeck & Hofford, 1994; Thatcher, 1996; Payne, 1995). The purpose of this investigation was to generate tentative nursing diagnoses with patients having SDS and general anesthesia at 24 and 72 hours postoperatively, using qualitative analysis.

Research Question

The overall research question for this study asked "What are the tentative, nursing diagnoses and defining characteristics at 24 and 72 hours after surgery for patients having same day surgery with general anesthesia?"

Identification of Variables

Within the context of this investigation, the terms perioperative experience, same day surgery, general anesthesia, nursing diagnoses, defining characteristics and postoperative follow up are defined. Table 1 presents these variables and operational definitions.

Literature Review

According to Rothrock (1990), there is a need for nursing to identify and document patient outcomes so the professional role of nurses within the perioperative experience can be clarified. Jones, Coakley, Dauphinee and Fernsebner (1996) found patients identified nursing knowledge, presense and touch as highly valuable factors throughout the perioperative experience.

Anxiety is a common response often associated with unfamiliar experiences. Research suggests (Levitt, 1980, Spielberger, 1972; Jones, 1986) when there is increased uncertainty, anxiety may intensify, especially when personal adequacy is being evaluated (e.g., testing situations). Jones, Coakley, Dauphinee and Fernsebner (1996) found preoperative stress on the day of surgery was significantly higher than postoperative stress in patients having SDS for breast biopsy. When these patients did not have an opportunity to find out the physician's initial impressions post-operatively, their stress increased. While high stress was reported in women scheduled for breast biopsy, other studies have suggested that the more information the patient has about the surgical experience, the less stressful the experience (Bader, 1988; Deriarain, 1990; Fitzmaurice, 1992).

The use of telephone follow-up calls has been described as an effective way to evaluate patients in the home. Worth and Tierney (1993) described the cost and time savings attributed to follow-up calls with the elderly after discharge. The researchers cited hearing impairments, difficulty with recall, and need for detail and advise on multiple issues, as difficulties in using the telephone interview particularly with this population. Oberle, Allen and Lynkowski (1994) reported follow-up phone calls for patients having SDS with selected health problems were helpful in identifying difficulty with pain management and unexpected fatigue. A limitation in telephone interviewing is inconsistency in communication skills of the interviewer, resulting in potential discrepancies about information obtained (Studdiford, Panitch, Synderman, & Pharr, 1996). Kleinbeck and Hafford (1994) used telephone interviews on second day postlaparoscopic cholecystectomy to uncover stories about patients recovery experiences. The University of North Carolina (UNC) at Chapel Hill (Same Day Surgery, March, 1995) found 71% of SDS patients suffered significant and unnecessary pain at home. Roberts, Peterson, Friesen and Beckette (1995) found that patients who had "open" surgery were often in significant pain up to 3 days post-operatively.

The literature supports the reality that surgery can be a stressful and painful event for patients. Stress is heightened by discomfort and uncertainty. Surgery can also affect self-care home and use of telephone calls may help to quickly address patient problems at home and reduce stress. While research studies have investigated function and the use of post-operative phone calls with patients after surgery, there has been limited research with the SDS population and nursing diagnoses.

Conceptual Framework

Nursing's interactions with clients seeking health care is central to empowering individuals and enhancing quality care. The transaction between the nurse and the client is unique and is focused on the meaning of the human experience for each individual. The caring presence of the nurse facilitates this identification of the person's response to an experience can enable the nurse to uncover knowledge embedded within clinical practice (BEnner, 1984) and enhance health care for all persons. The active involvement of the nurse with persons anticipating SDS with general anesthesia is critical to the entire perioperative experience. Through the careful assessment of each client, the nurse comes to know the person's unique response to surgery and generate clinical judgements (Gordon, 1994) that reflect the personhood of the individual. This can provide opportunities for the development of new knowledge and enable the nurse to empower patients and improve care outcomes.

Methodology

In order to answer the research question as stated, content analysis was used on data obtained from 95 telephone interviews at 24 and 72 hours post-operatively. The current study is part of a larger investigation which used a descriptive correctional methodology to study a number of variables and the same day surgery experience.

Table 2

Questions Asked at 24 Hours Post-Op

At 24 hours the patients were called by the nurse who met with the patient preoperatively and asked a series of questions. They included:

1. How have you been since your surgery?
2. Have you found that you need help since you have been at home?
3. Has there been someone with you since you have been home?
4. Did you have any questions after you got home?

Table 3

Questions Asked at 72 Hours Post-Op

At 72 hours patients were called by the clinical specialists on the research team and asked a series of questions, data were recorded. Questions included:

1. In general, how did you find the surgical experience?
2. Overall, how have you managed since you have been home?
3. How closely did your actual experience in day surgery match your expectations of how things would go?
4. Have you found it necessary to call anyone for help since your surgery?
5. How adequately were you prepared for the same day surgical experience?

Sample and Setting

Admission into the study included achievement of the following criteria: a) males or females over 18 and receiving general anesthesia for SDS such as hernia repairs, laporoscopy and arthroscopy; b) able to read, write and comprehend English; c) willing to participate in all aspects of the study as outlined in letter to the participant.

Ninety-five patients who had outpatient surgery under general anesthesia were recruited into the study sample. Ninety-five complete cases were included in the analysis. Ages of the participants ranged between 20 and 70 years.

The sample was obtained from an ambulatory Same Day Surgical Unit (SDSU) at a large medical center in the northeastern part of the United States. Patients coming to the setting predominantly lived within the state where the data were collected.

Instrumentation

Data to answer this research question were obtained using The 24 Hour/72 Hour Post Operative Interview Schedule. The tool contains a series of open ended questions asked of participants during the 24 and 72 hour postoperative phone calls. The questions included in the study were reviewed by a panel of experts (master's and doctorally prepared perioperative nurses) for content, clarity, accuracy and appropriateness. There was 100% consensus approval for all questions asked. In addition, a demographic information sheet was used to record age, gender and surgical procedure. Sample questions from the 24 and 72 hour interview schedule are included in Table 2 and 3.

Procedure

Data for this investigation were collected at 24 and 72 hours postoperatively. On the day of surgery, the nurse who initially met the patient in pre-admission attempted to meet with each patient in the SDSU. The nurse was also available to answer any questions, identify and document any problems and review surgical day experience. All information was recorded and included in a data collection envelope assigned to each patient with an individual code. This code number appeared on all of the study documents to protect patient anonymity.

Following the surgery, the preoperative nurse met with patients in the postoperative suite just prior to discharge. The patient was told that a nurse would be calling 24 and 72 hours after surgery to evaluate their health status and to ask questions to determine how they were managing at home. The nurse verified with the patient the phone number where they would be called post-operatively. A nurse then phoned the patient at 24 and 72 hours and recorded patient answers to the questions. All of the patient responses were recorded on appropriate data collection sheets.

Data Analysis

Descriptive responses from each patient at 24 and 72 hours were analyzed using content analysis. All responses to questions were reviewed by the investigators. Data and defining characteristics were then classified into the diagnoses from North American Nursing Diagnosis Association (NANDA) language. Tentative hypotheses (nursing diagnosis) were reviewed by an expert panel familiar with the diagnosis for agreement and content placement. There was 100% agreement by the panel.

Results

The research question under investigation asked: "What are the defining characteristics, and tentative nursing diagnoses at 24 and 72 hours after surgery for patients having selected same day surgery with general anesthesia?" A total of 95 cases were analyzed to arrive at findings.

Nursing Diagnoses

The tentative nursing diagnoses generated from patient data post surgery were identified through content anaysis of the 24 and 72 hour postoperative telephone interview. The top five nursing diagnoses at 24 and 72 hours after surgery are reported in Table 4 and 5 and used qualitative data only.

Self Care Deficit was described by patients as a difficulty performing activities of daily living (e.g., bathing, hygiene, toileting, dressing). Pain was validated by patient report of pain despite analgesic use. Knowledge Deficit was described by patient report as difficulty and confusion with instructions. Impaired Physical Mobility was described by patient report as difficulty maneuvering prescribed equipment, need for assistance with ambulating, and unsteady gait with movement. Sleep pattern disturbance as evidenced by patient report of interrupted sleep due to pain, difficulty falling asleep because of fear of injury to limb while asleep, and complaints of fatigue with increased hours of sleep (e.g., naps) beyond usual pattern.

Impaired physical mobility was described by patient's report of difficulty with ambulating with or without equipment and inability to perform exercises prescribed because of pain or stiffness on movement. Social Isolation was noted because patient lived alone and had no assistance or was left alone while the family or significant other worked. Pain was described verbally by patients as continued breakthrough pain despite medication use. Knowledge deficit

Table 4

Tentative Nursing Diagnoses and Defining Characteristics at 24 Post Surgery: Preliminary Results

Nursing Diagnoses at 24 Hours	*Defining Characteristics*
Self-Care Deficit (feeding, bathing, hygiene, toileting, dressing)	"Needed help for everything." "Needed help with washing, ambulating, dressing, and/or bathing."
Pain History	"I had difficulty managing pain secondary to substance abuse." "It hurts more than I thought." "I needed pain medication every three hours."
Knowledge Deficit	"I was confused by my instructions." "I did not see doctors and I thought I would – to hear what he found." "I was confused by what the doctor told me. I was so groggy when I saw him."
Impaired Physical Mobility	"I felt unsteady with crutches and/or brace." "I was much less mobile than expected." "I needed crutches." (unexpected) "I was unclear about the use of the crutches."
Sleep Pattern Disturbance (interrupted sleep, sleep onset difficulty)	"I woke up with pain." "My sleep was interrupted." "I cannot stay awake."

was described as confusion over instruction or believing the experience was minimized by physicians. Fatigue was described by patient report of irregular sleep or need for more sleep than usual.

Discussion

The preliminary results of this investigation indicated significant changes in patient life style and roles following SDS with general anesthesia.

The findings presented were evidenced by verbal dialogue with the patients and nurses during the 24 and 72 hours telephone follow up calls. Most (over 90%) of the patients reported calling physicians and emergency rooms for questions about postoperative care such as request for "stronger" pain medications. Many patients reported such things as "I am feeling exhausted" or "I'm supposed to exercise and I can't even get out of bed." There was an overall sense of lack of

Table 5

Tentative Nursing Diagnoses and Defining Characteristics at 72 Hours Post Surgery: Preliminary Results

Nursing Diagnoses	*Defining Characteristics*
Impaired Physical Mobility	"I had a hard time getting around." "I needed crutches."
Social Isolation	"I needed much more help than I thought." "I have children to care for and I was not going to be able to do so." "I had nothing to eat when I got home." "I did not have enough help."
Pain	"I continued to have pain beyond what I thought." "I am very uncomfortable."
Knowledge Deficit	"The whole experience was minimized." "There is a lack of closure on the discharge." "There's more to this than you've told." "I expected to feel better by now." "I feel terrified, nervous, like a burden." (Described unexpected feelings) "I feel uncertainty about the whole thing."
Fatigue	"I feel tired." "I haven't slept well." "I'm too exhausted to do exercise."

energy and a lack of "feeling like themselves" after surgery. In some instances patients reported being told "you should be back to work in a few days." However, at the 72 hour post-surgical period, many still felt unready to return to work.

For the elderly and those living alone, pain compromised the ability to eat, care for themselves (e.g., washing and toileting), or caring for the household. Regardless of age or gender, pain, fatigue, and sleep pattern disturbances and compromised self care were major problems following day surgery. These problems became more complex when the person had lack of support or care-taking in the home.

The nursing diagnoses generated at 24 and 72 hours post-surgery were obtained from descriptive/qualitative data and add a new dimension to the study of post-operative care. Results from this investigation not only documented and supported the potential for specific nursing diagnosis following same day surgery but also described the defining data that can help validate the phenomena observed. The findings are similar to other investigations studying adult orthopedic patients (Shappler, Fitzmaurice, Michaud, 1994). The data also supports the earlier discussion concerning nursing diagnoses such as pain management and responses related to sleep, activity and mobility, nutrition and self care management in this population (Kleinbeck & Hoffart, 1994).

Limitations of Study

The following limitations have been identified for this invetigation. They are: 1) the use of a convenience sample limited the ability to generalize findings; 2) the small sample size could affect the significance of findings; 3) differences in data collectors may have resuulted in influenc ed findings during the 24 and 72 hour telephone interviews; 4) data were generated from telephone inteview only and did not include quantitative data.

Conclusions and Recommendations

The preliminary results from this investigation suggest patients having same day surgery have a difficult postoperative course for at least the first 72 hours after surgery. Tentative nursing diagnoses included pain, impaired mobility, interrupted sleep and inability to fully care for themselves after surgery. Elderly patients experienced a difficult recovery at home and often stated "I wish I could have stayed at the hospital just one more night."

People who were either young or elderly and lived alone described a difficult recovery post-operatively. Both groups described the need for assistance and were unable to recruit the needed help on short notice. Within middle age adults there was a sense of being prepared because of a previous experience with the same surgery or because they were living with someone they were able to recruit the help needed.

Generally, people when initially aked about their experience responsed positively, stating: "It was a good experience." It was not until further probing that the researchers were able to unravel discontented feelings about the experience. These findings are similar to other satisfaction studies: e.g., in the 1996 Picker Commonwealth survey of over 23,000 who said care "in general was okay." It was not until probing that problems surfaced.

These results suggest the need for nurses to probe the availability of assistance post-operatively, fully inform patients of potential limitations postoperatively, and when calling probe to illicit precise feelings about the experience. The preliminary findings of this investigation require further replication and continued investigation with patients having other surgical procedures. Data from this study indicate patients do experience significant suffering and compromised function following same day surgery. In addition, it appears that when patients are elderly or live alone they need assistance from resources such as friends, home health aides or nurses. Increased preoperative teaching is needed with an emphasis on the use of relaxation techniques before surgery.

Better pain management is essential for patients during recovery at home. Ineffective pain management may be due to drug choice, or patients taking inadequate amounts of a medication because of fear of "taking to much." This should be reassessed early in the post-operative recovery period. It is apparent from this investigation that the same day surgical experience with general anesthesia is stressful for the individual.

It is equally apparent that the nurse can dramatically affect the pre- as well as the post-operative phases of same day surgery and influence the recovery trajectory of the patient in the home.

References

Abbott, C., & Rodriquez, W. (1989). Delegating intraoperative activities. *AORN, 50*(3), 338.

American Hospital Study (1996). *Patient satisfaction – Picker Commonwealth Survey.*

Association of Operating Room Nurses (1992). *Standards and recommended practice for perioperative nursing.* Denver: AORN, Inc.

Bader, M. (1988). Nursing care behaviors that predict patient satisfaction. *Journal of Nursing Quality Assurance, 2*(3), 11-17.

Benner, P. (1984). *From novice to expert: Excellence and power in clinical nursing practice.* Menlo Park, California: Addison-Wesley.

Derdiarian, A. (1990). Effects of using systematic assessment instruments on patients and nurses satisfaction with nursing care. *Oncology Nursing Forum, 17*, 95-100.

Fitzmaurice, J. (1992). *Evaluation of same day surgery program report* (Unpublished manuscript) Massachusetts General Hospital, QRD. Boston, MA.

Fitzmaurice, J.B. (1987). Nurses uses of cues in the clinical judgement of activity tolerance. In A.M. McLane (Ed.), *Classification of nursing diagnoses: Proceeding of the seventh conference.* (pp. 315-323). St., Louis: Mosby.

Gordon, M. (1987). Issues in nursing diagnoses. In A.M. McLane (Ed.), *Classification of nursing diagnoses: Proceeding of the seventh conference.* (pp. 282-289). St. Louis: Mosby.

Gordon, M. (1994). *Nursing diagnosis: Process and application.* St. Louis: Mosby.

Gordon, M., & Hiltunen, E. (1995). High frequency: treatment priority nursing diagnoses in critical care. *Nursing Diagnoses, 6*(4), 143-154.

Hackbarth, D., Haas, S., Kavanaugh, J., & Vlasses, F. (1995). Dimensions of the staff nurse role in ambulatory care: Part I – methodology and analysis of data on current staff nurse practice. *Nursing Economics, 13*(2), 89-98.

Jones, D. (1986). *The effects of an interactive information mapped textbook on mastery learning of physical examination and state anxiety of undergraduate student nursing student.* Dissertation: University Microfilms International, Ann Arbor, MI.

Jones, D., Coakley, A., Dauphinee, J., & Fernsebner, W. (1996). Patient response to same day surgery with local anesthesia. Final Grant Report, *AORN.*

Kleinbeck, S., & Hoffart, N. (1994). Outpatient recovery after laparoscopic cholecystectomy. *AORN, 60*(3), 396-402.

Leske, J.B. (1993). Anxiety of elective surgical patient's family members, *AORN, 57*(5), 1091-1093.

Levitt, E. (1980). *The psychology of anxiety.* Hillsdale, N.J.: Lawrence Earlbaum, Inc.

Lewis, S.M., & Collier, J.C. (1983). *Medical surgical nursing. Assessment and management of clinical problems.* St. Louis: McGraw-Hill Book Co.

Minton, J., & Creason, N. (1991). Evaluation of admission nursing diagnoses. *Nursing Diagnoses, 2*(3), 119-125.

Oberle, K., Allen, M., & Lynkowski, P. (1994). Follow-up of same day surgery patients: A study of patients concerns. *AORN, 59*(5), 1016-1025.

OR Manager Monthly Newsletter, (1992). 8(6), 8.

Payne, F. (1995). Same day surgery patients feel too much pain. Same Day Surgery, 19(7), 33-36.

Pfister, J. (1979). Suvey finds role being practiced. AORN, 30, 875.

Roberts, B., Peterson, G., Friesen, W., & Beckette, W. (1995). An investigation of pain experience and management following gynecology day surgery: Differences between open and closed surgery. Journal of Pain Symptom Management, 10(5), 370-377.

Rothrock, J.C. (1990). Perioperative nursing care planning. St. Louis, MO.

Shappler, N., Fitzmaurice, J., & Michaud, J. (1994). High frequency diagnoses in adult orthopedic patients. In R.M. Carroll-Johnson and M. Paquettel, (Eds.), Classification of Nursing Diagnoses. Philadelphia: J.B. Lippincott. pp. 255-256.

Spielberger, C. (1972). Anxiety: Current trends and in theory and research. New York: Academic.

Staddiford, J., Pavitch, K., Snyderman, D., & Pharr, M. (1996). The telephone in primary care. Primary Care, 23(1), 83-98.

Thatcher, B. (1996). Follow-up after surgery: How well do patients cope? Nursing Times, 11(92), 30-32.

Ware, J., Davies-Avery, A., & Stewart, A. (1978). The measurement and meaning of patient satisfaction. Health and Medical Care Services Review, 1, 2-15.

Worth, A., & Tierney, A. (1993). Conducting research interview with elderly people by telephone. Journal of Advanced Nursing, 18, 1077-1084.

Nursing Diagnoses in the Neonatal ICU (abstract)

Maria Helena Baena de Moraes Lopes

The aim of this paper was to survey the most frequent nursing diagnoses by means of a nursing history and medical procedure to help the assistance at the Oncology Nursing Service of women Health Whole Care (Centro de Atencao Integral a Saude de Mulher - CAISM). The five most common diagnoses were: risk for infection, risk for altered body temperature, risk for aspiration and colonic constipation of exchanging pattern, and risk for activity intolerance of moving pattern. Data collection was better geared to these patterns, data predominantly involving social, cultural, psychological and spiritual aspects were hardly interpreted, because they were poorly registered or omitted.

Secondary Data Analysis of Nursing Diagnoses in Post-Hospital Experiences of Ambulatory Surgical Patients

Jean A. O'Neil, EdD, RNC
Nancy J. Fairchild, MS, CAES, RN

Introduction

In 1961, the Butterworth Hospital in Grand Rapids, Michigan opened what is believed to be the country's first established ambulatory surgery program (Defazio-Quinn, 1997). Since then, ambulatory surgery has continued to increase. According to the American Hospital Association, approximately 16% of all surgeries performed in 1980 were performed on an outpatient basis. In contrast, 1993 reports revealed 53.8% of surgeries to be performed in the outpatient setting. Predictions for the year 2000 estimate that from 70% to 80% of all elective surgical procedures in the United States will be performed on an ambulatory surgical basis (Brockway, 1997). Successful surgical outcomes related to refined surgical techniques and advances in anesthesia are well documented.

Prior to this transition to ambulatory surgery, nurses had conducted research regarding the entire perioperative experience of the hospitalized patient. Since the transition, the professional nurse continues to be responsible for comprehensive management and monitoring of patients' response to the surgical experience. The nurse is concerned not only with the immediate perioperative care but also with the patient's post-discharge recovery. Now, the short-term surgical stay of the ambulatory surgical patient brings the nurse into a discharge planning obligation that follows only a brief interaction with the patient. Post-discharge recovery was less studied by the hospital unit-based nurse (Baker, 1989). The ambulatory surgery patient needs and may demand more information in the current health information media environment. Additionally, the nurse often needs to guide a family member who is replacing the nurse as the primary postoperative caregiver.

One method nurses used to address post-discharge needs of ambulatory surgery patients was the follow-up phone call. Some articles in the nursing literature discussed the timing of these calls. Several authors reported a telephone call on the day following surgery for purposes of assessing the patient's status and answering questions (Allen & Oberle, 1993; Dougherty, 1996; Kleinbeck & Hoffart, 1994). For the same reasons, two studies (Neal, 1996; Thatcher, 1996) described home visits on the day following surgery. A longer time frame ranging from 24 to 48 hours post surgery occurred in two additional research investigations (McGrory & Assman, 1994; Law, 1997) that used telephone surveys.

Other articles addressed the findings during post-discharge communication. One study of 72 cataract patients (McGrory & Assmann, 1994) found a good knowledge level overall on follow-up telephone calls while another study (Law, 1997) concluded that patients reported difficulty remembering verbal advice. This implied a need for written leaflets or audiotapes to accompany verbal instructions. A three-month study of 140 patients by Bostrom, Caldwell, McGuire & Everson, 1996 compared post-discharge phone calls with other methods of communication. These patients had been hospitalized for either medical or surgical treatments.

The investigators compared a group who received a phone call at 3-5 days after discharge with a second group who received a brochure describing a nurse-run phone service they could call and a third group who received no instruction about post-discharge contact. The study suggested that patients had educational needs but were unlikely to initiate communication to resolve their needs. Only nine patients called the number offered to them. Likewise, Kleinbeck and Hoffart (1994) inferred reluctance on the part of patients to call physicians or hospital nurses about questions not directly related to the hospital experience. They recommended follow-up calls to patients because of the prevalence of questions elicited during their telephone survey.

A few studies identified specific problems experienced by ambulatory patients. Kleinbeck and Hoffart (1994) described a theme in the recovery processes from ambulatory laparoscopic surgery to be a progression toward a "usual self" with patterns of increased activity and self-management. These authors also found patients requesting clarification of general advice such as "take it easy," yet unwilling to initiate phone calls to health care providers with these questions. Qualitative study of six patients (Thatcher, 1996) identified problems experienced post-discharge by patients to be pain, mobility and body posture, post-anesthesia effects of drowsiness with an intense desire to sleep, impaired cognitive and psychomotor function, and nausea and vomiting. Likewise, home health nurses visiting on the day of discharge and the following day after ambulatory orthopedic surgery for reconstruction of the anterior cruciate ligament found patients had many needs. These included pain control; evaluation of circulation, swelling and sensorimotor changes; use of ice packs; wound care, and progressive mobilization (Neal, 1996).

This recent nursing research encouraged careful analysis of data elicited by phone interview of patients experiencing recovery from ambulatory surgery.

Current Study

The current study proceeded in two steps. Originally, an investigation studied the post-discharge experience of the ambulatory surgery patient during the first twenty-four and the next seventy-two hours. Preliminary survey of the qualitative data (Jones, Flanagan & Coakley, 1996) led to nursing diagnoses. The current study used secondary data analysis to determine whether these nursing diagnoses would be validated.

Purpose

The purposes of this investigation were (1) to validate the nursing diagnoses and the cues that are manifestations of dysfunctional responses to the experience of ambulatory surgery and (2) to test the validation criterion used in nurse expert clinical validation studies.

Method

Doctoral students and nursing faculty expert in the use of diagnostic reasoning obtained the data by conducting home telephone calls at 24 and 72 hours to patients who had ambulatory surgery at a large urban medical center. They used an interview with open-ended questions and a symptom rating scale, the SF-36. Content analysis of the interviews produced cues for possible nursing diagnoses. That study compared content analysis data from the interview with published definitions and defining characteristics of the nursing diagnoses. Examples of the open ended questions used in the interview are: Overall, how have you managed since you have been home? Have you found that you have needed help since you have been at home? If yes: What did you need?

The current study used both interview and SF-36 was developed by Ware and associates and described in a 1978 publication in *Health and Medical Services Review*. This questionnaire has eight scales to measure patient function. The eight scales of the SF-36 questionnaire are Physical Functioning, Role-Physical, Bodily Pain, General Health, Vitality, Social Functioning, Role-Emotional and Mental Health. The scales vary in number of items but each has response categories allowing the subject to rate her or his function from negative to positive. The interviewer asks the person to rate how surgery interfered with each of these aspects of functioning. The following description of physical functioning illustrates the

content and scoring of the SF-36. Example: "The following items are about activities you might do during a typical day. Does your health now limit you in these activities? If so, how much?" Sample activities following this question are lifting or carrying groceries, climbing one flight of stairs, bending, kneeling or stooping, walking one block, bathing or dressing yourself. The scale invites one of three responses: Yes, limited a lot, Yes, limited a little, No, not limited at all.

Secondly, the investigators compared the diagnostic cues from interview and questionnaire with the defining characteristics in Gordon's Manual (Gordon, 1997). Published research results in Gordon's Manual of Nursing Diagnosis served as the criteria for validating the cues that were used to formulate nursing diagnoses. Judgment of diagnostic content validity was derived from consistency of responses to the open-ended interview questions and the SF-36 questionnaire ratings. Finally, the criterion for labeling high frequency cues and diagnoses was adapted from Gordon's nurse expert studies as those cues and diagnoses that were present in 75% of subjects in the sample.

Sample

Data were collected from a convenience sample drawn from patients having an arthroscopic surgical procedure under general anesthesia with discharge on the same day after a brief postoperative observation. The sample included 77 subjects ranging in age from 19-82. Thirty subjects were 50 years or older and 47 subjects were under age 50. The sample included 45 males and 32 females.

Definitions

For this study, the following definitions applied:
- Ambulatory surgery refers to a surgical

procedure performed on a non-hospitalized client under anesthesia, of short duration, with a short period of post-operative observation pre-discharge.

- The term "same day surgery" is often interchanged with the term "ambulatory surgery."
- Arthroscopy involves an arthroscope introduced into the knee joint to debride damaged cartilage or remove loose particles.

Data Analysis

Secondary data analysis yielded four high frequency nursing diagnoses at 72 hours post-surgery. The discussion reports adjusted percentages because data were unobtainable in certai areas from some subjects.

The first validated diagnosis was Acute Pain. The Gordon manual included both verbal report and presence of objective indicators in the definition of this diagnosis. The telephone interview technique for data collection in this study limited data to verbal report. Therefore, one diagnostic cue: Report of severe discomfort (pain), was used to formulate this diagnosis. Fifty-seven of 64 patients or 89% reported severe discomfort when responding to interview questions and the SF-36 bodily pain rating scale at 72 hours post-discharge.

Secondly, cues for dysfunctional mobility led to further examination of both a long standing and a newly proposed nursig diagnosis. The older nursing diagnosis, Impaired Mobility, defined as limitation of independent movement within the environment, could be formulated for 67 of 70 subjects (96%). This diagnosis asks specification of the level of impaired mobility. Eight subjects or 12% of the sample required only the use of equipment or device such as crutches, cane or walker. Nineteen subjects, or 28% of the sample, reported assistance from another person and did not use devices. Finally, 40 subjects or 60% of the sample required the help of both people and equipment.

A newly proposed dysfunctional mobility diagnosis described a specific mobility problem. The diagnosis "Impaired Ambulation," proposed by the Rehabilitation Nurses Association, specifically addresses ambulation as limitation of independent movement within the environment on foot. Forty-nine of 60 subjects, or 82% of the sample, on interview and in two items from the SF-36 scales, gave responses matching listed diagnostic cues for "Impaired Ambulation." These defining characteristics were: inability to climb stairs and inability to walk required distance. Elements of each diagnosis contributed to understanding how the surgical experience interfered with the person's mobility.

The fourth high-frequency nursing diagnosis was Social Isolation, defined as feelings of aloneness attributed to interpersonal interaction below the level desired or required for personal integrity. This diagnosis was formulated for 47 subjects, or 75% of the sample, The quoted statements about being alone or reporting interference with desired social activities matched listed diagnostic cues of verbalization of isolation, absence or limitation of contact with significant other or community. Two separate items on the SF-36 provided additional validation of this diagnosis. The first item asked, "To what extent has your physical health or emotional problems interfered with your normal social activities with family, friends, neighbors or groups?" A five-point scale offered responses ranging from not at all to extremely. The second item was, "How much of the time has your physical health or emotional problems interfered with your social activities (like visiting with friends, relatives, etc.)"? Again, a five-point scale ranged from none of the time to all of the time.

Three other nursing diagnoses were formulated for this sample but did not reach the criterion of 75% response. These were High Risk of Injury, Sleep Pattern Disturbance and Self Care Deficit: Bathing. This finding may be attributed to the convenience nature and size of the sample as limitations of findings as well as limiting generalizability.

Results indicated that Acute Pain and Impaired Physical Mobility from the initially hypothesized diagnoses met the validation criteria of cues manifested by 75% of the subjects. Cues were present for Sleep Pattern Disturbance and Self Care Deficit: Bathing for some subjects at 72 hours post-discharge but did not meet the validation criterion. One additional proposed diagnosis, Impaired Ambulation, meeting the criterion added more specific description of the mobility problem. The fourth high frequency diagnosis emerging from secondary data analysis was Social Isolation, based on interview data plus two items on the SF-36 that validated each other.

Discussion

This study encouraged continued use of secondary data analysis for validation of cues used to formulate a nursing diagnosis. The combination of interview and questionnaire data available at the 72-hour data collection point also aided validation. The more focused and efficient the designation of nursing diagnoses in the ambulatory patient population, the more proficient the nurse can be in meeting the needs of the patient.

The validated findings have clinical nursing implications for perioperative nurses. The report from this sample of high frequency diagnoses with valid cues could help nurses do focused and thorough assessment of areas of concern in ambulatory surgery patients. Likewise, in nursing education, the student would benefit from learning specific nursing diagnosis expected in this population of patients.

Areas for further study, especially in the formulation of definition and defining characteristics for nursing diagnoses, emerged from the data describing mobility problems. The two mobility diagnoses formulated were neither comprehensive nor mutually exclusive. A true description of the patients' problems required elements from each diagnosis.

Finally, the data variability demonstrated the importance of each data collector in using the same framework, probe short answers and document fully. The many reports in the literature of the use of follow-up telephone calls with the ambulatory patient mandates attention to orientation and training of telephone interviews.

References

Allen, M., & Oberle, K. (1993). Follow-up of day-surgery cataract patients. *Journal of Ophthalmic Nursing & Technology, 12*(5), 211-216.

Bostrom, J., Caldwell, J., McGuire, K., & Everson, D. (1996). Telephone follow-up after discharge from the hospital: Does it make a difference? *Applied Nursing Research, 9*(2), 47-52.

Brockway, P.M. (1997), The ambulatory surgical nurse. *Nursing Clinics of North America, 32*(2), 387-394.

Brumfield, V.C., Kee, C.C., & Johnson, J.Y. (1996). Preoperative patient teaching in ambulatory surgery settings. *AORN Journal,*

64(6), 941-952.

Clinch, C.A. (1997). Nurses achieve quality with pre-assessment clinics. *Journal of Clinical Nursing, 6,* 147-151.

DeFazio-Quinn, D. (1997). Ambulatory surgery: An evolution. *Nursing Clinics of North America, 32*(2), 377-386.

Dougherty, J. (1996). Same-day surgery: The nurse's role. *Orthopaedic Essentials, 15*(4), 15-18.

Gordon, M. (1997). *Manual of nursing diagnosis 1997-98,* St. Louis: Mosby-Yearbook, Inc.

Kleinbeck, S.V., & Hoffart, N. (1994). Outpatient recovery after laparoscopic cholecystectomy. *AORN Journal, 60*(3), 394-402.

Law, M. (1997). A telephone survey of day-surgery eye patients. *Journal of Advanced Nursing, 25,* 355-363.

Marley, R.A. (1996). Postoperative nausea and vomiting: The outpatient enigma. *Journal of PeriAnesthesia Nursing, 11*(3), 147-157.

McGrory, A., & Assmann, S. (1994). A study investigating primary nursing, discharge teaching, and patient satisfaction of ambulatory cataract patients. *The Journal of the American Society of Ophthalmic Registered Nurses, Inc., 19*(2), 8-13.

Neal, L.J. (1996). Outpatient ACL surgery: The role of the home health nurse. *Orthopaedic Nursing, 15*(4), 9-13.

Same-day hysterectomy beneficial for sompe patients. (1995). *OR Manager, 11*(7/8), 39-41.

Thatcher, J. (1996). Follow-up after day surgery: How well do patients cope? *Nursing Times, 92*(37), 30-32.

Implementation of Standardized Nursing Language Into Practice

Leann M. Scroggins, MS, RN, CRRN

This paper will present the process used at Mayo Medical Center to develop and implement patient care guidelines using standardized nursing language. The patient care guidelines discussed are designed for use in the inpatient setting and are available to registered nurses across Mayo Foundation regional practices.

Framework for Development

"Guidelines describe a process of client care management which has the potential of improving the quality of clinical and consumer decision making. Guidelines are systematically developed statements based on available scientific evidence and expert opinion." (ANA, 1991). They support standards of clinical nursing practice by defining specifically recommendations for care.

Patient care guidelines serve several purposes. They include assessment, nursing diagnoses, planning, interventions, evaluation, and outcomes. Patient care guidelines provide a reference for clinical nursing action and recommend the course of nursing action. They standardize nursing practice and convert science-based and expert knowledge into clinical nursing actions. In addition, patient care guidelines provide nursing information for integration into clinical pathways.

A patient care guideline committee was formed to oversee the development, implementation, and maintenance of patient care guidelines. The functions of the committee are to:

- establish and utilize a system for reviewing, developing, and revising patient care guidelines.
- assure the guidelines are reflective and supportive of the Department of Nursing Standards.
- approve patient care guidelines for internal use and distribution.
- coordinate a system of identifying patient care guidelines.
- establish and utilize a system of support to assure distribution of patient care guidelines and staff

awareness of such documents.

Membership on the committee includes registered nurses from all clinical specialties. These specialties include ambulatory care, cardiovascular, critical care, emergency/trauma, hematology/oncology, medical, neuroscience, orthopedic, pediatric, perinatal, perioperative, psychiatric, rehabilitation, and surgical.

Development Process

The development process began with selecting the most commonly used diagnoses across all clinical specialties. Initially, 40 diagnostic labels were identified for guideline development. Currently, 101 diagnoses have been developed into guidelines. Having identified diagnoses for guideline development, a format was developed to assure consistency of information on each guideline. Essential components of each guideline are the nursing diagnosis label, definition, defining characteristics, and related factors according to North American Nursing Diagnosis Association (NANDA, 1996); nursing intervention labels, definitions, and activities from the Nursing Intervention Classification (NIC) (McCloskey & Bulechek, 1996); and nursing outcome labels, definitions, and indicators from the Nursing Outcomes Classification (NOC) (Johnson & Maas, 1997). Permission for use of NANDA, NIC and NOC was obtained from the publishers prior to guideline development. Clinical resources, references, indexing terms, author names, and user panel members are also included in each guideline.

Principles which guided the development of guidelines include:

- maintaining consistency with NANDA for the nursing diagnosis label, definition, defining characteristics, and related factors.

- maintaining consistency with NIC for the intervention label, and definition. The activities are also consistent with NIC but may be adapted to reflect the inpatient practice at Mayo Medical Center.

- maintaining consistency with NOC for the outcome label and definition. The indicators may be adapted to reflect the inpatient practice at Mayo Medical Center.

A committee coordinator from the Patient Care Guideline Committee was designated for each diagnosis. The committee coordinator generated an initial draft of the proposed patient care guideline for committee review. The primary references for the development of each guideline are the most recent publications of the standardized nursing vocabularies of NANDA, NIC, and NOC. Prior to the publication of NOC, various nursing texts were utilized to select outcome statements for guidelines. The linkages between nursing diagnoses and interventions and nursing diagnoses and outcome recommended by the University of Iowa research teams are utilized in development of patient care guidelines and are extremely valuable (Johnson & Maas, 1997, McCloskey & Bulechek, 1996).

Formal review of guidelines occurs at three levels. The first level is that of peer review. Peer review occurs with review by registered nurses from various specialties who are expert in the use of the diagnosis. Peer review participants are typically staff nurses and clinical nurse specialists (CNSs).

The second level of review is by the Patient Care Guideline Committee. The committee reviews the guideline for consistency with NANDA, NIC, and NOC references, appropriate adaptation of activities, and indicators for practice at Mayo Medical Center and the usability and appropriateness of guidelines across clinical specialties.

Legal review is the third review. Guidelines are reviewed by legal advisers for identification of any legal implications in the terminology used within the guideline.

Implementation Process

Once through the formal review process, guidelines are ready for implementation. Guidelines are accessible to staff on the internal website (Intranet) and also in hard copy in a guideline manual. It is anticipated that in 1998 the manuals will be removed from patient care units and the guidelines will be accessible only on the Intranet web site.

When patient care guidelines were first introduced to staff, an extensive education program was implemented. All staff were requested to attend an inservice program to orient them to the guidelines. Although staff had been using NANDA nursing diagnoses for many years, the nursing intervention classification and established outcomes were new. The committee representative from each clinical specialty met with nursing staff in the practice area to discuss specialty issues/concerns. Guidelines have also been used in patient care rounds and are referenced extensively in staff development programs. Some units have designated a "guideline of the month" to increase staff awareness of less familiar diagnoses.

Patient care guidelines are referenced when documenting patient care. The nursing diagnostic label is entered in the plan of care as are the selected nursing activities for each diagnosis. When implemented, the activities are recorded on the patient care record with the outcome. More work is in progress to streamline documentation while assuring that the work of nursing is reflected in the record. Work is also being done to incorporate use of guidelines in the electronic medical record environment.

Providing accessibility to the guidelines has been an important component of implementation. Accessing the guidelines on the Intranet web site has promoted staff referencing guidelines to enhance patient care.

Continuous Improvement

Patient care guidelines have provided a framework for continuous improvement (CI) activities. Initially, CI activity focused on evaluating the extent to which the guidelines were used by nursing staff. The frequency by which nursing diagnosis labels are used in select patient populations has been measured both pre and post guideline implementation to evaluate the impact of the guidelines on nursing practice. Currently, continuous improvement initiatives are focusing more on accuracy of the diagnosis.

Lastly, patient care guidelines have been incorportaed into annual competency reviews. Case study scenarios are a framework used for evaluating staff competence in clinical decision making including diagnostic reasoning, care planning, and outcome evaluation.

Conclusion

Patient care guidelines have been an effective tool in facilitating the implementation of standardized nursing language into practice. They provide a consistent frame of reference for nursing staff across multiple clinical specialties.

References

American Nurses Association. (1991). *Standards of Clinical Nursing Practice.*

Kansas City: American Nurses Association.

North American Nursing Diagnosis
Association. (1996). *Nursing diagnoses:
Definitions & classification 1997-1998.*
Philadelphia: NANDA.

McCloskey, J.C., & Bulecheck, G.M., (Eds).
(1996). *Nursing intervention classification
(NIC)* (2nd ed.). St. Louis: Mosby.

Johnson, M., & Maas, M. (Eds). (1997).
Nursing outcomes classification (NOC). St.
Louis: Mosby.

Dehumanization of the Workplace: A Call for Nursing Diagnosis

Bonnie Wesorick, MSN, RN

It is important to stop and prevent dehumanization of the health care settings. The American Heritage Dictionary defines dehumanize (1993, p. 366) "To deprive of human qualities such as compassion. To render mechanical and routine." Consciously or unconsciously the providers know the impact of a dehumanized work culture on the quality of their lives and the quality of the people in their care. Many providers spend more waking hours in the work place than they do in their home, in the community, or in play. There is no one thing that will stop the dehumanization of the health care culture. It requires a fundamental understanding of the factors that are related to the dehumanization process as well as the factors that support the emergence of a healthy "humanized" culture. This paper will briefly address both and correlate these factors to the call for nursing diagnosis. The perspectives throughout this paper are based on 15 years of experience implementing the Clinical Practice Model (CPM) in over 40 sites, including rural, community and university settings across the United States and Canada. CPM was designed to stop dehumanization of the clinical setting and create a healthy culture, one that is the best place for providers and recipients of care (Wesorick, 1990, 1995, 1996, 1997).

A Brief Look At Culture

What is culture? What is this invisible but very tangible force that surrounds each person who walks into the work place? Quinn (1993, p. 41)defines culture as "a people enacting a story." Is it influenced by the presence of each human being? Is this invisible field nothing more than the presence of the unseen souls of the many who walk or have walked there? What are the characteristics of a dehumanized or unhealthy culture versus a humanized and healthy culture? (See Table 1 for a comparison.)

A Look At The Process of Dehumanization

The past not only gives insight into the insidious process of dehumanization of the health care culture but a sense of the direction needed to

Table 1

Comparison of a Healthy, Humanized Culture to an Unhealthy Dehumanized Work Cultures

Dehumanize: "To deprive of human qualities such as compassion. To render mechanical and routine." (American Heritage Dictionary, p.366.)

Culture: The invisible but tangible presence of the unseen souls of the many who work there.

Characteristics of Healthy Work Culture

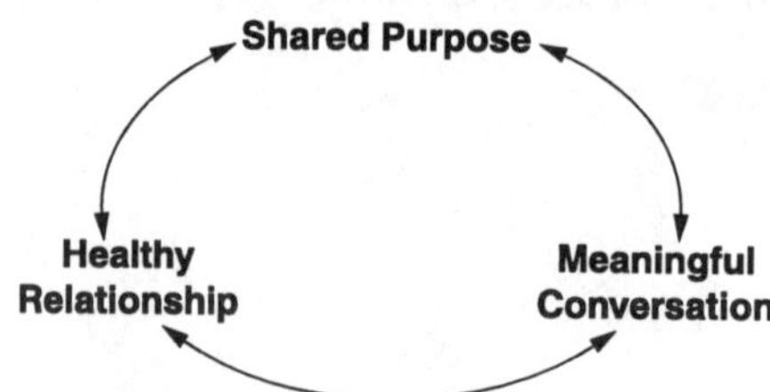

Healthy and unhealthy work cultures have similarities and differences.

Similarities: Both are very busy doing important work, and there is always much to be done. In a typical day there are unexpected events, problems, opportunities, challenges, successes and failures.

DIFFERENCE

Healthy Work Culture	Unhealthy Work Culture
Focus: Honoring the wholeness (BodyMindSoul) both provider and recipient of care.	Focus: The "tasks" to be done by provider for receipient of care.
Connection of the unseen souls of the many who carry out important work.	Lack of connection of the unseen souls of the many who carry out important work.
Shared meaning and purpose.	Shared accountability to get things done
Meaningful conversation-dialogue	Transactional conversations around tasks to be done.
Healthy relationships-partnerships.	Hierarchical relationships.

Adapted From:

Wesorick, B., Shiparski, L., Troseth, M., and Wyngarden, K. (1998) Partnership council field book – Strategies and tools for co-creating a healthy work place. Michigan: Practice Field Publishing.

stop it. Table 2 demonstrates the common thinking and behaviors that developed over the last 35 years of practice and the shift to new ways of thinking and behaviors that give hope for the future. During this time span, the practice arena transitioned from low technology to high technology. Sandelowski (1997) provides a 35 year literature overview which uncovers two opposing views about the impact of technology on nursing. She notes that major concerns surfaced with the introduction of technology including the ability to preserve the essence of nursing; the need to minimize depersonalizing, distancing and other deleterious effects of automation; and the need to prevent the subordination of nursing to medicine via time allocation for medical development rather than nursing development. Although there are many factors that impacted dehumanization of the health care setting, a closer look at one factor, the introduction and advancement of technology, will give insights into the overall process as it relates to nursing.

The focus of the health care provider in the sixties was "to fix" and the expectation of the consumers was "to be fixed." This accelerated the emergence of new and advanced technology. The focus on technology was driven by daily clinical evidence that the spirit of an individual will leave a body that cannot sustain life. Therefore, the natural focus of health care became the medical model. The desire to help people live or support physical status fueled the determination to use technology to uncover better diagnosis of disease, treatment, cures, and prevention.

In the typical hospital setting where the majority of nurses practiced, the focus on medical care and the introduction of technology shaped the norms that still exist today. Strong patterns emerged. The work to keep the patients alive required nurses to understand the people's physical condition, and to develop the competencies associated with new technology, procedures and treatments. Since nurses were the only professionals present and caring for the patients over the 24 hour day, they were accountable for the continuity of medical care. The demands of the new technology and the advancing medical science influenced every aspect of the patient's care. The credibility of a nurse's practice started to shift into an institutional service orientation as described in Table 2. The nurse's expertise was determined by the speed and accuracy in carrying out doctors' orders, the number of tasks competently completed according to hospital policy and procedure, and the ability to have everything done before the next shift arrived.

It was during this transition that dehumanization of the practice culture began. Compassion was not the expectation, rather completion of the task was the expectation. Nurses actually began to refer to their patients more by medical diagnosis or treatment than by name. The following comments were common: "I have the kidney in room 2 and the heart in 6." "Well, I have the ventilator in 4 and the liver in room 5." The focus was on the tasks, rituals, routines, procedures and treatments that needed to be accomplished to support the person's physical status. The daily routines and conversations rarely focused on the care related to the person's wholeness or human response. The professional scope of practice as delineated in Table 3 was dominated by "institutional service." Insidiously dehumanization took place. Just as patients were referred to by disease or body parts, nurses started to see their colleagues as FTE's (full-time equivalent) whose credibility was deter-

Table 2

Emerging Paradigms

Emerging Paradigms

Old Paradigm	*New Paradigm*
Newtonian View (Fragmentation)	Quantum View (Integration)
Medical Care Model	Health Care Model
"Absence of Disease"	"Body, Mind, and Spirit in Balance"
Physiological (objective)	Human Response (subjective)
Mechanical View	Wholistic View
Life Events: Medical	Life Events: Balance
Fix: "Power Over"	Ownership: "Power Releasing"
Passive	Partnership
Episodic (Short Term)	Continuous (Long Term)
Limited Strategies	Endless Possibilities
Institutional Service	Professional Service
Dependent, task-dominated practice wherein the nursing service is directed by physicians' orders and hospital policies and procedures. *"Doing things right."*	Independent, process-dominated practice wherein the nursing service is based on the individual's human response to the present health status or situation. *"Being there at the right time, intervening in the right way with the right resources to support healing."*
Hierarchy	Partnership

Table 3

Professional Services:

- *Delegated:* Services which enhance the health of a person and require a physician's order.
- *Interdependent:* Services which enhance health by assessing, monitoring, detecting, and preventing physiological complications associated with certain health situations or treatment plans.
- *Independent:* Services which enhance health by assessing, monitoring, detecting, diagnosing, and treating the human responses to health status or situation.

Human Response: A person's reaction emerging from the integration of physical, psychological, sociocultural, and spiritual dimensions.

The services are intended to potentiate the health (BodyMindSpirit) of patients, families and communities across the lifeline from birth to death.

Adapted From:

Wesorick, B. (1990). Standards of nursing care: A model for clinical practice. Philadelphia: J.B. Lippincott Co.

---

mined by what tasks or procedures they could do and the speed with which they could do them. Nurses looked more like medical extenders assuring medical services were given.

Ulrich (1992) noted that ironically Florence Nightingale spoke about patterns back in 1887 when she said, "The world, more especially this hospital world is so busy... that it is too easy to slip into old patterns before we are aware." Most importantly Nightingale warned that "nursing and medicine must never be mixed up, it spoils both." The concept of nursing diagnosis clearly differentiates the professional choice to serve as nurse. It clarifies that nurses have primary accountability to diagnose and treat the human response while physicians have primary accountability to diagnose and treat disease. One is not more important than the other. Both are essential.

The Call For Nursing Diagnosis

It was in the midst of this 35 year technical evolution of health care that the formation of NANDA emerged. It was NANDA that called for the profession to focus on the essence of nursing by clarifying the nursing diagnostic phenomena. NANDA (1996, p. 8) defines nursing diagnosis as "a clinical judgment about individual, family or community responses to actual and potential health problems/life processes. Nursing diagnoses provide the basis for selection of nursing intervention to achieve outcomes for which the nurse is accountable." It is a call to shift from a medical model to a nursing model of practice. NANDA's work from the first national conference (Gebbie and Lavin, 1975) to the present is to clarify, classify and support nursing's unique accountability to diagnosis and treat the human responses. This effort highlighted the human response and brought attention to a scope of practice very different from the clinical realities of a disease oriented, technological and task driven practice. (See Table 3.)

Joseph Campbell (1988) believed that every human being faces one challenge which is to "remain human regardless of the time born." The challenge is to remain human regardless of external circumstance, whether living during the times of caves, plagues, wars, famine, mergers, fiscal restraints, chaos, change or intense technology. The human response is a person's reaction that emerges from the integration of one's physical, psychological, sociocultural, and spiritual dimensions. It is a concept that honors the wholeness (BodyMindSpirit) of each person. It is a call for compassion. The work related to the diagnosis and treatment of the human response is nursing's professional accountability and commitment to "remain human" regardless of the circumstance. It is a commitment to never see a person as a body part, a DRG, a medical diagnosis, treatment, critical path — or to see a peer as a task master. The work related to the diagnosis and treatment of the human response is not only a decision to practice the essence of nursing but to stop the dehumanization process.

Dehumanization is an ageless concern. NANDA, along with ANA, focused the profession of nursing on this concern. The struggle to live the ANA (1980, 1995) definition of nursing to "diagnose and treat the human response to actual or potential health problems" got lost in the clinical patterns common in a medical model framework. However, the classification of nursing diagnosis and the defining of practice as the diagnosis and treatment of human response are not sufficient for the creation of clinical cultures that use nursing diagnosis in practice or stop dehumanization. Lunney, Karlik, Kiss, and

Murphy (1997) note that today there is still inconsistency in both the use of and accuracy of the psychosocial response. King, Chard, and Elliot (1997) note that the clinical realities interfering with the use of nursing diagnosis will continue without a framework to help nurses in practice. The CPM Framework emerged out of a conscious intention to stop the dehumanization of the work place and includes an infrastructure that supports the practitioner to diagnose and treat the human response.

Many lessons have been learned over the last 15 years implementing CPM in multiple, diverse settings including rural, community and university sites. One major lesson learned, related to nursing diagnosis, is: There will be no shift to the theory of nursing diagnosis in the reality of day-to-day practice unless there is a clinical infrastructure to support such practice. Diagnosing and treating the human response in a strong medical model culture takes great vision, clarity, work and an integrated infrastructure that supports each component of professional practice. There is no one thing, no quick fix, that will create a humanized culture that welcomes the souls of providers and recipients of care. Table 4 lists the fundamental leverage points of a clinical framework that supports the emergence of a humanized culture. These leverage points unfolded over a period of 15 years of work. Two year single-site pilots were followed by a six year multi-site pilot and seven years of work within a growing consortium of clinical settings. The fundamental work related to the leverage points is complex and cannot be discussed in this short overview.

The patterns of outcomes reported during implementation of CPM reflect the creation of a healthy, humanized culture. A few of those outcomes are listed in Table 5. No one leverage

Table 4

Leverage Points on an Integrated Health Care System

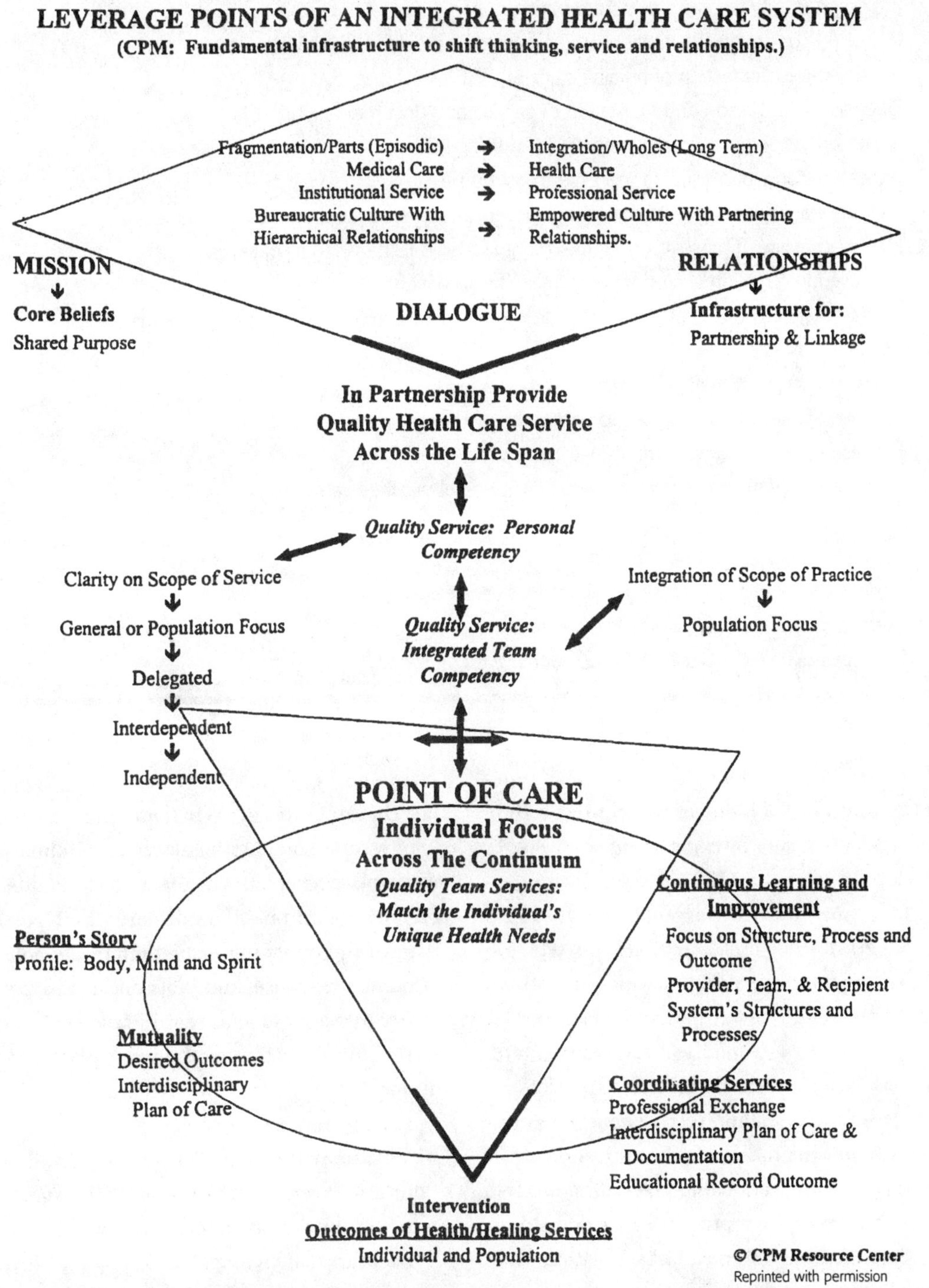

Table 5

Reported Patterns of Outcomes During Implementation of a Clinical Framework

1. Increased quality of care provided to patients.
2. Increased community perception of quality of care provided to patients.
3. Increased job satisfaction of nursing staff.
4. Decreased duplication and replication of service and documentation.
5. Increased sense of practice ownership for nursing staff.
6. Increased clarity of nurses on the essence of nursing.
7. Increased ability of nurses to describe their scope of practice and professional services.
8. Increased ability of nurses to describe the quality of care provided to patients.
9. Increased information shared by nursing staff with patients.
10. Increased willingness to plan and provide care according to patient priorities rather than provider priorities.
11. Increased focus on asking patients what they need.
12. Improved ability of nursing staff to participate in change processes.
13. Increased patient involvement in their own care.
14. Increased patient involvement in decision making about their care.
15. Greater self-awareness by staff.
16. Improved nurse-patient relationships.
17. Improved relationships across the disciplines.
18. Improved relationships across patient care units.
19. Improved connections with resources within the community.

point as listed in Table 4 can explain the listed outcomes. It is the integration of each that makes up the whole.

Outcomes have fiscal ramifications. It is easy to grasp the fiscal rewards related to increased patient satisfaction which is often associated with increased market share potential. It is easy to grasp the fiscal rewards related to increased staff satisfaction and the correlation to increased retention and recruitment benefits. There are obvious fiscal ramification associated with stopping duplication and replication of service. However, can you put a price tag on stopping the cycle of dehumanization within the

health care setting? What are the short- and long-term fiscal ramifications of a humanized work place that effects the quality of life for recipients and providers of care? Is it possible that nursing in its understanding of the concept of human response, and in its declared accountability to diagnose and treat it, hold the hope to stop dehumanization of the work place for this humanity?

References

American Nurses Association (1980). *Nursing: A social policy statement*. Kansas City: The American Nurses Association.

American Nurses Association (1995). *Nursing: A social policy statement.* Washington, DC: The American Nurses Association.

Campbell, J., & Moyers, B. (1988). *The power of myth.* New York: Doubleday.

Costello, R. (Ed.). (1993). *The American Heritage College Dictionary* (3rd ed.). Boston-New York: Houghton Mifflin Co.

Gebbie, K., & Lavin, M.A. (Eds). (1975). *Classification of nursing diagnosis: Proceedings of the first national conference.* St. Louis: Mosby.

King, V., Chard, M., & Elliot, T. (July-September, 1997). Utilization of Nursing Diagnosis in Three Australian Hospitals. *Nursing Diagnosis – The Journal of Nursing Language and Classification,* 8(3).

Lunney, M., Karlik, B., Kiss, M., & Murphy, P. (October-December, 1997). Accuracy of Nurses' Diagnosis of Psychosocial Response. *Nursing Diagnosis – The Journal of Nursing Language and Classification,* 8(4), p. 157.

North American Nursing Diagnosis Association. (1996). *Nursing Diagnosis: Definitions and classification.* Philadelphia: North American Nursing Diagnosis Association.

Quinn, D. (1993). *Ishmael.* New York: Bantan Hard Cover.

Sandelowski (1997) (IR) Reconcilable differences? The debate concerning nursing and technology. *Image: Journal of Nursing Scholarship,* 29(2), p. 169-174.

Ulrich, B. (1992). *Leadership and management according to Florence Nightingale.* Norwalk: Appleton and Lange.

Wesorick, B. (1990). *Standards of nursing care: A model for clinical practice.* Philadelphia: J.B. Lippincott Co.

Wesorick, B. (1995). *The closing and opening of a millennium, A journey from old to new thinking.* Michigan: Practice Field Publishing.

Wesorick, B. (1996). *The closing and opening of a millennium, A journey from old to new relationships in the work setting.* Michigan: Practice Field Publishing.

Wesorick, B., & Shiparski, L. (1997). *Can the human being thrive in the work place? Dialogue as a strategy of hope.* Michigan: Practice Field Publishing.

Wesorick, B., Shiparski, L., Troseth, M., & Wyngarden, K. (1998) *Partnership council field book – Strategies and tools for co-creating a healthy work place.* Michigan: Practice Field Publishing.

For further information, please contact the CPM Resource Center.

CPM Resource Center
100 Michigan NE (MC 166)
Grand Rapids, MI 49503
(616) 391-2017

Effect of a Critical Thinking Elective Course on Diagnostic Reasoning Ability

Margaret E. Briody, MSN, RN

The positive effect of a curriculum revision on improving the inferential ability of diagnostic reasoning between two different groups of senior baccalaureate nursing students before and after a curriculum change has been previously demonstrated (Briody, 1996). In addition, the positive effect of progressing through the revised curriculum has also been discussed (Briody, 1997). The study reported here demonstrates that an elective course developed for baccalaureate nursing students to augment general curricular instruction in critical thinking and diagnostic reasoning has a positive effect on diagnostic reasoning ability.

A thirteen week two credit course entitled "Critical Thinking and Diagnostic Reasoning" examined current concepts, processes, and models of critical thinking and diagnostic reasoning for application in nursing practice. An in-depth, active engagement in learning approach was used. Analyzing critical thinking and diagnostic reasoning skills in linking the steps of the nursing process was provided as well as opportunities to practice strategies to improve critical thinking, critical reading, critical speaking, critical listening, critical writing and diagnostic reasoning. The format emphasized an interactive approach to knowledge and skill development through nursing process applications and the extensive use of case studies, vignettes, videos, stories, and computer simulation exercises.

This elective course was offered for undergraduate nursing students who desired to intensively improve their critical thinking and diagnostic reasoning knowledge and skills. The course augmented the basic content already included in the baccalaureate curriculum. It was meant to supplement and enhance basic material so that students think at a higher level and exceed minimal expectations of the standard curriculum.

Purpose

The implementation of a new elective course in a bachelor of science in nursing program provided the opportunity to study its effectiveness.

The purpose of this study was to determine the effect of a critical thinking elective course on diagnostic reasoning ability.

Review of the literature

The National League for Nursing (NLN) organization in the US heralded the importance of critical thinking skills in nursing by requiring that programs be able to demonstrate evidence of the development of critical thinking skills as one outcome criterion for the accreditation of baccalaureate and master's programs (NLN, 1989). In addition, since 1986, the American Association of Colleges of Nursing has identified the development of critical thinking as essential for baccalaureate nursing education (AACN, 1986).

Currently there are four texts on critical thinking in nursing (Alfaro-Lefevre, 1995; Bandman & Bandman, 1995; Miller & Babcock, 1996; Rubenfeld & Scheffer, 1995). In addition, there is rapid growth about critical thinking in nursing in the periodical literature. A review of the recent literature pertinent to this study reveals four areas of focus:

1. the theoretical/conceptual approach to critical thinking in nursing,
2. measuring critical thinking in nursing,
3. strategies to teach/promote critical thinking in nursing, and
4. diagnostic reasoning in nursing.

Critical Thinking in Nursing

Despite a proliferation in critical thinking in nursing literature, there is no consensus on a definition of critical thinking in nursing nor agreement on accompanying skills and dimensions (Briody, 1996). Jones and Brown (1991) found varying understandings used by faculties of surveyed US schools of nursing. Definitions of critical thinking in the nursing literature have been primarily borrowed from Smith, Kurfiss, Watson and Glaser, Ennis, Meyers, Paul, McPeck, and Toulmin (Birx, 1993; Hickman, 1993; Miller, & Malcolm, 1990).

In 1990, the American Philosophical Association (APA) conducted a delphi survey and cross-disciplinary experts defined critical thinking as "purposeful, self-regulatory judgment which results in interpretation, analysis, evaluation, and inference, as well as explanation of the evidential, conceptual, methodological, criteriological, or contextual considerations upon which that judgment is based..." (APA, 1990, p.3). A major departure from previous understandings in this definition is the importance of both cognitive and affective domains in the critical thinking construct. This APA definition relates directly to the processes of diagnostic reasoning and clinical judgment required in nursing (Briody, 1996).

In addition to conceptualizing the nature of critical thinking, the nursing literature is now including conceptual models in order to communicate the specific perspective of nursing. Miller and Malcolm (1990) created a model based on attitudes, knowledge, and skill levels of critical thinking for the purpose of evaluating nursing curricula. Kataoka-Yahira and Saylor (1994) built upon this model, and included nursing experience, competencies, and standards to offer the Critical Thinking Model for Nursing Judgment. In a divergent view, Ford and Profetto-McGrath (1994) proposed a framework that goes beyond the discussion of critical thinking as a product and/or process to include action and reflection. Videbeck (1997) took the discussion one step further and described a model to inform curriculum development from the individual learner and course perspective as well as adding the overall program evaluation perspective.

Measuring Critical Thinking in Nursing

Reviews of the nursing literature for research on critical thinking by Beck and colleagues (1992), Hickman (1993), Kintgen-Andrews (1991), and Miller and Malcolm (1990) revealed conflicting results and major concerns about its measurement. Until the time of these reviews, there was an almost exclusive use of the Watson-Glaser Critical Thinking Appraisal as the measure. In later reviews, both Rane-Szostak and Robertson (1996), as well as Adams, Whitlow, Stover, and Johnson (1996) critiqued commercially available critical thinking tools and supporting research but made a strong argument for considering alternative measures or the development of a nursing specific critical thinking instrument tailored to a nursing definition and desired outcomes.

Strategies to Teach Critical Thinking in Nursing

The 1990's nursing periodical literature indicates an explosion in the area of critical thinking in general. One foci of this literature is in the area of strategies deemed helpful to teach and develop critical thinking skills. These strategies include argumentation/debate, ethnographic interviewing, ethical-decision making case studies (White, Beardslee, Peters, & Supples, 1990), writing-to-learn approach to course assignments and exams (Bowers, & McCarthy, 1993), thinking-out-loud, Socratic questioning, active involvement of the learner (Case, 1994; Cravener, 1997), critical incident debriefing, mind mapping, journaling, computer simulations (Baker, 1996; Dobrzykowski, 1994) and maternal interviewing (Callister, 1996), among others.

Using Paul's critical thinking framework, Chubinski (1996) creatively described teaching strategies appropriate to each of Paul's skills while Abegglen and Conger (1997) transformed a community health nursing course using a critical thinking perspective with many of the creative strategies listed above.

Diagnostic Reasoning in Nursing

As previously reported, diagnostic reasoning and its research remain scantily addressed in the nursing literature (Briody, 1996; Briody, 1997). Approaches in conceptualizing this process have contrasted from rationalist to information-processing paradigms, and from intuitive to mathematical to phenomenological models (Tanner, 1988). Meanwhile, Pesut and Herman (1992) presented a compelling argument for the metacognition aspect of critical thinking to be a framework for teaching and learning diagnostic reasoning. Gordon, Murphy, Candee, and Hiltunen (1994) proposed an integrated model of diagnostic-therapeutic and ethical reasoning as a framework for clinical judgment.

The literature discusses diagnostic reasoning as synonymous with (or at least closely related to) decision-making, problem-solving, and clinical judgment. Nursing research in this area continues to attempt to clarify these concepts (Benner, Tanner, & Chesla, 1996; Jenks, 1993; Jenny & Logan, 1992; Tanner, Benner, Chesla, & Gordon, 1993) building on research by Benner (1984) and on scholarship of Carnevali and others (1984) in the 1980's. A recent study by Aquilino (1997) examined cognitive development, knowledge, and clinical experience in relation to diagnostic reasoning ability. Her use of simulations is similar to the vignette approach used in the measurement tool and data reported here. Relatively few papers focused solely on strategies to teach the 'diagnostic reasoning process' to students have been described (Plunkett & Oliveri, 1989).

As yet, there is still no published tested measurement instrument specific for nursing diagnostic reasoning (Briody, 1997). The study reported here uses a portion of the second edition of the Diagnostic Reasoning Test by Gordon and Plunkett (1993).

To summarize the review of the literature on critical thinking and diagnostic reasoning, the critical thinking skills identified by the APA (1990) study are completely synonymous with the diagnostic reasoning process as described by Gordon (1994). Nursing care of patients requiring clinical judgments and decision-making skills demands that the critical skill of diagnostic reasoning be taught, measured, and evaluated in nursing students (Briody, 1996).

Method

For the purposes of measuring critical thinking in the context of nursing and for this study, critical thinking was operationalized as diagnostic reasoning.

Design

A pre/post descriptive design was used to evaluate the effect of an elective course on the diagnostic reasoning ability of generic junior, senior and registered nurse baccalaureate nursing students.

Sample

A convenience sample of 26 undergraduate junior, senior, and registered nurse students enrolled in the elective course in either Fall 1994 and 1995 was invited to participate. At the conclusion of the course, the same convenience sample was again invited to participate. All stu-

dents chose to participate. A matched pair of scores for each anonymous student pre/post the course was obtained and compared on diagnostic reasoning ability.

Instrument

This study uses a portion of the second edition of the original unpublished Diagnostic Reasoning Test by Gordon (1986). The second edition by Gordon and Plunkett (1993) is an objective-type tool and a sub-set, consisting of 10 vignettes, was used to measure the diagnostic reasoning ability of the students. This tool has since undergone a third revision and is now in the final stages of psychometric testing.

The tool includes vignettes from which correct priority nursing diagnoses and additional cues are identified. For each of 10 patient care vignettes, the test-taker was asked to identify 4 possible nursing diagnoses that should be assessed further, to select the "most likely" diagnosis, and to list the additional cues that must be present to confirm this most likely diagnosis. Frequency count scores were obtained by summing the number of correct choices on all 10 vignettes (total of 40 possible) as well as determining the correct number of diagnoses for each vignette. In addition, the number of vignettes with correct identification of the highest priority nursing diagnosis was tallied. Individual responses were matched anonymously; results are aggregate scores using t-tests for paired samples.

Results

Analysis of Gordon and Plunkett's Diagnostic Reasoning Test scores revealed that 20 students improved, 4 students remained the same, and 2 did worse on the post-test compared with the pre-course test in identifying the total number of correct nursing diagnoses. Before the course, the students achieved a mean of 13.34 of 40 correct nursing diagnoses. After the course, the same students increased the mean to 17.84 of 40 correct nursing diagnoses. Comparison tests show significantly improved diagnostic reasoning ability for the number of correct nursing diagnoses when measured at the end of the course ($t(25) = -5.43$, $p<.001$).

The Diagnostic Reasoning Test revealed a mean of 4.38 correct highest priority nursing diagnosis on 10 vignettes when measured before the course. After the course, the mean increased to 6.65 correct highest priority diagnosis on 10 vignettes. Comparison tests show significantly improved diagnostic reasoning ability for the most correct highest priority nursing diagnosis when measured at the conclusion of the course ($t(25) = -6.20$, $p<.001$). Each vignette was also analyzed but these data are too detailed for the scope of this paper.

Limitations

One of the major limitations to this study is validity and reliability issues related to the Diagnostic Reasoning Test, as discussed elsewhere (Briody, 1994). A second limitation is the possible effect of minimal teaching differences between the course teaching in 1994 and 1995. A third limitation is the assumption that these diagnostic reasoning scores are reflective of learning in this course and not a result of some other influence.

Although a year separated the two cohorts of students, there were no changes in the syllabus nor difference in offering of the course from one year to the next. There were no curricular changes in other courses taken simultaneously.

Discussion

This study evaluated the effects of a critical thinking elective course on diagnostic reasoning ability. The results demonstrated an improvement in diagnostic reasoning ability of 26 students after the course. Because of the necessary connection between critical thinking and diagnostic reasoning in nursing, critical thinking ability also improved.

Although significant improvement was demonstrated, the low scores in ability to identify the total number of correct nursing diagnoses (17.85 of 40 after the course) as well as moderate scores in ability to identify the highest priority nursing diagnosis (6.65 of 10) indicate that efforts must continue to further increase diagnostic reasoning content, processes, and teaching strategies in all nursing courses. In the clinical arena, the nurse needs to identify the highest priority nursing diagnosis 10 out of 10 times.

Despite the low scores, student feedback about the course demonstrated high valuing of the course and recognize it as an important contribution to their education. Direct quotes from the students include:

"I feel better prepared for clinical."

"I have a better grasp of the diagnostic process."

"This course helped me write my care plans."

"This has helped me prioritize diagnostic reasoning."

"I believe I will be able to use these concepts throughout my career as a nurse."

"I have progressed from road block thinking to being able to write and expand my thoughts more easily."

"My thought process is clearer and more consistent."

"I am able to think much more quickly 'on

my feet'; I constantly question my conclusions and adjust them accordingly now."

"As a result of this course, my thinking began to progess more logically."

Additional comments from the students focused on the value of the course in relation to other curriculum courses:

"This course was the most beneficial 2 credits of all."

"This course helped me synthesize all my learning."

"This course should be a required course."

"I am now able to tie previous knowledge with new data and reach conclusions."

"I am more self-aware of my perspective and biases; the course has improved my accuracy in assessing and diagnosing."

"I now take the time to reflect and see if all the angles are explored."

Conclusion

Preparing future professional nurses in the areas of critical thinking and diagnostic reasoning is imperative. These skills will be daily tools essential to the creation of new practice models providing nursing care to individuals, families, and communities in an increasingly complex and competitive health care arena.

References

Abegglen, J., & Conger, C. (1997). Critical thinking in nursing: Classroom tactics that work. *Journal of Nursing Education, 36*(10), 452-458.

Adams, M., Whitlow, J., Stover, L., & Johnson, K. (1996). Critical thinking as an educational outcome. An evaluation of current tools of measurement. *Nurse Educator, 21*(3), 23-32.

Alfaro-Levre, R. (1995). Critical thinking in nursing. Philadelphia: Saunders.

American Association of Colleges of Nursing. (1986). *Essentials of college and university education for professional nursing.* Washington, DC: Author.

American Philosophical Association. (1990). *Critical thinking: A statement of expert consensus for purposes of educational assessment and instruction. The Delphi report: Research findings and recommendations prepared for the committee on pre-college philosophy.* ERIC Document Reproductions Service No. ED 315-423.

Aquilino, M. (1997). Cognitive development, clinical knowledge, and clinical experience related to diagnostic ability. Nursing *Diagnosis, 8*(3), 110-119.

Bandman, E., & Bandman, B. (1995). *Critical thinking in nursing* (2nd ed.). Norwalk CT: Appleton & Lange.

Beck, S., Bennett, A., McLeod, R., & Molyneaux, D. (1992). Review of research on critical thinking in nursing education. In L. Allen (Ed.). *Review of research in nursing education,* V (p.1-30). New York: NLN.

Benner, P. (1984). *From novice to expert.* Menlo-Park, CA: Addison-Wesley.

Benner, P., Tanner, C., & Chelsa, C. (1996). *Expertise in nursing practice: Caring, clinical judgment and ethics.* New York, NY: Springer.

Birx, E. (1993). Critical thinking and theory-based practice. *Holistic Nursing Practice, 7*(3), 21-27.

Bowers, B., & McCarthy, D. (1993).

Developing analytic thinking skills in early undergraduate education. *Journal of Nursing Education, 32*(3), 107-114.

Briody, M. (1994). Measurement issues related to diagnostic reasoning ability. Abstract. In R. Carroll-Johnson & M. Paquette (Eds.). *Classification of nursing diagnosis: Proceedings of the tenth conference* (p. 351). Philadelphia: Lippincott.

Briody, M. (1996). Effect of curriculum change on student anxiety and diagnostic reasoning. *Nursing Diagnosis, 7*(4), 141-146.

Briody, M. (1997). Effect of progression through a revised curriculum on student anxiety and diagnostic reasoning. In Rantz, M., & LeMone, P. (Eds.). *Classification of nursing diagnosis: Proceedings of the twelfth conference* (p. 112-116). Glendale, CA: CINAHL.

Callister, L. (1996). Maternal interviews: A teaching strategy fostering critical thinking. *Journal of Nursing Education, 35*(1), 29-30.

Carnevali, D., Mitchell, P., Woods, N., & Tanner, C. (Eds.). (1984). *Diagnostic reasoning in nursing.* Philadelphia: Lippincott.

Case B. (1994). Walking around the elephant: A critical-thinking strategy for decision making. *Journal of Continuing Education in Nursing, 25*(3), 101-109.

Chubinski, S. (1996). Creative critical-thinking strategies. *Nurse Educator, 21*(6), 23-27.

Cravener, P. (1997). Promoting active learning in large lecture classes. *Nurse Educator, 22*(3), 21-26.

Dobrzykowski, T. (1994). Teaching strategies to promote critical thinking skills in nursing staff. *Journal of Continuing Education in Nursing, 25*(6), 272-276.

Facione, N., Facione, P., & Sanchez, C. (1994). Critical thinking disposition as a measure of competent clinical judgment: The development of the California critical thinking disposition inventory. *Journal of Nursing Education, 33*(8), 345-350.

Ford, J. & Profetto-McGrath, J. (1994). A model for critical thinking within the context of curriculum as praxis. *Journal of Nursing Education, 33*(8), 341-344.

Gordon, M. (1986). *Diagnostic reasoning test.* Unpublished manuscript. Boston College School of Nursing, Chestnut Hill, MA.

Gordon, M. (1994). *Nursing diagnosis: Process and application* (3rd ed.). St. Louis, Mosby.

Gordon, M., Murphy, C., Candee, D., & Hiltunen, E. (1994). Clinical judgment: An integrated model. *Advances in Nursing Science, 16*(4), 55-70.

Gordon, M., & Plunkett, E. (1993). *Diagnostic reasoning test* (2nd ed.). Unpublished manuscript. Boston College School of Nursing, Chestnut Hill, MA.

Hickman, J. (1993). A critical assessment of critical thinking in nursing education. *Holistic Nursing Practice, 7*(3), 36-47.

Jenks, J. (1993). The pattern of personal knowing in nurse decision making. *Journal of Nursing Education, 32*(9), 399-405.

Jenny, J., & Logan, J. (1992). Knowing the patient: One aspect of clinical knowledge. *Image: The Journal of Nursing Scholarship, 24*(4), 254-258.

Jones, S., & Brown, L. (1991). Critical thinking: Impact on nursing education. *Journal of Nursing Education, 33*(1), 529-533.

Kataoka-Yahiro, M., & Saylor, C. (1994). A critical thinking model for nursing judgment. *Journal of Nursing Education, 33*(8), 351-356.

Miller, M., & Babcock, D. (1996). Critical

thinking applied to nursing. St. Louis: Mosby.

Miller, M., & Malcolm, N. (1990). Critical thinking in the nursing curriculum. *Nursing & Health Care, 11*(2), 67-73.

National League for Nursing. (1989). *Criteria for the evaluation of baccalaureate and higher degree programs in nursing* (6th ed.). New York: Author.

Pesut, D., & Herman, J. (1992). Metacognitive skills in diagnostic reasoning: Making the implicit explicit. *Nursing Diagnosis, 3*(4), 148-154.

Plunkett, E., & Oliveri, R. (1989). A strategy for introducing diagnostic reasoning: Hypotheses testing using a simulation approach. *Nurse Educator, 14*(6), 27-31.

Rane-Szostak, D., & Robertson, J. (1996). Issues in measuring critical thinking: Meeting the challenge. *Journal of Nursing Education, 35*(1), 5-11.

Rubenfeld, M., & Scheffer, B. (1995). *Critical thinking in nursing*. Philadelphia: Lippincott.

Tanner, C. (1988). Curriculum revolution: The practice mandate. *Nursing & Health Care, 9*, 427-430.

Tanner, C., Benner, P., Chesla, C., & Gordon, D. (1993). The phenomenology of knowing the patient. *Image: The Journal of Nursing Scholarship, 25*(4), 273-280.

Videbeck, S. (1997). Critical thinking: A model. *Journal of Nursing Education, 36*(1), 23-28.

White, N., Beardslee, N., Peters, D., & Supples, J. (1990). Promoting critical thinking skills. *Nurse Educator, 15*(5), 16-19.

Educational Strategies for Integrating Diagnoses and Care Components

Sheila M. Sparks, DNSc, RN, CS
Virginia K. Saba, EdD, RN, FAAN, FACMI

Preparation of nurses for practice in the 21st century requires new educational strategies and maximal use of computer systems. The Georgetown University Nursing Model (GUNM) (Sparks, 1995) was developed using the Saba Home Health Care Classification (HHCC) system (Saba, 1997, Saba, 1995, Saba, 1994) as a framework for the nursing process. The 20 care components of the HHCC form the core elements of the assessment, care planning, and evaluation tools used in the undergraduate program of study. All of the instruments are accessible to students via the school's computer laboratory and university computer system. Faculty use the HHCC's care components along with other key elements of the GUNM to structure lectures, provide clinical examples, and evaluate student clinical performance. Key elements of the GUNM include the client and nurse in an interactive caring exchange; the use of critical thinking and the nursing process; and the elements of health, human development, technology, and collaboration. This paper describes the integration of the care components in teaching nursing science and gives examples from each instrument of implementation strategies for using this system. The teaching instruments developed for this system are available online or as computer printouts.

Overview of Teaching Strategies Using Care Components

A set of integrated teaching instruments and forms provide the structure for educating students about the nursing process. The 20 care components are organized using 5 patterns: Health Behaviors Components, Psychological Components, Functional Components, and Physiological Components. A Life-Cycle Component was added to address reproductive and developmental issues that were not part of the original HHCC model. Instructional forms used to teach the nursing process include: Client Assessment Instrument, Developmental Assessment, Data Collection Form for Client Assessment, Clinical Log, and Plan of Care.

"

Figure 1

Client Assessment Instrument

Georgetown University School of Nursing
Client Assessment Instrument

Demographic Data (Adapted Minimum Data Set)

Component	Normal	Findings
Health Behavior		
A. Medications		
B. Safety		
C. Health Behavior		
Psychological		
D. Cognitive		
E. Self-Concept		
F. Coping		
G. Role Relationship		
Sexuality		
Functional		
H. Activity and Rest		
Physical Assessment/Signs*		
Diagnostics*		
Interview*		
I. Nutrition		
J. Fluid Status		
K. Sensory		
Vision		
Hearing		
Taste/Smell		
Proprioceptive/Kinesthetic Status		
L. Self-Care		
Physiological		
M. Physical Regulation		
N. Skin Integrity		
O. Tissue Perfusion		
P. Cardiac		
Q. Respiratory		
R. Metabolic		
S. Bowel Elimination		
T. Urinary Elimination		
Life-Cycle		
U. Human Growth and Development		
V. Reproductive		

*categories included in each session

Forms to evaluate performance include a Clinical Evaluation Tool and Clinical Evaluation Guidelines which will not be described in this paper. Each of the nursing process instruments is described below.

Client Assessment Instrument

The Client Assessment Instrument (see Figure 1) begins with collection of demographic data and elements of the Nursing Minimum Data Set. It is then organized in 5 sections: Health Behaviors Components (Medication, Safety, Health Behavior), Psychological Components (Cognitive, Coping, Role Relationship, Self-Concept), Functional Components (Activity, Fluid Volume, Nutritional, Self-Care, Sensory), Physiological Components (Cardiac, Respiratory, Metabolic, Physical Regulation, Skin Integrity, Tissue Perfusion, Bowel Elimination, Urinary Elimination), and Life-Cycle Component (Human Development, Reproductive). Each of the sections is further subdivided to include relevant interview questions, physical examination, and diagnostic tests. There is a column that presents normal findings as well as one to record actual findings. Students are introduced to the GUNM as first-year students and in their second semester take a Health Assessment course where they use the Client Assessment Instrument throughout the semester. Because the instrument is very lengthy, a Data Collection Form for Client Assessment was developed for recording information. As skill develops in conducting client interviews, students use the Client Assessment Instrument as a reference.

Developmental Assessment

Because of the emphasis in the GUNM on development, a special form was developed to cover assessing human development across the lifespan. The Developmental Assessment (see Figure 2) consists of questions/cues, norms for age, and actual findings arranged in separate sections for children (infants, toddlers, early childhood, middle childhood, and adolescence) and adults (early adulthood, middle adulthood, and late adulthood). Students take a separate Human Growth and Development course and integrate knowledge of human development in assessing all clients. The Developmental Assessment form provides a quick overview of normal growth and development and enables students to be sensitive to developmental issues that impact on health care services and client responses to treatment.

Figure 2

Developmental Assessment		
U. Human Growth & Development		
Developmental Assessment		
Questions/Cues	Normal	Findings
Diagnostic Interview	*Children* Infants Newborns Toddlers Early Childhood Middle Childhood Adolescence	
	Adults Early Adulthood (18-40 years) Middle Adulthood (40-60 years) Late Adulthood (>60 years)	

Data Collection Form for Client Assessment

The Data Collection Form for Client

Assessment provides room for recording client data in a concise manner. It is comprised of columns for the 5 health patterns and blank spaces for recording interview/survey, physical exam/physical environment, and diagnostic tests/epidemiological biostatistical data. This information forms the basis for the Plan of Care.

Plan of Care

After students complete a client assessment, they use the Plan of Care (see Figure 3) to record all pertinent nursing diagnoses in one column and their scientific rationales (with references) in another column. This affords the student the opportunity to explain his/her choices and for faculty to respond to them. In some cases, students are advised to consider other diagnoses or to collect additional data to support their decisions. Students then select nursing diagnoses to develop into a plan of care. Although the focus of each course may vary, the usual expectation is to include diagnoses that represent physiological, psychological, as well as social and spiritual problems. Students are also encouraged to use different diagnoses throughout the semester so they can develop a broad knowledge base of health care problems. Students use a nursing diagnosis reference (Sparks & Taylor, 1998) to supplement their plan but must individualize the outcomes, interventions, and their evaluation to meet actual client needs.

The second page of the Plan of Care contains space to record the nursing diagnosis and related statement, outcomes, nursing interventions (classified into categories of assess [monitor], care [perform], teach [instruct], and manage [coordinate]), rationales, and evaluation. Students often need assistance in selecting different types of interventions. The HHCC nursing intervention data dictionary provides 160 home health nursing interventions linked to specific diagnoses. Students are provided with examples of interventions, e.g., assess or monitor blood glucose, provide bowel care, teach medication side effects, or coordinate schedule with other health care providers. This page can be reproduced for however many nursing diagnoses the student wishes to complete. The final page is used to record the references used in preparation of the plan of care. In most cases, students are required to list at least one reference from the current literature.

Figure 3

Plan of Care

Georgetown University
School of Nursing
Plan of Care

Student   Client Initials

Medical Diagnosis

Date   Course   Faculty

List Nursing Diagnoses in Priority Order:
Scientific Rationale
(Reference)
Nursing Diagnosis

Outcomes (Goals)	Nursing Interventions (classify into categories of assess, care)	Rationale (with references)	Evaluation (including revision, if appropriate)

Repeat nursing diagnoses and plan of care as many times as necessary

Clinical Log

The Clinical Log (see Figure 4) is organized around the components of the GUNM and includes the following sections: Health, Collaboration, Technologies, Caring, and Nursing Process/Critical Thinking. Once students have received their client assignment for clinical they are expected to complete the Preclinical Preparation column which includes the above mentioned sections and to develop a list of nursing care problems in priority order. Once in the clinical setting, students complete the Clinical Validation column which provides an opportunity for correction of information or

Figure 4

Clinical Log		

Georgetown University School of Nursing
Clinical Log

Student   Client Initials   Medical Diagnosis
Date   Course   Faculty

Nursing Model Components	Preclinical Preparation	Clinical Validation
Health		Reflection
Collaboration (other disciplines or community organizations)		Documentation
Technologies (e.g., fluids, medications, special feedings.)/Levels of Prevention		
Caring		
Nursing Process/Critical Thinking		
Assessment		
Interview/Survey		
Physical Exam		
Diagnostic Tests/ Epidemiological or Biostatistical Data		

revision of plans. At the conclusion of clinical, students use the area, Documentation, for recording their nursing note, and complete the section, Reflection, which provides a way to summarize the clinical experience and allows the faculty member to evaluate the student experience.

The other 2 forms, Clinical Evaluation Tool and Guidelines for Clinical Evaluation, are used to evaluate clinical performance and will not be discussed in this paper.

Summary

Use of the HHCC system provides a framework for the development of teaching strategies to prepare nurses for practice in the 21st century. The use of an integrated system of instruments accessible to students on-line allows for a smooth transition from course to course and later to nursing practice. Students and faculty use this conceptual approach to facilitate collaboration with other healthcare providers and to model professional behavior for students.

References

American Nurses Association. (1991). *Standards of clinical nursing practice.* Washington, D.C.: ANA.

Farley, J.N. (1995, Spring/Summer). *New conceptual framework. Vision for Nursing,* p. 11. Washington, D.C.: Georgetown University.

Saba, V.K. (1994). Twenty nursing diagnosis home health components. In R.M. Caroll-Johnson & M. Paquette, *Classification of nursing diagnoses: Proceedings of the tenth conference,* (p. 301). Philadelphia: J.B. Lippincott.

Saba, V.K. (1995). A new paradigm for computer-based nursing information systems: Twenty care components. In R.A. Greenes, et al. (Eds). *MEDINFO 95 Proceedings*. Amsterdam: IMIA.

Saba. V.K. (1997). *Home health care classification of nursing diagnoses and interventions*. Paper presentation at: Implementation of Nursing Vocabularies in Computer-based Systems. San Jose, CA: American Medical Informatics Association.

Sparks, S.M. (1995). Integrating nursing diagnosis in nursing education. In M.J. Rantz & P. LeMone, (Eds)., *Classification of nursing diagnoses: Proceedings of the eleventh conference of the North American Nursing Diagnosis Association*. Glendale, CA: CINAHL Information Systems.

Sparks, S.M., & Taylor, C.M. (1998). *Nursing diagnosis reference manual* (4th ed). Springhouse, PA: Springhouse Corporation.

The Power of Nursing Diagnosis: A Transcultural Experience "The Power of Having Words" (abstract)

Betty Ackley, RN, MSN

Gail Ladwig, RN, MSN, CHTP

T. Nakaki

K. Fujisaki

Nursing diagnosis has provided a universal language that transcends culture and language. This workshop will demonstrate group work on the clinical implementation of nursing diagnosis and critical thinking. The workshop will be based on two seminars that were given in Tokyo and Kyoto. The workshop will be presented by two Japanese and two American professors.

The four of us were able to communicate with each other and then with 600 and 1000 Japanese nurses because we spoke a common language of nursing and nursing diagnosis. We facilitated an activity that had these large numbers of nurses working in groups of 4-6 developing nursing diagnoses based on case studies. It was an impressive sight.

My colleague and I spoke about 20 words of Japanese; the Japanese professors understood more English than they could speak. (We had conference interpreters but that wasn't the entire explanation). How were we able to do group work with 600 and 1000 nurses? We had a common language that transcended cultures. The language of nursing and in particular the language of nursing diagnosis. Because everyone had a common language — the language of nursing diagnosis — we were able to work through a process and accomplish mutual goals. We will demonstrate this process in this workshop.

The promotion of the use of nursing diagnosis is supported by this wonderful experience in Japan where we were able to communicate across cultures. It is meaningful to NANDA that we could work together because of the existence of NANDA diagnoses. We could also understand each other when we explained related factors and defining characteristics.

What an impressive sight, the power of common language!

Validation of Select Terms of the International Classification for Nursing Practice (ICNP) Alpha Version

Amy Coenen, PhD, RN, CS
Madeline Wake, PhD, RN, FAAN
Funded by the International Council of Nurses

Background

The International Classification for Nursing Practice (ICNP) was initiated by the International Council of Nurses (ICN) to provide a vocabulary for nursing and a unifying framework into which existing vocabularies and classifications can be cross-mapped. The Alpha Version of the ICNP, first published in 1996, identified three elements: (a) classification of Nursing Phenomena, (b) Classification of Nursing Interventions, and (c) Classification of Nursing Outcomes. The elements were disseminated at early stages of development to stimulate feedback and evaluation.

This study focused on terms in the Classification of Phenomena. Nursing Phenomena are defined in the ICNP Alpha Version as: "phenomena which nurses diagnose." The term diagnosis, although familiar in the United States of America, was not universally acceptable. In the Webster's (1984) dictionary the term phenomenon denotes "a fact or occurrence that can be perceived or observed." The ICNP Alpha Version Classification of Phenomena is a hierarchy of 292 terms classified into two broad categories: Human Beings and Environment.

In accordance with classification principles, each term in the Alpha Version Classification of Phenomena is defined by the genus or higher category of placement in the classification and specific characteristics of the term (Neilsen & Mortensen, 1996). Some definitions are further developed than others. For example, the definition of fever needs further work. In the Alpha Version, the term fever is defined as follows:

Fever is a Nursing Phenomena pertaining to Hyperthermia with the following specific characteristics: Changes in the internal thermostat, with or without shivering, with or without flushed skin, increased respiratory rate and tachycardia.

"

Multinational efforts were seen as essential in ongoing work toward developing definitions.

Purpose

The project provided an in-depth examination of select terms using multiple methods to enhance global participation in the ongoing development of the ICNP, across nations and languages. The purpose of this study was to validate select terms in the Alpha Version of the ICNP Classification of Nursing Phenomena across various countries and three languages (English, French, and Spanish). A secondary purpose of the project was evaluation of validation methods for future work.

Sample

Eighteen countries were represented in the study. The nurse participants of the focus groups totaled 43 and represented 13 countries (Brazil, Canada, Finland, France, Japan, Pakistan, Spain, Sweden, United Kingdom, and United States of America). Over 1,300 surveys were distributed to nurses in 14 countries. To date, 596 surveys were completed and returned from 11 countries (Australia, Belgium, Canada, Chile, France, Indonesia, New Zealand, South Africa, Spain, Taiwan, and USA).

Methods

Multiple methods (content analysis, focus groups, surveys) were combined to validate terms and specific characteristics for select nursing phenomena in the ICNP Alpha Version. Six terms were selected for the study: dehydration, fever, anxiety, confusion, loneliness, and water pollution. This study was approved by the Marquette University Institutional Review Board for the protection of human subjects.

Content analysis was conducted using both literature review and nurses with expertise in the terms selected. Literature was analyzed in a systematic manner generating categories of definitions and specific characteristics. Experts provided clarification and enhanced interpretation of the findings from the literature.

Focus groups were conducted in English, Spanish, and French (the three ICN languages) at the ICN Congress in Vancouver, 1997. A standardized format was used to conduct each focus group, the format included using pilot surveys in the participants' language to facilitate communication.

Surveys were developed in English, based on results of the content analysis and focus group sessions. Surveys were distributed in the appropriate language to 14 countries. Each country had a site coordinator who facilitated the distribution and collection of surveys. In addition to other questions, the surveys incorporated the diagnostic content validation (DCV) model to obtain expert opinions from nurses on the degree to which each clinical characteristic is indicative of a given phenomenon (Fehring, 1987).

Findings

The complexities of cross-cultural sensitivity in an international classification were highlighted in the focus groups and survey responses. Overall, the findings supported the need of an international classification to attend to variation in meaning of terms by language, culture, and practice (settings, specialties, and roles). For example, several participants objected to the term "obesity" as judgmental and preferred the term "overweight." Other nurses stated that only patient-identified problems are nursing problems.

Many of the nurses involved in the study reported that they were not content with existing systems in nursing. However, they had invested efforts in using select systems, such as the North American Nursing Diagnosis Association taxonomy (NANDA), and were relieved that the ICNP was being developed to accommodate cross-mapping to these systems.

One Example – Fever: Analysis of survey data using the DVC method provided the rating of specific characteristics for each term. Along with rating characteristics, nurses identified synonyms for the terms examined and additional specific characteristics. There were 168 nurses who completed the survey examining the term fever. Nurses responded that they see fever "quite often" (M = 3.95 on a 5 point scale). The mean of years of professional nursing experience of nurses, in this subsample was 17.34 (range of 1 - 44 years). Educational preparation varied (41.6% technical or diploma, 31.1% baccalaureate or university, 24.2% master's, and 3.1% doctorate). Over 60% of the nurses were working in direct patient care.

An example of the findings for specific characteristics with DCV scores > 0.65 in the total sample, by select countries, are reported in Table 1. Additional terms nurses identified using instead of fever included: Febrile (New Zealand), Hyperthermia (Chile, France, Spain), and Pyrexia (New Zealand, South Africa).

Summary and Recommendations

The study provided participation of nurses from many countries. This participation enhanced nurses' exposure to the ICNP and to the different methods used in validation. This study provided results which will be used in the development and refinement of the ICNP. The following recommendations were provided:

1. Continue to use multiple methods in development and testing of the ICNP to promote participation of practicing nurses.

Table 1

Examples of diagnostic content validation (DVC) scores for clinical characteristics of FEVER by total sample and select countries

Characteristics	Total N = 168	France N = 39	Spain N=20	New Zealand N=16	Chile N=16	Taiwan N= 23	South Africa N=16
Lethargy	.679	.776	.612	.609	.518	.706	.703
Increased pulse	.803	.846	.712	.717	.844	.804	.859
Thirst	.659	.724	.587	.578	.641	.674	.850
Increased body temperature	.935	.968	.937	.953	.891	.978	.859
Chills	.739	.801	.850	.703	.609	.793	.672
Warm	.730	.704	.475	.734	.609	.837	.797
Increased respiratory rate	.697	.711	.575	.641	.750	.685	.683

2. Use focus groups to examine cultural variation.
3. Use survey methods for large studies or target groups at the multinational level.
4. Develop and test new methods for clinical validation.

References

Fehring, R. J. (1987). Methods to validate nursing diagnoses. *Heart & Lung, 16,* 625-629.

International Council of Nurses (1996). *The International Classification for Nursing Practice (ICNP): A unifying framework. The Alpha version.* Geneva Switzerland: Author.

Nielsen, G. H. & Mortensen, R. A. (1996). The architecture for an International Classification for Nursing Practice (ICNP). *International Nursing Review, 43*(6), 175-182.

Webster's II new Riverside dictionary. (1984). New York: Berkley Books.

Violence: A NANDA Nursing Diagnosis Targeted as a Universal Problem: One Proposal for Preventive Intervention

Marga Simon Coler, EdD, RN, CS, CTN, FAAN
Maria de Oliveria Ferreira Filha, MS, Enf
Gulten Ozalting, PhD, RN
Kim Lutzen, RN, PhD
Don Gorman, RN, DipNEd, BEd, MEd, EdD, FANZCMHN, FRCNA
Assumpta Rigol, MS, Enf
Nico Oud, RN, Dipl. N.Adm., MNSc

The concept of Violence had been targeted as a nursing diagnosis by the North American Nursing Diagnosis Association (NANDA) since 1980. It had undergone one revision in 1996 and is presently subdivided into two nursing diagnoses: Risk for Violence:Directed at Others and Risk for Violence: Self Directed

The focus of this paper will be on the further development of the diagnosis *Risk for Violence, Directed at Others*, with a proposition that the diagnosis should, once again, be studied, this time only two years after the revision of the original version. It is proposed, also, that the nursing diagnosis be expanded from its present definition: Behaviors in which an individual demonstrates that he/she can be physically, emotionally, and/or sexually harmful to others (NANDA, 1997). The diagnosis, the focus of nursing intervention, should also reflect, perhaps in an axis, or in the title, the client, i.e., the individual, family, group or community.

The challenge of this paper is to address the concept of violence in its entirety in the reality of 1998 by informing the audience of the work of a ten-member international group of leaders in psychiatric nursing. The conclusions of the ten-day conference are based on how violence is experienced and its global impact as an increasing mental health problem in all of the countries that were represented at the team residency (Argentina, Australia, Brazil, Chile, The Netherlands, Spain, Sweden, Turkey and the United States).

The Literature

Major sources in the identification of *violence* as a diagnosis of society were the empirical findings of international committees such as those which were published in two reports of the Pan American Health Organization (PAHO), entitled Development of Mental Health Nursing Services in the Countries of the Southern Cone (PAHO, 1995) and Analysis of the PAHO Mental Health Program (PAHO, 1995). The latter has been updated by the report resulting from the XL meeting of the Directing Council, entitled The Mental Health Program (PAHO, 1997).

The publication Development of Mental Health Nursing Services in the Countries of the Southern Cone (PAHO, 1995) lists violence as first in nine principle problems due to the socioeconomic, cultural and political conditioning factors which contribute to an increasing prevalence of mental health problems. The ensuing chronicity of persons with mental illness has led to the identification of multiple mental health problems among the mental hospital workforce which, in turn, has led to violence, born of frustration with the chronically mentally ill population as the scapegoat. The links in the chain of violence continue to rattle loudly, because of lack of continuing education/training programs for members of the mental health work force. This lack reinforces the traditional reliance on pharmacological restraining, continued long-term hospitalization, marginalization of the mentally ill with a denial of human rights, and continued chronification.

A review of the literature also showed that behavior (a key factor in defining the concept of violence), at the individual and collective level, has been de-emphasized for decades, probably because of the shift to a neurophysiological basis of mental illness. Still, individual and group behavior has recently been identified as a critical factor in four out of ten leading causes of death in developing countries and in six of the leading causes in the developed countries. (PAHO, 1997). As may be seen in the NANDA definition of the nursing diagnosis Risk for Violence, Directed at Others, "behaviors" is a key word in defining the NANDA concept.

A further look into violence literature shows that violence is a topic of utmost consideration at the societal level. "Collective violence" in the last few years of the twentieth century has been cited to be a disturbing universal reality by Desjarlais et al (1997). It is frequently directed at health care providers, and is a cause for the disruption of places and communities. Violence creates advere solidarity among the perpetrators thereby causing the victims to flee and abandon their community. This aggravates isolation and marginalization of the fleeing population causing a multiplicity of psychic trauma. Lost is the power of assertion and expression in society of the new refugee population (Desjarlais et al, 1997). Consequences are:

- Increased psychic trauma
- Loss of capacity to fend for self
- Deterioration of quality of life
- Disintegration of family
- Abandonment of children
- Displacement of population
- Dismemberment of social institutions

It may be noted that these phenomena are not Defining Characteristics, nor are they Risk Factors, nor Related Factors which are etiologic in nature. (Perhaps the word, Consequences, is missing from NANDA classification system!)

Desjarlais and his co-authors (1997) list "problems associated with Violence" that in NANDA protocol might be termed, Defining Characteristics. These are:

- Fear
- Loss of natural diversity (Deversa naturaleza)
- Feelings of guilt
- Anxiety
- Hatred
- Sadness
- Disintegration of daily social life

None of these appear as Defining Characteristics in the current NANDA diagnosis, Risk for Violence: Directed at Others.

Presently the NANDA listing focuses only on the individual, and is marked permanently by the qualifier "risk for." It is imperative to broaden the definition now, and to expand the hierarchy of violence diagnoses to include the concept of the aggregate.

According to the same authors, the methods of violence are directed toward an end of demoralizing and controlling a population. Examples are torture, terror, detention, creating the disappearances of individuals and/or groups, and disintegrating health services and educational institutions. Often, the adults affected by violence fight to maintain a sense of normalcy, well-being and social behavior; however, children, who have not yet developed sophisticated coping mechanisms, frequently suffer emotional illness, have frequent nightmares, and show signs of mental regression.

Violence begets violence. The children consequently often become aggressive, withdrawn, agitated, impatient, finally becoming aberrant, destructive adolescents and adults without a moral conscience (Desjarlais et al, 1997).

Development of the concept of violence

It is not surprising, then, in this decade of global turmoil and migration, that violence was targeted as one of three areas of need for the planning of pilot educational modules at the post-baccalaureate level by the international team of leaders in psychiatric/mental health nursing. The 10-day team residency, funded by the Rockefeller Foundation, was held in the Foundation's Study and Conference Center in Bellagio, Italy toward a goal of developing three post-basic educational modules that would meet the needs of all of the nine represented countries.

Figure 1

Violence, Societal (Turkey)		
Phenomena	Populations at Risk	Comments
Honor Saving (Punishment by DEATH)	WOMEN (considered property of family, husband)	Ex: *Marriage without consent of family * Extra-marital relationship
Blood Feuds (Punishment by DEATH)	MEN	Ex: *If a member of one family is killed, a member of that family has to kill the killer
Animal Sacrifice	ANIMALS (sheep, cows)	Ex: *Blood of an animal is smeared on the forehead of a person within full view of spectators to give thanks to God, protect from evil such as in marriage, business venture, buying of a new house, etc.

NOTE: Reactions to violence range from:
- TOLERANCE (Reaction thought to be due to feeling of HOPELESSNESS)
- REVENGE

Figure 2

Violence, Societal (Australia)		
Phenomena	Populations at Risk	Comments
Family violence	Women and children	Abuse of family members. There is increasing reporting of this but it is difficult to know if that equates to increased incidence.
Crimes involving violence	Homeowners, Shopkeepers	Burglary, robbery. This seems to be on the increase although police suggest it is not. There seem to be larger numbers of elderly homeowners being assaulted, often by young offenders and probably drug related.
Sexual violence	Women, girls	Rape [this includes incest but there is a growing preference to use the word rape as it more effectively describes the act].
Massacres	General public	Killing of numbers of people usually randomly chosen. This is relatively new in Australia but a recent event has raised social awareness enormously resulting in major gun law reform.

NOTE: Reactions to violence range from:
- TOLERANCE
- REVENGE
- SHOCK
- POLITICAL LOBBYING
- LAW REFORM

Figure 3

Violence, Societal (Spain)		
Phenomena	**Populations at Risk**	**Comments**
Abuse: 　Neglect 　Psychological 　Physical	Children: 　78.5% 　43.6% 　27.0%	Causes: 　Family disintegration, 20.3% 　Alcohol, 17.8% 　Drug addiction, 7.6%
Abuse in Marriage	Women (Decreased by 1100 (1990-1995)	•>200,000 are not respected as persons •Denied equality as prescribed by constitution •Physical violence seems to be giving way to verbal abuse (78.6% in 1995)
Abuse in Marriage	Men/Women	•Mistreatment of husband, 1.0% •Mutual aggression, 23.0% •Mistreatment of wife
Sexual Liberty	Women, Children	•Rape　29.72% •Sexual aggression　40.95% •Sexual provocation　17.69% •Corruption of children　1.75% •Incest　0.22% •Kidnapping　2.90%

NOTE:　Interpretation of Statistical Data must consider:

- Data analysis methodology of reporting institution
- Attitudes of the professional caregivers
- Violation of laws
- Discrimination
- Social environments (poverty, middle class, etc.)
- Politics
- Knowledge of laws
- Tolerance, attitudes of assessors toward social marginalization
- Intervention strategies (i.e., Teaching of prevention)
- Monitoring/Evaluating effects of intervention

Figure 4

Violence, Societal (Brazil)		
Phenomena	**Populations at Risk**	**Comments**
Attack with physical	All social classes, sexes, ages and mental aggression	•No official statistics on assaults available •Common knowledge that many people suffer everyday •A phenomenon that frightens everyone •Major victims are the middle class •The impunity that exists in majority of cases – >fear and insecurity
Homicide	All social classes, sexes, ages (especially youth)	•Statistics show more youths die by infliction from other youths (67%, <25 years old) •Homicides without reason ("pathological impotence") •65% due to arguments (husband and wife, neighbors, in street, in bars, collection of money)
Sexual violence	Women and children of any age and from all social classes	•One rape per hour •Statistics compiled from police registers only •Shame prevents victim from reporting violence •Increase in child prostitution (especially in the Northeast
Massacres	Rural workers without land, prisoners, homeless children	•Police massacres (clandestine and reported)

Figure 5

Violence, Societal (The Netherlands)*		
Phenomena	Populations at Risk	Comments
Violence:	Psychiatric Nurses	Perpetrator Population, Psychiatric Patients
•Aggressive behaviors	4%	Visitors
•Verbal aggression	80%	
•Threatening aggression	75%	
•Humiliating aggression	16%	
•Direct physical aggression with no or light injury	74%	
•Direct physical aggression with serious injury	8%	
•Destructive aggression	36%	

*Oud, N. (1997) *Information Brochure, "Aggression and psychiatric nursing."* (Unpublished manuscript)

After an orientation period where each member presented a profile of psychiatric/mental health nursing education and practice in their country (Figures 1-5), the team began its task of curriculum formulation. An analysis of the status quo of each country followed so that commonalties could be identified. Societal debilitating factors affecting community mental health were listed and tabulated by country. It was apparent that there was an increasing prevalence of mental health problems as a response to the changing social structure, and that the role of mental health nursing needed to change concurrently. The trend in all countries was shifting from an emphasis on the individual to that of a community, societal focus. New mental health nursing issues seemed to evolve in the context of a complex and rapidly changing political, economical and social world. Mental health nursing would increasingly focus on diagnosing and intervening in the ills of society such as political repression from which spring fear and violence. It was noted also that mental health nursing would be dealing with the increase of mental illness and substance abuse due to social violence. The diagnosis Violence became apparent as mental health issues were listed by country. At times violence was listed as such, at times it was shrouded by issues of homelessness, substance abuse, suicide, post-traumatic stress disorder, etc. The identification of universal problems continued as the group set out to order and prioritize their nine-country findings.

The findings were categorized into an umbrella category called "Epidemiological Status" which was subdivided into Conventional Categories (DSM-IV diagnoses) and Non-conventional Categories such as societal findings. From this small group work, the Social Mental Health Framework (Figure 6) with its theoretical Paradigm (Figure 7) were developed to guide the pilot graduate modules which were selected from a Lickert-type rating of the most prevalent identified issues in each country. Violence was identified as one. This module became the one which over the ensuing months of refinement was addressed by the majority of team members. The three identified modules were developed generically according to the curriculum formula developed by Burns,

Figure 6

Mental Health Social Paradigm

-THEORETICAL FRAMEWORK-
Bellagio International Group for Mental Health Nursing

INTRODUCTION

The Social Paradigm of Mental Health is a complex of concept, which emerged from the teamwork of ten scholars in mental health nursing representing nine countries from four continents, at the Bellagio Center of the Rockefeller Foundation. From this paradigm, three generic post-graduate curriculum modules for advanced practice nursing were developed which will be tailored to be culture-specific by each scholar.

In this framework, the Social Concept of Mental Health is defined as social processes developed toward sub-jective and intersubjective well being of individual, family, group and community within society. It is affected by natural and social factors, which are linked by specific operational components (biological, cultural, ecological, economic, educational, ethical, organizational, political, psychological, and scientific). These components are linked to the objectives on which the post-graduate educational modules are based. Mental Health is a vital component of Health, both of which are affected by society and the environment.

The goal of the Paradigm is to illustrate the promotion and protection of mental health, the prevention of mental problems and, finally, the promotion of the concept of caring by mental health nurses. It is defined by three structuring theoretical components: Society, Health, and Mental Health.

The Theoretical Components

SOCIETY

1. SOCIETY is not homogenous, nor uniform, nor an harmonic totality.
2. SOCIETY is characterized by several kinds of inequities related to life conditions in a particular time and space.
3. Consequently, SOCIETY is an integration of social groups with different styles and qualities of life, with different interests, ideas, capabilities and powers. Those differences produce contradictions and con-flicts, which are natural and central components of the structure and dynamic of social life.
4. SOCIAL PROCESSES are historic, dynamic, complex, discontinuous, uncertain, ambiguous, conflictive, contradictory and are determined by multiple interactive factors. SOCIAL PROCESSES are mobilized by power relationships. They determine the possibility of access to health services including those of health maintenance and illness prevention.

The complex of social factors that — with natural factors — influence health may be classified into *biological, environmental, ecological, historical, cultural, socio-economic, political, scientific, technical factors* and as *factors emerging from the organizing of health system and services.* These factors interact with and are mobilized by power relationships which, in turn, determine and condition the process of health and illness.

Figure 6 *(continued)*

HEALTH

1. HEALTH is social determined process and, from the individual perspective, is also a subjective state of being, influenced by society. Therefore, it is social, subject to societal politics in a particular time and in a particular culture.
2. HEALTH is a historical-social process, relative to style and quality of life of populations. It is linked to the conditions of accessibility, to various kinds of wealth (cultural, economical, political, geographic, affective, spiritual and others) in every place and at all times.
3. The "STATE OF HEALTH" of an individual, group or population is reflected in the scientific statements of, and influenced by the subjectivity of the individuals or groups defining this state. It is further a social expression of a complex of factors in a particular time and culture that also can be considered as indicators of the state of the health.
4. The PROCESS OF HEALTH-ILLNESS is expressed, not only in a variety of problems of illness and risk, but also in different conditions of daily life and social relationships.

MENTAL HEALTH

1. The FIELD OF MENTAL HEALTH is still unknown and unrecognized in many cultures. Therefore, it needs to be developed as a complex and transdisciplinary field focusing on the comprehension of subjectivity, singularity and differences within and between individuals and groups, thereby promoting an understanding of the complexity of healthy and unhealthy conditions of social life and processes.
2. From the perspective of quality of mental life, MENTAL HEALTH can be defined as a historically-determined social process characterized by the integration of the fundamental and conflictive elements of individuals and groups, with several kind of crises that can be subjectively and objectively assessed. Through this process individuals and groups actively participate in changes on themselves, their groups, and on the their social environment. MENTAL HEALTH is one components of holistic health of the individual, along with physical and social health.
3. From an etiologic point of view, MENTAL HEALTH may be defined as a process determined and conditioned by a complex of factors: biological, environmental, ecological, historical, cultural, socio-economic, political, scientific, technical factors, and as factors emerging from the organizing of health system and services. All of these factors are interrelated.
4. From the political point of view MENTAL HEALTH is a social subject which is reflected in the relations between State and Health. It is one of the principal points of political responsibility of a legal system that promotes citizenship, freedom, democracy and solidarity, and that condemns discrimination, exclusion and violation of human rights.
5. From a scientific and epistemological point of view, MENTAL HEALTH is comprised of elements of theory of many academic fields, especially those related to health and illness. Because of its integration, it is neither possible nor convenient to limit its field.
6. MENTAL HEALTH CARE is defined as a complex of activities based on cultural and scientific theory that has, as its principal goal, the promotion protection, destabilization and rehabilitation of individuals and groups. Ideally mental health care involves the participation of all actors involved in the process. MENTAL HEALTH CARE has as its focus the society that can be pointed as individuals, families, groups and communities.
7. MENTAL HEALTH CARE includes a complex of health, socio-cultural, scientific, political, economic and organizational measures. Its mission is oriented to link it with general health systems and services developing a net of community services, as opposed to the still existing custodial psychiatric hospitals. The MENTAL HEALTH SYSTEM has to be articulated and integrated with all other areas of social life.
8. QUALIFICATION AND EDUCATION of mental health professionals, technicians and workers, is a structuring and mobilizing factor in the provision of mental health services. They are vital components in generating and developing changes and transformation in mental health values concepts, practices and services.

Figure 7

Social Mental Health Paradigm

Processes determining
Mental Health (MH)/MH Problems

HEALTH / ILLNESS PROCESS

Processes
Factors
Objectives

Science

Natural Processes
Biological
/ 3,10
Environmental
/ 6,8,10,20
Ecological
/ 6,8,10,20

Social Processes
Existential
/ 6,10,12,18,19
Psychological
/ 9
Cultural
/ 8,9,14
Economical
/ 6
Political
/ 9,10,15,16,21
Scientific
/ 10,11,12,13,17
Educational
/ 4,6,7,11,12,13
Organizational
(Services)
/ 5

Focus
Individual
/ 4,5,9
Family → Groups
(developmental, other)
/ 4,5,9
Society
(Institutions)
/ 4,5,6,7,8,9,10,14,16,17,20

GOALS
Goals
Promoting
Mental Health
/ 3,4,5,6,7,10,14,20
Preventing
Mental Illness
/ 3,4,5,6,7,8,10,14,20
Caring
/ 4,6,9,13,14

Other Considerations
Attitudes
Beliefs
Human values/value system
Related to
mental illness

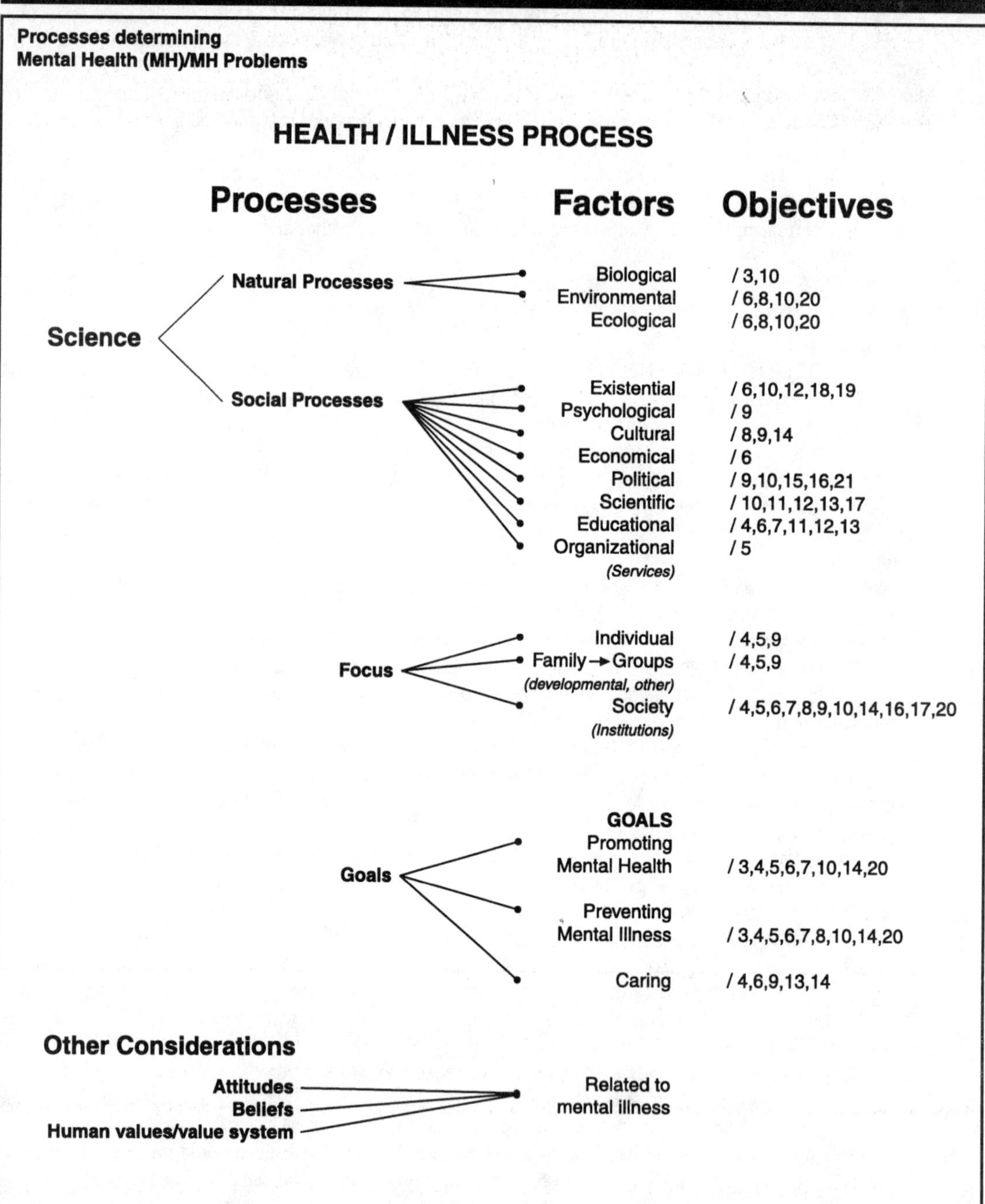

Figure 8

**Federal University of Paraiba
Master's Program
Health and Community Development
Chronogram of Classes**

Date	Subject
8/20/97	The community as a client • Definition of community • Concept of community • Concepts of population/subpopulation
8/27/97	•Identification of common health/mental health problems •Vulnerable subpopulations to the impacts of VIOLENCE; CHRONICITY; CULTURE
9/3/97	•Independent nursing practice •Health promotion, maintenance, illness prevention
9/17/98	•Nursing Diagnoses (NANDA/ICN) • Formulation • Validation • Communication (colleagues, community leaders, community as a client)
9/24/97	•VIOLENCE, a nursing diagnosis of an aggregate
10/1/97	•CHRONICITY...as a potential aggregate nursing diagnosis
10/08/97	•Transcultural Competence as an essential for Community/Aggregate focused nursing
10/15/97	•Population-based nursing interventions through nursing diagnoses •Defining Population/based Outcomes
10/22/97	•Evaluation Strategies • formative • summative
10/29-11/26/97	•Practica
12/3, 12/10	•Presentation of student projects

The authors gratefully acknowledge the contribution to the modules of the remainder of the BIGmh team: Prof. Silvina Malvarez, Argentina, Dr. Jeanne Clement, U.S.A., Prof. Sylvia Raffo, Chile, and the Rockefeller Foundation for its financial support, and the Bellagio staff for their "resource" support services.

Thompson & Ciccone (1993) before the team disbanded (Bellagio Notes, 1997).

The societal post-graduate curriculum module on violence has been culturally refined and translated into a free-standing module in Brazil and Turkey. Culture-specific violence factors are being identified by students, faculty and practicing nurses. Most of the team members have adapted the modular material into existing graduate course in a generic manner (see Figure 8). It is from these efforts and the proliferation of violence data in the literature the authors recommend to NANDA the expansion of the violence diagnoses into a major category called Violence, which might include a modification of the two existing individual-based diagnoses to include an aggregate and crisis-based focus to identify the many subpopulations who wake up to threats of violence every day. The aggregate might be a family, a specific group of persons or a community. The aggregate might be identified as an axis as was proposed by the 1992 NANDA Taxonomy Committee, perhaps as a segment of the title.

Ideally, the title of the existing NANDA diagnoses on violence should be stripped of the qualifiers "At Risk For" and toward whom it is directed. A diagnostic title should begin in a pure simple form, and then be built to qualify. With such thinking, the violence modules that are being multiculturally refined can contribute to the pure diagnostic concept of Violence. Because of the paradigm and framework that went into the development of the module the evolving diagnostic term will have a societal focus. As a nursing diagnosis, it could be titled Violence and qualified as Societal.

Somewhere in the development of aggregate-based nursing diagnoses the target population (the recipients of diagnosis-based nursing intervention) must also be identified, perhaps as the perpetrator population and/or perhaps as the victim population. Each population would have a different set of Defining Characteristics or Risk factors. Etiology/Related Factors could be the same; consequences would be decidedly different.

The definition of an aggregate-based, societal nursing diagnosis could, even at this juncture, be developed from what in the generic Bellagio module was termed Rationale, in which the terms, socially destructive, nonadaptive, frustration, anger, aggression, learned behavior, expression of conflictive social relationships or conditions. These could also be worked into an operational definition.

The title, definition and qualifiers provide cues to intervention protocol, which, according to the Bellagio group (BIGmhn) would be directed at three levels: the general population, the at risk population and the crisis population. The nurse (in case of the BIGmhn, the mental health nurse) has the social responsibility to intervene in government (social policy and legislation), community, institutions, the family and the individual (Bellagio notes, 1997) through primary, secondary and tertiary prevention. However, before the nurse focuses on the aggregate a special type of primary prevention must occur, that of educating the care providers. It is this facet the module on Violence will address in the nine countries through post basic graduate education.

In summary, the development, the synthesis, of an aggregate-based nursing diagnosis is a very multifaceted undertaking. Giving the diagnosis an international and multicultural perspective adds challenges. Yet, in the twenty-first century NANDA must begin thinking beyond "North American" and the "individual." Nursing diagnoses are and should be an important outcome of the Alma Ata Declaration of Health for all by the year 2000.

An offshoot of the culture-specific refinement of the generic BIGmhn modules would be for the team, or the NANDA members on the team to sort their new data into Defining Characteristics and/or Risk Factors. This will be a task for the future, for the team is still in the data-gathering stage. However, because of the many findings reported in the literature which relate to the global, societal concept of violence, and because of the rich representation of the 10 experts in mental health nursing working on the concept, it behooves the membership of NANDA to consider broadening and updating the two to specific individual-based nursing diagnoses on violence. Nursing as a profession must leave the comfort of a single institution (academia or the health center) to become actively involved in diagnosing and combating violence, locally, regionally, nationally and globally; to find and label infractions, to diagnose them and to intervene in them through prevention and support within the realm of the nursing profession.

References

Bellagio International Group for Mental Health Nursing. (1997). *Note of Meetings.* Bellagio, Italy

Burns, E., Thompson,A., & Ciccone, J. (1993). *An addictions curriculum for nurses and other helping professional (The graduate level: Advanced knowledge and practice)* (pp.1-11). New York: The Springer Publishing Co.

Desjarlais, R., Eisenberg, L., Good, B., Kleinman, A. (1997) *Salud Mental en el Mundo: Problemas y prioridades en poblaciones de bajos ingresos.* Washington, DC: PALTEX.

North American Nursing Diagnosis Association (NANDA). (1997). *NANDA nursing diagnoses: Definitions & classification, 1997-1998.* Philadelphia, PA: NANDA

Pan American Health Organization (PAHO). (1997). *The mental health program in the XL meeting of the directing council.* Washington, DC: PAHO.

Pan American Health Organization (PAHO). (1995). *Analysis of the PAHO mental health program.* Washington, DC: PAHO.

Pan American Health Organization (PAHO). (1995). *Development of mental health nursing services in countries of the southern cone.* Washington, DC: PAHO

Evolving Model of Clinical and Ethical Judgment (abstract)

Kate Sullivan Collopy
Joan M. Agretelis

The generation of patient phenomena of concern is a complex and evolving process. It includes the patient and nurse in dynamic interaction. Judgements resulting from assessment data obtained through this interaction reflect a synthesis of cues and concepts that have emerged both verbally and non-verbally through the experience.

Clinical and ethical decision-making models have traditionally been represented as linear in approach. Gordon, Murphy, Candee and Hiltmen (1994) described an integrative model of clinical and ethical judgment of hypothesis. The purpose of this paper is to expand upon Gordon et al.'s existing integrative model of clinical and ethical judgment to include an interactive nursing dimension focusing on intentional presencing with the patient.

The goal of nursing is to interact with the patient purposefully to understand the patient's experience. This added dimension of the interactive model is a logical extension of a more theoretical approach to decision making and information processing. The importance of adding this component is to explicitly articulate the fundamental nature of the patient-nurse relationship in mutual decision-making.

Use of this more intuitive, inductive model will foster linkage between theory and practice, with the potential for increasing accuracy of diagnostic and clinical judgments via purposeful engagement. Exemplars of the mutual information processing approach to diagnostic reasoning and clinical and ethical judgment will be presented to underscore the utility of the revised model in daily nursing practice.

Nursing Diagnosis Extension and Classification (NDEC) Report

*NDEC Research Team**
Principal Investigators:
Martha Craft-Rosenberg, PhD, RN, FAAN
Connie Delaney, PhD, RN
Janice Denehy, PhD, RN

The Iowa Nursing Diagnosis Extension and Classification team (NDEC) has been working in a collaborative agreement with NANDA for four years (Craft-Rosenberg & Delaney, 1997). The aims for the research are to: (a) refine the existing NANDA diagnoses; (b) extend the list of diagnoses; (c) validate the diagnoses; (d) classify the diagnoses; and (e) validate the classification. The purpose of this discussion is to report on the work completed as of Spring, 1998, the work in progress, and the work planned for the future.

Work Completed

The NDEC research team consists of 24 investigators with diverse clinical expertise and diverse research perspectives.* Investigators serve as chairs and members of 10 Diagnosis Work Groups (DWGs) for the diagnosis refinement process. During the past three years a total of 65 nurses who are considered experts on a certain patient phenomena (diagnosis) have participated in concept analysis of existing diagnoses. In turn, each of the three principal investigators has supervised and monitored a group of DWGs during the concept analysis process.

The protocol for concept analysis is a synthesis of methods proposed by Rogers and Knafl (1993) and Waltz, Strickland, and Lenz (1991). The step-by-step protocol ** was developed to: (a) state the criteria for literature (data) identification and selection for concept analysis; (b) describe the extent to which the selected literature (data) represented health across the health status continuum, populations, developmental stages, and units of care (individual, family, or community); and (c) assist the DWG members in the identification of a diagnosis label, a diagnosis definition, defining characteristics (which we are calling signs and symptoms upon agreement with the NANDA board), and related factors.

DWG members reviewed and synthesized the literature to formulate their recommendations for refinement. Refinement recommendations were sent to the NDEC Rules committee to be edited for conformity to language rules developed by the research team.** Following review and necessary modification, the entire team reviewed the refined diagnoses for: (a) validity; (b) clarity; (c) internal consistency; (d) relevance for clinical practice; and (e) utility for clinicians to identify outcomes and interventions.

The products of NDEC work at this point have been a protocol for refining diagnoses using concept analysis, language rules for refinement or development of nursing diagnoses, 77 refined and new diagnoses, and a pool of candidate diagnoses. A packet of diagnoses was submitted to the NANDA Diagnosis Review Committee in November, 1997.

Another very important "product" of our work has been the networking established with the International Classification of Nursing Practice (ICNP). The principal investigators have consulted with leaders in the ICNP work and will continue to meet with them as requested.

Work in Progress

Currently, the NDEC team is finishing the last refinement work on the existing NANDA diagnoses while the principal investigators are planning the next aim of research, which is to extend the list of diagnoses. This extension will be facilitated by the addition of several satellite DWGs working on diagnoses for: (a) clients of advanced practice nurses; (b) neonatal and perinatal patients; (c) patients who are elderly; (d) patients with neuromuscular conditions; (e) nutrition diagnoses; and (f) spiritual diagnoses. In addition, the first international NDEC satellite DWG has been established in England.

The methodology for development of candidate diagnoses is being discussed and developed. At this point the investigators have approved several steps. First, candidate diagnoses submitted by members of the satellite DWG will be added to the candidate pool consisting of diagnoses submitted by the DWGs and a list of candidate diagnoses developed during pilot research (Manuscript in progress). Second, the investigators will examine the resulting list (approximately 400) of candidate diagnoses, with investigators being assigned a group of labels to match their expertise. Redundancy will be identified and removed by team consensus. If the team is uncertain as to the extent to which diagnoses are redundant, simultaneous concept analysis (Haase, Leidey, Coward, Britt, & Penn, 1993) will be used.

The resulting list will then be compared to other diagnostic classifications in order to determine if the diagnosis already exists and does not need to be developed. These classifications will include the DSMIV, the ICD9, and the Omaha (Martin & Sheet, 1992) and Saba (Saba, 1992) lists. This comparison will be done on a computerized data base when possible, using word search capabilities. Last, the linkage of NIC (Iowa Intervention Project (1996) and NOC (Iowa Outcomes Project, 1997) to NANDA diagnoses that has been completed and the relationship of NANDA labels to the CPT code will be studied to identify other possible diagnostic labels. The candidate diagnoses that remain after determination that they do not already exist and that they are independent phenomena from existing diagnoses will be developed by the research team using the same concept analysis methods that were used for refinement of diagnoses.

While the NDEC team is finishing Aim 1 and planning for Aim 2, expert validation and clinical validation of the refined NANDA diagnoses is beginning. The questionnaire for expert validation is being tested for reliability and validity with expert clinicians who are in the graduate program at The University of Iowa College of

Nursing. Data are being collected over E-mail. In addition, expert validation of diagnosis concepts for the elderly and their linkage to NIC interventions and NOC outcomes is being planned during this next year.

One site for clinical validation is already testing the revised NANDA diagnoses and three other sites have been identified. These sites include two large teaching hospitals, a community hospital, and a public health nursing setting. The methodology for clinical validation will be that proposed and tested by Delaney, Memhert, and colleagues (Delaney & Mehmert, 1990; Delaney & Mehmert, 1991).

Work Panned for the Future

Work planned for the future includes the completion of refinement, the extension of the diagnosis list, the validation of the diagnosis concepts, the classification of the extended list of diagnoses, and the validation of the classification.

This next year the NDEC research team will determine the psychometric properties of our questionnaire for expert validation and then collect data using a Web site. The team also plans to move forward with clinical validation and the identification of candidate diagnoses which need to be developed. The development of candidate diagnoses can be done with team and satellite DWGs. The satellite DWGs will work together with other NDEC investigators with a Web Chat Room for satellite DWGs who have Web access, or through e-mail, which is being used currently.

The NDEC work has been funded by a small internal seed grant from the University of Iowa and the University of Iowa College of Nursing. Therefore, work for the future will also include submission of grant proposals for external funding.

In summary, the NDEC work that began with the negotiation between a large research team and a professional organization is beginning to become visible. The methods, procedures, and relationships that have developed through the processes of the past five years will be the repository of knowledge and skills required for the next five years of work.

*Investigators on the NDEC research team include Joanne Chapman, M.A., R.N.; Judith Collins, M.A., R.N.; Dame June Clark, Ph.D., R.N.; Mary Clarke, M.A., R.N.; Carolyn Crowell, M.A., R.N.; Mary Pat Donahue, Ph.D., R.N., F.A.A.N; Orpha Glick, Ph.D., R.N.; Cyd Graff, M.S., R.N.; Jone Johnson, M.S.N., R.N.; Kathleen Hansen, Ph.D., R.N.; Deborah Jensen, Ph.D., R.N., Leslie Marshall, Ph.D., R.N.; Meridean Maas, Ph.D., R.N., F.A.A.N; Sandra Powell, Ph.D., R.N.; Colleen Prophet, M.S., R.N.; Jean Reese, Ph.D., RN., LaVonne Ruther, M.A., R.N.; Lu Sheehy, B.S.N. with research assistants Jane Tang, B.S.N. and Joseph Greiner, M.A., R.N.

**Available from the investigators upon request.

References

Craft-Rosenberg, M., & Delaney, C. (1997). Nursing diagnosis extension and classification (NDEC). In M. Rantz & P. LeMone (Eds.). *Classification of nursing diagnoses: Proceedings of the twelfth conference, North American Nursing Diagnosis Association.* Glendale, CA: CINAHL.

Delaney, C., & Mehmert, P. (1990). *Electronic transfer of clinical NMDs facilitates nursing diagnosis validation. {Paper}. In Proceedings of the Fourteenth Annual Symposium on Computer Applications i Medical care*

(*SCAMC*). Washington, DC: IEEE Computer Society Press.

Delaney, C., & Mehmert, P. (1991). Utility of NMDS is validation of computerized nursing diagnoses. In R. Carroll-Johnson (Ed.), *Classification of nursing diagnoses: Proceedings of the ninth conference, North American Nursing Diagnosis Association.* Philadelphia: Lippincott.

Haase, J.E., Leidy, N.K., Coward, D.D., Britt, T., & Penn, P.E. (1993). *Simultaneous concept analysis: A strategy for developing multiple interrelated concepts. In Concept development in nursing: Foundations, techniques, and applications.* Philadelphia: W. B. Saunders Company.

Iowa Intervention Project. (1996). *Nursing interventions classification (NIC).* J. McCloskey & Bulecheck, G. (Eds.) (2nd. ed). St. Louis: Mosby.

Iowa Outcomes Project (1997). *Nursing outcomes classification (NOC).* M. Johnson & M. Maas (Eds). St. Louis: Mosby.

Rodgers, B.L., & Knafl, K.A. (1993). *Concept development in nursing: Foundations, techniques, and applications.* Phildadelphia: W. B. Saunders.

Waltz, C. F., Strickland,O., & Lenz, E. (1991). *Measurement in nursing research.* Philadelphia: F.A. Davis.

Conceptual and Structural Issues Related to Implementation of Nursing Diagnoses, Interventions, and Outcomes Classifications in Clinical Nursing Information Systems (abstract)

Connie Delaney, PhD, RN

Nursing's need to have data repositories representative of client care delivered by nurses is unequivocal. Major efforts to develop and implement standardized nursing languages to describe this contribution make the reality of large data repositories tangible. Likewise, the initial work of Delaney, Ryan, Coenen, and Moorhead to develop methods for retrieving and analyzing nursing data from large computerized repositories supports nursing's long-term goal of using clinical data to support policy development and evaluation. The purpose of this paper is to discuss the conceptual and structural issues related to the nurse diagnoses (NANDA), interventions (NIC), and outcomes (NOC) classifications; issues that have become apparent as these nursing classifications are refined and implemented within computerized clinical nursing information systems. Conceptual issues include diagnosis, intervention and outcome definitions, interdisciplinary access and use, health/wellness/prevention foci, and global applicability. Structural issues focus on clinical information system design, associations within each classification, and linkages and associations among the classifications.

Categorization of States According to Trendsetting, Contemporary, or Traditional Definitions of the Practice of Professional Nursing

Mary Ann Lavin, ScD, RN, CS, ANP, FAAN

Geralyn Meyer, MS(N), RN, CS

Judith H. Carlson, MSN, RN, CS, GNP

This study was supported by the Saint Louis University School of Nursing Research Fund.

Since Florence Nightingale began her work to improve the quality of health care, the status of the nursing profession has made great strides. One example of its growth is the legal acceptance of nursing as a distinct profession. In their analysis of the legal aspects of nursing, Lesnik and Anderson (1947) report that nursing licensure was proposed in 1899. The first state to enact a licensure law was North Carolina in 1903. Lesnik and Anderson did more than report history, however. They also provided a critique of what nursing is not. At that time, it was common for nursing licensure laws to state that nurses do not diagnose. Lesnik and Anderson (1947) challenged this practice by stating, "Although diagnosis has been long regarded as the province of the physician, there is current belief, and support for that belief, that this province warrants clarification insofar as the activities of nursing are concerned" (p. 157).

Legislative clarification began in 1972 with the passage of a revised nurse practice act in state of New York. This act defined nursing as "diagnosing and treating human responses to actual or potential health problems through such means as case finding, health teaching and counseling" (Bullough, 1975, p. 160). The New York State Practice Act became a prototype for many of the state practice acts that followed.

This view of nurses as diagnosticians was echoed in the move to more effectively communicate nursing's domain by means of labeling and classifying nursing diagnoses. The systematic organization of these diagnoses began in 1973 when Gebbie and Lavin of Saint Louis University called the First National Conference on the Classification of Nursing Diagnoses. The major goals of the first conference were to generate labels or names of diagnoses and to begin ordering them in a framework.

The North American Nursing Diagnosis Association (NANDA) grew out of the National Clearinghouse for Nursing Diagnoses formed at the First National Conference. NANDA's mission was to develop, refine, and promote a taxonomy of nursing diagnoses to be used by the professional nurse. In concert with that mission, the organization established a definition of nursing diagnosis: "Nursing diagnosis is a clinical judgment about individual, family or community responses to actual or potential health problems/life processes. Nursing diagnosis provides the basis for selection of nursing interventions to achieve outcomes for which the nurse is accountable" (NANDA, 1996, p. 8).

One measure of the success of NANDA's mission is the growing number of nursing diagnosis associations in Asia, Europe, and Latin America. Another measure of its success is the fact that nursing diagnosis is a legally recognized concept, incorporated into the definition of nursing or into the definition of the practice of professional nursing within the nurse practice acts of 33 of the 50 states of the United States. An examination of these definitions revealed that newer trends in terminology were emerging also. The purpose of this study was twofold. The authors sought to: (a) categorize state nurse practice acts according to their trendsetting, contemporary, or traditional approach to nursing; and (b) examine variations in the focus of nursing diagnosis in the states in which it is used.

Methods

Nurse practice acts from the 50 states were studied. A preliminary review revealed: (a) inclusion of the term "diagnosis" within the context of the practice of professional nursing in many of the acts, and (b) considerable variation in how the term was used. Differences were also apparent in the use of related terms such as "treatment" and "prescribe." To capture these similarities and differences, the practice acts were divided into three operational categories: trendsetters, contemporary, or traditional.

Trendsetters were defined as practice acts

that employed the term "nursing diagnosis" (or the term "diagnosis" within a nursing context) along with concepts relatively new to nursing. These newer concepts included the terms: (a) treatment in lieu of interventions, (b) prescribe in lieu of words such as, institute or implement, and (c) disease as an object of nursing diagnoses.

Contemporary nurse practice acts included the term "diagnosis" within the framework of nursing but did not include trendsetting concepts.

Traditional nurse practice acts did not use the term "diagnosis" in a nursing context.

Using these definitions, three nurse researchers independently categorized the state practice acts. Full agreement among all three researchers was evident in the categorization of 40 of the 50 practice acts. Ratings on the 10 remaining practice acts were negotiated among the researchers until 100% consensus was reached. In this manner, interrater agreement was established.

Contemporary and trendsetting practice acts were further subdivided according to variations in their descriptions of the focus of nursing diagnosis and their use or nonuse of NANDA-based terminology.

Results

Trendsetters

Using the previously described criteria, 13 or 26% of the state nurse practice acts were identified as trendsetting: Alaska, California, Colorado, Kansas, Iowa, Maine, Nevada, New Jersey, New York, Oklahoma, Oregon, Pennsylvania, and Vermont. Except for California, all included the term "diagnosis" within the definition of the practice of professional nursing. California included the term under a statement on the standards of competent performance of registered nurses.

In addition to incorporating nursing diagnosis into their nurse practice acts, trendsetting states also used the terms "treatment" or "prescribing" within a nursing context or identified disease as an object of nursing diagnosis. Eleven of the 13 trendsetting states used the term "treatment" within a nursing context: California, Colorado, Kansas, Iowa, Maine, Nevada, New Jersey, New York, Oklahoma, Oregon, and Pennsylvania. An example is Iowa's Nurse Practice Act, which states that registered nurses "formulate nursing diagnosis and conduct nursing treatment of human responses to actual or potential health problems" (Iowa Board of Nursing, 1997, p. 1334).

Two of the 13 trendsetting states used the term "prescribing" within the context of nursing. Vermont speaks of "prescribing nursing interventions to implement the strategy of care" (Vermont Board of Nursing, 1994, p. 1). In Alaska's Nurse Practice Act, a listing of professional acts of service performed by registered nurses includes "the prescription of medical therapeutic or corrective measures under regulations adopted by the board" (Alaska Division of Occupational Licensing, 1996, p. 12).

Two of the 13 trendsetting states (Alaska and Colorado) used the term "disease" as the object of nursing diagnosis. Colorado's Practice Act (Colorado Board of Nursing, 1995, p. 2) defines the professional practice of nursing as including the performance of "independent nursing functions and delegated medical functions in accordance with accepted practice standards." Among other activities this includes the "diagnosis and treatment of human disease, ailment, pain, injury, deformity, and physical or mental conditions." Alaska's states that the practice of registered nursing includes "performance of acts of medical diagnosis... under regulations adopted by the board" (Alaska Division of Occupational Licensing, 1996, p. 12).

Contemporary

Of the 50 nurse practice acts, 20 or 40% used the term "diagnosis" within a nursing context, but avoided terms such as "nursing treatment" or "prescribing" nursing therapy. None considered disease to be an object of nursing diagnoses. These 20 practice acts, categorized as contemporary, are: Connecticut, Delaware, Florida, Georgia, Illinois, Indiana, Kentucky, Louisiana, Maryland, Mississippi, Missouri, Nebraska, New Hampshire, New Mexico, North Dakota, South Carolina, South Dakota, Texas, Washington, and Wyoming. An example of a contemporary definition includes New Hampshire's definition of registered nursing as the "assessment and diagnosis of people's physical and psychosocial health status" (New Hampshire Board of Nursing, 1997, 326-B:2). Illinois' definition of registered professional nursing, amended during the State's 1997-1998 Ninetieth General Assembly, includes "the assessment of health care needs, nursing diagnosis, planning, implementation and nursing evaluation" (Illinois Department of Professional Regulation, Amended 1997-1998, LRB9001265LDcw, line 159).

Traditional

Seventeen (34%) of the practice acts were categorized as traditional because they did not use the term "nursing diagnosis" nor recognize diagnosis as a nursing act: Alabama, Arizona, Arkansas, Hawaii, Idaho, Massachusetts, Michigan, Minnesota, Montana, North Carolina, Ohio, Rhode Island, Tennessee, Utah, Virginia, West Virginia, and Wisconsin.

Several of the acts, identified as traditional, actually substituted another term for "diagnosis," thus forming a subcategory called "ambivalently traditional" by the researchers. Eight practice acts fell within this subcategory: Alabama, Idaho, Massachusetts, Michigan, Montana, North Carolina, Ohio, and Utah. Two examples serve to illustrate the word or phrase substitution employed. Massachusetts' act substitutes the phrase "clinical decision making" for diagnosis. It states that "nursing practice involves clinical decision making leading to the development and implementation of a strategy of care" (Massachusetts Board of Registration in Nursing, 1994, p. 86). Montana's act substitutes "nursing analysis" for nursing diagnoses. It states that the practice of professional nursing means the use of "assessment, nursing analysis, planning, nursing interventions, and evaluation in the promotion of health" (Montana State Board of Nursing, 1996, p. 42).

A few of the "ambivalently traditional" practice acts incorporated newer nursing terminology but were classified as ambivalently traditional because they avoided the use of the term "diagnosis." For example, had "diagnosis" been included, Michigan's definition of nursing practice would have been categorized as a trendsetter because it employs the term "treatment" in its definition of professional nursing. Likewise, Idaho's practice act, which substitutes "identifying" for "diagnosing," would have been categorized as a trendsetter because it uses the term "prescribe" within a nursing context.

Practice acts in nine states did not reflect the concept of nursing diagnosis in any manner. This subcategory of traditional practice acts was called "traditionally traditional" by the researchers. Wisconsin's definition of the practice of professional nursing typifies the content in these acts. It states:

The practice of professional nursing within the limits of this chapter means the performance for compensation of any act in the observation or care of the ill, injured or infirm, or for the maintenance of health or prevention of illness of others, which act requires substantial nursing skill, knowledge or training, or application of nursing principles based on biological, physical and social sciences... (Wisconsin Statutes, 1995, p. 3856).

There is no attempt in this definition to use substitute words for "diagnosis" nor is there reference to the nursing process nor newer nursing terminology, such as "treatment" or "prescribe." It is representative of the other eight traditionally traditional practice acts unchanged by the nursing diagnosis movement: Arizona, Arkansas, Hawaii, Minnesota, Rhode Island, Tennessee, Virginia, and West Virginia.

Language Issues Surrounding Nursing Diagnosis

The "who and what" of a diagnosis may be called the diagnostic focus. Physicians diagnose the disease states of individuals; nurses diagnose the "responses of the individual, family, or community responses to actual or potential health problems and/or life processes" (NANDA, 1996, p. 8). Using this logic, the "what" of medical diagnosis is disease and the "what" of nursing diagnosis is response. In like manner, the "who" of medical diagnosis is the individual, while the "who" of nursing diagnosis is the "individual, family, or community. This section examines the focus of nursing diagnosis in trendsetting and contemporary nurse practice acts, looking first at variations on NANDA's themes and secondly at other variations.

The "what" of nursing diagnosis. A review of the trendsetting and contemporary practice acts revealed that several relied, at least in part, upon the NANDA definition when describing the "what" or the grammatical object of nursing diagnosis. Practice acts were operationally defined as NANDA-based insofar as they identified the object of nursing diagnoses to be responses to actual or potential health problems. Of the 13 trendsetting nurse practice acts, seven (Iowa, Maine, New Jersey, New York, Oklahoma, Oregon, and Pennsylvania) were categorized as having NANDA-based objects of nursing diagnosis.

Of the 20 contemporary nurse practice acts, five were considered to have NANDA-based objects of nursing diagnosis (Connecticut, North Dakota, South Carolina, South Dakota, and Wyoming). The majority of the contemporary practice acts used the following terms for the "what" or object of diagnosis: health care needs (Georgia, Illinois, Louisiana); needs (Delaware, Indiana, and Nebraska); health concerns (Kentucky); health status (New Hampshire, New Mexico, Texas); and responses to illness, injury or infirmity (Mississippi). Four states (Florida, Maryland, Missouri, Washington) did not specify any particular object of nursing diagnosis.

The "who" of nursing diagnosis. The "who" or the recipients of nursing diagnoses, according to NANDA, are individuals, families, and communities. None of the trendsetting practice acts utilized the terms individual, family, and community, however. Many modified the word "responses" only by the term "human" (Iowa, Maine, New Jersey, New York, Oklahoma, Oregon, Pennsylvania).

Contemporary practice acts demonstrated more variation in specifying the "who" of nursing diagnosis. Eight of these acts (Delaware, Georgia, Illinois, Louisiana, Nebraska, New Mexico, South Carolina, South Dakota) more closely conformed to the NANDA-based "who." For five of the states (Florida, Kentucky, Maryland, Missouri, Washington), the ill and the injured constituted the "who." Connecticut and North Dakota modified the word "responses" by the word "human." Mississippi and Texas implied that the focus of nursing diagnosis is the individual and client, respectively. People are the focus of nursing diagnosis for New Hampshire. Two of the states (Indiana and Wyoming) did not specify for whom nursing diagnosis were made.

Discussion and Implications

Thirty-three of the 50 state practice acts include the term "diagnosis" in their definitions of professional nursing practice. The fact that two-thirds of the nurse practice acts utilize the term "diagnosis" speaks to the legislative impact of the nursing diagnosis movement. Nursing has made important strides in its attempt to identify and label its domain.

The extent to which nursing diagnosis is incorporated within nurse practice acts has important legal and policy implications. It can be argued that nurses who practice in states that include nursing diagnosis as part of the responsibilities of the registered nurse are legally obligated to derive and document nursing diagnoses for the clients they serve. Failure to do so implies a less than fully professional level of practice.

There are research and educational implications that flow from these findings. Historical study of other professional language variations among the states and the tracking of language changes over time would contribute to greater understanding of nursing's own language development. Another avenue of research is to question whether differing definitions of professional nursing practice, as articulated in state practice acts, translate into differences in practice and, ultimately, patient outcomes. Educationally, students need to be taught that the use or nonuse of nursing diagnosis is not optional when the act of diagnosis helps define professional practice in their states.

Given the differences among states' definitions of nursing, nurses themselves need to be aware of the definition of nursing in the state in which they practice. This will become especially important if the mutual recognition model for nursing regulation as proposed by the National Council of State Boards of Nursing (1997) is adopted. Under the model, a nurse will hold a license in a state of residency and will be able to practice in any state that has signed onto the interstate compact, provided the nurse follows the laws and regulations of the state in which he or she practices. With or without the mutual recognition model, differences in the definitions of professional practice need to be recognized by nurses who practice in more than one state or who relocate in another state. Alterations in nursing practice may need to be made accordingly.

In summary, nursing language is changing. The majority of states now define the practice of professional nursing as including the diagnostic act. A smaller but important number of practice acts speak of the professional nurse prescribing nursing treatments.

The issue of disease diagnosis remains ambiguous within the practice of nursing. Despite statements that physicians diagnose disease and nurses diagnose responses to actual or potential health problems, practicing professional nurses know that the boundaries surrounding the diagnosis of human disease lack precise definition. Physiologic science and disease are overlapping domains shared by both medicine and nursing. Both nurses and physicians are responsible for diagnosing abnormal physiologic responses such as hypokalemia, or the constellation of signs and symptoms that constitute a disease manifestation such as, clonic-tonic seizure activity. Modifying the word "disease" by the word "medical" is, therefore, misleading; but equally misleading is the attempt by some nurses to deny saying they are diagnosing physiologic responses or disease. By incorporating disease diagnosis into their definitions of the practice of professional or registered nursing, Colorado and Alaska have addressed this issue in a forthright manner. Although considerable progress has been made in the 50 years since Lesnik and Anderson (1947) called for more clarity in this province of diagnosis, it is time to renew the call.

References

Alaska Division of Occupational Licensing Statutes and Regulations: Nursing. (1996). *Article 6, General Provisions*, Section 410, Definitions, Sec. AS 08.68.410, 8(F).

Bullough, B. (1975). *The law and the expanding nursing role*. New York: Appleton-Century-Crofts.

Colorado Board of Nursing. (1995). *Nurse Practice Act*, Article 12, §12-38-03, Definitions (10)(a).

Illinois Department of Professional Regulation: *Nursing Act of 1987, Amended. (1997-1998)*. LRB9001265LDew.

Iowa Board of Nursing. (1997). *Chapter 152, Nursing, §152.1, 6a.*

Lesnik, M. J., & Anderson, B. E. (1947). *Legal aspects of nursing*. Philadelphia: Lippincott.

Massachusetts Board of Registration in Nursing. (1994). *Nurse Practice Act. §80B. Practice of Nursing Defined*.

Montana State Board of Nursing. (1996). *Statutes and Rules Relating to Nursing, Chapter 8, Nursing, Part I, §37-8-102, (5)(b)*.

National Council of State Boards of Nursing, Inc. (1997). Boards of nursing approve proposed language for an interstate compact for a mutual recognition model of nursing regulation. *Issues, 18*(4), 3.

New Hampshire Board of Nursing. (1997). *Statutes, Chapter 326-B, Section 326-B:2, Definitions, XVIII(a)*.

North American Nursing Diagnosis Association. (1996). *Nursing diagnosis: Definitions and classification 1997-1998*. Philadelphia: Author.

Vermont State Board of Nursing. (1994). *Title 26 V.S.A., Chapter 28, Nursing, §1572, b.*

Wisconsin Statutes. (1995). *Chapter 441, Board of Nursing, §441.11 (4)*.

Classification Schemes for Nursing Language (abstract)

Harry John Tillman, RN, PhD

In discussing nursing knowledge and practice, Clark and Lang (1992) have noted that "if we cannot name it, we cannot control it, finance it, teach it, or put it into public policy." Establishing a standard language could benefit nursing by providing for: a) validation of existing diagnoses, b) testing of interventions, and c) measurement of the effectiveness of these intervention as nursing outcomes of care. Recent developments in standardizing nursing language include: a) the Nursing Minimum Data Set (NMDS) proposed as a structure for a unified nursing language, b) revisions in the North American Nursing Diagnosis (NANDA) taxonomy, c) the publication of the Nursing Intervention Classification (NIC). These developments have moved nursing closer to realizing a standardized language. This language system, however, would need to work in roughly six thousand hospitals in this country, and this study will assist in evaluating whether these classification systems have the potential to do so.

The purposes of this study were to examine the availability of the NMDS elements in acute care patient records and to determine how reliably the data elements can be translated and coded according to the NANDA taxonomy and the NIC. Data that did not these language systems were examined for patterns that suggest revisions in the classification schemes. This descriptive, ethnomethodologic field study used content analysis as an investigative strategy within an interpretive research design to examine 92 randomly selected medical admissions to a university medical center.

There were 686 text phrases captured in this study describing nursing diagnoses, of which 508 (74%) could be coded according to the NANDA taxonomy. Eleven categories emerged from the remaining text phrases, nine of which may be potential concepts consistent with NANDA. A total of 34,230 text phrases were abstracted and 88 percent (30,117) were able to be coded according to the NIC. Twenty-seven categories emerged from the remaining text phrases that may suggest addition classification work to be done.

Implications for improving the exclusivity of the NANDA and NIC labels are discussed. Current diagnostic and intervention labels that could be expanded to be more inclusive of the "natural language" of the generalist registered nurse are discussed. Finally adjustments to the NMDS instrument, modifications of the coding categories, and refinements to the definitions are offered

The International Classification For Nursing Practice (ICNP): Toward The Beta Version

Madeline Wake, PhD, RN, FAAN
Amy Coenen, PhD, RN, CS

In 1989 the International Council of Nurses (ICN), a non-governmental organization comprised of member national nursing associations (NNA), authorized the development of an international nursing nomenclature. In 1991, a development team initiated work resulting in publication of working papers in 1993 and an Alpha Version of the International Classification for Nursing Practice (ICNP) in 1996. The ICNP is a classification of nursing phenomena, interventions and outcomes which provides a unifying framework into which terms from other classifications may be cross-mapped. Because it is intended for all nurses, the ICNP is inclusive of all terms existing in other nursing classification systems.

Nurses from over 120 nations have been invited to participate in development of the ICNP. Participation was promoted by written invitation to all NNA members of ICN, by meetings in many parts of the world, and by communication to interested audiences. The Alpha Version was published at an early stage in order to provide a basis for discourse. In this presentation, we will summarize feedback on the Alpha Version and report on progress to date on the Beta Version. It should be noted that international classification work is long-term work. In working on the Beta Version, it is important to remember that there are 26 letters in the Greek alphabet, Alpha through Omega. ICN is committed to disseminating ongoing work to engage the global nursing community in creating the ICNP.

Feedback

Feedback has been received from both NNAs and individuals. The feedback was submitted using the feedback form in the Alpha Version or by means of an in-depth report on issues and elements. The NNAs responding included Australia, Canada, Columbia, Finland, France, Germany, Guyana, The Netherlands, Samoa, Sweden, Taiwan, Trinidad-Tobago, and the United Kingdom. In addition, ICN has been notified that a number of other NNAs, including

"

the American Nurses Association, are preparing official responses.

Some general themes in the Alpha Version feedback demonstrating positive support for ICN involvement in nursing classification include:

1. Desire for continued participation in development
2. Focus on application to the electronic patient record
3. Need for more clarity of relationships with other classifications
4. Concern about the ease of use
5. Need for clear statement of the priority purpose(s)
6. Problems with the level of detail in some sections, and
7. Translation and grammar problems.

Two NNA responders decided that the Alpha Version was too premature for clinical testing. Several responders commented on the Phenomena Classification. Concerns included discomfort with the top term "phenomena," insufficiency of wellness and community terms, and inconsistency of the quality of definitions and principles of division. Many specific recommendations also were provided.

Emerging Beta Version

Feedback, as described above, as well as results from other development and evaluation initiatives, have been utilized in shaping the Emerging Beta Version. Noteworthy initiatives include the European Union funded Telenurse project (ICNP in Europe, 1996) and the W. K. Kellogg Foundation funded country-level projects in community based/primary health care (ICN, 1997). This report is current to the January 1998 meeting of the ICNP Development Team. The work in progress will be referred to as the "Emerging Beta Version" and there will be further refinement prior to the release of the ICN Beta Version planned for 1999.

The Emerging Beta Version, similar to the Alpha Version, continues to have three components: Nursing Phenomena, Nursing Actions, and Nursing Outcomes. The top terms have been clarified in the Emerging Beta Version. Current, working definitions include:

Nursing Phenomena: Factors influencing health status, which are concerns of nursing.

Nursing Diagnosis: Label given by a nurse to the decision about a phenomenon which is the focus of nursing interventions. For the ICNP, a nursing diagnosis is composed of concepts contained in the Classification of Phenomena axes.

Nursing Actions: Behaviors of nurses in practice.

Nursing Interventions: The action taken in response to a nursing diagnosis in order to produce a nursing outcome. For the ICNP, a nursing intervention is composed of concepts contained in the Classification of Actions axes.

Nursing Outcomes: The measure of status in a nursing diagnosis at a point in time, after a nursing intervention.

The three ICNP Classifications (phenomena, actions, and outcomes) are multi-axial. In the multi-axial approach, the diagnoses and interventions are "combinatorial" terms, concepts which are developed by combining terms from the different axes in a classification. This approach enhances the expressive power of the classification and supports the concept of a uni-

Figure 1.

Example of Combined Terms from the ICNP Classification of Nursing Phenomena Axes to Create	
Axis	**Terms**
Focus	Sleep
Judgment	Disturbed
Chronicity	Chronic
Likelihood	Risk for
Diagnosis: Disturbed sleep Chronic disturbed sleep Risk for disturbed sleep	

fying framework. A further description of the multi-axial architecture may be found in Nielsen and Mortensen (1997).

Classification of Nursing Phenomena

The move in the Classification of Nursing Phenomena from a mono-axial to a multi-axial classification has resulted in a number of proposed axes. The following axes are being further developed in the Emerging Beta Version:

- focus of nursing practice
- judgment
- degree
- frequency
- chronicity
- topography
- body site
- likelihood

An in-depth explanation of each axes is beyond the scope of this paper. Examples are of using the axes to create diagnoses are provided (Figure 1). The focus of nursing practice axis is similar to the Alpha Version Classification of Phenomena with modifiers of the terms removed. These modifiers now appear in the other axes. Many of the modifiers are included

in the second axis, the judgment axis. For example, the user may combine terms from these two axes, or other axes, to express nursing diagnoses. Combined terms are displayed in Figure 1.

In addition to the shift to a multi-axial approach, there were changes proposed in the structure of the Classification of Nursing Phenomena foci of nursing practice axes. These included two major changes: (a) shifting of Family, Community, and Society categories from under the Environment to under a category of "Groups" of Human Beings (see Figure 2) and (b) reclassifying the category of "Sensations" as a Function.

Classification of Nursing Actions

A major change in the Emerging Beta Version is the title of this classification, previously titled Classification of Nursing Interventions. The revision in the title represents the classification of actions. Again, in using the multi-axial approach, terms from the different axes are combined, in this case terms are combined to create interventions. A language-based approach, using grammatical categories as a framework, is being tested in the development

Figure 2.

ICNP Nursing Phenomena Classification

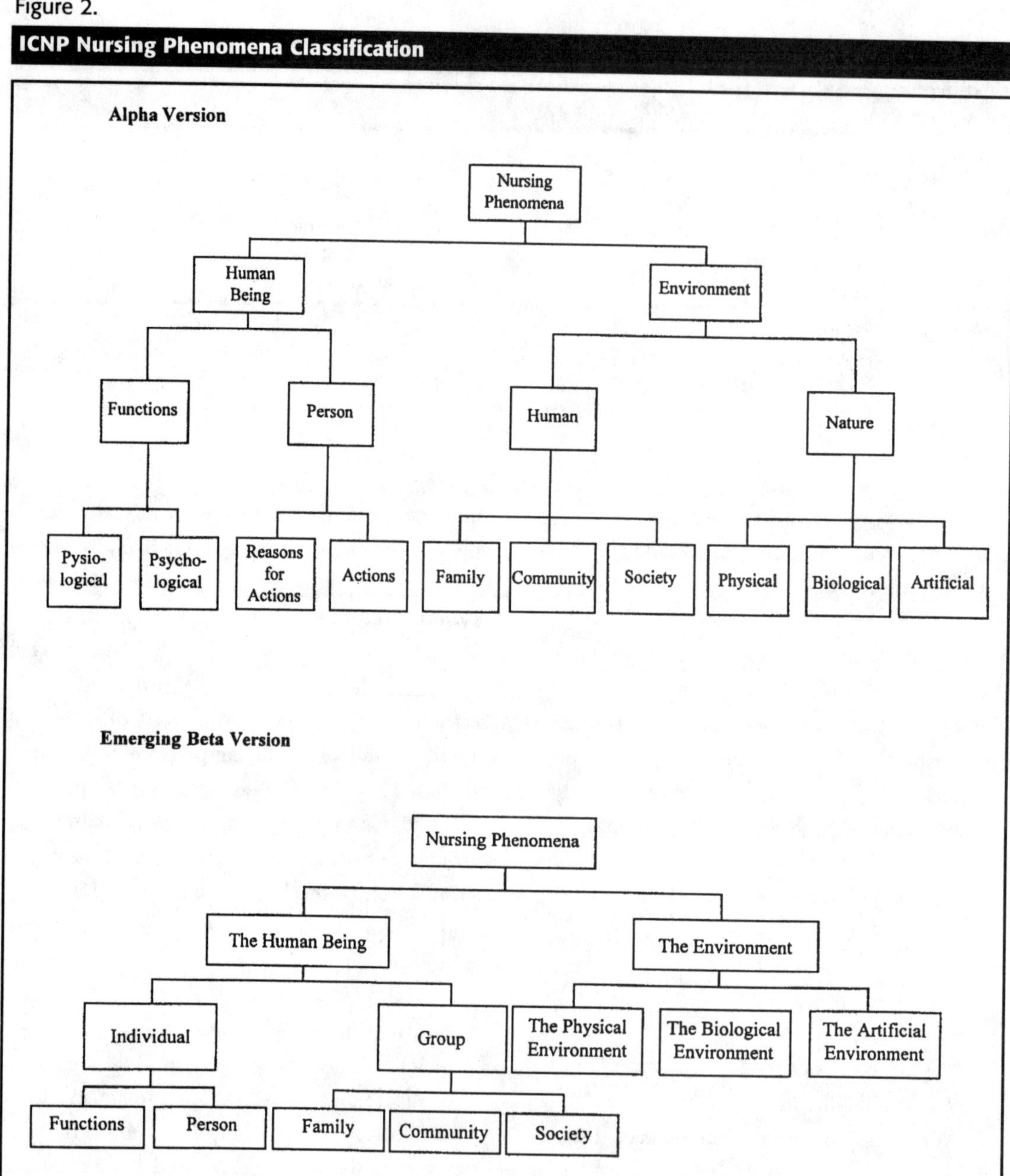

of the Classification of Nursing Actions. A number of different axes have been proposed. The major axis would classify the action types and be composed of verbs. The list of proposed axes under consideration includes:

- action types
- objects
- targets or recipients
- methods
- instruments

Using the ICNP

Feedback on the Alpha Version included concern regarding ease of use of the ICNP. In the ICNP field tests, developers are exploring systems which provide pre-combined terms. Therefore, the atomic level terms may be combined for a specific group and not demand combination of terms each time the concepts are named by clinicians. The development of logical combination of terms will enhance the use of the ICNP as a unifying framework to cross-map with other nursing systems.

Summary

Plans are to incorporate ongoing Alpha feedback as well as feedback on the Emerging Beta into a Beta Version to be published for the 1999 ICN Centennial. The ICN invites comments from all interested in classification. We share a common goal of making nursing visible in world health care.

References

ICNP in Europe: Telenurse (1996). *International Nursing Review, 43*(6). 188-189.

International Council of Nurses (1997). *ICNP News*. Geneva Switzerland: Author.

International Council of Nurses (1996).). *The International Classification for Nursing Practice (ICNP): A unifying framework. The Alpha version*. Geneva Switzerland: Author.

International Council of Nurses (1993), *Nursing's next advance: An International Classification for Nursing Practice (ICNP): A working paper*. Geneva, Switzerland: Author.

Nielsen, G. H., & Mortensen, R. A. (1996). The architecture for an International Classification for Nursing Practice (ICNP). *International Nursing Review, 43*(6), 175-182.

Nielsen, G. H., & Mortensen, R. A. (1997). The architecture of ICNP: A time of outcomes - Part 1. *International Nursing Review, 44*(6), 182-188, 176.

Nielsen, G. H., & Mortensen, R. A. (1997). The architecture of ICNP: A time of outcomes - Part 2. *International Nursing Review, 45*(1), 27-31.

Hopelessness and Depression: Separate or Connected Phenomena

Beverly J. Bartlett, PhD, RN

Acknowledgements

The author wishes to thank Alexandra M. Jennings for her initial work on this research and her continued support as an angel on my shoulder. Additional thanks go to Karen Lumia, MSN, RN, for her role as primary data collector. I was fortunate to have a senior nursing student Hali Jo Frost working with me as part of an Undergraduate Research Award. Finally, I thank Gannon University for Faculty Development Grants and Research Grants.

Hopelessness is a nursing diagnosis category label accepted by the North American Nursing Diagnosis Association (NANDA) for clinical use and study. Some of the major questions generated around nursing diagnoses involve the appropriateness of the concepts as appropriate labels. Is hopelessness, the concept, appropriate as a nursing diagnosis category label?

This research project is the last of three phases. The first phase, a concept analysis, was part of the process of validating hopelessness as a diagnostic category. The conclusion of that research was no clear differentiation between hopelessness and depression (Bartlett, 1992). Based on the results, the researcher believed that it was imperative to pursue this with further study.

The second phase was descriptive study, which looked at hopelessness and depression as separate or connected phenomenon. In this pilot study, Beck's Hopelessness Inventory (BHI) and Beck's Depression (BDS) were administered to a purposive sample of 26 sub-jects. The sample consisted of two groups of 13 subjects. Group I was composed of clients with a medical diagnosis of depression, who were members of a community based support group. Group II was composed of clients with chronic obstructive pulmonary disease who was clients of an outpatient clinic of a local medical center. obstructive pulmonary disease (COPD) clients were chosen for this study since they are at high risk for depression (Gift & McCrone, 1993).

The NANDA definition of hopelessness used is "a subjective state in which an individual sees limited or no alternatives or personal choic-es available and is unable to mobilize energy on own behalf" (NANDA, 1994).

Depression was defined by the character-istics of depression according to the APA (1987):

persistent sad, anxious, or "empty" mood
feelings of hopelessness, pessimism
feelings of guilt, worthlessness,
   helplessness
loss of interest or pleasure in hobbies or

activities that were once enjoyed, including sex; insomnia, early morning awaking, or oversleeping

appetite and/or weight loss or overeating or weight gain

decreased energy, fatigue, being "slowed down"

thoughts of death or suicide: suicide attempts

restlessness, irritability

difficulty in concentrating, remembering, making decisions

persistent physical symptoms that do not respond to treatment, such as headaches, digestive disorders and chronic pain (p.218-224)

The Beck Depression Inventory (BDI) and Beck Hopelessness Scale (BHS) were the tools utilized in this study. The BDI assesses the severity of depression in adults and adolescents. (Beck & Steer, 1993, p. 1). It has been determined to have good to excellent reliability. The BHS also addresses adults and adolescents and the extent of their negativism (pessimism) about the future (Beck & Steer, 1993, p. 2).

Test-retest reliability varied between a Pearson product moment correlation of .69 (p less than .001) and .66 (p .001) (Beck & Steer, 1993, p. 12). Beck, Shuyler, and Herman (1974) studied the relationship between the BHS and the BDI for seven normative samples. "The BHS was significantly related to the BDI beyond the .001 level, one-tailed test in all seven samples" (Beck & Steer, 1993, p. 15).

Twenty males and six females were in the study. The mean age of the participants was 56 with a range of 19-81. There was a moderate degree of hopelessness and depression in the sample, as reflected in the mean scores on the BDI and BHS. The mean score on the Beck's Hopelessness Scale was 9.65 with a mean score on the Beck's Depression Inventory of 23. There was a significant correlation between the Beck's Hopelessness Scale and the Beck's Depression Inventory with a Pearson Product Moment Correlation value of .8003, p value of .0000. The significance of findings led into the third and current phase of research on hopelessness.

The Current Study
Design, Setting, and Sample

Based on the pilot study results, a third study was undertaken. The problem remained the differentiation between hopelessness and depression. Are hopelessness and depression the same or are they different? Is hopelessness a core characteristic of depression, rather than independent phenomena? When nurses are diagnosing hopelessness, is it the depression that is being addressed? If hopelessness is an inherent component of depression can a treatment be successful if just focused on hopelessness? If the attempt is to just treat hopelessness without treating the depression, will the result be a successful treatment?

The research question was "Does hopelessness occur without depression?" This was a descriptive study again using the BHS and BDI. The primary setting was a 450-bed medical center in Northwestern Pennsylvania. The secondary setting was an outpatient pulmonary rehabilitation center. The purposive sample of 55 clients included 26 men and 29 women. Group One were 26 clients who are diagnosed with COPD and were either in-patients on a pulmonary unit or outpatients in a pulmonary rehabilitation center. Group Two consisted of 29 clients with the primary diagnosis of depression. These clients were from the in-hospital psychiatric setting. Inclusion criteria for all participants would be willingness to participate and age between 18-80. Exclusion criteria would include not being able to read or write English or having additional psychiatric diagnoses.

The research assistant explained the study to all potential participants. There were three research assistants used to collect the data. A script was used for consistency. Informed consent was obtained from all participants. Confidentially and anonymity was maintained by numbering the inventories and eliminating identifying data from the forms.

Instrumentation

The Beck Depression Inventory (BDI) and Beck Hopelessness Scale (BHS) were the tools utilized in this study.

Data Collection Procedures

Research Assistants made specific provisions in each area for the administration of the BHS and BDI. The procedure for administering them was as follows: introduction of the study through reading a script; obtaining informed consent; and administering the BHS and BDI. Additional data was reviewed in the charts, such as secondary diagnosis and current medical regimen. If a participant was found to have a secondary psychiatric diagnosis, he or she was excluded from the study.

Data Analysis

The BHS and BDI were scored according to specified instructions. A Pearson Product-Moment Correlation Coefficient was determined regarding the BHS scores and the BDI scores. Descriptive statistics included age, diagnosis, and gender.

Results

The sample consisted of 55 clients, 26 males and 29 females with a mean age of 61. The mean age of the males was 65, and the mean age of the females was 57. Group I consisted of 37 clients diagnosed with COPD. The 18 clients in Group II were diagnosed with depression. Table 1 summarizes the sample.

Table 1

Sample Summary	
Gender	Mean Age
Females	57
Males	65

Sample mean age was 61 (60-76)

Descriptive Statistics

The sample means on theBDI and BHS indicate mild hopelessness and depression. The sample mean of the BDI was 15.65 with the BHS sample mean of 5.90. Table 2 summarizes the results of the BHS and BDI.

Table 2

Results of the BDI and BHS
Sample mean of BDI=15.65 standard dev 12.34
Sample mean of BHS=5.90 standard dev 5.02

As expected, Group II, the depressed sample, scored higher on both the BDI and BHS, indicating moderate depression and hopelessness (BDI mean = 29.61, BHS mean = 11.05. Minimal hopelessness and depression were found in Group I, the COPD sample (BHS mean = 3.40, BDI mean =8.86). Table 3 summarizes these results.

Table 3

BDI and BHS Results by Diagnosis

Group I, COPD sample:
    BDI mean 8.86   BHS mean 3.40

Group II, depressed sample:
    BDI mean 29.61   BHS mean 11.05

Pearson Product Moment Correlation

There is a positive correlation between the BHS and BDI with a correlation of .806 p value of .0000. Table 4 summarizes the results of the Pearson Product Moment Correlation.

Table 4

Pearson Product Moment Correlation

	BDI	BHS
Pearson Correlation BDI	1.000	.806**
Pearson Correlation BHS	.806**	1.000

Correlation is significant at the 0.01 level (2-tailed).

Discussion

The results of this study show that there is a positive correlation between hopelessness and depression. The research question was "Does hopelessness occur without depression?" The answer is that the coefficient of determination of .64 shows the two variables, depression and hopelessness, share 64% of the variability or that the other can explain 64% on one. So only 37% of the time hopelessness and depression occur independently.

Research in clinical practice determined a relationship between depression and three nursing diagnosis category labels, specifically hope- lessness, powerlessness, and chronic low self- esteem (Zauszniewski, 1994). Beck's (1973) cog- nitive theory of depression supports the rela- tionship between chronic low self-esteem, pow- erlessness, hopelessness, and depression.

Professional nurses cannot diagnose depression, nor can they treat it independently. As a nursing diagnostic category label, hopeless- ness, is a phenomenon that can be addressed and treated independently by professional nurs- es. However, if the nursing diagnosis hopeless- ness is being used to address depression, it is an improper use of the diagnostic category label. Nurses treating hopelessness, without the over- lying depression being treated is like medically treating the edema of congestive heart failure without treating the heart itself (the overlying problem resulting in the edema). Therefore, treatment will not be effective. Hopelessness can occur transiently in everyone's life. When it is pathological and needs to be treated, it is a major symptom of the overlying problem, depression.

Conclusion

There is a strong correlation between hopelessness and depression. Since hopeless- ness and depression are so highly correlated, hopelessness should not be considered a nursing diagnostic category label.

References

American Psychiatric Association (1987). *Diagnostic and statistical manual of mental disorders* (3rd ed.). Washington, DC : Author

Bartlett, B.J. (1994). A concept analysis of hopelessness. In R. M. Carroll-Johnson & M. Paquette (Eds.), *Classification of nursing diagnoses* (p.393). Philadelphia: J.B.

Lippincott Company.

Bartlett, B.J. (1996, April). *Hopelessness and depression: Separate or connected phenomena?*. Poster presentation at the 12th Biennial Conference on the Classification of Nursing Diagnoses, Pittsburgh, PA.

Beck, A.T., & Steer, R. A. (1993). *Beck depression inventory manual*. San Antonio, Texas: The Psychological Corporation.

Beck, A.T., & Steer, R. A. (19937). *Beck hopelessness scale*. San Antonio, Texas: The Psychological Corporation.

Gift, A.G., & McCrone, S.H. (1993). Depression in patients with COPD. Heart & Lung: *Journal of Critical Care,* 4 (22), 289-297.

North American Nursing Diagnosis Association (1994). *Nursing diagnoses: Definition & classification, 1995-1996*. Philadelphia: Author.

Zausniewski, J.A. (1994). Nursing diagnosis and depressive illness. *Nursing Diagnosis, 5*, 106-114.

Self-Efficacious Skills Helpful to Battered Women to Remain Battered-Free (abstract)

Judy Carlson-Catalano, MSN, RN

This paper is the report of a qualitative study of battered women who have remained battered-free for at least a year. The objectives of this study were to: 1) develop a conceptual framework of self-efficacy for the battered women; 2) determine the cognitive, social, and behavioral sub-skills needed for development of self-efficacy in the battered women; and 3) validate these sub-skills with battered women who have moved to a protected lifestyle for a period of at least one year. The significance of this study cannot be overstated because the prevalence and incidence of the battering of women continues to be a major societal and health care issue as we enter the 21st century (Campbell, 1992). In August of 1995, the battering of women received significant international focus as women from every nation came forward with the details of the abuses occurring in their homelands and the International Women's Conference held in Huairow, China. The battering of women appears to cut across every nation, ethnic category, religious branch, socioeconomic strata, educa-

tional level, and adult age grouping (Blair, 1986; Tilden & Shepherd, 1987). A question often asked is, "Why don't women leave these abusive relationships?" In some countries leaving spouses in a sentence to death (e.g., public stoning) or outcasting. In America, where our society seemingly protects women from such overt consequences, it is often less understood as to the women's reasons for staying. This study will serve to provide the basis for a new nursing diagnosis, low self-efficacy, and a nursing intervention, self-efficacy, enhancement.

A self-efficacy theory as described by Bandura (1986) has relevance for battered women. Research has indicated that battered women have gone back to the abuser because of perceptions that they could not make it on their own (Newman, 1993). According to Bandura (1986), efficacy involves a generative capability in which cognitive, social and behavioral sub-skills must be organized into integrated courses of action to serve innumerable purposes. Bandura (1986) suggests that these sub-skills

"

can be learned.

This study developed a self-efficacious conceptual framework for battered women and a tool detailing sub-skills needed to enhance self-efficacy which was validated by experts. In addition, the tool was further validated by 9 battered women who have remained battered free for at a least a year, in two-hour individual sessions. Retrospectively, low self-efficacy scores were revealed by the women while in battering situations, and higher self-efficacy scores were present when these women were battered free for at least one-year. The author will present the conceptual framework and the sub-skills that were determined to be helpful to enable battered women to move to a more protected lifestyle. Nursing interventions to enhance self-efficacy will also be presented.

Caregiver Role Strain: It's Not Just for Caregivers of Persons with Dementia

Jessie Daniels, MA, RN

Sharon Ridgeway, PhD, RN

Acknowledgements

National Center for Nursing Research & Mayo Foundation for funding the Family Caregiver Study, Sigma Theta Tau, Int., Kappa Phi Chapter for funding the doctoral dissertation.

One hundred and ten million people require some form of home care (O'Connor, Vander Plaats, & Betz, 1992). The family home caregiver is defined as a member of the person's informal support system (family/friend) who accepts the duty of management at home and is not paid for that service (Wilson, 1989).

The caregiving process has a multidimensional impact on the caregiver, causing high risk of emotional, physical, financial, and social problems (Farran, Keane-Hagerty, Tatorowitz, & Scorze, 1993). Researchers conclude that the providers of care and the setting in which care is given best predict the multidimensional impact of caregiving (Brody, Litvin, Hoffman, & Kleban, 1995; Burns, Archbold, Stewart, & Shelton, 1993; George & Gwyther, 1986; Schulz, O'Brien, Bookwala, & Fleissner, 1995).

If context and multidimensionality are significant factors, then it is important to investigate the caregiver's perception of caregiving, using a multidimensional framework. A multidimensional framework was provided by the North American Nursing Diagnosis Association (NANDA) nursing theorists who defined health as a fluctuating field of person-environment interaction (Newman, 1984; Roy, 1984). This subjective perspective of health, each person's view of their own pattern of person-environment interaction, became the focus of nursing.

The theorists then developed a framework for assessing patterns in person-environment interaction. They clustered practicing nurses' phenomena of concern into nine groupings and chose an interactive conceptual label to describe each grouping. These interactive concepts were labeled the nine dimensions. The nine dimensions were then synthesized into three groupings: interaction, action, and awareness. The nine dimensions, dimension definitions, and the phenomena are listed in Table 1. This paper will examine how to use the NANDA taxonomy to assess for caregiver multidimensional patterns that indicate caregiver role strain or the risk for caregiver role strain.

Caregiver role strain/risk for caregiver role

Table 1

Parallels of dimensions and diagnostic phenomena

Dimension	Definition	Phenomena
1. Interaction Characteristics		
Exchanging	Mutual giving and receiving.	Nutrition, elimination, oxygenation, circulation, physical regulation, physical integrity.
Communicating	Sending messages.	Communication.
Relating	Establishing bonds.	Role, socialization, family processes, sexuality patterns.
2. Action Characteristics		
Valuing	Assigning of relative worth.	Spirituality.
Choosing	Selection of alternatives.	Coping, participating, judgment, health seeking.
Moving	Activity.	Activity, rest, recreation, activities of daily living, self-care, growth and development, relocation.
3. Awareness Characteristics		
Perceiving	Reception of information.	Sensory perception, self-concept, meaningfulness.
Feeling	Subjective awareness of information.	Comfort, emotional integrity, emotional state.
Knowing	Meaning associated with a world view or with information.	Knowledge, thought processes.

Adapted from Roy, 1984, p. 29-33, England, 1989, p. 353, & Taxonomy I – Revised (1992), Carroll-Johnson & Paquette, 1994, p. 481-483.

strain is defined as "a family-oriented diagnosis, which occurs when the caregiver feels difficulty performing the family caregiver role" (Burns et al., 1993, p. 70). Students should be aware of this diagnosis because of the number of family caregivers in the general population. Burns et al. (1993) assert that "approximately 31% of all children under the age of 18 have one or more chronic illness, 7.5% of adults between 45 and 64 years of age are limited in the kind of work they do because of chronic illness, and 37% of people older than 65 years report some limitations" (p. 71). These statistics provide evidence for the occurrence of family caregiving throughout the lifespan.

Survey of Nursing Textbooks

Because the diagnosis of caregiver role strain was accepted by NANDA in 1992, a sample of medical-surgical, mental health-psychiatric,

Table 2

Review of medical-surgical texts for the diagnosis of caregiver role strain

Adult Medical-Surgical Textbooks	Identification of Caregiver Role Strain Diagnosis	Identification of Care Recipient
Black & Matassarin-Jacobs, 1997	Present	Clients with Alzheimer's disease
Beare & Myers, 1998	-------	-------
Ignatavicius, Workman, & Mishler, 1995	-------	-------
LeMone & Burke, 1996	Present	Clients with Alzheimer's disease
Lewis, Collier, & Heitkemper, 1996	Present	Nonspecific
Monohan & Neighbors, 1998	-------	-------
Phipps, Cassmeyer, Sands, & Lehman, 1995	Present	Clients with senile dementia

Table 3

Review of mental health/psychiatric texts for the diagnosis of caregiver role strain

Mental Health/Psychiatric Nursing Textbooks	Identification of Caregiver Role Strain Diagnosis	Identification of Care Recipient
Antai-Otong & Kongable, 1995	-------	-------
Carson & Arnold, 1996	-------	-------
Frisch & Frisch, 1998	Present	Clients with mental illness
Johnson, 1997	Present	Clients with dementia & delirium disorders
Rawlins, Williams, & Beck, 1993	Present	Clients with dementia
Stuart & Sundeen, 1995	Present	Elderly clients
Townsend, 1996	-------	-------
Wilson & Kneisl, 1996	-------	-------

Table 4

Review of pediatric nursing texts for the diagnosis of caregiver role strain		
Pediatric Textbooks	Identification of Caregiver Role Strain Diagnosis	Identification of Care Recipient
Ashwill & Droske, 1997	------	------
Ball & Bindle, 1995	Present	Children with acute & chronic conditions
Betz, Hunsberger, & Wright, 1994	Present	Children with genetic disorders, chronic illnesses, and all newborns
Wong & Wilson, 1995	Present only in the appendix	Nonspecific

Table 5

Review of nursing texts for the diagnosis of caregiver role strain		
Fundamental Textbooks	Identification of Caregiver Role Strain Diagnosis	Identification of Care Recipient
Bolander, 1994	------	------
Craven & Hirnle, 1996	Present	Persons across the lifespan with chronic illnesses
Kozier, Erb, Blasi, Wilkinson, Van Leuven, 1998	Present	Persons across the lifespan with chronic illnesses
Potter & Perry, 1997	Present	Spouse with dementia
Taylor, Lillis, & LeMone, 1997	------	------

pediatric, and fundamental nursing textbooks published from 1993 through 1998 were reviewed for presentation of caregiver role strain across the life span. Tables 2, 3, 4, and 5 outline the findings from that survey.

Four of the seven adult medical-surgical textbooks presented the diagnosis of caregiver role strain. However, discussion of this nursing diagnosis was limited to family caregivers of person's experiencing Alzheimer's disease.

In a sample of eight mental health-psychiatric textbooks, four identified the diagnosis of caregiver role strain. Care recipients were the elderly and those suffering from delirium disorders, mental illnesses, and dementia.

The diagnosis was included in three of the four pediatric textbooks. One text listed the diagnosis in the appendix only, while the other two texts referred to caregiver role strain in the context of caring for a child with an acute or chronic illness, genetic disorder, or as a diagnosis for parents preparing for a newborn child.

Of the five fundamental nursing texts surveyed, three discussed caregiver role strain in chapters on home management, families and their relationships in the home and community, and stress and adaptation. Two texts considered caregiving as occurring with care recipients across the lifespan and one sample care plan in the third textual discussion referred to a caregiver managing a spouse with dementia.

In summary, 14 of the sample survey of 24 nursing textbooks presented the nursing diagnosis of caregiver role strain. The nursing diagnosis was in the context of caring for persons experiencing Alzheimer's disease and related disorders (ADRD) in six of the textbooks, three of the texts were nonspecific in their identification of the care recipient, while the remaining five texts referred to care recipients across the life span

with a variety of patterns of health. This review indicated that the scope of textbook presentations of the diagnosis of caregiver role strain is limited in terms of discussion of the diagnosis in general as well as consideration of care recipients across the lifespan with a variety of patterns of health. In view of this finding, the nurse educator must supplement textbook resources by guiding the nursing student through a holistic assessment process that would help identify those individuals who are experiencing caregiver role strain/risk for caregiver role strain.

NANDA Framework for Assessment

The NANDA dimensions of person-environment interaction provide a holistic framework for assessing for caregiver role strain or risk for caregiver role strain. Two approaches that students may use to diagnose caregiver role strain are described. First, viewing caregiver descriptions of the caregiving experience through the lens of the nine dimensions is outlined. In contrast, the second approach delineates the use of a form based on the nine dimensions which guides the interview.

Unstructured Interview

Ridgeway (1995) analyzed daughter/daughter-in-law caregivers' descriptions of caring for parents with Alzheimer's disease and related disorders (ADRD) using the NANDA dimensions of person-environment interaction. The descriptions culminated from one question: What is the caregiving experience like for you? Findings indicated that the NANDA dimensions were evident in the data. The dimensions were further synthesized to describe individual daughter/daughter-in-law caregiver person-environment interactional patterns. See Figure 1 for an illustration of the process of pattern identification.

Figure 1.

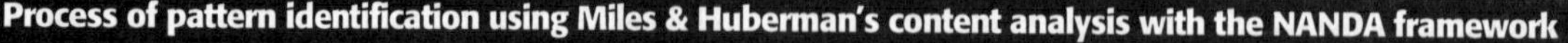

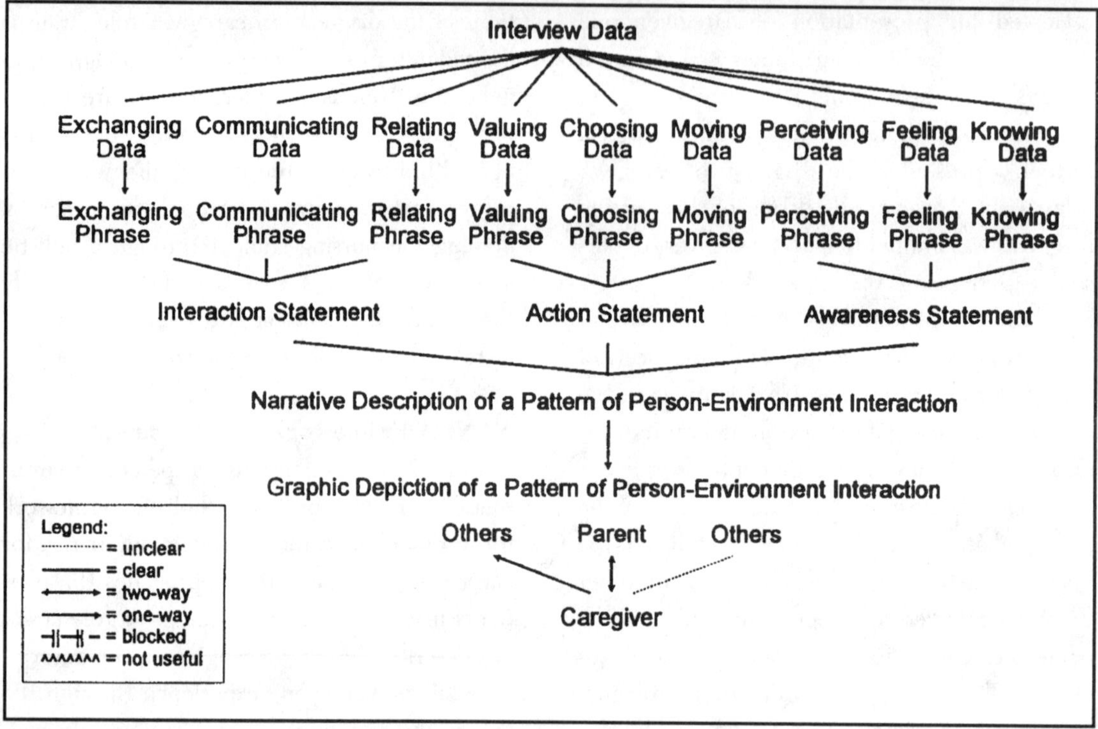

Figure 2.

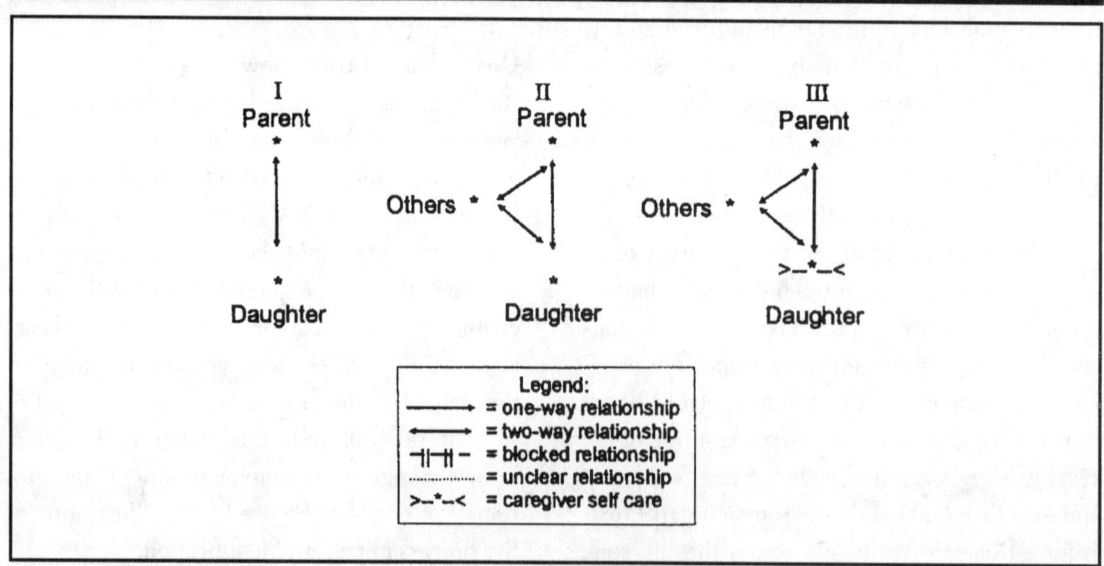

Caregiver patterns of person-environment interaction are clustered into three common groupings: (a) unconnected caregiver interactional patterns, (b) connected caregiver interactional patterns, and (c) interconnected caregiver interactional patterns. See Figure 2 for a graphic depiction of the three patterns.

In the first group of caregiver interactional patterns, daughters cared for their parents unconnected to others in their environment and provided no description of caring for themselves. The second group described connecting with others to help with caregiving, but also gave no description of caring for themselves. The third group described caring as a natural, interconnected process in which the family and community participated. These daughters indicated they cared for themselves as part of the process. Caregivers with connected and unconnected interactional patterns may experience caregiver role strain/risk for caregiver role strain.

For example, Susie is a 44-year-old daughter caregiver who completed 18 years of education. She lives with her 84-year-old father who was diagnosed a year ago with an irreversible dementia. Her father has severe cognitive impairment. Susie provides 18 hours of care per day for her father and receives 6 hours of professional and informal help per day.

In her interview, Susie is hearing the confusion in her father's messages when he asks her, "Did you know you tied me in bed last night? I had one heck of a time getting out of that" (communicating). Susie illustrates that her relationship with her father is one of intensive caregiving: "He is up all night and wandering and he'd fall. He'd pull out the catheter. We didn't know if we were going to make it the first couple of weeks" (relating). Susie did not talk about receiving any benefits for the intensive caregiv-

ing she is providing, therefore no data were indexed according to the exchanging dimension.

Susie assigns worth to the (a) humor in the situation when she exclaims: "Oh, you'll love my posey story!" and (b) ability to rest because "as we started getting sleep at night we could handle more of what he presented" (valuing). Even though "it was really bad," Susie is still caring for her father at home (choosing). Susie goes on to explain "I am up at two, three, or four o'clock in the morning because he has days and nights totally mixed up. He pulls out his catheter. We take him to Dr. ---- to try to help him" (moving).

Additionally, Susie is interpreting that the physician's help is not useful because "Dr. gave us some medication to give him at night, the pill did nothing. Then he told us we needed to see a psychiatrist who prescribed some more medication that made him weak. So we haven't been giving him anything and he started sleeping nights" (perceiving). Susie senses that caregiving has been "nerve racking, exhausting," and that "it was really bad" (feeling). "Additionally, we have not known what to do at times, we didn't know if we were going to make it at times, but as we started getting sleep at night, we could handle more of what he presented" (knowing).

Figure 3 includes a graphic description of Susie's pattern of person-environment interaction based on a synthesis of data clustered under each of the dimensions. Susie's pattern is described as an intensive one-way expenditure of energy in caring for her father with no helpful interventions from physicians. She does not describe mutuality in other relationships in her life, or awareness of how to care for herself, but is aware that her interventions are effective.

Structured Interview

The second method of assessing for caregiver

Figure 3.

Example of a graphic depiction of caregiver interactional pattern

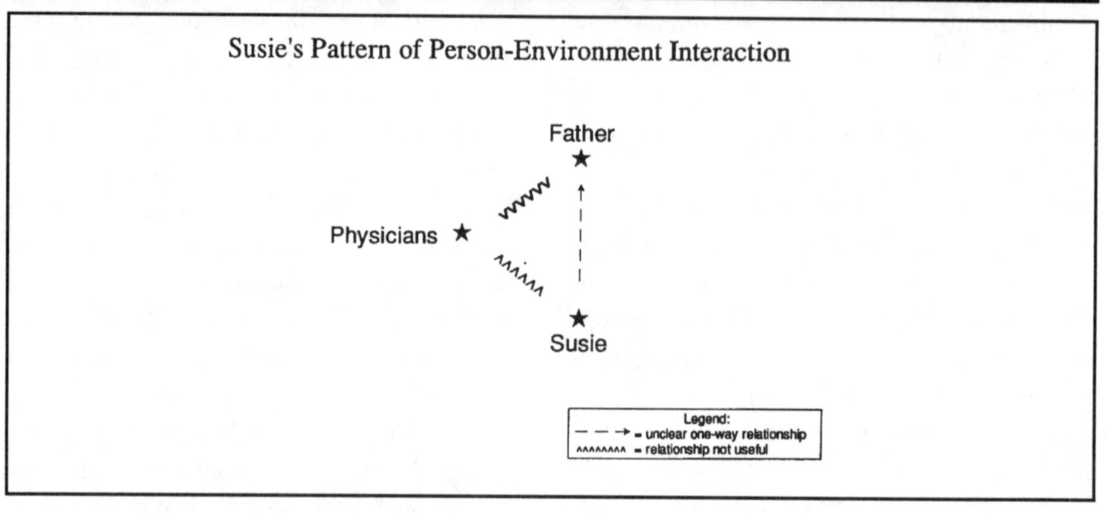

role strain/risk for caregiver role strain utilizes an assessment guide. Nursing students at the University of Minnesota School of Nursing use an assessment guide which is a modification of Guzzetta, Bunton, Prinkey, Sherer, and Seifert's (1989) clinical assessment tools. These clinical assessment tools are organized according to the NANDA dimensions and nursing diagnoses are clustered under each of the dimensions. The modified assessment guide, in conjunction with a nursing diagnosis text, and a medical-surgical text enables the students to do a holistic assessment of the individual/family. The following case study exemplifies the use of these resources to identify caregiver role strain.

Mrs. P is a 37-year-old white married female and has one eight-year-old daughter. Mrs. P's history includes a kidney transplant seven years ago, a pancreas and kidney transplant for Type I diabetes two years ago, seizures related to hypoglycemia, depression for the past two years treated with elavil, macular vitrectomy of the left eye one year ago, and an ankle fusion one year ago. Mrs. P is in the hospital with symptoms of fever, nausea, vomiting, and possible urinary tract infection/urosepsis. She is wearing bilateral braces on her lower extremities for foot drop.

Using the assessment guide to direct the interview, the student asks about Mrs. P's role, which is included under the relating dimension. Role information recorded would be that patient states she has difficulty caring for her eight-year-old daughter and there is family stress because of her frequent hospitalizations. The daughter is curious about her mom's condition. Mrs. P has other roles such as wife and worker outside the home. Her husband cleans the house and washes dishes.

When addressing the choosing dimension, the student asks about participation with past/current health regimens and Mrs. P does comply with the medical regimen for the pancreas/kidney transplant. The information about

Mrs. P's depression and her statement about family stress due to her frequent hospitalizations are included under the feeling dimension, specifically under the category of emotional integrity/status.

The nursing student's nursing diagnosis is that Mrs. P is experiencing caregiver role strain related to health impairment secondary to urosepsis as manifested by communication of unfulfilled roles due to hospitalization. Mrs. P's identification of herself as being unable to care for her daughter is consistent with one of the defining characteristics of caregiver role strain.

Nurse educators must take opportunities like this, when students use the diagnosis of caregiver role strain, to point out that caregiving occurs for persons across the lifespan with a variety of patterns of health. Using this example helps to clarify for students that care recipients are not just the elderly with ADRD.

Conclusion

The NANDA framework for assessment may be used with students in two ways, to organize their interview holistically or to view unstructured interview data holistically. Students should be exposed to both methods of assessment.

Secondly, the textbooks nursing students use tend to be narrow in scope in terms of discussion of caregiver role strain. Nurse educators must supplement these resources by helping students to understand that families care for persons across the life span with a variety of patterns of health.

References

Antai-Otong, D., & Kongable, G. (Eds.). (1995). *Psychiatric nursing: Biological and behavioral concepts*. Philadelphia: Saunders.

Ashwill, J.W., & Droske, S.C. (1997). *Nursing care of children*. Philadelphia: Saunders.

Ball, J., & Bindler, R. (1995). *Pediatric nursing: Caring for children*. Norwalk, CT: Appleton & Lange.

Beare, P.G., & Meyers, J. H. (Eds.). (1998). *Adult health nursing*. St. Louis: Mosby.

Betz, C.L., Hunsberger, M.M., & Wright, S. (1994). *Family-centered nursing care of children*. Philadelphia: Saunders.

Black, J. M., & Matassarin-Jacobs, E. (1997). *Medical-surgical nursing: Clinical management for continuity of care*. Philadelphia: Saunders.

Bolander, V.B. (1994). *Sorensen's and Luckmann's basic nursing: A psychophysiologic approach*. Philadelphia: Saunders.

Brody, E.M., Litvin, S.J., Hoffman, C., & Kleban, M.H. (1995). Marital status of caregiving daughters and co-residence with dependent parents. *The Gerontologist, 35*(1), 75-85.

Burns, C. Archbold, P. Stewart, B., & Shelton, B.S. (1993). New diagnosis: Caregiver role strain. *Nursing Diagnosis, 4*(2), 70-76.

Carroll-Johnson, R.M., & Paquette, M. (Eds.). (1994). *Classification of nursing diagnosis: Proceedimgs of the tenth conference*. Philadelphia: Lippincott.

Carson, V.B., & Arnold, E.N. (1996). *Mental health nursing*. Philadelphia: Saunders.

Craven, R.F., & Hirnle, CJ. (1996). *Fundamentals of nursing: Human health and function*. Philadelphia: Lippincott.

England, M. (1989). Nursing diagnosis: A conceptual framework. In J.J. Fitzpatrick & A.L. Whall (Eds.), *Conceptual models of nursing* (pp. 348-369). Norwalk, CT: Appleton & Lange.

Farran, C.J., Keane-Hagerty E., Tatarowicz, L.,

& Scorza, E. (1993). Dementia care receiver needs and their impact on caregivers. *Clinical Nursing Research, 2*(1), 86-97.

Frisch, N.C., & Frisch, L.E. (1998). *Psychiatric-mental health nursing: Understanding the client as well as the condition*. Albany: Delmar.

George, L.K., & Gwyther, L.P. (1986). Caregiver well-being: A multidimensional examination of family caregivers of demented adults. *The Gerontologist, 26*(3), 253-259.

Guzzetta, C., Bunton, S.D., Prinkey, L.A., Sherer, A.P. & Seifert, P.C. (1989). *Clinical assessment tools for use with nursing diagnoses*. St. Louis: Mosby.

Ignatavicius, D.D., Workman, M.L., & Mishler, M.A. (1995). *Medical-Surgical nursing: A nursing process approach*. Philadelphia: Saunders.

Johnson, B.S. (1997). *Psychiatric-mental health nursing: Adaptation and growth*. Philadelphia: Lippincott.

Kozier, B, Erb, G., Blasi, K., Wilkinson, J.M., & Van Leuven, K. (1998). *Fundamentals of nursing*. Menlo Park, CA: Addison-Wesley.

LeMone, P., & Burke, K.M. (1996). *Medical-surgical nursing: Critical thinking in client care*. Menlo Park, CA: Addison-Wesley Nursing.

Lewis, S.M., Collier, I.C., & Heitkemper, M.M. (1996). *Medical-Surgical nursing: Assessment and management of clinical problems*. St. Louis: Mosby.

Miles, M.B., & Huberman, A.M. (1994). *Qualitative data analysis*. Thousand Oaks, CA: Sage.

Monahan, F.D., & Neighbors, M. (1998). *Medical-surgical nursing: Foundations for clinical practice*. Philadelphia: Saunders.

Newman, M.A. (1984). Nursing diagnosis: Looking at the whole. *American Journal of Nursing, 84*(12), 1496-1499.

O'Connor, P., Vander Plaats, S., & Betz, C.L. (1992). Respite care services to caretakers of chronically ill children in California. *Journal of Pediatric Nursing, 7*, 269-275.

Phipps, W., Cassmeyer, V.H., Sands, J.K., & Lehman, M.K. (Eds.). (1995). *Medical-surgical nursing: Concepts and clinical practice*. St. Louis: Mosby.

Potter, P.A. & Perry, A.G. (1997). *Fundamentals of nursing*. St. Louis: Mosby.

Rawlins, R.P., Williams, S.R., & Beck, C.K. (Eds.). (1993). *Mental health-psychiatric nursing: A holistic life-cycle approach*. St. Louis: Mosby Year Book.

Ridgeway, S.A.P. (1995). *Rural daughter/daughter-in-law caregivers' interactional patterns*. Unpublished doctoral dissertation, University of Minnesota, Minneapolis.

Roy, S.C. (1984). Framework for classification systems development: Progress and issues. In M.J. Kim, G.K. McFarland, & A.M. McLane (Eds.), *Classification of nursing diagnoses: Proceedings of the fifth national conference*. St. Louis: Mosby.

Schultz, R., O'Brien, A.T., Bookwala, J., & Fleissner, K. (1995). Psychiatric and physical morbidity effects of dementia caregiving: Prevalence, correlates, and causes. *The Gerontologist, 35*(6), 771-791.

Stuart, G.W., & Sundeen, S.J. (1995). *Principles and practices of psychiatric nursing*. St. Louis: Mosby.

Taylor, C., Lillis, C., & LeMone, P. (1997). *Fundamentals of nursing: The art and science of nursing care*, (2nd ed).. Philadelphia: Lippincott.

Townsend, M.C. (1996). *Psychiatric mental health nursing: Concepts of care.* Philadelphia: F.A. Davis Company.

Wilson, H.S. (1989). Family caregiving for a relative with Alzheimer's dementia: Coping with negative choices. *Nursing Research, 38*(2), 94-98.

Wilson, H.S., & Kneisl, C.R. (1996). *Psychiatric nursing.* Menlo Park, CA: Addison-Wesley Nursing.

Wong, D.L. ,& Wilson, D. (1995). *Whaley and Wong's nursing care of infants and children.* St. Louis: Mosby.

Measuring Acute Care Functional Status of the Older Adult

Gail C. Davis, RN, EdD
Mildred O. Hogstel, RNC, PhD

This study was supported by an award from the Texas Christian University Research and Creative Activity Fund. The invaluable assistance of Katy Scherger, RN, APN, who assisted in coordinating the project, and the nurses who collected the data made this study possible.

The major aim of this study was to develop a precise, valid, and reliable clinical index for assessing the functional status of acutely-ill hospitalized patients, age 65 and older. Since older adults may have diminished physical, cognitive, and/or social resources, their overall condition can decline rapidly when an acute illness or the need for surgery occurs. The rapidity of this decline makes the close monitoring of functional status of hospitalized older adults extremely important. Thirty-four to fifty percent of older persons lose function unrelated to their primary medical diagnosis while hospitalized (Inouye et al., 1993).

Acute care functional status was conceptually defined as the level of the older adult's functional independence during hospitalization for an acute condition. Nursing diagnoses accepted by the North American Nursing Diagnosis Association (NANDA) were examined to determine which might provide an appropriate basis for assessing this status. Those identified by the investigators as most related to this definition were Toileting: Self-care deficit, Urinary Incontinence, Bathing/Hygiene: Self-care deficit, Dressing/Grooming: Self-care deficit, Feeding: Self-care deficit, Impaired Physical Mobility, Knowledge Deficit, Powerlessness, Altered Thought Processes, Relocation Stress Syndrome, Activity Intolerance, Sensory/Perceptual Alterations, and Risk for Injury. Indicators of these nursing diagnoses were then selected as possible measures of the concept, i.e., acute care functional status.

Introduction to the Problem

Persons age 65 and older are estimated to constitute 50% to 70% of the hospitalized patient population, and the average number of hospital days for each hospitalization of this age group is 8.6 (AARP, 1993). This "average length of stay for older people has decreased 5 to 6 days since 1968 and 2.1 days since 1980" (AARP, p. 14). Shorter hospital lengths of stay (LOS) require that increased attention be given to maintaining function and preventing the decline of functional status. "Many frail older adults are discharged from hospitals weaker, more confused, and more dependent than they were before admission" (Trella, 1994, p. 316). Failure to address the diminished functional capacity of older patients along with the use of potentially harmful interventions (e.g., indwelling catheters for incontinence) may lead to longer hospitalization and/or discharge to a setting that can provide a dependent level of care (Hirsch, Sommers, Olsen, Mullen, & Winograd, 1990).

Health care delivery decisions today are increasingly influenced by cost, and this places an ever greater emphasis on attempts to quickly measure the relevant indicators that will have a major impact on the outcomes of care. In an attempt to lower hospitalization costs, hospital LOS are continuing to decrease for all age groups. This presents a special issue for the nursing care of older persons who may be frail and have several coexisting conditions. Loss of function during hospitalization may occur related to the illness, the plan of treatment, inattention to aspects of care that promote the maintenance of function, and because older patients generally do not regain their previous levels of functioning as quickly as younger people.

The older adult is also more susceptible to experiencing disorientation and confusion during the course of treatment that often involves bedrest in a strange environment with either sensory deprivation or sensory overload. Early hospital discharge associated with these added obstacles to regaining pre-hospitalization functional status becomes a major issue for the older person. Functional decline may be due to the hospitalization itself, as well as to the illness that caused hospitalization in the first place (Keating, 1992). Negative factors that often cause unnecessary functional decline in hospitalized older patients are indiscriminate use of restraints (Sullivan-Marx, 1994), overmedication, lengthy response to call lights causing nurse-induced incontinence, lack of satisfactory communication with health care providers, and absence of essential nursing interventions such as normal range-of-motion exercises.

A number of functional status tests exist for use with older adults, such as the Katz ADL Scale, Barthel Index, Kenny Self-Care Scale, and Instrumental ADL Scale (Applegate, Blass, & Williams, 1990). These include measures of activities of daily living (ADL) and instrumental activities of daily living (IADL). ADL scales are helpful in providing information about assistance the person needs in performing basic activities (bathing, dressing, toileting, transferring, continence, and feeding) (Katz et al., 1963). IADL scales provide added information about such activities as telephone use, travel, shopping, meal preparation, housework, taking own medicine, and handling personal finances (Fillenbaum, 1985). While these provide valuable information for planning rehabilitative services, the intent of the development of the Acute Care Functional Status Index (ACFSI) was to provide assessment and monitoring of functional status during hospitalization. As opposed to most existing measures, it is hoped that this tool will require little training of raters, provide very specific information that can impact ongoing treatment, and will require minimal assessment time.

Research Objectives

The major objective of this study was to develop

a valid and reliable measure of the functional status of hospitalized older adults. The specific objectives related to the measure's psychometrics were to (a) select a range of clinical indicators for measurement that meet specified criteria (i.e., represent selected nursing diagnoses, simple to observe, measurable using a simple rating scheme, and relevant to the study's definition of acute care functional status), (b) estimate content validity of the selected functions (i.e., items), (c) estimate interrater reliability, and (d) estimate test-retest reliability (i.e., stability). Such estimates of validity and reliability are essential documentation for any instrument that is to be used in the process of clinical decision making (Davis, 1994). In keeping with the intent to develop a tool that is precise, accurate, and easy to use, simple scaling is needed to provide the nurse with a method for rating the perceived level of the individual patient's independence in performing each function. The professional nurse's judgment provides the data source.

Methods
Design
This methodological study focused on item development and psychometric estimations deemed appropriate for this index: content validity, interrater reliability, and test-retest reliability. A recognized limitation of the study is that there are other unmeasured variables (e.g., mental status and social activity) contributing to functional status when it is more broadly defined as including these components (Rubenstein et al., 1989).

Sample
Study participants (n=34) were selected from older adults admitted to one of two participating medical-surgical units in a university-affiliated hospital. The mean age of the sample that included 25 females and 9 males was 80.5 years (s.d.=4.9). Subjects met the following criteria for participation: at least 75 years of age and admitted to the hospital for an acute condition (e.g., respiratory infection, surgical procedure, fracture, stroke, and complication of a chronic condition).

Instruments
Acute Care Functional Status Index (ACFSI). The instrument under development was used for the purpose of psychometric testing. It was estimated to have a content validity index (CVI) of 1.00. Each of the eight content experts rated all of the items as relevant to the concept measured using the procedure suggested by Lynn (1986). The ACFSI is a tool used by the nurse to rate the individual patient's level of independence in performing each of the identified clinical indicators related to the selected nursing diagnoses (see Figure 1). Two subscale scores and a total score may be computed by summing the ratings and dividing that total by the number of items rated, first for the 12 indicators/items on each subscale and then for the 24 combined. This scoring method adjusts for situations where a zero (0) rating may be used. It should also be noted that if the item scores are averaged, the 0 rating should not be included. Subscale 1 (Physical Function) uses the following rating scale:

0 = not applicable/no opportunity to assess
    (e.g., patient sleeping)
1 = not able to perform alone; needs
    maximum assistance
2 = able to partially perform; needs
    moderate assistance
3 = performs with only minimal assistance
4 = performs, but needs standby
    assistance/supervision

Figure 1

Nursing diagnoses and related clinical indictors selected to measure acute care functional status of the older adult

Nursing Diagnoses	Clinical Indicators
	Subscale I: Physical Function
Toileting: Self-Care Deficit	Uses commode in bathroom or uses bedpan/urinal or bedside commode
Urinary Incontinence	Uses toilet, bedpan, or urinal when needed or reports need to urinate
Bathing/Hygiene: Self-Care Deficit	Bathes self in bed, chair, tub, or shower
	Carries out oral hygiene
Dressing/Grooming: Self-Care Deficit	Removes and/or puts on gown or other clothing
	Puts on own hose, slippers, and/or shoes
	Combs/brushes hair
	Applies cosmetics/shaves
Feeding: Self-Care Deficit	Cuts food/opens cartons
	Moves food from plate to mouth
Impaired Physical Mobility	Moves in and out of bed or chair
	Walks with or without assistive devices
	Subscale II: Physiological/Psychosocial/Cognitive and Sensory Function/Risk for Injury
Knowledge Deficit	Identifies the correct reason(s) for hospitalization (e.g., specific diagnoses, surgery, or tests) when asked. Asks questions/seeks information as appropriate (e.g., "What time does the doctor usually come?")
Powerlessness	Verbalizes positive feelings about gaining control over current life situation (e.g., any comments that demonstrate a sense of having self-control)
Altered Thought Processes	States own first and last name when asked
	States current month and year when asked
Relocation Stress Syndrome	States current location when asked (e.g., "in hospital"). Follows simple instructions (e.g., uses call system correctly)
Activity Intolerance	Verbalizes feeling weak or fatigued (when appears to be) without being asked. Remains alert during activities (e.g., eating, talking)
Sensory/Perceptual Alterations	Identifies a small object (not furniture, etc.) at least 5 feet away when asked to do so. Identifies words whispered at least 1 foot away when asked to do so
Risk for Injury	Uses appropriate judgment (e.g., does not attempt to get out of a bed that is raised)

5 = needs no assistance/performs independently

Due to the different nature of the indicators, Subscale 2 (Physiological/Psychosocial/Cognitive & Sensory Function/Risk for Injury) uses a 0 to 3 rating scale:

0 = no opportunity to assess (e.g., patient sleeping)
1 = does not identify/demonstrate/respond to questions
2 = identifies/demonstrates/responds to questions only with considerable prompting
3 = independently identifies/demonstrates/responds to questions

Demographic Form. An individual data sheet provided descriptive data related to each patient.

Procedure

Prior to data collection, interrater reliability was estimated with the ratings of 12 patients by the 8 nurse raters. Participants who met the study criteria gave informed consent prior to entering the study. Functional status was measured, using the ACFSI, at 3 different times: (a) within the first 12 hours of admission, (b) 24 hours following the first measurement, and (c) within 12 hours of discharge. All assessments were done by one of 8 registered nurses (RNs) (i.e., 4 on each unit) prepared to use the ACFSI. In-hospital assessments were done within 12 hours of admission, 24 hours following the first measurement, and within 12 hours of discharge.

Data Analysis

Estimation of the ACFSI's reliability focused on testing interrater reliability and stability (test-retest from admission to 24 hours). Due to the preciseness desired for a clinical instrument, a simple computation of the proportion of observed interrater agreements in the same classification by the two different raters provided the interrater reliability estimate (Waltz, Strickland, & Lenz, 1991). In addition to evaluating the percentage of agreement, the agreement/disagreement of individual items was also examined (Washington & Moss, 1988). Stability of the instrument was estimated by correlating the first two assessment scores (i.e., at admission and within 24 hours of admission).

Results

The psychometric estimations of the ACFSI are high. Experts (i.e., nurses specializing in care of older adults) indicated that all of the indicators/items demonstrated content validity (CVI=1.00). Stability was also high when the first two ratings (admission and 24 hours later) were correlated (r=.96). Likewise, the interrater reliability was high when tested prior to data collection with the study sample. Rater agreements across the items ranged from 61 percent to 100 percent. Items that appeared to be the most troublesome were (a) "uses toilet, bedpan, or urinal when needed or reports need to urinate," (b) "carries out oral hygiene," and (c) "puts on own shoes." These first two will need to be further evaluated for consistency; the problem ratings were primarily related to the lack of opportunity to assess. The third item was revised prior to actual testing to include hose and slippers, as well as shoes.

Discussion

Continuing psychometric estimates with other samples of hospitalized older adults are needed to determine whether these findings replicate.

Additionally, it will be interesting to assess the sensitivity of the instrument to change. It will be important to statistically compare the ACFSI scores at the times of hospital admission and discharge as the tool is used with various samples. Since a visual examination of these scores with this sample showed limited variation within or between patients, such comparisons will be of interest for determining the sensitivity of the instrument to change. Meanwhile, the ACFSI should provide a precise clinical measure of the older adult's functional status that is useful for ongoing assessment of the individual.

References

American Association of Retired Persons (AARP). (1993). *A profile of older Americans: 1993* (DHHS Publication No. PF3049 [1293]. D996). Washington, DC: Program Resources Department.

Applegate, W. B., Blass, J. P., & Williams, T. F. (1990). Instruments for the functional assessment of older patients. *The New England Journal of Medicine, 32*, 1207-1214.

Davis, G. C. (1994). Measurement and clinical decision making: Focus on instrument development. *Nursing Diagnosis, 5*, 121-126.

Fillenbaum, G. G. (1985). Screening the elderly: A brief instrumental activities of daily living measure. *Journal of the American Geriatrics Society, 33*, 698-706.

Hirsch, C. H., Sommers, L., Olsen, A., Mullen, L., & Winograd, C. H. (1990). The natural history of functional morbidity in hospitalized older patients. *Journal of the American Geriatrics Society, 38*, 1296-1303.

Inouye, S.K., Wagner, D.R., Acampora, D., Horwitz, R.I., Cooney, L.M., & Tinetti, M.E. (1993). A controlled trial of a nursing-centered intervention in hospitalized elderly medical patients: the Yale geriatric care program. *Journal of the American Geriatrics Society, 41*, 1353-1360.

Katz, S., Ford, A. B., Moskowitz, R. W., Jackson, B. A., Jaffe, M. W., & Cleveland, M.A. (1963). Studies of illness in the aged: The Index of ADL: A standardized measure of biological and psychosocial function. *Journal of the American Medical Association, 185*, 94-99.

Keating, H.J. (1992). Major surgery in nursing home patients: Procedures, morbidity, and mortality in the frailest of the frail elderly. *Journal of the American Geriatrics Society, 40*, 8-11.

Lynn, M.R. (1986). Determination and quantification of content validity. *Nursing Research, 35*, 382-385.

Rubenstein, L. V., Calkins, D. R., Greenfield, S., Jette, A. M., Meenan, R. F., & Nevins, M. A. (1989). Health status assessment for elderly patients: Report of the Society of General Internal Medicine Task Force on Health Assessment. *Journal of the American Geriatrics Society, 37*, 562-569.

Sullivan-Marx, E.M. (1994). Delirium and physical restraint in the hospitalized elderly. *Image, 26*, 295-300.

Trella, R. (1994). From hospital to nursing home: Bridging the gaps in care. *Geriatric Nursing, 15*, 313-316.

Waltz, C. F., Strickland, O. L., & Lenz, E. R. (1991). *Measurement in nursing research* (2nd ed.). Philadelphia: F.A. Davis.

Washington, C. C., & Moss, M. (1988). Pragmatic aspects of establishing interrater reliability in research. *Nursing Research, 37*, 190-191.

Analysis of the Nursing Diagnosis Altered Growth and Development

Janice A. Denehy, RN, PhD
Cyd Q. Grafft, RN, MSN, ARNP

The growth and development of infants and children is of primary concern to nurses who work with children and families. When children visit their primary health care provider for child health maintenance appointments, the first assessment data collected is the child's height and weight which is subsequently plotted on standardized growth charts which quickly reveal patterns of growth and comparisons of the child's height and weight to established norms. During these visits, developmental screening is also performed routinely to determine if the child is achieving expected developmental milestones. When these assessments indicate a deviation from the norm in either growth or development, Altered Growth and Development (NANDA, 1996) is the nursing diagnosis of choice.

After working with experienced pediatric nurses and advanced nurse practitioners over the years, it became apparent this nursing diagnosis was not reflective of what actually was seen in clinical practice. The first concern related to the fact that the diagnostic label, Altered Growth and Development, indicates there is a problem with both growth and development which is not the case in many instances where the diagnosis is used. Many children for whom this diagnosis is selected have either altered growth or altered development. For example, many children with failure to thrive or growth disorders exhibit normal development; conversely, many children with developmental delays or disabilities may be growing appropriately for their age. Therefore, this becomes problematic when both altered growth and altered development do not coexist. The existing diagnosis, Altered Growth and Development, lacks the specificity needed to differentiate between these two populations of children (See Table 1).

Second, the major defining characteristics of the nursing diagnosis Altered Growth and Development lack the precision needed to trigger early intervention services needed by children with altered development. The major char-

Table 1

Altered Growth and Development*

6.6 ALTERED GROWTH AND DEVELOPMENT (1986)

DEFINITION:

The state in which an individual demonstrates deviations in norms from his/her age group.

DEFINING CHARACTERISTICS:

Major: Delay or difficulty in performing skills (motor, social, or expressive) typical of age group; altered physical growth; inability to perform self-care or self-control activities appropriate for age.

Minor: Flat affect; listlessness, decreased responses.

RELATED FACTORS:

Inadequate caretaking; indifference; inconsistent responsiveness; multiple caretakers; separation from significant others; environmental and stimulation deficiencies; effects of physical disability; prescribed dependence.

NANDA Nursing Diagnoses: Definitions and Classification 1997-98. (1996). St. Louis: North American Nursing Diagnosis Association (p. 65-66).

---

acteristics (delay or difficulty in performing skills and inability to perform self-care or self-control activities appropriate for age) are vague and do not add much to what is already stated in the definition. The only defining characteristic that relates to altered growth (altered physical growth) again does not state specific criteria needed to make this diagnosis. The minor defining characteristics (fiat affect, listlessness and decreased responses) are not useful in characterizing children with either altered development or altered growth. The related factors, while more complete in the psychosocial domain, need to include physiological factors that contribute to altered growth and altered development. Many children with altered development experience prematurity or serious illness after birth. For other children, a traumatic head injury or brain tumor may be contributing factors to developmental delay. Abnormal growth is frequently a result of genetic conditions, physical or metabolic disorders which need to be included in the list of related factors. An earlier validation study by Coviak (1987) identified the need for a separate diagnosis for children with nonorganic failure to thrive and suggested maternal child nurses adopt a common term for children who display developmental delay.

Third, nursing diagnoses are used to give direction to the selection of nursing interventions and outcomes. The Iowa Intervention Team has linked all of the NANDA nursing diagnoses to the interventions in the Nursing Interventions Classification (NIC) (Iowa Intervention Project, 1996). The NIC interventions linked to Altered Growth and Development include a wide scope of interventions, ranging from Developmental Enhancement to Nutrition Therapy (p. 635).

From this list it is evident that interventions used to treat altered growth and altered development are very different. In fact, interventions designed to treat altered growth may not be appropriate for altered development and visa versa. Nursing diagnosis also give direction to the choice of interventions used to achieve desired outcomes. The Iowa Outcome Project (1997) has developed 10 outcomes related to child development from infancy through adolescence and one outcome labeled Growth which are included in the Nursing Outcomes Classification (NOC). The NOC outcomes also have been linked to each NANDA nursing diagnoses. Linkages for the diagnosis Altered Growth and Development include the outcomes related to child development and growth, as well as outcomes developed for the adult and elderly population (p. 335).

Finally, nurses frequently see children who are at risk for altered growth and development. For example, nurses who work in high-risk infant follow-up clinics monitor infants for a number of years post discharge from a neonatology unit following a premature birth or other serious health problem which put them at risk for altered growth or altered development. Therefore, there is a need for additional nursing diagnoses to reflect this risk status that triggers regular vs. enhanced follow up and other interventions designed to promote optimum growth and development.

Methods and Results

The purpose of this study was to analyze the NANDA nursing diagnosis Altered Growth and Development. The researchers are members of the Nursing Diagnosis Extension and Classification (NDEC) research team at The University of Iowa College of Nursing.

Procedures developed by the NDEC team (Craft-Rosenberg & Delaney, 1997) were pilot tested to analyze this diagnosis. To begin the concept analysis process, an exhaustive literature review was done on the concepts of growth and development. This review of research and practice literature in nursing and related disciplines was essential in identifying the defining characteristics and related factors of these two concepts. From the vast body of literature identified, the five to ten most relevant empirically-based articles were selected based on requirements for clear concept attributes (defining characteristics) and antecedents (related factors). Each article was reviewed and data regarding the diagnostic label, definition, defining characteristics and related factors were recorded. The concept analysis validated the need for two separate diagnoses, Altered Growth and Altered Development, based on the fact that two distinct bodies of literature existed for the two concepts and there were different and distinct defining characteristics and related factors for each concept.

After the review of the literature was completed, a synthesis of the data was done to formulate diagnostic labels based on terminology used in current practice and to develop definitions to clearly articulate the phenomena of concern. A list of defining characteristics (labeled signs and symptoms by the NDEC team) and related factors was formulated and referenced for each diagnosis. The new diagnoses were worded clearly to insure identification of individuals who meet requirements for special education services, supported living or environmental adaptations available for children with developmental disabilities. At the same time the new diagnoses were developed, diagnoses to reflect the risk status, At risk for Altered Growth and At risk for Altered Development, were developed from the literature (Grafft, 1996).

After the new diagnoses were completed, they were submitted to the Parent/Infant/Child Diagnosis Work Group Chairman of the NDEC team for review. During this process, the diagnoses were reviewed by others in the work group with content expertise in the area for clarity, comprehensives and usefulness in clinical practice. Wording and format changes were suggested, including organizing related factors into clusters, such as prenatal factors, postnatal factors and environmental factors, for ease of retrieval. In addition, the defining characteristics and related factors were organized into vertical lists that contributed to ease in scanning and identifying content of the diagnosis and making it more visually pleasing and readable for the user. These lists were then placed in columns so each diagnosis could be produced on one page, including references. These procedures were then adopted by the NDEC team for their further diagnosis refinement work.

After review by the Diagnosis Work Group, the refined diagnoses were submitted to the NDEC Rules Committee where they were reviewed for conformity to language structure and format developed by the principal investigators and Rules Committee members. At this point, the diagnosis labels were reworded to Growth Alteration, Development Alteration, Growth Alteration Risk and Development Alteration Risk to be consistent with NDEC conventions for the wording of diagnostic labels. After revisions and approval by this committee, the diagnoses were sent to the entire NDEC team for review and subsequent final approval (See Tables 2 & 3). The approved diagnoses have been staged and submitted to NANDA for review and acceptance in the classification. The need for two additional or candidate diagnoses, Potential for Enhanced Development and Potential for Normal/Optimal Growth, was identified (Grafft, 1996). These diagnoses will be useful in ambulatory settings, schools and communities where the focus is health promotion and wellness.

Implications for Practice and Research

Although nursing diagnoses have been a part of nursing practice for over 20 years, there still is a lot of exciting and challenging work ahead of us as a profession to update, validate and make the NANDA classification more reflective of the wide scope of nursing practice in all specialties. Particularly needed are diagnoses to promote the health of children and families in the community. The researchers at The University of Iowa College of Nursing have embraced this challenge and have assembled a large research team composed of nursing educators, researchers and clinicians to evaluate, revise, validate and extend the existing NANDA nursing diagnoses classification. This study is an example of the first aim in the research program, concept analysis of one nursing diagnosis, Altered Growth and Development, and presentation of the resulting refinement and development of four new nursing diagnoses, Growth Alteration, Development Alteration, Growth Alteration Risk, and Development Alteration Risk.

The refined nursing diagnoses will assist nurses who work with children and families in more clearly diagnosing problems related to growth and development. In addition, more precision in the diagnoses will lead to selection of specific interventions designed to treat the problems identified and to achieve desired outcomes. Hopefully, the work of the NDEC team

Table 2

Growth Alteration

<u>DEFINITION</u>:

Growth above the 97th percentile or below the 3rd percentile for age, crossing two percentile channels; disproportionate growth pattern.

<u>SIGNS AND SYMPTOMS</u>:

Weight above 98th percentile or below the 3rd percentile the 1st 2 years of life [2,3,6,7]
Growth of less than 2-2.5 inches/year ages three to ten years [4,5]
Growth above or below 3 standard deviations from the mean [1,4,5,7]
Failure to maintain consistent pattern of growth [5,7,8,9]
Bone age greater or less than chronological age [1,3,6]
Delay or absence of puberty [2,4,6,7]
Precocious puberty [1,3,6]
Learning problems [1,4,5,7]
Behavioral difficulties [1,4,5,7,9]
Depression [5,9]

<u>RELATED FACTORS</u>:

<u>Prenatal Factors</u>:
   Infection [2,5,8]
   Congential/genetic disorders [1,2,3,4,5,7,8]
   Maternal nutrition [4,5,8]
   Multiple gestation [5,8]
   Teratogen exposure [2,3,4,5,8]
   Substance use/abuse [3,4,5,6,8]

<u>Postnatal Factors</u>:
   Prematurity [3]
   Malnutrition [2,3,4,5,6,7,8]
   Organic and inorganic factors [2,5,6,8]
   Caregiver and/or individual maladaptive feeding behaviors [2,3,5,7,9]
   Anorecia [5,7]
   Insatiable appetite [7,9]

<u>Individual Factors</u>:
   Infection [1,2,3,7]
   Chronic Illness [2,3,4,5,7,8]
   Substance Abuse [1,5]
<u>Caregiver Factors</u>:
   Abuse [3,5,7,8,9]
   Mental illness, mental retardation, or severe learning disability [3,5,8]

<u>Environmental Factors</u>:
   Deprivation [7,8]
   Teratogen exposure [8]
   Lead poisoning [3,7]
   Poverty [3,7,8]
   Violence [3,7]

References:

1. Connaughty, M. S. (1992). Accelerated growth in children. *Journal of Pediatric Care, 6*(5), 316-324.
2. Denniston, C.R. (1994). Assessing normal and abnormal patterns of growth. *Primary Care, 21*(4), 637-654.
3. Frank, D.A., Needlman, R., & Silva, M. (1994). What to do when a child won't grow. *Patient Care, 28*(5), 107-110, 113, 117-120. 125-128, 135.
4. Giordano, B.P. (I (1992). The impact of genetic syndromes on children's growth. *Journal of Pediatric Health Care. 6*(5), 309-315.
5. Henry, J.J. (1992). Routine growth monitoring and assessment of growth disorders. *Journal of Pediatric Health Care, 6*(5), 291-261.
6. Lobo, M.L., Barnard, K.E., & Coombs, J.B. (1992). Failure to thrive: A parent-infant interaction perspective. *Journal of Pediatric Nursing, 7*(4),251-261.
7. Parker, S.H. (1992). The school nurse's role: early detection of growth disorders. *Journal of School Nursing, 8*(3), 30-32, 34, 36-38, 40-41.
8. Pinyerd, B.J. (1992). Assessment of infant growth. *Journal of Pediatric Health Care, 6*(5), 302-308, 333-334.
9. Stanhope, R., Wilks, Z., & Hamill, G. (1994). Failure to grow: Lack of food or lack of love? *Professional Care of Mother & Child, 4*(8), 231-233.

Table 3

Development Alteration

<u>DEFINITION</u>:

A delay in one or more of the areas of social or self-regulatory behavior, or cognitive, language, gross or fine motor skills.

<u>SIGNS AND SYMPTOMS</u>:

Delay of 25% or more or failure to achieve developmental milestones [1,15]

Permanent loss of skills [1,5,10]

<u>RELATED FACTORS</u>:

<u>Prenatal Factors</u>:

Maternal age <15> 35 years [4]
Substance Abuse [1,4,8,11,12,13]
Infections [1,4,8,11,12,13]
Genetic/endocrine disorders [1,4,8,9,12]
Unplanned/unwanted pregnancy [8]
Lack of, late or poor prenatal care [3,4,6,8,9]
Inadequate nutrition [6,8]
Illiteracy [6,7,9]
Poverty [4,6,8,9,12,14]

<u>Postnatal Factors</u>:

Prematurity [1,4,8,9,11,12,13]
Seizures [1,5,6,8,9,12,14]
Congenital/genetic disorders [1,4,5,8,9,11]
Positive drug screening test [8]
Brain damage, e.g., hemorrhage in postnatal period, shaken baby, abuse, accident, infection [4,5,8,9,10]
Vision impairent [1,4,6,8,14]
Hearing impairment/frequent otitis media [1,4,6,8,9]
Chronic illness [1,4,6,8,9,12]
Technology dependent [1,3,4,8,9]
Failure to thrive/inadequate nutrition [1,4,8,11,12]
Foster or adopted child [2]
Lead poisoning [4,8]

<u>Caregiver Factors</u>:

Abuse [3,4,6,8]
Mental illness [3,6,8,9]
Mental retardation or severe learning disability [1,3,4,6,8,9]

<u>Individual Factors</u>:

Behavior disorders [2,3,6,7,10,15]
Substance abuse [4]

<u>Environmental Factors</u>:

Poverty [4,6,8,9]
Violence [8,9,12]

References:

1. Batshaw, M.L., & Perret, Y.M. (1992). *Children with handicaps: a medical primer.* (3rd Edition.) Baltimore: Paul H. Brookes.
2. Brodzinky, D.M., & Steiger, C. (1991). Prevalence of adoptees among special education populations. *Journal of Learning Disabilities, 8*(10), 484-489.
3. Child, A.A., Murphy, C.M., & Rhyne, M.C. (1980). Depression in children: Reasons and risks. *Pediatric Nursing, 6*(4), 68-72.
4. Curry, D.M., & Duby, J.C. (1994). Developmental surveillance by pediatric nurses. *Pediatric Nursing, 29*(l), 40-44.
5. Dam, M. (1994). Children with epilepsy: The effect of seizures, syndromes, and etiological factors on cognitive functioning. *Epilepsia, 31*(Supp. 4), S26-S29.
6. Davidhizar, R., & Frank, B. (1992). Understanding the physical and psychosocial stressors of the child who is homeless. *Pediatric Nursing, 86*, 559-562.
7. Glascoe, F.P, Alterneier, W.A., & MacLean, W.E. (1989). The importance of parents' concerns about their child's development. *American Journal of Diseases in Children, 143*(8), 955-958.
8. Kimmel, S.R., Quinn, E.A., & Phelps, KA. (1994). Assessing child development. *Primary Care, 21*(4),673-692.
9. King, E.H., Logsdon, E.A., & Schroeder, S. (1992). Risk factors for developmental delay among infants and toddlers. *Child Health Care, 21*(l), 39-52.
10. Koskiniemi, M., Kyykka, T., & Jarho, L. (1995). Long-term outcome after severe brain injury in preschoolers is worse than expected. *Archives of Pediatric and Adolescent Medicine, 149*(3), 249-245.
11. Little, B.B., Snell, L.M., Rosenfeld, C.R., Gilstrap, L.C., & Grant, N.R. (1990). Failure to recognize fetal alcohol syndrome in newborn infants. *American Journal of Diseases in Children, 144*(10), 1142-1146.
12. Lipsi, K, Clements-Shafer, K., & Rushton, C.H. (1991). Developmental rounds: An intervention strategy for hospitalized infants. *Pediatric Nursing. 17*(5), 433-436.
13. Singer, L., Arendt, R., Song, L.Y., Warshawsky, E., & Skiegman, R. (1994). Direct and indirect interactions of cocaine with childbirth outcomes. *Archives of Pediatric and Adolescent Medicine, 148*(9), 959-964.
14. Sran, S.K., & Baumann, R.J. (1988). Outcome of neonatal strokes. *American Journal of Diseases in Children, 142*(10), 1086-1088.
15. Stone, W.L., Hoffman, E.L., Lewis, S.E., & Ousley, O.Y. (1994). Early recognition of autism. *Archives of Pediatric and Adolescent Medicine, 148*(2), 174-179.

will inspire other nurses to identify additional nursing diagnoses that are needed in an ever changing health care arena. Lastly, existing and refined nursing diagnoses need to be validated through research in clinical settings with children representing a wide range of socio-economic, cultural, racial, and geographic groups. Such research will provide an empirical base for the practice of professional nursing.

References

Coviak, C.P., (1987). Alteration in growth and development: A nursing diagnosis validation study. In A.M. McLane (Eds.). *Classification of nursing diagnoses: Proceedings of the seventh conference North American Nursing Diagnosis Association.* (pp. 212-216.). St. Louis: The C.V. Mosby Company.

Craft-Rosenberg, M., & Delaney, C. (1997). Nursing diagnosis extension and classification (NDEC). In M.J. Rantz & P. LeMone (Eds.). *Classification of nursing diagnoses: Proceedings of the twelfth conference North American Nursing Diagnosis Association.* (pp. 26-31.). Glendale, CA: Cinahl Information Systems.

Grafft, C.Q. (1996). *Validation of Nursing Diagnosis: Altered Growth and Development.* Unpublished master's thesis. The University of Iowa, Iowa City, IA.

Iowa Intervention Project (1996). *Nursing interventions classification (NIC).* (2nd ed.). St. Louis: Mosby Yearbook.

Iowa Outcomes Project (1997). *Nursing outcomes classification (NOC).* St. Louis: Mosby Yearbook.

NANDA nursing diagnoses: Definitions and classification 1997-1998. (1996). St. Louis: North American Nursing Diagnosis Association.

Nursing Interventions and Outcomes for the Nursing Diagnosis Decreased Cardiac Output

Cynthia M. Dougherty RN, PhD, ARNP

The inability of the heart to supply the amount of oxygenated blood needed for the body's metabolic requirements is termed pump failure or decreased cardiac output. Decreased cardiac output has been defined by the North American Nursing Diagnosis Association (NANDA) as "a state in which the blood pumped by an individual's heart is sufficiently reduced that it is inadequate to meet the needs of the body's tissues" (NANDA, 1995). For decreased cardiac output, defining characteristics were developed at the second conference on the classification of nursing diagnosis by the panel of nurses who were present. Etiologies were not developed until the fifth national conference, at which time changes were made in the definition and defining characteristics as well. Subsequent NANDA publications now have eliminated etiologies for decreased cardiac output, with no further changes made in the other structural components of the diagnosis since 1982. (See Table 1.)

Since its original listing in the NANDA taxonomy in the 1970's, there have been a number of clinical papers describing nursing diagnoses associated with varying cardiac conditions, including decreased cardiac output (Brooks-Brunn, 1987; Cardin, 1985; Buman & Speltz, 1989; Contrades, 1987; Kelly, 1991; Rossi, 1979; Russell & Blake, 1989; Teplitz, 1990, 1991; Whitman & Hicks, 1988). Two papers have described the design of assessment tools for measuring the nursing diagnosis of decreased cardiac output (Contrades, 1987; Dougherty, 1986). A number of validation studies have been published since the early 1980's that suggest the need for revision in the original definition, etiologies, and defining characteristics as listed by NANDA (Burke et al, 1986; Dalton, 1985; Hubalik & Kim, 1984; Kern & Omery, 1992; Kim et al, 1984; Lazure & Cuddigan, 1987; Miller & Helander, 1979; Roberts, 1992; Scanlon, 1992). Investigations have used descriptive methods, contained small sample sizes, primarily focused on critically ill individuals, relied on medical records for data gathered, and used a variety of definitions of the concept.

"

Table 1

Diagnosis, Interventions, and Outcomes

DIAGNOSIS	INTERVENTIONS	OUTCOMES
Decreased Cardiac Output	**Cardiac Care**	**Cardiac Pump Effectiveness**
	Circulatory Care	Circulation Status
	Hemodynamic Regulation	*Vital Sign Status*
Defining Characteristics	*Activities*	*Indicators*
Variations in hemodynamic readings	**Monitor vital signs frequently**	***BP IER**
		Vital signs IER
	***Recognize presence of BP alterations**	CVP IER
	Monitor SVR & PVR	Free of orthostatic hypotension
	Place in trendelenberg position	
	Monitor pulmonary artery pressures	PWP IER
	Administer positive inotropic agents	
	Evaluate negative effects of inotropic agents	
Elevated pulmonary artery pressures	*Monitor cardiac output and cardiac index*	Cardiac Index IER
Arrhythmias; ECG changes	***Document cardiac dysrhythmias**	Free of dysrhythmias
	Monitor for cardiac dysrhythmias	***Heart rate IER**
	Monitor pacemaker functioning, if applicable	
	Evaluate response to ectopy or dysrhythmias	
	Provide anti-arrhythmic therapy	
	Monitor response to anti-arrhythmic medications	
Decreased peripheral pulses	Perform appraisal of peripheral circulation	***Peripheral pulses strong**
Color changes, skin & mucous membranes	*Evaluate peripheral pulses	Skin color normal
Cold, clammy skin	Inspect skin for stasis ulcers & wounds	**Free of diaphoresis**
	Palpate limb with caution	Peripheral tissue perfusion IER
	Assess degree of discomfort or pain	Peripheral pulses symmetrical
	Lower extremity to improve arterial circulation	Free of large vessel bruits
	Apply anti-embolism stockings	
	Elevate limb above heart for venous circulation	
	Administer antiplatelet medication	
	Change position every 2 hours	
	Use therapeutic mattress	
	Instruct on importance of prevention of stasis	
	Instruct on importance of foot care	
Weight gain	***Monitor fluid balance**	24 hour I/O balanced
	Monitor abdomen for decreased perfusion	Free of ascites
	Monitor electrolyte levels	
	Insert urinary catheter	
Edema	*Evaluate peripheral edema	***Free of peripheral edema**
Oliguria	*Monitor fluid status	
Jugular vein distention (JVD)	*Maintain adequate hydration	***Free of neck vein distension**
Dyspnea	**Monitor respiratory status for heart failure**	Free of pulmonary edema
Orthopnea	**Monitor for dyspnea, fatigue, tachypnea, orthopnea**	Blood gases IER
Wheezing	*Auscultate lung sounds*	A-V O2 difference IER
Increased respiratory rate	*Elevate head of bed*	Free of adventitious breath sounds
Use of accessory muscles for breathing		
Abnormal heart sounds S3 and S4		Free of abnormal heart sounds
Abnormal chest x-ray (congestion)		Heart size normal
Chest pain	Evaluate chest pain	***Free of angina**
	Instruct on immediate reporting of angina	
Ejection fraction < 40%		Ejection fraction IER
Elevated cardiac enzymes		
Abnormal heart sounds (S3, S4)		Free of abnormal heart sounds
Restlessness	Recognize psychological effects of condition	
	Establish supportive relationship	
	Offer spiritual support	
Altered mental status	*Promote stress reduction	Cognitive status IER
Fatigue	Instruct on activity restrictions	Activity tolerance IER
	Arrange exercise and rest periods to avoid fatigue	Free of fatigue
	Monitor activity tolerance	
	Encourage passive or active ROM exercises	
	Encourage exercise as tolerated	
Other	Note S&S of decreased cardiac output	
	Monitor cardiovascular status	
	Restrict smoking	

*= appears in all categories
IER = In Expected Range.
Black Bolded = Cardiac Care/Cardiac Pump Effectiveness
Black = Circulatory Care/Circulation Status
Italics = Hemodynamic Regulation/Vital Sign Status
d:\cindy\cindy\dconandatable.doc

Despite these issues, research results reflect that NANDA's efforts at defining decreased cardiac output had good beginnings. Recommended revisions in the definition and defining characteristics have been presented but not yet incorporated into the NANDA taxonomy (NANDA, 1995).

Although much has been written about decreased cardiac output, little of the work so far has explicated a conceptualization of cardiac output that reflects physiological and pathophysiological concepts within a framework that is workable for nurses. This concept is challenging and complex in delineation given that both the right and left heart are connected by two complex vascular systems. In clinical practice cardiac output is rarely allowed to fall below normal levels when individuals are hospitalized, so more information is required regarding defining characteristics in order for nurses to detect and adequately treat decreases in cardiac output effectively. The purpose of this paper is to present a model of altered cardiac output, with links to nursing interventions and nursing sensitive outcomes that are specific for clinical practice.

Altered Heart Rate

Cardiac rate and rhythm are regulated by the rate of discharge from the sinoatrial (SA) node, discharges from the sympathetic and parasympathetic nervous systems, metabolic demands, and other neural mechanisms. Stimulation of the sympathetic nervous system will cause increases both in heart rate and in the strength of contraction by releasing norepinephrine at nerve-ending sites throughout the heart muscle (Guyton, 1981). An increase in heart rate alone can increase cardiac output threefold within a limited time frame. Stimulation of the parasympathetic nervous system produces a decrease in heart rate only. Bradycardia does not always produce a decrease in cardiac output because stroke volume will increase to compensate for the drop. In patients with fixed stroke volume, decreases in heart rate will produce reductions in cardiac output, as in the patient who has suffered a myocardial infarction (Braunwald, 1988).

Heart rates that are too slow, too fast, or irregular may cause decreased cardiac output in patients with compromised cardiac function. Tachycardia (HR > 100 bpm) results in decreased atrial and ventricular filling time and emptying. During diastole the coronary arteries fill with blood, with increased heart rates producing reduced oxygen supply to the myocardium. Bradycardia (HR < 60 bpm) may result in decreased cardiac output if not compensated with increases in stroke volume. Arrhythmias produce a loss in atrial-ventricular sequencing and may decreased cardiac output by as much as 30%. Individuals may manifest alterations in heart rate by complaining of palpations, dizziness, lightheadedness, or syncope.

Altered Stroke Volume

Preload is the volume of blood that fills both ventricles during diastole, the right heart receiving blood from the systemic circulation and the left heart from the pulmonary circulation. Factors affecting preload include systemic venous return, venous pressure or tone, pulmonary venous volume, intrathoracic pressure, pericardial pressure, and atrial contraction (Braunwald, 1988).

Increases in preload occur when venous system pressure rises. The patient may experience edema in dependent body parts such as the sacrum and lower extremities and a weight gait of 10 pounds or more. With advancing decreases in cardiac output, fluid may accumulate in pericardial cavities. As the work and forcefulness of the right ventricle (RV) decreases, a lifting or heave in the chest wall along the sternal border may be produced. In either RV or left ventricle (LV) failure, rising pressure within the heart produces apposition of valves, resulting in murmurs. Preload of the right heart is assessed by central venous pressure (CVP, normal 2-6 mm Hg), right ventricular stroke work index (RVSWI normal, 7-12 g/m2/beat), and pulmonary artery systolic pressure (PAS, normal 20-30 mm Hg). Preload of the LV is reflected as afterload of the RV. Alterations in RV function are manifested in the patient by peripheral edema, hepatomegaly, cool extremities, jugular venous distension, nausea and vomiting, abdominal fullness and pain, fatigue and weakness.

Increases in pulmonary artery (PA) pressures will affect the right heart, resulting in decreased output from the right heart. As pressure in the right heart rises, congestion in the venous system, abdominal organs, and capillary interstitial spaces occurs. This rising pressure causes an increase in right ventricular end diastolic pressure (RVEDP), increasing right atrium (RA) pressure, increasing CVP, and backup of blood from the right heart into the venous system (Braunwald, 1988). Jugular venous distention (JVD) can be used to determine a general estimate of right heart venous return and RA pressure. An elevation of the JVD more than 1 to 2 cm above the Angle of Louis at 45 degrees signals increased RA pressure and may even produce observable venous pulsations. Increased pressure in the inferior vena cava causes the liver and spleen to become enlarged and congested. The patient may complain of abdominal pain, and the hepatojugular reflux may be positive. Ascites, edema of the bowel,

nausea, vomiting, anorexia, and abdominal distention may also accompany venous congestion (Loeb & Gunnar, 1981).

Myocardial contractility is the inherent ability of the cardiac muscle to contract and is explained by the Frank-Starling Law of the Heart (Starling, 1926). Contractility is not readily measurable at the bedside but is indicative of LV function. The ability of the heart to contract is decreased by factors causing increased myocardial oxygen consumption, such as tachyarrhythmias, an enlarged ventricular diameter, high afterload, primary myocardial disease (cardiomyopathy), coronary artery disease, and myocardial infarction, all of which can cause myocardial ischemia with a secondary decrease in contractility. Ventricular contractility is also affected by factors that decrease myocardial oxygen delivery such as hypoxemia, acidosis, narrowing of the coronary arteries, and low arterial pressure. Drugs known to affect the contractile state of the ventricle include lidocaine, quinidine, propranolol, pronestyl, and disopyramide (Loeb & Gunnar, 1981). Within certain limits, the heart will pump whatever amount of blood that flows into it without significant changes in cardiac output, unless contractility is severely affected.

A decreased pumping efficiency of the left ventricle causes both backward and forward effects. The forward effect is decreased tissue perfusion to organs, and the backward effect is increased volume and pressure in the pulmonary circulation. As the ventricle becomes less able to empty completely and effective cardiac output falls, blood remains in the left ventricle at the end of systole. In an attempt to augment the amount of blood ejected from the left ventricle, the heart enlarges and increases its rate and force of contraction (Starling, 1926).

This compensatory mechanism, primarily governed by the sympathetic nervous system, can maintain cardiac output for a time but eventually becomes ineffective and the heart decompensates. As decompensation progresses, more blood accumulates in the left ventricle and causes further dilation and hypertrophy (Guyton, 1981). Tachycardia and pulsus alterans (alternation of one strong beat with one weak beat during sinus rhythm) may be noted. Consequently, left ventricular end diastolic pressure (LVEDP) increases and a third heart sound (S3) appears. The fourth heart sound (S4) is produced late in diastole and is created when the atria contract with resistance to ventricular filling, indicating decreased myocardial compliance and rising left ventricular pressure (Braunwald, 1988).

As pressure continues to increase in the left ventricle and blood backs up from the left ventricle to the left atrium, a rise in LA pressure will be noted. Eventually pulmonary artery and venous pressures will increase, pulmonary artery wedge pressure will increase above plasma oncotic pressure in the lung, and signs of pulmonary vascular congestion develop. As fluid begins to accumulate in the lungs, more specific symptoms such as dyspnea, orthopnea, paroxysmal nocturnal dyspnea, and Cheyne-Stokes respirations will appear (Poole-Wilson, 1988).

A dry cough develops early in the failure phase of decreased cardiac output as fluid acts as an irritant in the interstitial spaces. As the alveoli become filled with fluid, the cough will become productive, and occasionally pulmonary vessels will rupture, producing hemoptysis. Rales develop when pulmonary capillary pressure has exceeded normal plasma osmotic pressure, and fluid moves from the pulmonary capillary to the alveoli (Chapman & Mitchell, 1965). Chest pain, wheezing, and pleural effusion may

also be noted. Rales are first noted in dependent lobes of lung tissue. As pulmonary edema develops, they will gradually become diffuse and bilateral. Myocardial contractility is indirectly measured by stroke volume index (SVI, normal 35-70 ml/beat/m2 or SV/BSA), left ventricular stroke work index (LVSWI, normal 50-60 g/m2/beat or (MAP-PAD)SVI x 0.0136), and ejection fraction (EF, normal 50-60% or SV-EDV x 100).

Afterload is the resistance against which the heart must pump to eject blood. It is determined by the diameter of arterioles in the pulmonary and systemic circulations (Parmley, 1989). Factors determining left ventricular afterload include cold temperatures or any substance that causes vasoconstriction and increases systemic vascular resistance; drugs such as levophed, aramine, epinephrine, and dopamine in high doses; pulmonary artery hypertension; aortic valvular disease; or high mean arterial pressure (Dahlen & Roberts, 1996).

Right ventricular afterload is determined by the pulmonary circulation. If pulmonary vessels constrict or obstruction to pulmonary blood flow is present, an increase in pulmonary vascular resistance occurs with subsequent increase in afterload of the right ventricle (RV). This will in turn decrease preload of the left heart (Braunwald, 1988). Factors affecting right ventricular afterload include any condition causing pulmonary constriction such as an increase in alveolar p02 or decrease in arterial p02, pulmonary embolism that causes obstruction to blood flow, pulmonary vascular defects, and vasoactive substances such as histamine, which will increase pulmonary vascular resistance.

Afterload of the RV is determined by pulmonary vascular resistance (PVR, normal 150-250 dynes/sec/cm-5 or PA mean - PAW/CO x

80). PVR is the ratio of pressure drop across the pulmonary vascular system to total flow in the pulmonary circulation. An increase in intravascular volume or increase in venous return can overfill the LV and cause increased PVR and pulmonary edema. Pulmonary artery diastolic pressure (PAD, normal 10-20 mm Hg) and pulmonary artery wedge pressure (PAW, normal 4-12 mm Hg) are determinants of pulmonary vascular dynamics.

The forward effects of decreased cardiac output are primarily the result of decreased blood flow to organs and tissues and usually appear early in the cycle. A decrease in blood flow to the musculoskeletal system produces complaints of fatigue, weakness, and restlessness. The patient may complain that his or her energy level is gone and may exhibit changes in posture, gait, and speech. Blood flow to the heart and brain will be maintained by the sympathetic nervous system at the expense of the skin, kidneys, and muscle. Central nervous system signs of decreased perfusion are manifested by confusion, agitation, decreased attention span with memory lapse, and anxiety. The patient may complain of insomnia. As blood flow is decreased to the skin in response to vasoconstriction produced by the sympathetic nervous system, the skin becomes cold and clammy with slow capillary refill, diaphoretic, cyanotic, and pale. This redistribution of blood to the core organs will cause a decrease in skin temperature in peripheral areas, while the trunk remains warm (White & Roberts, 1992).

Afterload of the LV is determined by systemic vascular resistance (SVR, normal 900-1200 dynes/sec/cm-5 (MAP-CVP/CO x 80). SVR reflects resistance to LV emptying and is affected by blood pressure and autonomic stimulation producing catecholamines and angiotensin.

Increased SVR is often an automatic response stimulated in an attempt to maintain BP in patients with falling LV function. The patient with alterations in afterload with increased PVR and increased SVR will manifest SOB, dyspnea, peripheral edema, anxiety, increased respiratory rate, confusion, cool skin, cyanosis, pallor, and fatigue.

As cardiac output becomes more severely decreased, the patient may begin to move toward the cardiogenic shock, representing the most severe impairment of cardiac output. The exact cause is not known but can be predicted when greater than 40% of the heart muscle has become dysfunctional (White & Roberts, 1992). There are usually profound decreases in stroke volume and arterial pressure; therefore, organs and tissues are severely deprived of oxygen. As a result, cells divert to anaerobic glycolysis, producing metabolic acidosis. For survival, the sympathetic nervous system maintains perfusion to vital organs, with widespread arteriole and venule constriction, tachycardia, increased forcefulness of contraction, and dilation of coronary arteries. When cardiogenic shock is allowed to ensue and continue over an extended time period, compensatory mechanisms fail and death results.

Nursing Interventions

Nursing interventions for the treatment of decreased cardiac output have been described in clinical papers that outline nursing care for patients with coronary artery disease. Two research investigations (Dougherty, 1985; Wessel & Kim, 1984) have identified nursing interventions associated with decreased cardiac output by critical care nurses. These investigations are descriptive in nature. Clinical trails testing nursing interventions related to decreased cardiac output with their associated outcomes have not been conducted.

In congestive heart failure and cardiogenic shock, Dougherty (1985) identified both independent and collaborative interventions used by nurses when treating decreased cardiac output. Independent interventions included monitoring activity, responses to oxygen, arterial blood gases, IV fluids and intake, environment and laboratory values; planning frequent rest periods; bathing; feeding; assisting with deep breathing exercises; performing CPR and emergency drug administration; reassuring family members; changing dressings; providing positive support and frequent patient contact; starting IV fluids; encouraging rest; and allowing the patient to participate in care. Collaborative nursing interventions include calculating intake and output, daily weights, monitoring hemodynamic parameters, administering medications and oxygen, treating chest pain, and initiating bedrest.

Wessel and Kim (1984) outlined nursing interventions in a sample of 21 patients with congestive heart failure and decreased cardiac output. Twenty-six nursing interventions were developed from questionnaire data provided by staff nurses caring for this sample. Interventions were then classified as independent, collaborative, or dependent based on nurses opinions. Independent interventions included: cardiovascular assessment, pulmonary assessment, physical assessment, interpretation of laboratory data, nutrition, activities of daily living (ADL), skin care, therapeutic positioning, deep breathing/coughing, aseptic environment, intravenous (IV) therapy, patient teaching, psychological support, family teaching and psychological support, therapeutic environment, written communication, overall evaluation.

Collaborative interventions included vital signs, Swan-Ganz readings, ECG monitoring, fluid management, therapeutic activity, oxygen therapy, collaboration with other health care providers. Dependent interventions included medication administration and regulating medications.

The goals of treatment for a person with decreased cardiac output are to: 1) optimize the availability of oxygen and other nutrients to tissues, 2) optimize cardiovascular function, and 3) minimize fear, anxiety, and stress (Bumann & Speltz, 1989). Treatment strategies can be directed at determinants of cardiac output, namely heart rate and rhythm, preload, afterload, and contractility. Four categories of nursing interventions described by Bumann and Speltz (1989) included 1) rhythm monitoring and treatment, 2) hemodynamic monitoring and treatment, 3) reducing the workload of the heart, and 4) psychosocial interventions. The goal of rhythm monitoring and treatment is the establishment of an effective heart rate and rhythm to maintain cardiac output. Specific nursing interventions would include ECG monitoring, administration of anti-arrhythmic treatments, monitoring activity, treating chest pain, and patient and family education (Bumann & Speltz, 1989; Futrell, 1990; White & Roberts, 1992).

The goal of hemodynamic monitoring and treatment is early detection and treatment of changes in cardiac output and prevention of complications. Astute observations as well as accurate interpretations and clinical judgments by the nurse are needed in order to maintain a stable cardiac output. This includes the technical expertise in set up, maintenance, and trouble shooting of hemodynamic monitoring systems. Monitoring of blood pressure, pulmonary artery pressures, calculating cardiac output, cardiac index, and other parameters are required. These hemodynamics must be correlated with physical data such as mentation, heart sounds, peripheral pulses, urine output, peripheral capillary refill, breath sounds, skin color/temperature, and fluid volume status in order to make correct judgments about the state of the heart. When hemodynamic parameters are abnormal, other nursing interventions are instituted such as titrating medication drips and fluids and monitoring side effects.

Reducing the workload of the heart is achieved by the monitoring of preload, afterload, and contractility. When preload is assessed to be reduced, crystalloids, colloids, and blood products will be used, depending on the needs of the person. Preload is reduced by the use of diuretics and vasodilating agents that the nurse must monitor. When afterload is elevated, the workload of the heart increases. Afterload is reduced by vasodilating agents and intra-aortic balloon pumping, both of which require expert monitoring skills. Myocardial contractility must be maintained in order to improve ventricular emptying. This is achieved with titration of inotropic agents and monitoring clinical indicators of contractility. Reducing the workload of the heart is also achieved by eliminating activity and stressors that increase myocardial oxygen demands. Some of these interventions include planning rest periods, administering oxygen, positioning to optimize ventilation and bowel elimination, and evaluating the impact of activity.

Psychological interventions will influence all other physiological parameters of cardiac output. Cardiac related illness produces cognitive and emotional responses that need to be assessed and monitored as well. Reducing stress associated with the critical care environment,

assessing illness perceptions, and recognizing emotional responses will lead the nurse to facilitation of the expression of concerns and anxiety. Crisis management may be necessary for both patients and their family members (Bumann & Speltz, 1989; Futrell, 1990; White & Roberts, 1992).

A number of suggested nursing interventions have been linked to decreased cardiac output in the most recent Nursing Intervention Classification (McCloskey & Bulechek, 1996). The three nursing interventions categories most salient for decreased cardiac output cardiac care, circulatory care, and hemodynamic regulation. Cardiac care has been defined as a limitation in complications resulting from an imbalance between myocardial oxygen supply and demand for a patient with symptoms of impaired cardiac function (McCloskey & Bulechek, 1996, p. 156). Cardiac care also includes the activities associated with acute cardiac care and cardiac precautions. Acute cardiac care interventions are implemented in order to limit complications for a patient experiencing a recent cardiac event while cardiac precautions are used in order to prevent an acute episode of impaired cardiac function. Circulatory care is defined as the promotion of arterial and venous circulation. Hemodynamic regulation is defined by the NIC as the optimization of heart rate, preload, afterload, and contractility (McCloskey & Bulechek, 1996). Nursing activities associated with these nursing interventions can be found in Table 1.

Other nursing intervention categories relevant to the nursing diagnosis decreased cardiac output include fluid management, shock management: cardiac, circulatory care: mechanical assist device, dysrhythmia management, vital sign monitoring, and electrolyte management.

Any or all of these interventions can be applied depending on the severity of the impairment. The majority of the nursing activities within each intervention category contain monitoring interventions. Monitoring the defining characteristics of decreased cardiac output include both the collection of data and the judgments made about the data that then leads the nurse to implement other interventions. The anticipation and prevention of complications in patients with acute cardiac disorders can be aided by these interventions.

Nursing Sensitive Outcomes

Outcomes associated with the diagnosis decreased cardiac output will include a return to normal values in the defining characteristics found to be present when the diagnosis was made. Some of these outcomes could be associated with actions taken by the nurse when implementing nursing interventions, but others can be attributed to adaptive mechanisms in the body or medical interventions. As with nursing interventions associated with decreased cardiac output, outcomes have been generally described (AACN, 1990), but not systematically studied in populations with varying cardiovascular conditions.

From the Nursing Sensitive Outcomes Classification (Maas & Johnson, 1998), the two categories of outcomes most salient to decreased cardiac output are cardiac pump effectiveness and circulation status. Cardiac pump effectiveness is defined as the amount of blood ejected from the left ventricle per minute to support systemic perfusion pressure and includes the indicators of BP, cardiac index, ejection fraction, heart rate, activity tolerance all within expected range; peripheral pulses strong; free of neck vein distension, dysrhythmias, angi-

na, abnormal heart sounds, peripheral edema, pulmonary edema, and diaphoresis; and normal skin color and heart size (Maas & Johnson, in press). Circulation status is defined as the extent to which blood flows unobstructed, unidirectionally, and at an appropriate pressure through large vessels of the systemic and pulmonary circuits. Indicators for circulation status that are in addition to those for cardiac pump effectiveness include a normal pulse pressure, mean BP, CVP, PWP, blood gases, A-V O2 difference, peripheral tissue perfusion and cognitive status; being free of orthostatic hypotension, adventitious breath sounds, large vessel bruits, ascites, and fatigue; balanced 24 intake and output; and strong and symmetrical peripheral pulses (Bumann & Speltz, 1989; Futrell, 1990; White & Roberts, 1992). (See Table 1.) Depending on the etiology and severity of the heart condition, any or all of these outcomes could be monitored and recorded.

Summary

Decreased cardiac output was first listed in the nursing diagnosis taxonomy in 1975. Since that time, discussions have focused on whether or not this diagnosis should continue to be included in the NANDA taxonomy. Current discussions now demonstrate that decreased cardiac output is a nursing diagnosis frequently encountered by nurses in a variety of patient care settings. Interventions used by nurses to stabilize and treat decreased cardiac output have been outlined using descriptive research methods. A conceptual model that links clinical and theoretical concepts was proposed. Nursing sensitive outcomes associated with decreased cardiac output have been described in clinical papers but have not been systematically tested. Future research should be focused on the systematic testing of components of the conceptual model, linking the diagnosis with interventions and outcomes.

References

American Association of Critical Care Nurses (1990). *Outcome standards for nursing care of the critically ill.* Laguna Niguel, CA: AACN.

Braunwald, E. (1988). *Heart disease: A textbook of cardiovascular medicine.* (3rd ed.). Philadelphia: WB Sanders Co.

Brooks-Brunn, J. A. (1987). Formulating appropriate nursing diagnoses for the patient receiving tissue-type plasminogen activator. *Heart and Lung, 16*(6), 787-791.

Buman, R., & Speltz, M. (1989). Decreased cardiac output: A nursing diagnosis. *Dimensions of Critical Care Nursing, 8*(1), 6-15.

Burke, L.J., Gabriel LM, Fischer LE, & Zemke SL (1986). Nursing diagnoses, indicators, and interventions in an outpatient cardiac rehabilitation program. *Heart and Lung, 15*(1), 70-76.

Cardin, S. (1985). A nursing diagnosis approach to the patient awaiting cardiac transplantation. *Heart and Lung, 14*(5), 499-504.

Chapman, C.B., & Mitchell J.H. (1965). *Starling on the heart.* London: Dawsons of Pall Mall.

Contrades, S. (1987). Altered cardiac output: An assessment tool. *Dimensions of Critical Care Nursing, 6*(5), 274-283.

Dahlen, R., & Roberts, S.L. (1996). Acute congestive heart failure: Preventing complications. *Dimensions of Critical Care Nursing ,15*(5), 226-241.

Dalton, J. (1985). A descriptive study: Defining characteristics of the nursing diagnosis

cardiac output, alterations in: decreased. *Image, 17*(4), 113-117.

Davies, M.J. (1992). Pathology of the aging heart. In J. C. Brocklehurst , R.C.Tallus, & H. M. Fillit (Eds.). *Textbook of geriatric medicine and gerontology*, (4th ed.) (pp. 181-187). Edinburgh: Churchill Livingstone.

Dougherty, C.M. (1985). The nursing diagnosis decreased cardiac output. *Nursing Clinics of North America, 20*(4), 787-799.

Dougherty, C.M. (1986). Decreased cardiac output: Validation of a nursing diagnosis. *Dimensions of Critical Care Nursing, 5*(3), 182-188.

Futrell, A. (1990). Decreased cardiac output: Case for a collaborative diagnosis. *Dimensions of Critical Care Nursing, 9*(4), 202-209.

Guyton, A.C. (1981). The relationship of cardiac output and arterial pressure control. *Circulation, 64*(6),1079-1088.

Harizi, R.C., Bianco, J.A., & Alpert, J.S. (1988). Diastolic function of the heart in clinical cardiology. *Archives of Internal Medicine, 148*, 99-109.

Hubalik, K., & Kim, M.J. (1984). Nursing diagnoses associated with heart failure in critical care nursing. *Classification of nursing diagnoses Proceedings of the fifth national cnference*, p. 139-149.

Hurst, J.W. (1986). *The heart.* (7th ed.), New York: McGraw Hill Co.

Kaminsky, A., & Molitor, M.. (1987). Validation study of the nursing diagnosis decreased cardiac output. In A. McLane, (Ed). *Classification of nursing diagnoses: Proceedings from the seventh national conference.* (pp. 275). St. Louis: C.V. Mosby.

Kelly, D.J. (1991). The identification and clinical validation of the defining characteristics of alteration in cardiac tissue perfusion. In R.M. Carroll-Johnson (Ed), *Classification of nursing diagnoses Proceedings of the ninth national conference*, (pp.105-111). Philadelphia: J.B. Lippincott Co.

Kern, L .,& Omery A (1992). Decreased cardiac output in the critical care setting. *Nursing Diagnosis, 3*, 94-106.

Kim, M.J., Seritella, R.A., Gulanick, M., Moyer, K., Parsons, E., Scheberel, J., Stafford, M.A., Suhayda, R.M., & Yocum, C. (1984). Clinical validation of cardiovascular nursing diagnoses. *Classification of nursing diagnoses Proceedings of the fifth national conference*, 128-138.

Kitzman, D.W. (1988). Age-related changes in normal human hearts during the first 10 decades of life. Part II: Maturity: A quantitative anatomic study of 765 specimens from subjects 20 to 99 years old. *Mayo Clinic Proceedings, 63*, 137-146.

Lakatta, E.G. (1990). Cardiovascular disorders: Normal changes with aging. In W.B.Abrams & R. Berkow (Eds). *Merck manual of geriatrics*. (pp. 309-325) Rahway, NJ: Merck, Sharp, & Dohme Research Laboratories.

Lazure ,L.L., & Cuddigan, J. (1987). (Abstract). Clinical validations of decreased cardiac output: Differentiation of defining characteristics according to etiology. In A. McLane. (Ed). *Classification of nursing diagnoses: Proceedings from the seventh national conference*. (p. 274). St. Louis: C.V. Mosby.

Loeb, H., & Gunnar, R.M. (1981). Treatment of pump failure in acute myocardial infarction. *JAMA, 245*, 2093-2096.

Maas, M., & Johnson, M. (1997). *Nursing outcomes classification (NOC)*. St. Louis: C.V. Mosby Co.

McCloskey, J.C., & Bulechek, G. (1996). *Nursing intervention classification*. St. Louis: C.V. Mosby

Miller, J.C.,, Helander, M (1979). The 24-hour cycle and nocturnal depression of human. cardiac output. *Aviation Space Environmental Med, 50,*1139-1144.

NANDA (1995). *NANDA nursing diagnoses: Definitions and classification 1995-96*. Philadelphia: North American Nursing Diagnosis Association.

Parmley, W.W. (1989). Pathophysiology and current therapy of congestive heart failure. *American College of Cardiology, 13*(4), 771-785.

Poole-Wilson, P. (1988). Current therapeutic principles in the acute management of severe congestive heart failure. *American Journal of Cardiology, 62*, 4C.

Roberts, S. (1992). Common nursing diagnoses for pulmonary alveolar edema patients. *Dimensions of Critical Care Nursing, 11*(1), 13-26.

Rossi, L.P. (1979). Nursing diagnoses related to acute myocardial infarction. *Cardiovascular Nursing, 15*(3), 11-15.

Russell, A.C., & Blake, S.M. (1989). Aortic valvuloplasty: Potential nursing diagnoses. *Dimensions of Critical Care Nursing, 8*(2), 72-82.

Scanlon, L.M. (1992). The nursing diagnosis decreased cardiac output: A clinical diagnosis validation study. *Military Medicine, 157*, 166-68.

Starling, E.H. (1926). Regulation of the energy output of the heart. *J Physiol, 62*, 243-261.

Swan, H.J.C. et al (1970). Catheterization of the heart in man with use of a flow-directed balloon-tipped catheter. *New Eng Journal of*

Med, 283, 451-477.

Teplitz, L. (1990). Patients with ventricular assist devices: Nursing diagnoses. *Dimensions of Critical Care Nursing, 9*(2), 82-87.

Teplitz, L. (1991). Nursing diagnoses for automatic implantable cardioverter defibrillator patients. *Dimensions of Critical Care Nursing, 10*(4), 188-201.

Wessel, S., & Kim, M.J. (1984). Nursing functions related to the nursing diagnosis decreased cardiac output. In M.J.Kim G. McFarland, & A. McLane. *Classification of nursing diagnoses: Proceedings of the fifth national conference,* (pp.192-98), St. Louis: C.V. Mosby.

White, B.S., & Roberts, S.L. (1992). Pulmonary alveolar edema: Preventing complications. *Dimensions of Critical Care Nursing, 11*(2), 90-103.

Whitman, G.R., & Hicks, L.E. (1988). Major nursing diagnoses following cardiac transplantation. *Journal of Cardiovascular Nursing, 2*(2), 1-10.

Wong, W.F., Gold, S., Fukuyama, O., & Blanchette, F.L. (1989). Diastolic dysfunction in elderly patients with congestive heart failure. *American Journal of Cardiology, 63,* 1526-28.

Anxiety in Adult, Intubated, Mechanically Ventilated Patients: An Expert Validation Study

Susan A. Ford, RN, MSN, CCRN

The author wishes to express sincere appreciation to Dr. Lorys Oddi, Dr. Georgia Whitley, Joanne O'Donnell, and Nicole Haley for their assistance in the preparation of this manuscript. I also thank my fellow critical care staff nurses, pulmonologists, and respiratory therapists and Glen Oaks Medical Center.

Patients who require mechanical ventilation exhibit signs and symptoms of the stress response and anxiety that require immediate nursing interventions to prevent an unplanned extubation, a potentially life-threatening situation. This study explored the objective signs and symptoms of anxiety in adult, intubated, mechanically ventilated patients. The conceptual model of nursing diagnosis provided the framework for this study.

Background and Significance

Severe ventilatory compromise and insufficiency require immediate airway access for the delivery of supplemental oxygen, whether it be delivered by a mask or by a mechanical ventilator. This life-threatening situation elicits the stress response to prepare the body for "fight-or-flight" (Robinson, 1990). The stress response may, and often does, continue for the duration of mechanical ventilation and is exhibited physiologically and behaviorally. An intubated patient who is exhibiting this response is often labeled as "agitated" or "anxious." Once hypoxia due to an adverse change in the patients condition or an equipment malfunction has been ruled out as the potential etiology of the anxiety, "adequate sedation" is required to reduce the agitation or anxiety (Maguire, DeLorenzo, & Maggio, 1994; Pesiri, Stewart, Kobe, & Stewart, 1990; Taggert & Lind, 1994). If the stress response is not managed with timely interventions, it can lead to an unplanned extubation (Pesiri, 1994).

Unplanned extubation is a significant problem in mechanically ventilated patients because it can lead to laryngeal edema, laryngospasm, respiratory failure, cardiopulmonary arrest, and death. The incidence of unplanned extubation has been reported to be as high as

"

21% (Ellstrom, Brenner, & Williams, 1991). Nurses can play a role in helping to prevent these unplanned extubations by promptly identifying the exhibited stress response and providing interventions to mitigate its effects. The significance of managing this response and preventing unplanned extubation is recognized by the American Association of Critical-Care Nurses (AACN). This national organization identified as a first priority of clinical practice research in the 1990's "techniques to optimize pulmonary functioning and prevent pulmonary complications" (Lindquist, Banasik, & Barnsteiner, 1993).

Problem Statement

What objective signs or symptoms in adult, intubated, mechanically ventilated patients operationally define anxiety that may lead to an unplanned extubation?

Conceptual Framework

The conceptual model of nursing diagnosis provided the framework for this study. Nursing diagnostic categories within this model have three components: the label, the etiological and contributing factors, and the defining characteristics (Carpenito, 1983). Specifically, this study was guided by the defining characteristics component of the model nursing diagnosis. The North American Nursing Diagnosis Association (NANDA) defines nursing diagnosis as "a clinical judgment about individual, family, or community responses to actual or potential health problems/life process. Nursing diagnoses provide the basis for selection of nursing interventions to achieve outcomes for which the nurse is accountable" (Carroll-Johnson, 1990, p. 50).

The purpose of utilizing nursing diagnosis is to identify actual or potential human responses to stressors that adversely affect the patient's attainment of optimal health. Additionally, utilizing nursing diagnosis may help identify nursing's independent domain by providing nurses with a common frame of reference (Carpenito, 1983). Nursing intervention is directed toward causes of the response or the factors influencing it.

Nursing diagnosis is based on a framework that assumes that nursing practice is guided by an holistic model representing the dynamic interrelationships of the mind and body. The framework conveys unity of the individual and suggests that psychologic changes accompany physiologic changes (Guzzetta & Dossey, 1983). This model also suggests that man and environment are open systems that interact, exchange, and create patterns, processes, and organizations.

The nursing diagnosis format consists of the label, the etiology and contributing factors, and the defining characteristics. The label, or problem, is a statement of the patients actual or potential health problem. The etiology refers to the physiologic and/or psychologic factors that influence the problem. The defining characteristics are specific patient behaviors that can be observed through assessment; the defining characteristics lead the nurse to conclude that the patient has a specific problem. Defining characteristics must be present to enable a specific nursing diagnosis to be determined.

Review of the Literature
Unplanned Extubation: Definition and Sequelae

An unplanned extubation can be defined as an inadvertent, unexpected, or accidental removal of the patient's endotracheal tube. It can happen at any time, any place, or under any circumstance with or without the assistance of the patients hands, mouth, or cough reflex (Pesiri, 1994).

Sequelae of unplanned extubation include not only upper airway injury and aspiration of oral or gastric contents, but also the exacerbation of respiratory failure, hypoxemia, and death (Maguire, DeLorenzo, & Maggio, 1994). Such complications result in the patient requiring reintubation. The reintubation rate has been reported in some studies to range from 31-52% (Coppolo & May, 1990; Taggart & Lind, 1994). One study indicated that a patient who was severely ill with respiratory failure experienced a recurrent unplanned extubation that resulted in the patient's death (Maguire, DeLorenzo, & Maggio, 1994). Coppolo and May (1990) reported that 25% of the subjects who experienced an unplanned extubation in their study suffered respiratory failure and 17% suffered from an acute cardiac arrhythmia. Subsequently, these patients required reintubation.

Contributing Factors

Numerous compounding factors increase the incidence of unplanned extubation, including the route of assisted ventilation (oral versus nasotracheal), the duration of placement of the endotracheal tube (fewer than 24 hours), the time of day (morning versus night), and the degree of agitation of the patient (severe) (Taggart & Lind, 1994). Taggart and Lind also found that the unplanned extubation rate varied with the type of intensive care unit. In this study, the following units are listed with their respective unplanned extubation rates: Surgical Intensive Care Unit (SICU)=2% or 7/336, Medical Intensive Care Unit (MICU)=11% or 15/133, Neurosurgical/General Surgical Intensive Care Unit (NS/GSICU)=14% or 8/57, Burns Intensive Care Unit (BICU)=17% or 1/6. Therfore, the incidence of unplanned extubation not only varies in this sample's different units, but it also varies in different patient populations.

Additional contributing factors include ineffective mechanical restraining, inadequate securing of the endotracheal tube, improper length of the endotracheal tube, improper support of the ventilator circuit, underinflation of the endotracheal cuff, and inadequate sedation (Pesiri, 1994). The Pesiri study helped to establish protocols to prevent unplanned extubations: order and reorder "adequate sedation," employ "adequate" mechanical restraints, remove excess water from the ventilator circuit, monitor proper endotracheal cuff pressure, enforce the double-teaming method when giving oral care or releasing the tube fixation system, and consider early tracheostomy in those patients who will probably need prolonged mechanical ventilation.

The most significant factor contributing to unplanned extubation is inadequate sedation. All of the studies reviewed listed inadequate sedation as a major factor and cited it as the basis for the unplanned extubation. The inadequately sedated patient can frequently self-extubate despite other precautions such as physical restraints and vigilant monitoring by the nurse (Pesiri, 1994). A positive relationship exists between the degree of agitation and the likelihood of unplanned extubation (Coppolo & May, 1990; Lamb, Vogelson, & Tack, 1989). In the cited studies, nursing assessments of the patients as they were experiencing an unplanned extubation indicated that the patients were "restless," "agitated," or "anxious."

Findings from selected studies describe numerous interventions to manage agitated, intubated patients. Carroll and Magruden (1993) documented the need for administering medicinal sedation, applying physical restraints, and therapeutically communicating with the intubated patient. However, they did not describe the objective signs that the patient exhibited that led the nurse to describe the patient as "agitated" or "restless." Laing (1992) developed a scale to assess the level of sedation in an agitated, mechanically ventilated patient but did not provide specific, objective cues associated with this condition. Clearly, if inadequate sedation is the major reason for unplanned extubation, and nurses are identifying and interpreting but not defining agitation in the intubated patient, then further investigation to attempt to describe those behaviors that define the agitation is necessary.

Linking Agitation and Anxiety

Some general clinical manifestations of agitation have been described as "disorganized thinking, rambling, incoherent thought' (Crippen & Ermakov, 1992). These clinical manifestations are difficult to assess in the intubated patient because the patient cannot speak. Doherty (1991) defined agitation as a general syndrome of "confusion" and "altered cognitive function" but did not address behaviors specifically observed in the intubated patient. Thus, no available studies operationally defined agitation, which may impair the nurse's ability to identify specific agitated behaviors and provide appropriate interventions to alleviate he behaviors.

Another general definition of agitation is "psychomotor excitement with purposeless, restless activity that may serve to release tension associated with anxiety or fear" (Urdang, 1983). This general definition indicates that agitation is one expression of anxiety. Anxiety, as a nursing diagnosis, was established in 1973, based on the work of Peplau (Gebbie & Lavin, 1975). Peplau (1952) described anxiety as a subjective energy that cannot be observed. The subjective energy is then transformed by thought processes into

behavior, known as "relief behavior." Some subjective categories of anxiety include: feelings of uncertainty, dread, brooding, fear, doubt, apprehension, helplessness, powerlessness, and tension (Whitley, 1992). With intubated patients, these subjective categories are difficult to assess because the placement of the endotracheal tube impairs the patients' ability to communicate.

Nurses must rely on objective signs of anxiety expressed through relief behaviors. A relief behavior is indicated by random motor activity and body gestures that define objective anxiety. Examples of physiologic objective categories of anxiety that are initiated by the autonomic nervous system include: tremors, sweating, tachycardia, tachypnea, dyspnea, restlessness, and paralysis. Thus anxiety, which is perceived in the nursing literature as agitation in the intubated, mechanically ventilated patient, gives rise to observable behaviors. If certain objective behaviors denoting anxiety are specific to intubated, mechanically ventilated patients, operationally defining them can help nurses to diagnose this condition.

Application to Nursing Diagnosis

Important components that enable the nurse to diagnose any condition include operationally defining it by describing its defining characteristics. Once the nursing diagnosis has been made, appropriate nursing interventions can be implemented to help alleviate the condition and prevent the associated sequelae. The condition, once operationally defined, can also be clinically studied and measured.

However, because no operational definition of anxiety in the adult, intubated, mechanically ventilated patient exists, it is difficult to measure. Existing instruments that attempt to measure anxiety, such as the State Trait Anxiety

Inventory, the Trait Anxiety Scale, the Institute of Personality and Ability Test Anxiety Scale, and the Taylor Manifest Anxiety Scale, are inappropriate because of the intubated patients impaired ability to communicate feelings. This is due to the placement of the endotracheal tube, fatigue, disorientation from medicinal sedation, and ultimately, therapeutic paralysis (Dreger, 1983; Spielberger, 1983). Thus, if certain objective behaviors denoting anxiety are specific to intubated patients, operationally defining them can help nurses to diagnose the condition. Early, appropriate interventions could then be designed to reduce and potentially prevent an unplanned self-extubation which can have fatal consequences.

Methodology

Design

The present study was based on the Nurse Validation Model initially proposed by Gordon and Sweeney (1979) and expanded by Fehring (1986). This study employed a survey design in which the respondents (expert nurses) validated a list of objective defining characteristics of anxiety as applied to adult, intubated, mechanically ventilated patients. These experts rated each characteristic with respect to its importance for the diagnosis. This process is known as the expert validation phase of a clinical validation methodology (Hoskins, 1989).

Population and Sample

The target population for this study was the aggregate of all registered nurses employed in critical care who were members of AACN and were certified in adult critical care nursing (CCRN); these respondents are experienced in providing nursing care to adult, intubated, mechanically ventilated patients. Requirements

for certification in adult critical care nursing include a minimum number of hours per year in critical care practice and the successful completion of a multibody systems 200-item test. The certification is valid for three years and may be renewed by earning continuing education credits or rewriting the test. The accessible population was a random sample of CCRNs who were members of AACN.

A random sample of 100 CCRNs was invited to participate. Criteria for inclusion in the study consisted of (a) licensure as a registered nurse, (b) experience in an adult critical care unit, (c) certification in adult critical care nursing, and (d) experience in providing nursing care to adult, mechanically ventilated patients.

Procedures

Access to the sample was provided by the AACN Research Committee through a third-party mailing house. The investigator delivered 100 postage-stamped envelopes, each containing a cover letter, demographic data sheet, survey, and self-addressed, postage-stamped envelope to the mailing house. The mailing house attached the AACN membership labels to the outer envelopes and mailed the packets. Responses were returned to the investigator via the self-addressed stamped envelopes. Voluntary completion of the survey by the anonymous respondent indicated informed consent. Results are reported in the aggregate.

Instrument

The instrument that was used and modified with the author's permission was a version of the "Questionnaire on Anxiety: Anxiety 11" (Whitley, 1994). The 68 defining characteristics and corresponding operational definitions included in the instrument were the result of an extensive concept analysis of anxiety (Whitley, 1992). Forty-two items were eliminated from the original survey by the investigator because they describe subjective characteristics of anxiety. This modification of the original instrument was necessary because the subjective characteristics cannot be directly observed by the nurse. The intubated, mechanically ventilated patient cannot adequately express subjective, anxious feelings because of the impaired verbal communication. Additional items reflecting specific observable behaviors exhibited by intubated patients that were added to the survey were developed from a review of the literature.

The respondents were asked to indicate the degree to which the listed defining characteristics of anxiety and corresponding definitions describe a characteristic of anxiety in adult, intubated, mechanically ventilated patients. The degree of correspondence was indicated by rating on a 5-point Likert scale. The scale ranged from 1 (indicating the characteristic is almost never present with anxiety) through 5 (indicating the characteristic is almost always present with anxiety). The rating design was modeled from previously conducted work on methods to standardize and validate nursing diagnoses (Fehring, 1986; Gordon & Sweeney, 1979).

Reliability and Validity

A pilot study with a panel of six expert nurses was conducted to determine the clarity of items and directions for completion and to identify gaps or repetitions in the content of the items. Another purpose of the pilot study was to establish content validity by asking the experts to evaluate each of the listed defining characteristics as they applied to the adult, intubated, mechanically ventilated patient. Experts were asked to evaluate the operational

definitions and add or delete any of the defining characteristics or operational definitions. Finally, the pilot study evaluated the surveys reliability through a test/retest.

All of the respondents in the pilot study agreed that all defining characteristics and associated operational definitions were appropriate indicators for anxiety in the adult, intubated, mechanically ventilated patient. All of the respondents also agreed that the instructions were clear and the questions were easy to understand. Only one comment was made from one respondent indicating that confusion was "difficult to assess because of the impaired communication." The test/retest scoring was computed and resulted in a Pearson's correlation of .82 (p=.004). However, this must be viewed with caution because of the small sample size.

Analysis of Data

A total of 44 of the 100 distributed instruments was completed and returned for a response rate of 44%. All of the surveys had all of the items completed by all of the respondents.

Table 1

Subject's Level of Education		
Description	N	%
Baccalaurate	21	48
Master's	12	27
Doctorate	1	2
Diploma	7	16
Associate's	3	7

Means were calculated on the respondents' levels of education (see Table 1), types of

Table 2

Subject's Types of Units of Employment (N=44)		
Unit	N	%
ICU/CCU	18	41
SICU	9	20
CCU	8	18
MICU	6	14
Unspecified	2	5
Trauma	1	2

Table 3

Subject's Types of Positions Held (N=44)		
Position	N	%
Staff Nurse	31	70
Clinical Nurse Specialist	5	11
Educator	5	11
Unit Manager	3	7

Table 4

Subject's Approximate Number of Intubated Patients Cared For Per Month (N=44)		
Number of Patients	N	%
5-15	19	43
15-30	10	23
1-5	5	11
30-45	5	11
>45	5	11

units of employment (see Table 2), and positions held (See Table 3). Means were also calculated on the respondents' approximate numbers of intubated patients cared for per month (See Table 4).

Findings

Defining Characteristics of Anxiety

In accordance with the Diagnostic Content Validity (DCV) model, respondents rated each of the established, objective defining characteristics of anxiety according to the relevance of the characteristic to the adult, intubated, mechanically ventilated patient. Each characteristic was rated on a Likert-type scale ranging from 1 to 5, with 1 being not at all indicative of anxiety, 2 seldom indicative, 3 sometimes indicative, 4 frequently indicative, and 5 very indicative. According to the DCV model, each rating was then assigned a weight: 5=1.0, 4=0.75, 3=0.50, 2=0.25, and 1=0. A weighted response for each characteristic was calculated by summing the weights assigned by each of the respondents to each of the characteristics and then dividing this value by the total number of respondents. The mean represented the DCV score for each characteristic and was interpreted according to the criteria specified by the DCV model: Those characteristics scoring 0.80 or higher were classified as major characteristics; those scoring between 0.50 and 0.79 were considered minor characteristics; those scoring below 0.50 were considered not validated.

Major Characteristics of Anxiety

Four (13%) of the 30 objective defining characteristics of anxiety listed on the survey were categorized as major defining characteristics (See Table 5). The corresponding operational definitions included: Restlessness: an expressed feeling or an observed state of motion characterized by an inability to remain at rest or to be perpetually in motion; Teeth and Mouth Activity: patient biting the endotracheal tube or exerting pressure on the endotracheal tube with the tongue to attempt to push it out of the mouth;

Table 5

Major Defining Characteristics of Anxiety in Adult, Intubated, Mechanically Ventilated Patients	
Characteristic	Mean DCV Score
Restlessness	0.85
Teeth and Mouth Activity	0.85
Increased Pulse	0.81
Fight Behavior; Aggressive	0.80

Increased Pulse: a rise of greater than ten beats per minute from the baseline; Fight Behavior, Aggressive: a coping response to a threat which results in arousal, mobility, and offensively oriented actions that are directed at the feared object or fear source.

Minor Characteristics of Anxiety

Eighteen (60%) of the 30 defining characteristics listed on the survey were categorized as minor defining characteristics of anxiety in the adult, intubated, mechanically ventilated patient. These minor defining characteristics and the corresponding mean DCV scores are presented in Table 6.

Not-Validated Defining Characteristics of Anxiety

Eight (27%) of the 30 objective defining characteristics of anxiety listed on the survey were categorized as not validated. The not-validated characteristics and the corresponding mean DCV scores are presented in Table 7.

Additional Characteristics Not Included in Survey

Four behaviors not included in the survey were identified by each of five respondents as being indicative of anxiety in the intubated patient: pounding siderails with hands, attempting to get

Table 6

Minor Defining Characteristics of Anxiety in Adult, Intubated, Mechanically Ventilated Patients	
Characteristic	Mean DCV Score
Increased Respiration Rate	0.78
Insomnia	0.78
Increased Blood Pressure	0.75
Respiratory Difficulties	0.75
Synchronicity Mismatch	0.74
Confusion	0.72
Facial Tension	0.70
Wide-Eyed	0.69
Extraneous Movements	0.68
Increased Perspiration	0.66
Increased Alertness	0.64
Cough	0.63
Glancing About	0.57
Increased Reflexes	0.56
Forgetfulness	0.52
Arterial Pulse Oximeter Change	0.51
Dry Mouth	0.51
Poor Eye Contact	0.50

Table 7

Not-Validated Defining Characteristics of Anxiety in Adult, Intubated, Mechanically Ventilated Patients	
Characteristic	Mean DCV Score
Fight Behavior, Withdrawal	0.49
Flushed Face	0.46
Twitching	0.43
Weakness	0.43
Tremors	0.42
Pupil Dilation	0.39
Superficial Vasoconstriction	0.36
Diarrhea	0.34

hands out of wrists restraints, turning head from side to side, and attempting to sit up in bed. Behaviors mentioned only once included: attempting to talk around the endotracheal tube, attempting to hit or kick staff, stiffening extremities, and clenching hands.

Summary, Conclusions and Recommendations

Conclusions

The response rate may have been higher if postcard reminders had been sent or a second mailing of surveys had been done. A strength of this study is that 54% of the respondents were employed in either a combined ICU/CCU or SICU. This is significant because such units typically have mechanically ventilated patients with a wide variety of diagnoses. The diversity of diagnoses yields a varied amount of time a patient spends on mechanical ventilation. Typically, the mechanically ventilated patient in the SICU is extubated shortly after surgery, whereas the patient with a medical diagnosis in the ICU/CCU may spend more time intubated on mechanical ventilation. Therefore, the respondents who provided nursing care in these different critical care units may see a variety of signs they interpret as anxiety.

Having respondents experienced in caring for patients with a wide variety of diagnoses may provide a more comprehensive pool of signs of anxiety that can be used to identify this nursing diagnosis and prevent an unplanned extubation.

The demographic data also suggest that all of the respondents had extensive experience providing nursing care to the intubated patient. This extensive experience strengthened their ability to identify signs of anxiety in intubated patients.

The major characteristics "restlessness" and "increased pulse" are similar to the findings of previously conducted studies involving psychiatric/mental health and medical-surgical patient populations (Levin, Krainovich, Bahrenburg, & Mitchell, 1989; Whitley, 1994; Whitley, 1988; Whitley & Tousman, 1996). While Fadden, Fehring, and Kenkel-Ross (1987) did not clarify anxiety by the DCV scoring method, restlessness, extraneous movements, poor eye contact, facial tension, and glancing about were seen in the patients the experts observed.

Teeth and mouth activity was not found to be a major or minor characteristic of anxiety in any previously conducted studies. This item was included by the investigator in the modification to specifically address anxiety observed in patients with endotracheal tubes. This major characteristic that has been found in this study of the intubated patient population supports the debate for population-specific defining characteristics (Vincent-Goyette, 1991).

The major defining characteristic "fight behavior; aggressive" was not identified as a major characteristic in any other study. A similar concept of "attack behavior" was not validated in an earlier study of anxiety in psychiatric/mental health and medical-surgical patient populations (Whitley, 1994). A possible explanation for the variation in scoring characteristics as major or minor may be the difference in the patient populations studied. Intubated patients on mechanical ventilation are dependent upon proper endotracheal tube placement for the delivery of life-sustaining oxygen. The endotracheal tube can be very uncomfortable and frustrating because the patient cannot speak and will attempt to pull at the endotracheal tube to remove it. Therefore, most of these patients require physical, bilateral wrist or even ankle restraints. The use of physical restraints, the patients impaired ability to communicate, and the discomfort of the endotracheal tube may contribute to the expression of fight behavior that is elicited by the stress response more than that seen in patients who are not intubated.

A number of characteristics that were classified as major in other studies were not identified as major in this study: increased tension, apprehension, worried, and distressed (Whitley, 1988, 1994). These characteristics are subjective in nature, thus they would not be directly reported with intubated patients because they must be communicated by the patient.

The minor characteristics are similar to those identified in earlier studies of anxiety in other patient populations, with the exception of synchronicity mismatch, cough, and arterial pulse oximeter change. These characteristics were added to the original survey when modified to use with intubated patients.

Additional minor characteristics that were identified in other studies that were not observed in the present study included distressed, focus on self, uncertainty, fearful, scared, jittery, feelings of inadequacy, rattled, and increased wariness (Whitley, 1988). These subjective characteristics were deleted when modifying the instrument because of the intubated patient's inability to communciate subjective feelings.

Tremors and twitching were also found to be not-validated characteristics of anxiety in a previous study of psychiatrictmental health nurse experts (Whitley, 1994). The remaining not-validated characteristics were not specified in previous studies as being either not-validated minor or major characteristics.

It is not surprising that critical care nurse experts indicated that withdrawal and weakness were not indicators of anxiety in the intubated patient. A patient who cannot speak because of the placement of an endotracheal tube, cannot move the arms or legs because of the placement of physical restraints, and cannot sleep because of the multiple incessant noises emitted from the life-sustaining equipment is usually frantic without receiving intraveneous anxiolytics and/or analgesics. Thus withdrawal and weakness would not specfically indicate the nursing diagnosis anxiety when observed in intubated patients. However, withdrawal and weakness do not necessarily exclude the patient from possessing some degree of anxiety.

The respondents' additional characteristics of anxiety observed in intubated patients that were not included in the survey could easily be incorporated into existing operational definitions. These characteristics include restlessness; teeth and mouth activity; and fight behavior, aggressive.

A tentative operational definition of anxiety in the adult, intubated, mechanically ventilated patient can be suggested from the analysis of this data. The patient is observed by the nurse to exhibit the classic "fight behavior, aggressive," demonstrated by restlessness, teeth and mouth activity, increased pulse, blood pressure, respirations, perspiration, alertness and reflexes. The patient may also exhibit respiratory difficulties that may be indicated by a synchronicity mismatch between the ventilator-delivered breaths and the patients spontaneously initiated breaths, coughing, and a decreased arterial pulse oximeter. Additionally, the anxious, intubated, mechanically ventilated patient may exhibit confusion, forgetfulness, insomnia, wide-eyes, poor eye contact, glancing about, and extraneous body movements.

Limitations

The following limitations of this study are acknowledged. The responses of nurses participating in the study were recall descriptions and may not have represented behaviors as they actually occurred at the bedside. This limitation may have posed a threat to external validity because the respondents may have forgotten or exaggerated some experiences. The sample included only critical care nurses who are members of AACN and are certified in adult critical care nursing. The responses of this sample may differ from those of other nurses who care for intubated patients because not all critical care nurses are members of AACN or are CCRN certified.

Recommendations

Practice and Education

Findings from this study have relevance for nursing practice with intubated patients. The

Figure 1

Decisional flowchart depicting the identification of major and minor characteristics of anxiety leading to appropriate nursing interventions

extraneous movements

tachypnea

dyspnea

restlessness

tachycardia

fight behaviors

INTUBATED PATIENT

synchronicity mismatch

increased blood pressure

insomnia

=

=

DIAGNOSIS: ANXIETY

Rule out physiologic and/or mechanical etiologies

=

=

NURSING INTERVENTIONS

Educate Reassure Medicate Reassess

identification of these major and minor characteristics may be helpful to both the novice and experienced critical care nurse. These specific behaviors should be presented in didactic courses on critical care and the care of mechanically ventilated patients. And then when the novice critical care nurse is at the mechanically ventilated patient's bedside and the patient begins to exhibit these signs, the nurse would process the cues and provide immediate, appropriate interventions that would help to alleviate the anxiety and prevent an unplanned extubation.

These findings, especially the major characteristics, can improve patient outcomes by expediting the identification of an accurate nursing diagnosis and the initiation of timely nursing interventions before extubation occurs. For example, when the patient is exhibiting even one of the major defining characteristics, the nurse must first rule out any physiologic or mechanical problems as the source of the exhibited characteristic. Next, the nurse must confidently diagnosis the anxiety and provide interventions such as providing education, reassurance, and administering analgesics and anxiolytics (see Figure 1). The nurse could identify these signals of anxiety because they are based on empirical research. It would help to confirm what practicing critical care nurses have known for a very long time by placing a label on the cues.

Research

This study has implications for future nursing research: (1) The modified survey instrument should be revised to incorporate additional behaviors contributed by the respondents. Specifically, the following operational definitions should be revised to include the respondent's comments: restlessness, teeth and mouth activity, and fight behavior; aggressive (see Table 8).

Table 8

Revised Operational Definitions Incorporating Respondents' Comments

Characteristic	Revised Operational Definition
Restlessness	an expressed feeling or an observed state of motion characterized by an inability to remain at rest as evidenced by attempts to get hands out of wrist restraints, stiffens extremities, clenches hands, or turns head from side to side
Teeth and Mouth Activity	biting the endotracheal tube or exerting pressure on the endotracheal tube with tongue to attempt to push it out of the mouth or attempting to talk around the tube
Fight Behavior, Aggressive	a coping response to a threat that results in arousal, mobility, and offensively oriented actions such as pounding siderails with hand, attempting to hit or kick staff, or attempting to sit up in bed, that are directed at the feared object or fear source

Additionally, characteristics that were found to be not validated may need to be eliminated from the instrument after further refinement to shorten it. (2) The revised instrument should be used in a replication of the present study using a larger, more focused sample of master's prepared, pulmonary, clinical nurse specialists, possibly utilizing the Delphi technique. (3) Future studies should extend the DCV model to the second component: direct observation in the clinical setting. (4) Correlation studies should identify possible relationships between the defining characteristics and how the characteristics are rated. (5) Future studies should be undertaken to establish which behaviors occur early in anxiety in this patient population. (6) Future studies should be undertaken to establish if some signs are more predictive of unplanned extubation than others.

References

Carpenito, L. (1983). *Nursing diagnosis: Application to clinical practice*. Philadelphia: Lippincott.

Carroll, K., & Magruden, C. (1993). The role of analgesics and sedatives in the management of pain and agitation during weaning from mechanical ventilation. *Critical Care Nursing Quarterly, 15*, 68-77.

Carroll-Johnson, R. (1990). Editorial: Reflections on the ninth biennial conference. *Nursing Diagnosis, 2*, 49-50.

Coppolo, D., & May, J. (1990). Self-extubation: A 12-month experience. *Chest, 98*, 165-169.

Crippen, K., & Ermakov, S. (1992). Stress, agitation, and brain failure in critical care medicine. *Critical Care Nursing Quarterly, 15*, 52-74.

Doherty, M. (1991). Benzodiazepine sedation in critically ill. *AACN Clinical Issues in Critical Care Nursing, 4*, 48-763.

Dreger, R. (1983). State-trait anxiety inventory. In 0. Buros. (Ed.), *The eighth mental measurements yearbook*. (pp. 166-174). Highland Park, NJ: The Grypton Press.

Ellstrom, K., Brener, M., & Williams, J. (1991). Incidence and factors related to unplanned extubations. *Heart Lung, 20*, 23-26.

Fadden, T., Fehring, R., & Kenkel-Ross, E. (1987). Clinical validation of the nursing diagnosis anxiety. In A. Mclane (Ed.), *Classification of nursing diagnosis: Proceedings of the seventh conference*. (pp.32-34). St. Louis, MO: Mosby.

Fehring, R. (1986). Validating diagnostic labels: Standardized methodology. In M. Hurley (Ed.), *Classification of nursing diagnoses: Proceedings of the sixth conference*, (pp.44-49). St. Louis, MO: Mosby.

Gebbie, K., & Lavin, M. (Eds.). (1975). *Classification of nursing diagnoses: Proceedings of the first national conference*. (pp.189-194). Philadelphia, PA: Lippincott.

Gordon, M., & Sweeney, M. (1979). Methodological problems and issues in identifying and standardizing nursing diagnosis. *Advances in Nursing Science, 2*, 1-7.

Guzzetta, C., & Dossey, B. (1983). Nursing diagnosis: Framework, process, and problems. *Heart & Lung, 12*, 281-291.

Hoskins, L. (1989). Clinical validation methodologies for nursing diagnosis research. In R. Carroll-Johnson (Ed.), *Classification of nursing diagnoses: Proceedings of the eighth conference*. (pp.41-43). Philadelphia, PA: Lippincott.

Laing, A. (1992). The applicability of a new sedation scale for intensive care. *Intensive and Critical Care Nursing, 8*, 149-152.

Lamb, B., Vogelson, M., & Tack, K. (1989). Incidence of unplanned extubation. *Critical Care Medicine, 17*, 96-100.

Levin, R., Krainovich, B., Bahrenburg, E., & Mitchell, C. (1989). Diagnostic content validity of nursing diagnoses. *Image, 21*, 40-44.

Lindquiest, R., Banasik, J., & Barsteiner, J. (1993). Determining AACN's research priorities for the 90's. *American Journal of Critical Care Nursing, 2*, 110-117.

Maguire, G., DeLorenzo, L., & Maggio, R. (1994). Unplanned extubation in the intensive care unit: A quality of care concern. *Critical Care Nursing Quarterly, 17*, 40-47.

Peplau, H. (1952). *Interpersonal relations in nursing*. New York: Putnam's Son

Pesiri, A. (1994). Two-year study of the prevention of unintentional extubation. *Critical Care Nursing Quarterly, 17*, 35-39.

Pesiri, A., Stewart, K., Kobe, E., & Stewart, W. (1990). Protocol for preventions of unintentional extubation. *Critical Care Nursing Quarterly, 12*, 87-90.

Robinson, L. (1990). Stress and anxiety. *Nursing Clinics of North America, 4*, 935-943.

Spielberger, C. (1983). *State-trait anxiety inventory*. Palo Alto, CA: Consulting Psychologists Press, Inc.

Taggart, J., & Lind, M. (1994). Evaluating unplanned endotracheal extubations. *Dimensions of Critical Care Nursing, 13*, 114-120.

Urdang, L. (Ed.). (1983). Mosby's medical and nursing dictionary. St. Louis: Mosby.

Vincent-Goyette, K. (1991). Defining characteristics: General or population specific. In R. Carroll-Johnson (Ed.). *Classification of nursing diagnoses: Proceeding of the ninth conference.* (pp. 20-30). Philadelphia, PA: Lippincott.

Whitley, G. (1988). A validation study of the nursing diagnosis anxiety. *Florida Nursing Review, 2*, 1-7.

Whitley, G. (1992). Concept analysis of anxiety. *Nursing Diagnosis, 3*, 107-116.

Whitley, G. (1994). Expert validation and differentiation of the nursing diagnoses anxiety and fear. *Nursing Diagnosis, 5*, 143-150.

Whitley, G., & Tousman, S. (1996). A multivariate approach for validation of anxiety and fear. *Nursing Diagnosis, 7*, 116-123.

Decisional Conflict in Families Making End of Life Treatment Decisions

Elizabeth F. Hiltunen, MS, RN, CS

Susan K. Chase, EdD, RN, CS

Cynthia Medich, PhD, RN

This research was partially funded by the Robert Wood Johnson Foundation.

The Study to Understand Prognoses and Preferences for Outcomes and Risks of Treatments (SUPPORT) was designed to improve communication between patients and physicians in making end of life treatment plans. As part of this 5-year national study, nurses intervened with patients at 5 medical centers over a 2-year period (The SUPPORT Principal Investigators, 1995; Hiltunen, 1995). Reports of SUPPORT have focused on quantitative outcomes including those which showed no improvement in physician understanding of patient preferences for treatment and no decrease in time to make a do not resuscitate (DNR) decision or time to death in an intensive care unit. There has been a lack of description of the experience of those facing end of life decisions and the process of their decision making.

Seriously ill patients and families face difficult decisions about treatment near the end of life. Understanding the way these difficult treatment decisions are made and the experience of decisional conflict in these patients and families may help care providers to improve end of life care and decision making.

Purpose

The overall purpose of our qualitative study was to describe the difficult decisions of seriously ill patients near the end of their lives, the context of those decisions, and the SUPPORT nurse's role. The specific question to be explored in this paper is: What is the experience and meaning of decisional conflict faced by seriously ill patients in SUPPORT?

Methods

The data available for this analysis came from the 18 SUPPORT nurses' narrative accounts that they wrote of their patient experiences. As part of the 2-year intervention phase of the SUPPORT study, these specially trained nurses intervened with 2,519 patients. During this time the nurses recorded 476 critical incident narratives. Seventy five were classified by the nurses as representing decisional conflict. From these,

5 critical incidents were selected from each study site (n=25), allowing equal representation by site, SUPPORT nurse and both years of the intervention. Two narratives lacked sufficient detail, yielding 23 narratives for analysis.

The narratives were analyzed using interpretive hermeneutics (Spigelberg, 1982; Cohen & Omery, 1994) which allowed for interpretation of the meaning of the patient situation to the nurse, and through her narrative, to the patients and families. The narratives were coded independently for content. Categories were then compared and clustered into themes. Alternative explanations were explored. Descriptions of the themes were written and rewritten and linked to individual exemplars which best illustrated the essence of the themes. To strengthen validity the description of decisional conflict was shared with the SUPPORT nurses. They validated the findings and added nuances to our interpretations.

Results

The majority of the end of life treatment decisions were made by family members because of the severity of illness of the patients. Decisional conflict was experienced by the families as a somewhat predictable series of stages as they lived through the decision making process for their relative. The stages involved recognition of a dilemma, a period of vacillation, moving to a turning point and letting go.

A dilemma exists where there are no acceptable options. The dilemma sets the stage for decisional conflict in response to the choices presented. The following is an example of one family member's dilemma: "He knew his wife would not want the type of treatment she was receiving, but it was very difficult for him to be the one to make the decision to stop."

Vacillation among treatment options, sometimes described as ambivalence, was frequently exhibited by family members. This was evidenced by movement between the options, uncertainty and questioning. For example: "The family would alternate between accepting the rationale that withdrawing treatment would relieve the patient's suffering and a real reluctance to decide because of the patient's fear of death."

Moving to a turning point is an event which allows a plan to develop or a decision to evolve. This process requires time and, as in this example, learning about new options: "I asked if it would be helpful if the doctors made a recommendation ... One of them asked, 'Will they do that?'...(he) looked as if a great burden had been lifted from his shoulders."

Letting go is the ultimate turning point and the completion of the decision making process. Letting go took time and represented a readiness to accept the loss. "After this time had passed the husband summoned me and said, 'I'm ready, it'll be okay now.' 'We should stop the machine.'" Some nurses described the process of letting go as lifting the burden of decision making.

Reaching a turning point and letting go involved a process of "hearing" medical information and learning new perspectives, a process of gaining a deeper understanding, and then making new meaning. To move through this process, families needed to reframe the choice, try out new options and understand their meaning. Nurses facilitated this process by being present in the process, providing information, helping in reframing the choice, and in some cases, giving permission to let go. As one nurse observed: "empowering this family to make the difficult decision led to the actual decision and action of withdrawing care... The biggest component of this seemed to be letting them know that it was okay to stop, and okay to let go." With these steps most were able to move beyond vacillation and to resolve their decisional conflict.

An additional finding was the complexity of decision making for end of life treatment. Multiple decisions, not a single decision, were required. In the 23 narratives there were 83 decisions described, ranging from 2 to 10. In the 14 cases where withdrawal of treatment was considered, there was an average of five decisions. Beyond a DNR order, family members initially considered surgery, intubation, aggressive/invasive procedures and "placement." Subsequent decisions considered included home care, comfort/hospice care, nursing home placement, testing/trials/consultations, feeding/hydration, medications, withholding information and transfer. The type of decision being made affected the intensity of the experience of conflict, the most intense being the decision to withdraw treatment and allow death.

Multiple perspectives contributed to the complexity of decision making. Family patterns that were in place before the patients illness affected the decision making experience. The decision was not an individual choice but a family choice. Family members frequently were at different phases of the decision making process. Individual family members also had differing ways of specifying doing the best thing, or the goal. Differing perspectives between the family and the health care team were another source of conflict in decision making.

Discussion and Implications

Descriptions in the narratives gave evidence of the following NANDA (1996) defining characteristics: vacillation, delayed decision making,

verbalized uncertainty about choices, verbalization of undesirable consequences, verbalized feeling of distress, questioning personal values and beliefs, and self focusing. Frequent defining characteristics identified in a national survey of critical care nurses, including delayed decision making, expressed distress, vacillation and uncertainty (Hiltunen, 1994), were also supported. The defining characteristics of decisional conflict, originally identified for the individual, in this study applied to the family as well. Although the conflict was an internal and individual process, our data shows evidence that families experience conflict consistent with that described for individuals. We recommend this diagnosis be extended to include the family as client for care.

Although we anticipated describing the decisional conflicts of patients, we found that families have a major role in decision making for seriously ill patients. When decisional conflict was present there was a predictable process experienced by families making end of life treatment decisions. Decisional conflict was most intense in withdrawal of treatment decisions and was manifest as burden.

Clinicians can help in guiding families and patients through the complex process of decision making by: 1) anticipating family decisional conflict in seriously ill patient situations and identifying families at risk, 2) preparing families for the potential stages of decision making, 3) expecting the decision making process to take time, and 4) expecting vacillation.

Concurrent naturalistic studies need to be conducted, utilizing such methods as participant observation, interviews of health care providers, families and, if possible, patients, to more closely examine and describe the actual process of making decisions near the end of life. It will be important to compare and contrast decision making in seriously ill individuals and families both with and without decisional conflict, as well as to describe decisional conflict in other populations. Preventing excessive conflict and burden by identifying high risk situations, validating assessment strategies and interventions to support decision making are important goals of future research.

References

Cohen, M.Z., & Omery, A. (1994). Schools of phenomenology: Implications for research. In J.M. Morse (Ed.) *Critical issues in qualitative research methods*. Thousand Oaks, CA: Sage Publications.

Hiltunen, E.F. (1994). Validation of decisional conflict by critical care nurses. In R.M. Carroll-Johnson and M. Paquette (Eds.), *Classification of nursing diagnoses. Proceedings of the tenth conference* (pp. 213-217). Philadelphia: J. B. Lippincott.

Hiltunen, E.F., Puopolo, A.L., Marks, G.K., Marsden, C., Kennard, M.J., Follen, M.A., & Phillips, R.S. (1995, April). Research connections: The nurse's role in end of life treatment discussions: Preliminary report of the SUPPORT project. *The Journal of Cardiovascular Nursing*, 9(3), 68-77.

North American Nursing Diagnosis Association. (1996). *NANDA Nursing diagnoses. Definitions and classification 1997-1998*. Philadelphia: Author.

Spiegelberg, H. (1982). *The phenomenological movement* (3rd ed.). Boston: Martinus Nihjoff.

The SUPPORT Principal Investigators. (1995, November). A controlled trial to improve care for seriously ill hospitalized patients: The study to understand prognoses and preferences for outcomes and risks of treatments (SUPPORT). *Journal of the American Medical Association*, 74(20), 1591-1598.

Further Development and Testing of a Functional Health Pattern Assessment Screening Tool

Dorothy A. Jones, EdD, RNC, FAAN

Frances Barrett Foster, MS, RN, CS

**Study funded in part by Boston College Research Expense Grant*

Nursing assessment is an integral component of nursing care. It is the means by which nurses describe the initial and continued observations evaluated during patient/nurse interactions. Gordon (1994) defined nursing assessment as a deliberate and systematic process whereby clinical information is synthesized and hypotheses generated and tested. The way the nurse obtains data about the patient is critical to linking nursing contributions and patient care outcomes.

An assessment framework provides an important vehicle to facilitate the organization and focus of nursing data. The use of a structured assessment framework creates a data base from which the nurse can describe patient phenomena, generate nursing diagnoses, and evaluate interventions and outcomes.

Background

The need for a structured assessment framework in nursing has been documented since the 1950s (Smith, 1968). In 1959, the Public Health Department funded a study to research the effects of nursing interventions on patient care (McCain, 1965). The results of this investigation supported the need for a structured assessment framework to be incorporated into nursing practice. Over the years, the lack of a standardized assessment framework has resulted in inadequate and inconsistent clinical information about the patient care experience. According the McCain (1965), without a data base, clinical judgments are often based on intuition and difficult to validate.

Nursing's early response to standardize data collection was to adapt medicine's systems approach to assessment. This proved to be a serious mistake, as focusing on describing disease states organized around the body's systems, led to the generation of medical hypothesis, not nursing diagnoses. As a consequence, nursing became further enmeshed in the medical domain of practice rather than moving toward clearly delineating nursing's contribution to patient care.

It wasn't until 1974, when Gordon devel-

"

Table 1

Functional Health Patterns and Number of Items within FHPAST

Functional Health Patterns within Scale	Number of Items
Health Perception - Health Maintenance	13
Nutrition - Metabolic	4
Elimination	2
Activity - Exercise	4
Sleep - Rest	2
Coping - Stress	6
Self Perception - Self Concept	7
Cognitive - Perceptual	8
Role - Relationship	8
Sexual - Reproductive	2
Value - Belief	2

oped a nursing assessment framework within the Functional Health Pattern typology, that nursing began to bring the assessment process into nursing's practice domain of reasoning and decision making. This contribution moved clinical judgments from an intuitive process, to one based on rational thought and evidence. The development of the functional health pattern framework helped to further define nursing science and articulate a disciplinary contribution to patient/client care outcomes.

Gordon (1994) has described pattern as a sequence of behaviors developed over time. A functional pattern is depicted as the manifestation of each individual's interaction with their environment, influenced by human growth and development (Gordon, 1994, p. 73-75). Health within the functional health pattern framework is viewed as optimal level of functioning for an individual, family, or community.

There are 11 functional health patterns (named in Table 1), which capture unique responses of person, family, or community

(Gordon, 1994). Each of the 11 functional health patterns are interrelated, yet mutually exclusive. Every pattern must be assessed and all patterns synthesized before any clinical judgment (nursing diagnoses) can be made. Assessment of a pattern includes both subjective and objective information. The assessment data within each pattern is open to revisions and integrates new observations and reevaluation.

A complete assessment incorporates data into a narrative description of the individual's functional health status. The nurse analyzes the data from all 11 functional health patterns to isolate patient/client strengths, determine pattern function and identify nursing diagnoses or potentially dysfunctional patterns. The FHP framework may also be used to delineate overall health status or provide an overview of one's lifestyle (Gordon, 1994).

There are many advantages to using the functional health pattern framework to assess a client's health state. They include a) presenting a holistic focus of the human experience; b) validating clinical judgments through the evaluation of a patient/client assessment data base; c) generating testable hypothesis (diagnoses); d) providing clinical utility within the context of multiple conceptual practice frameworks across clinical setting, population, age, or health status; and e) creating a basis for organizing assessment data in research and publications (Gordon, 1994).

The value of a functional health pattern assessment framework has been extensive and well documented. However, its use has been inconsistent in practice, with the most common reason being nurses' lack of adequate time to complete the full assessment (Rossi, 1987, Wilson, Halkola, and Jones, 1989; Corrigan, 1986, Hirschfield-Bartek, Dow, and Craton, 1990).

Purpose of Current Investigation

The Functional Health Pattern Assessment Screening Tool (FHPAST) was developed to establish a reliable and valid instrument that could screen the functional health patterns, reduce assessment data collection time and potentially increase the utilization of a nursing assessment framework. By expanding the documentation of nurse judgments, it is anticipated that nursing's contribution to care can be better articulated.

There have been several tools described in the literature that screen the FHP framework; however, none have had rigorous psychometric testing (Jones & Barrett, 1997). Therefore, the purpose of this study was to continue to establish the psychometric properties of a screening tool (FHPAST).

DEVELOPMENT of FHPAST
Tool History

The Functional Health Pattern Assessment Screening Tool has been developed as a patient/client-completed screening tool. The tool screens all 11 functional health patterns and the nurse evaluates the responses for potential problems and identifies when additional assessment data is needed. Further evaluation is then conducted on selected areas of concern.

The FHPAST was originally an 83-item tool. Currently, after testing and refinement, the tool now contains 58 items. Each functional health pattern is represented within the 58 items. A declarative sentence structure is used for each test item and the patient/client selects responses from a 4-point Likert scale that includes the adjectives: a) never (1), b) sometimes (2), c) often (3), and d) routinely (4). A value is weighted for each adjective is described in a set of the directions on the tool. The item responses are to be considered by the patient/client as occurring during the past four weeks in the patient/client's life. If the patient/client responds with a 1 or 2 for items 1-42, it is a predictor of a potential problem within one or more functional health patterns. If the client answers 3 or 4 for items 43-58, the same is equally true.

Three studies have been conducted to further develop the Functional Health Patterns Assessment Screening Tool psychometric properties. Content validity and interrater reliability were established prior to clinical testing for each study (Jones & Barrett, 1997). The procedures for data collection have been consistent across studies which will enable merging data and further analysis.

Psychometric Testing - Study 1

The initial study to establish the instrument's psychometric properties was conducted with a nonrandom, convenience sample at an eye clinic of a medical center in the northeastern United

Table 2

Alpha Correlations on Total Scale across Studies			
Study Cases	Alpha Coefficient	# of Items	Sample
S1	.92	83	214
S2	.89	58	204
S3	.92	58	171

States. A population of adults with acute and chronic ocular diseases formed the study sample. The sample age ranged between 18 to 90 years with the mean age of 51 years. There were 275 females and 209 males in the final sample.

The FHPAST was administered to participants entering a selected clinical setting and they were informed about the use of the tool and the data use at the outset. Informed consent was given and confirmed upon data completion. All data was anonymous and assessment forms were coded. The tool was self completed by each participant. Each completed tool was then retained for psychometric testing.

Item analysis was performed on tool data using a corrected item total correlations and inter-item correlations. A total of 9 items were eliminated based upon study results (Jones & Barrett, 1997). Reliability testing using alpha coefficient was performed on the total scale

(alpha = .92, see Table 2). These scores are considered acceptable for use in human studies (Devellis, 1991). Factor analysis was not computed on study data, because significant missing data (Jones and Barrett, 1997).

History and Psychometric Testing - Study 2
In the second study, data were obtained on a well adult population. Again, a nonrandom convenience sample was used with adults from a university in the northeastern United States. The sample population consisted of undergraduates, graduate students, and staff. The age ranged between 18 to 82 years with the mean age of 20 years. There were 361 cases in the study sample, with 81 males, 137 females, and 51 with unidentified gender.

Item analysis was performed on data from the second study sample. Corrected item total correlations and inter-item correlations were

Table 3

Factors Identified on Study Two			
Factor	Alpha	Name	Items
1	.9055	General Well-being	18
2	.7590	Health Behaviors and Perceptions	13
3	.6721	Threats/Limitations to Function	7
4	.7324	Psycho-social Well-being	8
5	.4597	Risk Behaviors	3

used and 16 items were eliminated. Reliability testing using alpha coefficient was performed on the total scale. The alpha of the second study was 0.89 (Table 2), which again was an acceptable score for use in human studies (Devellis, 1991).

Factor analysis was completed on a 58-item FHPAST, the total number of items remaining after item elimination. Items loaded on five factors, using principal axis factoring with oblique rotation. Internal consistency was measured for each factor using alpha coefficient. The alpha scores ranged from .91 to .45 (Table 3). The fifth factor contained only 3 items and had a weak alpha coefficient of .45. However, a decision was made not to exclude the factor or related items, because the data clustered around risk behaviors such as smoking and the use of recreational drugs.

Current Investigation
Methodology
The third and most recent study was conducted with the goal of norming the instrument in this age group. A nonrandom convenience sample was used to collect data at a university in the northeastern United States. The sample consisted of graduate and undergraduate students and employees. There were 235 cases with an age range between 18-61 years and a mean age of 20. The sample included 81 males and 167 females with 5 missing responses. Data collection procedures as aforementioned remained the same as in the first two studies. All tools were coded, completed by the individual and returned into an empty "return" box.

Scoring
The scoring of the subscales was completed using the mean score of each scale. In computing the total score, reversed coding was used for items 42-58. The mean score of greater than 3 delineated functional health within that factor. A mean score of 3 for the total scale infers desirable functional health.

Results and Discussion
Response frequencies were analyzed. In the study, the response frequencies fell across the Likert scale with the majority of participants answering the most desired item responses. Item analysis was performed using corrected item total correlations and inter-item correlations. The coding for items 42-58 were reversed for psychometric testing, resulting in a score of 3 or 4 being the desirable response.

In this study, it was noted that items pertaining to sensitive content, such as sex, recreational drugs, and alcohol had low correlations. One item related to caretaking and annual exam also had similar results. It was thought that the later items tested poorly because the content was not relevant for this age group.

For other items, individuals may have been inhibited in an academic setting to answer such sensitive items even though anonymity was assured. A decision was made not to eliminate any test items until further psychometric testing with other populations is completed.

Reliability testing was conducted on the entire instrument to evaluate internal consistency. The use of alpha coefficient was used and yielded a score of a = .92 for the total instrument (Table 2). These results supports data from previous psychometric testing (Jones and Barrett, 1997) and is considered a reliable instrument for use with humans (Devellis, 1991).

Factor analysis was also performed on the data. Two hundred and fifty-three cases were analyzed. An initial scree plot generated, suggesting the presence of a three factor instru-

Table 4

Factors Identified in Current Study (1998)			
Factor	Name	Items	Alpha
1	General Well-Being/Perception	27	.93
2	Health Behaviors	17	.79
3	Risk/Threat to Function	12	.72

ment. After running an initial factor analysis, a principal axis factor with varimax rotation was used, forcing the data into three factors. The factors that resulted were: a) General Well-being and Perception; b) Health Behaviors; c) Risk/threat to Function.

The factors identified were consistent with the factors isolated during the previous study, with the following changes: a) the majority of the items under the factor Psychosocial Well-being combined with General Well-being; b) Perception of Well-being combined with General Well-being instead of Health Behaviors; and c) Risk Behaviors combined with Threats to Function, which were two separate factors in a previous investigation. The forcing of items into three factors eliminated the two weak factors and preserved the conceptual themes identified in the previous studies.

Internal consistency was tested for each factor using the alpha coefficient. The results were acceptable, ranging from a = .93 to .72 (Table 4). Two items did not factor, one related to use of recreational drugs and the other to annual exam. Again, these items were not eliminated form the tool until results from subsequent studies support removing them.

In analyzing each factor, it was noted that data from each functional health pattern did not fall into the conceptual factors, according to their content, but rather by the wording of the item. For example, within the pattern category Coping-Stress Tolerance the item "I feel stress, tension, and pressure" fell into the Factor 1, General Well-being and Perception. However, the item "I have a usual routine that helps me relax," also under Coping-Stress Tolerance, fell into Factor 2, Health Behaviors.

These results do not change the pattern typology of the functional health patterns, but rather transform the interpretation of function to a higher level of conceptualization. It also renders the tool applicable for use in research pertaining to the content areas of each factor, namely: 1) General Well-being and Perception, 2) Health Behaviors, and 3) Risk/Threat to Function.

CONCLUSION

In summary, the FHPAST is a valid and reliable 58-item screening tool that contains three subscales measuring the following factors: Health: General Well-being and Perception, Health Behaviors, and Risks/Threats to Function. The tool, based on Gordon's Eleven Functional Health Patterns, and can be completed independently by the patient. The nurse is able to evaluate the patient/client responses as a measure of function or predictors of cures suggesting a potential nursing diagnoses.

The FHPAST can direct the patient/client assessment for both the novice and the expert nurse by providing cues for further exploration. Results can lead to identification of potential pattern dysfunction based upon evidence. Early results suggest the emergence of an instrument with three factors to measure health perception and lifestyle, behaviors used to maintain health, and risk behaviors. The FHPAST will continue to under go psychometric testing and evaluation. The goal is to norm the tool across the lifespan and within a variety of clinical populations.

The development of a reliable and valid assessment screening tool is an important advancement for nursing practice. Through its use, a comprehensive patient data base can be generated in less time, without jeopardizing quality of care. The results can then be used to guide further assessment, nursing interventions and articulate care outcomes that describe patient responses to nursing care.

References

Corrigan, J.O. (1986). Functional health pattern assessment in the emergency department. *Journal of Emergency Nursing* 12(3), 163-167.

Devellis, R. (1991). *Scale development: Theory and applications*. Newbury Part, CA: Sage Publications Inc.

Gordon, M. (1987). *Nursing diagnosis: Process and application*. New York: McGraw-Hill Inc.

Gordon, M. (1994). *Nursing diagnosis: Process and application*. New York: McGraw-Hill Inc.

Hirschfield-Bartek, J., Dow, K.H., & Craton, E. (1990). Decreasing documentation time using a patient self-assessment tool. *Oncology Nursing Forum. 17*(2), 251-255.

Jones, D., & Barrett, F. (1997). Development and testing of a functional health pattern assessment screening tool. In M. Rantz & P. LeMone (Eds.). *Classification of nursing diagnoses: Proceedings of the twelfth conference*. Glendale, CA: Cinahl Informations Systems.

McCain, R.F. (1965). Nursing by assessment-Not intuition. *American Journal of Nursing, 65*(4), 82-84.

Rossi, L. (1987). Organizing data for nursing diagnosis using functional health patterns. In A. McCiane (Ed.). *Classification of nursing diagnoses: Proceedings of the seventh conference*. St. Louis: Mosby.

Smith, D. (1968). A clinical nursing tool. *American Journal of Nursing, 68*(11), 2384-2388.

Wilson, C., Halkola, P., & Jones, D. (1989). Validation of a screening assessment tool and generation of diagnostic hypotheses. In R.Carrol-Johnson (Ed.). *Classification of nursing diagnoses: Proceedings of the eighth conference*. Philadelphia: J.B. Lippincott.

Concept Development: Altered Sexuality in Chronically-Ill Women

Priscilla LeMone, RN, DSN, FAAN

The purpose of this presentation is to describe an overview of a three-stage design to clarify and clinically validate the concept of altered sexuality in women with chronic illnesses. Alterations in sexuality in women with chronic illnesses are known to occur, but have been less investigated that those occurring in men. However, chronic illnesses continue to increase and are a major health problem, with the incidence of many illnesses greater in women than in men. To provide appropriate interventions and achieve measurable outcomes of care, nurses must be able to identify and label problems such as altered sexuality. Concept validation of this altered response will begin with analysis and end with clinical validation. Clinical validation is a critical component of the project, providing the necessary base for further research.

Purposes of the Study

1. To clarify the meaning and identify defining characteristics of altered sexuality in women with chronic illness through concept analysis.
2. To determine if the identified characteristics, with operational definitions, are represented in women with chronic illness through validation by a panel of nurse experts.
3. To describe the representativeness of the identified defining characteristics for altered sexuality in women with selected chronic illnesses through clinical validation.

The Diagnoses of Altered Sexuality

Altered sexuality is labeled by two diagnoses (sexual dysfunction and altered sexuality patterns) in the NANDA taxonomy (NANDA, 1994). As has been the case with other diagnoses, alterations in sexuality diagnoses are abstract, do not permit differential diagnosis, and are not useful for outcome projection (Gordon, 1990). They are also not gender-specific, and represent an incomplete and overlapping set of descriptors (See Table 1). The rationale for the inclusion of

Table 1

The Two NANDA Nursing Diagnoses Related to Sexuality	
Sexual Dysfunction	**Altered Sexuality Patterns**
Definition: The state in which an individual experiences a change in sexual function that is viewed as unsatisfying, unrewarding, inadequate.	*Definition:* The state in which an individual expresses concern regarding his/her sexuality.
Defining Characteristics: — verbalization of problem — alterations in achieving perceived sex role — actual or perceived limitations imposed by disease and/or therapy — conflicts involving values — alterations in achieving sexual satisfaction — inability to achieve desired satisfaction — seeking confirmation of desirability — alteration in relationship with significant other — change in interest in self and others	*Defining Characteristics:* — reported difficulties, limitations, or changes in sexual behaviors or activities
Related Factors: — biopsychosocial alteration of sexuality — ineffectual or absent role models — physical abuse — psychosocial abuse (e.g., harmful relationships) — vulnerability — values conflict — lack of privacy — lack of significant other — altered body structure or function (pregnancy, recent childbirth, drugs, surgery, anomalies, disease processes, trauma, radiation) — misinformation or lack of knowledge	*Related Factors:* — knowledge/skill deficit about alternative responses to health-related transitions — altered body function or structure — lack of privacy — lack of significant other — ineffective or absent role models — conflicts with sexual orientation or variety preference — fear of pregnancy or of acquiring a sexually transmitted disease — impaired relationship with significant other

these two diagnoses in the NANDA taxonomy is difficult to determine, but according to Kim and Moritz, in a report of a 1978 4th conference workgroup, the diagnosis of sexual dysfunction arose from group consensus. The diagnosis of altered sexuality patterns was accepted for review and development at the 7th NANDA conference in 1986. At that same conference, further development and refinement were recommended, but no further work has been identified (although a workgroup has reviewed these diagnoses prior to this conference).

Rationale and Significance

The experience of sexuality differs in men and women (Bernhard & Dan, 1986; Unsain, Goodwin, & Schuster, 1982). Men primarily experience physiologic sexuality, concentrating on physical sexual satisfaction, while women experience sexuality as both physical satisfaction and as a sense of self as a woman within the context of day-to-day life, relationships, and emotions. While alterations in sexuality in men are manifested as objective and focused, women's experiences are essentially subjective and diffuse. Chronic illness threatens gender and sexual identity, self-concept, control of personal functions, intimate relationships, and may necessitate adjustments in roles and relationships...all of which may threaten a woman's sense of personhood as a woman (Anderson & Wolf, 1986; Burckhardt, 1986; Packard, Haberman, Woods, & Yates, 1991).

It has been well documented that nurses do not assess or plan interventions for alterations in sexuality. Although a variety of reasons are given, it may well be that a lack of clear understanding of the defining characteristics of this altered response in women makes it more difficult to make this diagnosis. The development of this concept will facilitate the construction of a middle-range theory that links diagnosis, interventions, and outcomes to support nursing practice.

Stage 1: Concept Analysis

The evolutionary method described by Rogers (Rogers, 1989; 1993) will be used for concept analysis. In this inductive method of inquiry, concepts are considered to be abstractions, formed by identifying and clustering characteristics common to a class of objects or phenomenon, along with some means of expressions such as words. Examination of the common use of a concept through words provides a way to explore the concept and to identify its attributes (in NANDA terminology, its defining characteristics).

The primary activities in this method of concept analysis are:

1. Identify the concept of interest and associated expressions.
2. Identify and select an appropriate setting and sample for data collection.
3. Collect data about the attributes of the concept, along with surrogate terms, references, antecedents, and consequences.
4. Identify concepts related to the concept of interest.
5. Analyze data regarding the characteristics of the concept.

The sample of literature will be selected from English language literature published during the years 1970 through 1998, and will include the disciplines of nursing, medicine, counseling, and psychology. A sample of the indexed literature will be chosen from each discipline, using a table of random numbers, with the minimum sample being 30 items. Each article will be read and data coded; frequency counts of surrogate terms and related concepts will be maintained. All records will be kept in computer files, accompanied by a reflexive journal of methodological decisions, thoughts and perceptions to assist in grouping and labeling major themes. Records provide an audit trail to substantiate credibility, and allow review by another investigator to ensure consistency and decrease potential bias. Major themes will be identified through qualitative content analysis to generate a comprehensive and relevant system of descriptors. The descriptors will be labeled and will become the defining characteristics for the diagnostic label of altered sexuality in women with chronic illnesses.

Stage 2: Expert Validation

In stage 2 the content validity of the defining characteristics, with their operational definitions, will be examined by a panel of nurses considered experts in the area of sexuality and women's health. The formulation of operational definitions is necessary to specify the activities or procedures necessary for the measurement of the characteristics (Grant & Kinney, 1991). They provide a consistent frame of reference in making assessments and indicate criteria for the evaluation of outcomes when nursing interventions are tested.

This stage of the inquiry will be conducted by using a modified 3-round Delphi survey method (Grant & Kinney, 1992; Notter, 1983). A panel of nurse experts will be selected from masters or doctorally prepared nurses who care for women with chronic illnesses, who have a clinical practice that focuses on sexuality, or who have published and/or made presentations about the topic from 1990 to 1998. As a minimum of 25 nurse experts are recommended, 30 will initially be chosen to allow for attrition.

The first round will consist of a demographic data sheet, a content validity questionnaire, and a form that includes the defining characteristics and operational definitions with a methods of indicating if each is appropriate and clear, as well as space for additional comments and the addition of other characteristics and def-

initions. Statistical analysis of percent agreement will be conducted to determine retention or elimination of defining characteristics, using a 90% agreement as the standard.

In round 2 the participants will be mailed the same proposed defining characteristics and definitions, and a summary of individual and grouped data about findings from round 1. The panel members will be asked to again rate the characteristics and definitions, and to also provide rationale for responses that were less than 90% agreement in round 1. Statistical analysis of results will be conducted, using a 70% agreement standard, and comments and rationale for responses less than 90% in round 1 will be aggregated and summarized.

If consensus has been reached, round 3 will be a final report of a statistical summary of individual and grouped responses from round 2. If consensus has not been reached, the survey from round 2 will be repeated.

The final outcome of stage 2 will be a list of defining characteristics with operational definitions for altered sexuality in women with chronic illnesses. The list will have achieved at least 70% agreement on appropriateness and clarity by the panel of nurse experts.

Stage 3: Clinical Validation

Stage 3 will be conducted to determine if the defining characteristics developed in stage 1 and validated by experts in stage 2 are experienced by women with chronic illness known to alter sexuality (coronary artery disease, cancer of the breast, and diabetes mellitus). Although most clinical validation studies have used quantitative methods, a qualitative approach is particularly suited to the discovery subjective phenomenon, such as sexuality.

A grounded theory study (Glaser, 1978;

Glaser & Strauss, 1967; Strauss, 1989) will be conducted to identify the experiences of sexuality in women with the selected chronic illnesses. A purposive sample of women will be used, with a minimum of 10 women with each illness.

Theoretical sampling based on theoretical purpose and relevance will be used for data collection. Selection of subjects is governed by the emerging theory as data is collected, coded, and analyzed, with the purpose of this sampling method to test and refine categories, allowing verification of the validity of each category. Subjects will be recruited through referral by advanced practice nurses and physicians, snowball technique, posting flyers, and speaking to support groups.

Data will be collected through tape-recorded interviews, observations, and review of written documents. The interviews will be transcribed, and subjects will be asked permission for a follow-up telephone call to answer any questions following review of the transcriptions. The interview will begin with collection of demographic data, followed by a brief discussion of sexuality as being more than just physical responses. The initial question will be "Tell me about your experience with sexuality as a woman since being diagnosed with this illness." Other questions that are more specific will then be asked. It is estimated that interviews will last from 60 to 90 minutes, but the woman is allowed to talk as long as she wishes.

Data will be analyzed using Glaserian methodology for constant comparison (Glaser, 1978). The strategies to be used are coding, writing memos, and categorizing. As data accumulates and is coded and categorized into clusters of data, theoretical memos will be written to build categories and develop conceptualization. Data will be collected, analyzed, coded and clus-

tered until no new data are collected and the categories are considered saturated. Throughout data collection and analysis, the literature will be reviewed and used as data to support the emerging theory. With continued comparisons and conceptualization, the core category emerges that is grounded in the data and accounts for patterns of behavior relevant to those involved (Glaser & Strauss, 1967).

As the clinical validation is the final stage of the concept analysis, it will be critical for the investigator to identify assumptions (in this case, the previously identified defining characteristics) and then to bracket or suspend these preconceptions in order to fully understand the women's experiences and not impose a priori analysis on the conceptualization.

The substantive theory derived from stage 3 will then be used to evaluate if the defining characteristics developed in stage 1 and 2 are represented in this group of women with chronic illnesses.

Following completion of the project, if findings support revision of the current NANDA diagnoses related to sexuality, recommendations for revision will be submitted to the Review Committee. The study findings will also provide a base for the development of nursing interventions and outcomes for altered sexuality in this population. Finally, additional knowledge will be gained about the experience of sexuality in chronically-ill women, a little-studied phenomenon.

References

Anderson, B., & Wolf, F. (1986). Chronic physical illness and sexual behavior: Psychological issues. *Journal of Consulting and Clinical Psychology, 54,* 168-175.

Bernhard, L., & Dan, A. (1986). Redefining

sexuality from women's own experiences. *Nursing Clinics of North America, 21,* 125-136.

Burckhardt, C. (1987). Coping strategies of the chronically ill. *Nursing Clinics of North America, 22,* 543-550.

Glaser, B. (1978). Theoretical sensitivity. Mills Valley, CA: Sociology Press.

Glaser, B., & Strauss, A. (1967). *The discovery of grounded theory: Strategies for qualitative research.* Chicago: Aldine Publishing.

Gordon, M. (1990). Toward theory-based categories. *Nursing Diagnosis, 1*(1), 5-10.

Grant, J., & Kinney, M. (1992). Using the Delphi technique to examine the content validity of nursing diagnoses. *Nursing Diagnosis, 3,* 12-22.

Grant, J., & Kinney, M. (1991). The need for operational definitions for defining characteristics. *Nursing Diagnosis, 2,* 181-185.

North American Nursing Diagnosis Association [NANDA]. (1994). *Nursing diagnoses: Definitions & Classification 1995-1996.* Philadelphia: NANDA.

Notter, L. (1983). *Essentials of nursing research.* (3rd ed.). New York: Springer.

Packard, N., Haberman, M., Woods, N., & Yates, B. (1991). Demands of illness among chronically ill women. *Western Journal of Nursing Research, 13,* 434-457.

Rogers, B. (1989). Concepts, analysis and the development of nursing knowledge: The evolutionary cycle. *Journal of Advanced Nursing, 14,* 330-335.

Rogers, B. (1993). Concept analysis: An evolutionary view. In B. Rogers & K. Knafl, *Concept development in nursing: Foundations, techniques, and applications.* (pp. 73-106). Philadelphia: Saunders.

Strauss, A. (1989). Grounded theory's applicability to nursing diagnosis research. In *Monograph of the invitational conference on research methods for validating nursing diagnoses.* Palm Springs, CA: NANDA.

Unsain, I., Goodwin, M., & Schuster, E. (1982). Diabetes and sexual functioning. *Nursing Clinics of North America, 17,* 387-393.

Refinement of Anxiety/Fear Nursing Diagnoses

Rona F. Levin, PhD, RN

Barbara Krainovich-Miller, EdD, RN, CS

Workgroup participants: Priscilla Adams, Marga Coler, Judy Collins, Terry Cotteta, Connie Delaney, Judie Much

Introduction

The nursing diagnostic categories of anxiety and fear both appeared in the very first system of diagnostic nomenclature developed by The National Conference Group on the Classification of Nursing Diagnoses in 1973. It is of historical interest that the diagnosis of Anxiety initially contained modifiers that specified the degree to which the problem was present, i.e., mild, moderate, severe and panic. Fear also contained modifiers ("Functional fear, mild" and "Nonfunctional fear, panic") when it was first identified as a nursing diagnosis. At the fourth conference in 1980, Anxiety was deleted from "the list" and Fear was accepted without any modifiers (Kim & Moritz, 1982). Anxiety was reinstated as a nursing diagnosis in the NANDA Taxonomy at the fifth NANDA conference; yet the modifiers were not returned. Fear has remained undeveloped beyond a definition and one defining characteristic since 1973.

Although research on the content (Levin, Krainovich-Miller, Bahrenber, & Mitchell, 1986; Whitley, 1992a, 1992b) and clinical validity of the diagnoses of fear (Taylor-Loughran, O'Brien, LaChapelle, & Rangel, 1989; Whitley, 1994) and anxiety (Krainovich-Miller, 1988) exists, it has not been synthesized in a way that has led to the development of the Fear diagnosis or the refinement of the Anxiety diagnosis. In 1996, prior to the Eleventh NANDA Conference, a workgroup was convened in an attempt to begin this work. Today's presentation on the refinement of the diagnostic categories of Fear and Anxiety is based on the efforts of the Anxiety/Fear Workgroup.

Methods

Prior to our meeting in April of 1996, each workgroup member was assigned to review at least five publications on each nursing diagnosis and fill out two forms for each publication. The first form was either a Research Critique Worksheet or a Conceptual Analysis Worksheet, depending on the nature of the publication. The second form was a Reference Rating Instrument which

"

Table 1

Comparison between the Components of Nursing Diagnoses Anxiety and Fear		
Component	Anxiety	Fear
Definition: Operational	1. Presence of vague uneasy feeling of discomfort or dread accompanied by autonomic response [1,5,6] 2. Source/cause unknown or nonspecific [2,5,6] 3. Subjective responses that act as energizers but cannot be directly observed are present [2] 4. Objective signs that are the result of transformation of energy into relief behaviors and responses are present [2]	1. Presence of immediate feeling of apprehension and fright [9] 2. Source known and specific [9] 3. Subjective psychological/behavioral responses are present [9] 4. Objective psychological/behavioral, physiologic, and cognitive responses are present [9] 5. Fight or flight behaviors are present [9]
Definition: Conceptual	Anxiety is: 1. An unpleasant feeling [2] 2. A feeling of apprehension caused by anticipation of danger (internal/external) [1,2] 3. An altering signal that warns of impending danger and enables a person to take measures to deal with threat [1,2]	Fear is: 1. Feeling of dread [5,6] 2. Anxiety caused by consciously recognized and realistic danger [1] 3. A perceived threat, real or imagined [3]

Sources: 1. Kaplan, Sadock & Grubb, 1994; 2. Whitley, 1992a; 3. Sarafino, 1986; 4. Scruton, 1986; 5. NANDA, 1992; 6. NANDA, 1994; 7. APA, 1994; 8. Kagan & Schulkin, 1995; 9. Whitley, 1992b; 10. Young, 1986; 11. Peplau, 1963; 12. Irving, 1973

evaluated the usefulness of the publication.

At its meeting the Workgroup first listed the definitions, defining characteristics (dcs) and related factors for each diagnosis found in the 1995-1996 edition of *Nursing Diagnoses: Definitions & Classification* (NANDA, 1994), hereinafter referred to as NANDA's Taxonomy. The literature that each group member had reviewed was then combed for agreement with what existed in the NANDA Taxonomy and for additional definitions, defining characteristics and related factors. After this step was accomplished, the defining characteristics for Anxiety were clustered into the broader categories of affective, physiological (sympathetic and parasympathetic), behavioral, and cognitive, and those for Fear were classified as subjective or objective.

In reviewing the intial work of the group for this presentation, the authors revisited the literature to substantiate the dcs for anxiety that the work group presented at the 12th Conference (Rantz & LeMone, 1997). References for anguish, rumination, and tendency to blame others were not found and were therefore deleted from the list in Table 3. Although a reference for fidgeting was not found, Webster's Dictionary (1983) indicated that it was a synonym for jittery and thus is indicated as such in Table 3.

Outcomes

Tables 1, 2 and 3 reflect the results of the Workgroup's deliberations. The definitions of both diagnoses were expanded and divided into conceptual and operational components. The major difference in the operational definitions is that the source of Anxiety is "unknown or nonspecific" while the source of Fear is "known and specific." This notion is a truism in nursing as well as in other disciplines. The conceptual definitions are differentiated in a similar fashion; that is, an impending or anticipated danger is

Table 2

	Anxiety/Fear: Related to Factors	
Component	Anxiety	Fear
Related to Factors (Etiology)	Anxiety is related to: 1. Unconscious conflict about essential goals & values of life [2,6] 2. Threat to self concept [2,6] 3. Threat of death [2,6] 4. Threat to or change in health status [6,7] 5. Threat to or change in role function [2,6] 6. Threat to or change in environment [2,6] 7. Threat to or change in interaction patterns [2,6] 8. Situational/maturational crises [2,6] 9. Interpersonal transmission/contagion [2,6] 10. Unmet needs [2,6] 11. Threat to or change in role status [2] 12. Threat to or change in economic status [2] 13. Substance abuse [7] 14. Exposure to toxins [7] 15. Stress [7] 16. Familial association/heredity [7]	Fear is related to: 1. Natural/innate origins [9] 2. Learned response [9] 3. Knowledge deficit [9] 4. Language barrier [9] 5. Sensory impairment [9] 6. Separation from support system in potentially stressful situation [9] 7. Phobic stimulus/phobia [9,4] 8. Environmental stimuli [9] 9. Classical conditioning [8] 10. Innate releasers [8] 11. Ideas [8] 12. Discrepancy [8] 13. Physical/social conditions [4] 14. Fear for others [4]

Sources: 1. Kaplan, Sadock & Grubb, 1994; 2. Whitley, 1992a; 3. Sarafino, 1986; 4. Scruton, 1986; 5. NANDA, 1992; 6. NANDA, 1994; 7. APA, 1994; 8. Kagan & Schulkin, 1995; 9. Whitley, 1992b; 10. Young, 1986; 11. Peplau, 1963; 12. Irving, 1973

related to Anxiety, whereas a "consciously recognized and realistic danger" is related to Fear.

Six additional related factors for Anxiety were found in the literature (APA, 1994; Whitley, 1992a) that are not currently listed in NANDA's Taxonomy. Also, 14 initial related factors were identified for Fear. Regarding dcs, 36 additional ones (not listed in NANDA's Taxonomy) were identified for Anxiety, and 42 initial dcs were gleaned for Fear in addition to the one previously included in the Taxonomy.

A comparison of the dcs for both diagnoses reflects considerable differences, an interesting but unexpected outcome. Only three dcs listed as affective for Anxiety and subjective for Fear were found to be identical: apprehension, jittery and scared. Two other, wariness and worried, were almost identical; they were listed as "increased wariness" and "worried" for Anxiety

and simply "wariness" and "worry" for Fear. Also, three dcs listed under the category of Physiological, Sympathetic for Anxiety and as objective for Fear were identical: anorexia, blood pressure-increased and pupil dilatation. A fourth dc was almost identical in wording; it was listed as "respiration increased" for Anxiety and as "respiratory rate increased" for Fear. Although "cardiovascular excitation" appears as a dc for Anxiety, but not Fear, other, more concrete indicators of such a physiologic state appear as dcs for both diagnoses. These are, for example, "pulse-increased" for Anxiety and "heart rate-increased" for Fear as well as "blood pressure-increased" cited above.

Discussion and Recommendations

Two of the sources reviewed (Taylor-Loughrain, O'Brien, LaChapelle, & Rangel, 1989; Whitley,

Table 3

Defining Characteristics: Signs and Symptoms Anxiety/Fear

Categorization	NDx Anxiety	Categorization	NDx Fear
AFFECTIVE [17]	anxious [1,6] apprehension [1,6,2] distressed [6,2] fearful [6,2] focus on self [6,2] helplessness, painful and persistent increased [6,2] inadequacy, feeling of [6,2] irritability [7,11] jittery [6,2] [synonym = fidgeting] overexcited [6] rattled [6,2] regretful [6] scared [6,2] shakiness [6] uncertainty [6,2] wariness-increased [6,2] worried [6,2]	SUBJECTIVE [16]	ability to verbalize object of fear [6] afraid [9] alarm [9] apprehension [9,4] dread [9] frightened [9] horror [4] impulsiveness [9] jittery [9] panicky [9] scared [9] self-assurance-decreased [9] terrified [9] tension-increased [9] wariness [4] worry [4]
PHYSIOLOGICAL Sympathetic [17]	anorexia [2] blood pressure-increased 2/hypertension [1] cardiovascular excitation [6] dry mouth [2,11] facial flushing [2] facial tension [6,2] palpitations 1 [synonym = heart pounding] perspiration-increased [1,6,2] pulse-increased [2] pupil dilation [6,2] respiration-increased [2] respiratory difficulties [2] reflexes-increased [2] twitching [2] vasoconstriction-superficial [6] voice quivering [6,2] weakness [2]	OBJECTIVE [27]	alertness-increased [9] anorexia [9] asthma [3] attack behavior [9] bedwetting [3] blood pressure-increased [9] concentration on the source [9] diaphoresis [9] diarrhea [9] fatigue [9] fight behavior-aggression [9] flight behavior-withdrawal [9] focus on "it" out there [9] heart rate-increased [9] identifies object of fear [9,5] immediate response to object of fear [9] muscle tightness [9] nausea [9] pallor [9] physical arousal [4] pupil dilation [9] respiratory rate-increased [9]

Sources: 1. Kaplan, Sadock & Grubb, 1994; 2. Whitley, 1992a; 3. Sarafino, 1986; 4. Scruton, 1986; 5. NANDA, 1992; 6. NANDA, 1994; 7. APA, 1994; 8. Kagan & Schulkin, 1995; 9. Whitley, 1992b; 10. Young, 1986; 11. Peplau, 1963; 12. Irving, 1973

Table 3 continued

Defining Characteristics: Signs and Symptoms Anxiety/Fear

Categorization	NDx Anxiety	Categorization	NDx Fear
PHYSIOLOGICAL Parasympathetic [13]	blood pressure-decreased [2] diarrhea [1,2] faintness [1,2] fatigue [7] nausea [2] pain-abdominal [2] pulse-decreased [2] sleep disturbance [7,11] tension-increased [2] tingling in extremities [1] urinary-frequency [1,2] urinary-hesitancy [1] urinary-urgency [1,2]	OBJECTIVE [27] continued	SOB [9] shunting of blood from ski & GI track to heart, CNS & skeletal muscles [9] urinary frequency [2] vomiting [2] wide-eyed [2]
BEHAVIORAL [8]	extraneous movements (e.g., foot shuffle, hand/arm movements) [6,2] eye contact-poor [6,2] glancing about [6,2] insomnia [6,2] productivity-diminished restlessness [1,6,2] scanning & vigilance [2] trembling/hand tremors [1,6,2]		
COGNITIVE [13]	attention-impaired [2] awareness of physiologic symptoms [1] blocking of thought [2] concentrating-difficulty [1,2] confusion [1,2] expressed concerns due to change in life events [6,2] fear of unspecific consequences [6,2] focus on self [5,62,] forgetfulness [2] learning ability-diminished [2,10] perceptual field-diminished [2,11] preoccupation [2] problem solving ability diminished [2]		

Sources: 1. Kaplan, Sadock & Grubb, 1994; 2. Whitley, 1992a; 3. Sarafino, 1986; 4. Scruton, 1986; 5. NANDA, 1992; 6. NANDA, 1994; 7. APA, 1994; 8. Kagan & Schulkin, 1995; 9. Whitley, 1992b; 10. Young, 1986; 11. Peplau, 1963; 12. Irving, 1973

1994) recommended exploring Fear/Anxiety Syndrome as a new diagnosis to be developed. Their rationales are based on their research which demonstrates "apprehension" and "cardiovascular excitation" as two critical dcs identified by nurses for both diagnoses. In addition, there may be a "...progressive and interactive...relationship" between Anxiety and Fear (Whitley, 1994). Taylor-Loughrain et al. provide an example of such a situation: "It is easy to imagine a preoperative patient being fearful of surgery (knowing the object of fear) and feeling anxious about the unknown consequences" (p. 184).

Other recommendations have to do with the refinement of the current diagnostic categories of Anxiety and Fear. It is essential that intensity or degree of each of these phenomena be considered in future validation studies. Peplau proposed a schema for assessing levels of anxiety in 1963. The purpose of formulating nursing diagnoses is to direct nursing action. If, in fact, nursing action would differ on the basis of the degree to which a client is experiencing Anxiety or Fear, then we must be able to be more precise about the intensity of the phenomenon present.

Also, consideration needs to be given to how the manifestations of Anxiety and/or Fear might differ in relation to age, developmental level and cultural background. For example, crying may be a critical indicator in a young child experiencing anxiety even though research has not shown it to be one for adults. We are learning more and more each day about the cultural influences on health, health beliefs and health values. Surely, culture plays a role in determining how one responds to real, anticipated or imagined danger.

Work To Be Done

The authors reviewed the literature that individual workgroup members submitted in 1996 and found several publications that had not been considered in the group's initial synthesis. In addition, the workgroup did not have sufficient time at the 1996 meeting to accomplish the following tasks that members agreed were needed:

1. Cluster the signs/symptoms if too numerous (NANDA, Instructions for Diagnosis Work Group, 1996); and

2. Cluster defining characteristics (signs/symptoms) into conceptually consistent levels of abstraction.

In order to accomplish these two tasks the authors propose conducting a Q-Sort to recategorize all the defining characteristics that were identified in 1996 and from the subsequent literature review as a next step in this ongoing work.

Summary

Anxiety and Fear have been included in NANDA's system of diagnostic nomenclature since 1973. Although research exists in nursing and other disciplines on these phenomena, the diagnostic categories have not been refined to reflect this work. The Anxiety/Fear Workgroup constituted by NANDA in 1996 began a synthesis of literature intended to refine these diagnoses. The Workgroup identified additional definitions, related factors and dcs for Anxiety and initial ones for Fear from a preliminary literature review. Recommendations for further refinement of these nursing diagnoses are presented.

References

American Psychiatric Association. (1994). *Diagnostic and statistical manual of mental disorders* (4th ed.). Washington, DC: author.

Irving, S. (1973). *Basic psychiatric nursing.* Philadelphia: Saunders.

Kagan, J., & Schulkin, J. (1995). On the

concepts of fear. *Harvard Review of Psychiatry, 3,* 231-134.

Kaplan, Sadock, & Grebb. (1994). *Kaplan & Sadock's synopsis of psychiatry behavioral sciences clinical psychiatry.* Baltimore: Williams & Wilkins.

Kim, M.J., & Moritz, D.A. (1982). *Classification of nursing diagnoses: Proceedings of the third and fourth conferences.* St. Louis: McGraw-Hill.

Krainovich-Miller, B. (1988). *Clinical validation of the nursing diagnosis pre-operative state anxiety.* Unpublished doctoral dissertation, Columbia University, New York.

Levin, R.F., Krainovich, B.C., Bahrenburg, E., & Mitchell, C.A. (1988). Diagnostic content validity of nursing diagnoses. *Image, 21,* 40-44.

North American Nursing Diagnosis Association. (1992). *Definitions and classification 1992-1993.* Philadelphia: Author.

North American Nursing Diagnosis Association. (1994). *Nursing diagnoses: Definitions & classification.* Philadelphia, PA: Author.

Peplau, H. (1963). A working definition of anxiety. In S. F. Burd & M. A. Marshall (Eds.), *Some clinical approaches to psychiatric nursing.* New York: MacMillan.

Rantz, M.J., & LeMone, P. (Eds.). (1997). *Classification of nursing diagnoses: Proceedings of the twelfth conference.* Glendale, CA: Cinahl.

Sarafino, E. (1986). *Fears of childhood.* New York: Human Sciences Press.

Scruton, D. (1986). *Sociophobics: The anthropology of fear.* Boulder: Westover Press.

Taylor-Loughran, A., O'Brien, M., LaChapelle, R., & Rangel, S. (1989). Defining characteristics of the nursing diagnoses fear and anxiety: A validation study. Applied *Nursing Research, 2,* 178-186.

Webster's deluxe unabridged dictionary (2nd ed.) (1983). New York: Simon & Schuster.

Whitley, G. (1994). Expert validation and differentiation of the nursing diagnoses anxiety and fear. *Nursing Diagnosis, 5,* 143-150.

Whitley, G. (1992a). Concept analysis of anxiety. *Nursing Diagnosis, 3,* 107-116.

Whitley, G. (1992b). Concept analysis of fear. *Nursing Diagnosis, 3,* 155-161.

Clinical Validation of Characteristics of the Alcoholic Family (abstract)

Marlene G. Lindeman, MSN, RN, CS
Jean Krajicek Bartek, PhD, ARNP, CARN
Jane Hokanson Hawks, DMSc, RN, C

Delivery of quality nursing care for alcoholic families depends on professional nurses' abilities to assess and diagnose potential health problems, stablish effective and efficient nursing interventions, and continuously reassess movement toward optimal health. The aims of this study were to 1) validate from a client and family perspective the defining characteristics for the nursing diagnosis, Altered family processes: Alcoholism, and 2) identify demographic, family, and selected treatment information from clients and family members. Subjects (n=150) were adult clients participating in five Midwestern treatment/recovery programs, and adult family members. Only adult clients whose primary drug of choice was alcohol were invited to participate, along with adult family members. Family members had lived within the family of the person in treatment and were wives, husbands, adult sons or daughters, mothers, fathers, adult siblings, or significant others. In this study, previously determined defining characteristics for the nursing diagnosis, Altered family processes: Alcoholism were tested using Fehring's (1987) clinical diagnostic validation (CDV) index to see if they are actually found in clinical practice. Examination of findings indicates that alcoholic families display behaviors of alcohol abuse, loss of control of drinking, denial of problems, nicotine addiction, impaired communication, inappropriate expression of anger, enabling behaviors, inability to meet emotional needs of members, inability to express or accept wide range of feelings, and harsh self-judgement. Examination of family feelings indicates the presence of unhappiness, hurt, frustration, tension, guilt, moodiness, repressed emotions, powerlessness, loneliness, mistrust, anger, anxiety, distress, insecurity, emotional isolation, hopelessness, and decreased self-esteem. Demographic findings indicate that the majority of subjects were employed full-time, 26-45 years of age, married or divorced, and high school or college graduates. Fifty-nine percent of subjects reported that they were adult children of alcoholics. A majority of the subjects participated in self-help support groups and reported that they viewed alcoholism as a family disease. Knowledge of these clinically validated characteristics will scientifically complete the assessment phase of this research and direct the path to future studies to determine appropriate goals/outcomes and interventions related to alcoholic families.

Clinical Validation of Signs/Symptoms, Related Factors and Interventions, and Outcomes of the Nursing Diagnosis Anxiety (abstract)

Sue Moorhead, PhD, RN

Anxiety is consistently ranked as one of the 10 most frequently occurring nursing diagnoses across populations and specialties. The majority of the research from a nursing perspective to date have been nurse validation studies using Ferhing's methodology. A recent review of the literature identified only two validation studies based on clinical data. This paper examines the clinical validation of the signs and symptoms and related factors of anxiety across a population of over 28,000 computerized patient discharge records from a Midwestern 500-bed medical center over a five-year period. Further, the paper examines the clinical validation of nursing interventions and nursing outcomes for this diagnosis. The nursing intervention validation was completed using mapping protocols to the Nursing Interventions Classification (NIC) as well as direct documentation of the NIC interventions by clinicians. The patient outcomes validation was completed using mapping protocols to the Nursing-sensitive Outcomes Classification (NOC). The following issues will be highlighted: 1) issues related to the use of these classifications for validation purposes, 2) issues related to the linkages among these standardized languages that support clinical decision making, and 3) issues related to the nursing Minimum Data set (NMDS) will be highlighted.

Validation of the Defining Characteristics of Body Image Disturbance

Chie Ogasawara, PhD, RN

Takako Egawa, PhD, RN

Eiko Masutani, MSEd, RN

Yasuko Kume, MSN, RN

Mitsuko Matsuki, PhD, RN

Yuko Ohno, PhD, RN

Yuko Yamamoto, MSN, RN

The defining characteristics of diagnoses on the NANDA list are used by nurses to identify accurate diagnoses (North American Nursing Diagnosis Association [NANDA], 1972). The defining characteristics of body image disturbance, however, were not previously validated for use in Japan. Body Image Disturbance (BID) is defined as a "disruption in the way one perceives one's body image" and there are twenty-one defining characteristics listed by NANDA (1992). In Japan, there is anecdotal evidence that nurses use a variety of defining characteristics that differ from those listed by NANDA.

Another reason to conduct this study is that the influence of culture should be considered to determine the validity and reliability of defining characteristics. Generally, Japanese adults do not verbally express themselves in terms of self-concept. This cultural trait may mean that some defining characteristics listed by NANDA are not valid for use with persons from the Japanese culture.

According to NANDA, the defining characteristics of "verbal response to actual or perceived change in structure and/or function" or "non-verbal response to actual or perceived change in structure and/or function" must be present to justify the diagnosis of BID. These defining characteristics are not observable. It was unknown how they would present in Japanese patients.

Considering the need to develop valid diagnoses for use, the authors surveyed Japanese nurses to determine which defining characteristics they use to diagnose BID. The purposes of this study were to describe the validity of nursing diagnosis of BID for use in Japan and to specify major and minor defining characteristics of BID as it relates to the Japanese culture.

Methods

Subjects

An initial sample (N=554) was drawn from ten hospitals in Japan in June 1996. The subjects were Registered Nurses (RNs) with more than three years of clinical experience who had learned about nursing diagnosis through continuing education in hospital settings and nursing associations and had used nursing diagnosis in hospitals. The purpose was to select from this sample a group of practicing nurses who had sufficient general knowledge of nursing diagnosis, frequently used the diagnosis of BID, and had sufficient clinical experience to be a considered as expert judges. This information was determined through a mailed questionnaire. The sample for the study was 149 nurses who stated that they diagnose BID "often" or "very frequent," indicated that they had knowledge of nursing diagnosis, and had an average of 10 years clinical experience.

Questionnaire

The questionnaire consisted of 21 items representing the NANDA defining characteristics and 8 additional items from literature and two distracting characteristics based on Fehring (1991). A Likert scale was used to rank each item (5 = very frequent, 4 = often, 3 = sometimes, 2 = seldom, 1 = never). We asked subjects to check each item that they use in clinical practice and to add other signs and symptoms, and to identify the physical condition of their clients for which they were most likely to use BID. The seven categories of physical conditions available were: loss of body part, post-operative, receiving chemotherapy and/or radiation, critical injury, chronic illness, eating disorder and other physical conditions. Nurses were able to select more than one condition. Nurses were asked to identify any defining characteristics in the list that were difficult to understand. Subjects were asked to document what they found from clients with BID related to "verbal response to actual or

perceived change in structure and/or function" and "non-verbal response to actual or perceived change in structure and/or function."

Data analysis

Fehring's Diagnostic Content Validation Model (1987) was used in this research of defining characteristics for the diagnosis BID. Defining characteristics that received DCV scores of 0.75 or above were considered to be major defining characteristics. Minor defining characteristics were determined by scores from 0.60 up to 0.75 following DCV score evaluation by Sparks (1994).

Results

The results of this study are reported below considering five categories. These are frequency of use of the nursing diagnosis BID by expert Japanese nurses, the DCV scores of 21 defining characteristics, variations in ratings of defining characteristics according to types of physical conditions, understanding the wording of defining characteristics listed by NANDA, and additional defining characteristics identified by subject to clarify the defining characteristics of non-verbal and verbal responses to actual or perceived changes in structure and/or function.

The frequency of use of BID by 149 Japanese nurse experts was: very frequent (9.3%), often (34.9%), seldom (51.9%), never (3.9%). The nursing diagnosis of BID was used by 76% of nurses for clients with loss of body part, by 66% of nurses for post-operative clients, by 40% of nurses for clients who were having radiation and/or chemotherapy treatment, by 32% of nurses for clients in critical condition, by 20% of nurses for clients with chronic diseases, by 13% of nurses for psychiatric clients with eating disorders and by 11% of nurses for clients in other physical conditions.

The DCV scores of 21 possible defining characteristics ranged from 0.51 to 0.81 (see Figure 1). In this study, four items were found to be major defining characteristics with DCV scores over 0.75: "inability to accept body changes," "missing body part," "actual change in structure and/or function" and "verbal response to actual or perceived change in structure and/or function." Fifteen items were found to be minor defining characteristics. The remaining ten items did not reach the designated score of 0.60 for consideration as defining characteristics. The minor defining characteristic, "verbalization of negative feelings about body" had an overall DCV score of 0.74 and DCV scores were over 0.75 in six separate situations.

There were variations in ratings of defining characteristics according to the types of physical conditions that nurses treated. In the case of psychiatric patients with eating disorders, there were eight defining characteristics with DCV scores above 0.75. The DCV scores of five defining characteristics were, however, considered minor characteristics for the total sample. These were verbalization of negative feeling about body; verbalization of feeling of helplessness, hopelessness, or powerlessness; focus on past strength, function, or appearance; preoccupation with change or loss; and verbalization of fear of rejection or of reaction by others. Another variation that is worthy of consideration occurred in reference to clients with critical conditions or chronic disease. With these two types of physical conditions, the DCV scores for "feeling of helplessness and hopelessness" were 0.82 and 0.80, respectively.

The findings indicated that the wording of defining characteristics listed by NANDA and other sources are difficult to apply in Japan. The percent of nurses who were unclear about the meaning of "change in ability to estimate spatial relationship of body to environment" was 43.9%; "extension of body boundary in incorporate environmental objects" was 31.0%; "unable to discriminate if the source of stimuli is internal or external" was 24.2%; "personalization of part or loss by name" was 20.4%.

In response to requests to list additional evidence of BID, especially nonverbal and verbal responses to actual and perceived changes in structure or function. One hundred and one nurses (67.8%) provided 182 free descriptions in response to the request to list nonverbal responses they see with BID. The most frequent descriptions were: clients do not want to see changed body part (n = 37), change in interpersonal relationship (n = 34), negative attitude and behavior (n = 18), concealing changed body part (n = 17), behavior and attitude that cannot accept appearance of body change (n = 11), unable control self emotion (n = 11), sleeplessness (n = 9), clients don't want to touch changed body part (n = 8).

One hundred seventeen nurses (78.5%) gave 184 free descriptions of types of verbal responses. Most of the free descriptions were similar to the defining characteristics of the 21 items. Verbal responses that were described but were not one of the 21 listed items were anger, envy jealousy were new descriptors, anxiety, frustration, low self-esteem with negative feelings to self. One descriptor that was difficult to translate into English was "shikataganai." This Japanese expression refers to a feeling that the person can do nothing except accept the situation as is.

Discussion

In this study, four defining characteristics were

Figure 1.

DCV Scores of ND: Body Image Disturbance

Defining characteristics	A	B	C	D	E	F
Client condition / Nurses	149	113	97	60	47	29	20

Item Number

	Defining characteristics	A 149	B 113	C 97	D 60	E 47	F 29	20
1	Inability to accept body change	0.81	0.85	0.84	0.84	0.86	0.81	0.80
2	Missing body part	0.78	0.79	0.81	0.81	0.85	0.78-	0.76
3	Actual change in structure and/or function	0.77	0.78	0.78	0.79	0.78	0.78	0.71
4	Verbal response to actual or perceived change in structure and/or function	0.75	0.77	0.75	0.79	0.79	0.74	0.82
5	Verbalization of negative feelings about body	0.74	0.76	0.75	0.75	0.78	0.77	0.83
6	Verbalization of feelings of helplessness, hopelessness, or powerlessness	0.72	0.75	0.73	0.74	0.82	0.80	0.75
7	Hiding body part	0.70	0.73	0.73	0.75	0.76	0.69	0.71
8	Nonverbal response to actual or perceived change in structure and/or function	0.70	0.72	0.72	0.72	0.78	0.71	0.74
9	Sleeplessness	0.69	0.69	0.70	0.68	0.74	0.73	0.68
10	Not looking at body part	0.67	0.70	0.72	0.69	0.72	0.67	0.68
11	Focus on past strength, function, or appearance	0.67	0.70	0.67	0.70·	0.71	0.71	0.79
12	Not touching body part	0.67	0.70	0.71	0.70	0.72	0.65	0.68
13	Inability to accept change in body boundary	0.65	0.66	0.67	0.64	0.72	0.74	0.64
14	Preoccupation with change or loss	0.65	0.68	0.66	0.68	0.70	0.67	0.78
15	Change in social involvement	0.65	0.67	0.65	0.69	0.66	0.70	0.63
16	Verbalization of change in lifestyle	0.64	0.65	0.64	0.65	0.68	0.68	0.66
17	Difficulty to control emotions	0.64	0.66	0.65	0.66	0.72	0.67	0.68
18	Verbalization of fear of rejection or of reaction by others	0.63	0.64	0.65	0.67	0.73	0.72	0.76
19	Guilt, shame	0.60	0.63	0.62	0.61	0.68	0.70	0.60
20	Self-destructive behaviors	0.53	0.55	0.54	0.58	0.63	0.66	0.69
21	Indifference, apathy	0.51	0.55	0.54	0.51	0.60	0.56	0.56

FIGURE 1 DCV Scores of ND: Body Image Disturbance

*The percent of the sample that said they utilized BID in clinical settings for patients in these conditions. Client Conditions: A = loss of body part; B=post-operation; C = receiving chemotherapy and/or radiation; D = critical condition; E= chronic disease; F = eating disorder

Major   Minor

identified as major (see Figure 1), with DCV scores over 0.75 (Sparks, 1994). The authors believe, however, that some defining characteristics identified as minor defining characteristics may be observable characteristics of the major defining characteristics. For example, numbers 5 and 18 as verbal responses and numbers 7, 10, 11, 12, and 20 as non-verbal responses (see Figure 1)could be considered subcategories of the defining characteristic "inability to accept body change." This indicates a need for concept clarification of body image disturbance for use of this diagnosis in Japanese culture.

With additional research, it may be shown that the defining characteristic of "verbalization of negative feeling about body" may meet the requirements as a major defining characteristic. This minor defining characteristic had a DCV score over 0.75 in six separate physical conditions; however, the overall DCV score was lower because of the responses in the "other physical conditions" category. In addition, 26 subjects in the study also wrote this defining characteristic in the free description of the questionnaire. Gordon (1997) also included this defining characteristic in the *Manual of Nursing Diagnosis*. Therefore, this "negative feeling about body" should be included as a major defining characteristic of BID.

Based on other case studies (Ohira, et al. 1993) and this research, some minor defining characteristics were upgraded to major defining characteristics for psychiatric clients and critical condition clients. This result suggests that these minor defining characteristics change depending on the client's condition. Further study is required here to distinguish the relationships of defining characteristics to the types of physical conditions.

Some of the defining characteristics of

BID identified by NANDA and other research were difficult for Japanese nurses to understand. The nurses in this study used more informal terminology and more observable evidence than the abstract concepts used by NANDA. This may be explained by the nature of nursing education in Japan. Japanese nurses have limited opportunities to learn the meaning of psychological terms such as BID. Based on case studies (Moriyama, 1992) (Horita, 1993) and this research, NANDA should consider revision of the defining characteristics of BID so that they are more concrete and observable for use by practicing nurses.

Some Japanese expert nurses also identified anxiety, frustration, low self esteem with negative feeling to self as defining characteristics for body image in the free descriptions. It seems that Japanese see self concept and body image as the same. Champion, Austin and Tzeng (1982) reported that body image and self concept may be interrelated. Further study such as clinical validation studies and factor analysis is needed to explain these perceptions.

In studies such as this, translation of diagnosis, definitions and defining characteristics from one language to another may explain some of the findings. This is especially relevant with psychosocial concepts/diagnoses such as body image disturbance. For example, the free description "Shikataganai" could not easily be translated in English. Besides language, other cultural differences need to be considered in order that diagnoses such as BID are valid and reliable for use by nurses from Japan and other cultures. The feeling of shame in Japan is expressed frequently and may have to be in a separate category from guilt, although Gordon (1997) lists shame and guilt in the same defining characteristic category.

In conclusion, four major defining characteristics and fifteen minor defining characteristics for BID met the criteria as defining characteristics. There was strong evidence that one of the minor defining characteristics may be a major defining characteristics. This study provides a foundation for further study of culturally appropriate defining characteristics for use in Japan.

References

Carpenito, L. J. (1993). *Nursing Diagnosis Application to Clinical Practice*, (5th ed.), Philadelphia: J. B. Lippincott Company.

Champion, V. L., Austin, J. K., & Tzeng, O. (1982). Assessment of Relationship between Self-Concept and Body Image Using Multivariate Techniques, *Issues in Mental Health Nursing, 4*, 299-315.

Fehring, R. J. (1987). Methods to validate nursing diagnosis. *Heart and Lung, 16*(6), 625-629.

Gordon, M. (1997). *Manual of Nursing Diagnosis 1997-1998*. Mosby -Yearbook, Inc.

Gordon, M. (1997). *Manual of Nursing Diagnosis 1997-1998*. (Japanese ed.) Mosby -Year book , Inc.

Horita,U.,Tsukahara,I. and Takamune,Y. (1993). Nursing for recurrent breast cancer having chemotherapy and hormone treatment. (Trans.) *Japanese Journal of Nursing Arts, 38*(5), 57-60.

Kim, C.J. (1993). *Pocket Guide to Nursing Diagnosis*, The C. V. Mosby Company.

Kim, C.J. (1990). A study on the development of standardized nursing care plans for computerized nursing service. *Kanho-Hakhoe-Chi., 20*(3), 368-380.

Moriyama, K., Ohta, H., Fujisawa, K., & Hatagami, T. (1992). Nursing of unmarried patients with mal-adaptation after mastectomy; Analysis of Nursing in a Crisis. (Trans.) *Japanese Journal of Nursing Arts, 38*(5), 53-56.

Musante,M.W. and Fehring, R.J. (1991). Multinational Validation of Anxiety, Hopelessness, and Ineffective Airway Clearance. *Nursing Diagnosis, 2*(2), 57-65.

NANDA (1992). *NANDA Nursing Diagnosis; Definition & Classification 1992-1993*, NANDA. (Japanese ed.)

NANDA (1992). *NANDA Nursing Diagnosis; Definition & Classification 1992-1993*, NANDA.

Ohira, S., Tanaka, T., Kobayashi, R., Matsutake, S., & Kita, Y., (1993). Nursing of Body Image Disturbance: Patients with lower leg amputations due to sarcoma. (Trans.) *Japanese Journal of Nursing Arts, 39*(15), 67-70.

Pokess-Vawter, S. (1998). *Assessment of positive and negative body image in normal weight and overweight females, Classification of nursing diagnosis*; Proceedings of the Eight Conference, 313-319.

Sparks, S. M. (1994). Modification of the Diagnostic Content Validity Model. *Nursing Diagnosis, 5*(1), 29-35.

Thompson, J. M., McFarland, J. K., Hersch, J. E., Tucker, S. M., & Bowers A. C. (1986). *Clinical Nursing*. (Japanese ed.) St. Louis: Mosby.

How do Expert Nurses Engage with Clients Who Present with Challenging Behaviors? (abstract)

Ivor Pattison, RN, MScN

Background: We live in an increasingly violent society and are confronted daily by media accounts of violent scenarios of all types, a fact which simple serves to poignantly underscore this harsh reality. The increase in violence in society at large has had parallel implications for all healthcare settings. Today, challenging patient behaviors, which were once almost the exclusive preserve of psychiatric treatment facilities and emergency rooms, are now being encountered with ever increasing frequency in all areas of the healthcare delivery system. The term "challenging behavior" describes patient/client behaviors which are either the precursors to, or the actual defining characteristics of, the nursing diagnoses Potential for Violence; Self Directed Physical Trauma, or Potential For Violence; Other Directed Physical Trauma. The term "challenging behavior" describes, but is not exclusively limited to, disorganized, disruptive, asocial and antisocial behavior, verbal threats, verbal and physical assaultiveness, non-lethal self destructiveness and, in extreme cases, frank suicidal and homicidal ideation. Such behaviors not only potentially threaten the welfare and the safety of responding nurses but also challenge their clinical expertise.

Aim: To identify the nuances of behavior and the clinical decision making processes which are utilized by nurses who are deemed to be Experts in engaging with individuals who manifest challenging behaviors.

Method: Using a nominated, purposive, snowball sampling methodology, in-depth audiotaped interviews were conducted with fifteen (15) nurses (research in progress) who were identified by their colleagues as being Experts in interacting with individuals who manifest challenging behaviors. Using a constant comparative, grounded theory methodology, data from these interviews were analyzed into open, axial and selective codes.

Findings: A preliminary review of the data gathered to date (research in progress), reveals that the clinical skills of nurses who effectively engage with individuals who present with challenging behaviors fall predominantly into five broad areas:

1. Reliance upon past experience and the clinical insight facilitated by that experience.
2. Trusting clinical intuitions.
3. The effective operationalization of "people skills."
4. Recognition on the part of the Expert that it is very important to be "present" for the individual patient/client.
5. Maintaining focus while retaining a "larger perspective" situational overview.

Although this is a "work in progress," it is anticipated that a new model of nurse-patient/client interaction will emerge as data analysis proceeds.

Implications: To observe the clinical actions of an Expert Nurse engaging with a patient/client who is manifesting challenging behaviors is to witness the artful application of know-how knowledge to an uncertain but ever unfolding, fluid and dynamic scenario in which the interpersonal behavioral and verbal dialogue between the patient/client and the nurse is seemingly skillfully and subtly structured by the nurse. An improved understanding of the essential essence of this interaction may make it possible to tease-out, and then teach to less experienced staff, the specific clinical skills of this particular area of Expert Nursing Practice. This in turn may promote the more timely delivery of focused clinical interventions to patient populations who present with challenging behaviors while helping to nurture the creation of safer healthcare environments.

Children's Spiritual Response: Validation of Two Nursing Diagnoses

Shelley-Rae Pehler, RN, MSN

This study was partially funded by a grant from the University of Iowa Student Government Association. The study was conducted in partial fulfilment of the MSN at the University of Iowa College of City, Iowa. Sincere appreciation goes to Dr. Martha Craft-Rosenbert, Dr. Leslie Marshall, Dr. Ann-Marie McCarthy, and Reverend Diane Wasson MSN, RN, for their assistance in the study.

The dimensions of spirituality are woven into client phenomena which nurses diagnose and treat. Two nursing diagnoses, "Spiritual Distress" and "Potential for Enhanced Spiritual Well-being," have been accepted by NANDA (1994) for further testing and refinement. The research problem is that nurses who work with children do not know the spiritual response in children and whether these two nursing diagnoses describe the spiritual response(s) found in children. The purpose of this study was to validate the two nursing diagnoses related to spirituality and determine the level of confidence with which the defining characteristics, label definitions, and related factors of the two nursing diagnoses can be used in clinical practice as indicators of spiritual distress and spiritual well-being in children.

Spirituality is defined as a dynamic state of being in which the individual seeks connectedness: interpersonally, intrapersonally and transpersonally. There is a developmental component to a person's spirituality, based on that person's individual characteristics, cognitive and emotional development, and interpretations of life experiences, events and questions. Spirituality is a broader concept than religion (Emblem, 1992; Farran, Fitchett, Quirring-Emblen, & Burck, 1989; Lane, 1987; Nagai-Jacobson & Burkhardt, 1989; Reed, 1992; Sommer, 1989).

The report of the research findings from the validation of the diagnosis of Spiritual Distress was previously published (Pehler, 1997) and will not be discussed in this paper. This paper will report the findings from the second component of the study which researched the validation of the diagnosis of Potential for Enhanced Spiritual Well-being.

Framework

The Neuman Systems Model was used as the theoretical framework for this study. Neuman Systems Model is based on open systems theory which supports that when one area of a person's life is affected, all areas are affected. Neuman identifies the core of her model as the client. The core is made up of those things that are common to all and are attributes for survival. These include normal temperature range, genetic structure, response pattern, organ strength, weakness, ego structure, known or commonalties (Neuman, 1989).

The core is supported by five variables: spiritual, developmental, psychological, physiological and sociocultural. The physiological variable refers to body structure and function, and the psychological variable refers to mental processes and relationships. The sociocultural variable refers to combined social and cultural functions, the developmental variable refers to life development processes, and the spiritual variable is broadly defined as the spiritual belief influence. The spiritual variable permeates all the other variables, whether or not it is acknowledged or developed by the client. Persons are felt to be energized by their spirit, resulting in a move toward optimal health. When a stressor such as illness, loss, or pain affects a person, energy is depleted and one's spirit is affected. This evokes spiritual needs and concerns (Clark, Cross, Deane, & Lawry, 1991).

The empirical literature does support that a child's life has a spiritual variable. Spiritual growth interacts with the child's physical and psychosocial growth and development. How a child interprets the experiences that happen to him or her is as important to that child's spiritual growth as the experience itself (Coles, 1990; Ebmeier, Lough, Huth, & Autio, 1991; Farran et al, 1989; Fowler, 1981; Harms, 1944; Heller, 1986; Nagy, 1951; Pehler, 1997; Webb-Mitchell, 1993).

Methods

Fehring's (1987) methodology for diagnostic content validity was used in this descriptive study to determine the validity of the defining characteristics, related factors and definitions for the two spiritual diagnoses found in NANDA. From the College of Chaplains, 70 Board Certified Chaplains identified their interest in pediatric clients, and could be classified as 'experts' using Fehring's validation model expert rating system (Fehring, 1994).

Instrument

The 16 defining characteristics for the nursing diagnosis of Potential for Enhanced Spiritual Well-being were listed separately. A Likert scale with values related to the responses of 1=Not Present, 2=Rarely Present, 3=Occasionally Present, 4= Frequently Present, and 5=Nearly Always Present were listed for each of four age groups (3 to 5, 6 to 10, 11 to 12, and 13 to 18 year olds) which correlated with Fowler's (1981) work on faith (spiritual) development. The chaplains were also given the opportunity to identify why a particular defining characteristic was inappropriate or unclear and offer suggestions for revision under the Comment section of the survey tool. Open-ended questions were asked to determine the reliability and validity of the definition and related factors to both diagnoses.

Procedure

The Total Design Method (Crosby, Ventura, & Feldman, 1989; Dillman, 1978) was implemented for data collection. Responses to the open-ended questions on the survey were analyzed through content analysis by the researcher and an independent rater. Content validity of the themes was ensured by an average interrater reliability of 94% (Glaser & Strauss, 1967; Lincoln & Guba, 1985). Weighted ratios were assigned to the Likert scale responses for the validation of the defining characteristics. Major

Table 1

Weighted Ratios for Defining Characteristics of Nursing Diagnosis: Potential for Enhanced Spiritual Well-Being (N=23)

Defining Characteristics	3-5 Years Average	6-10 Years	11-12 Years	13-18 Years	
Inner strengths: Sense of awareness	.45	.58*	.70*	.79*	.63*
Inner strengths: Self-consciousness	.34	.53*	.68*	.75*	.58*
Inner strengths: Sacred Source	.42	.52*	.61	.68*	.56*
Inner strengths: Unifying force	.24	.31	.41	.49	.36
Inner strengths: Inner core	.33	.46	.53*	.62*	.49
Inner strengths: Transcendence	.43	.51	.55*	.64*	.53*
Unfolding Mystery: Life's purpose and meaning	.20	.42	.58*	.74*	.49
Unfolding mystery: Mystery	.41	.47	.57*	.65*	.52*
Unfolding mystery: Uncertainty	.30	.43	.59*	.72*	.51*
Unfolding mystery: Struggles	.31	.43	.60*	.77*	.53*
Harmonious interconnectedness: Relatedness	.43	.53*	.61	.69*	.56*
Harmonious interconnectedness: Connectedness	.38	.46	.55*	.66*	.51
Harmonious interconnectedness: Harmony with self	.45	.45	.49	.56*	.49
Harmonious interconnectedness: Harmony with others	.40	.50*	.55*	.60*	.52*
Harmonious interconnectedness: Harmony with Higher Power	.48	.55*	.59*	.63*	.56*
Harmonious interconnectedness: Harmony with environment	.49	.54*	.55*	.61	.55*

*Designates a Minor Characteristics, **Designates a Major Characteristic

Table 2

Additional Characteristics Identified by Chaplains to be included for Potential for Enhanced Spiritual Well-Being (N=9)	
Characteristic	Number of Chaplains
Optimism/Hope	3
Energy/Resiliency	2
Playfulness as a spiritual quality	1
Willingness to experiment	1
Willingness to imagine	1
Trust	1
Faith	1

defining characteristics were those that received a weighted ratio of greater than or equal to 0.80. Minor defining characteristics were those that received a weighted ratio of between 0.50 through 0.79.

Results

The response rate was 57% (40 questionnaires out of the 70 sent). Thirty-seven percent of the 40 questionnaires returned were usable in the data analysis. The other 20% were not filled out because the chaplains either did not feel qualified, no longer worked with children, or had time constraints. The mean age of the chaplains responding was 51, the mean number of years the subject worked as a chaplain was 13.75, and the mean number of years that the chaplains had worked with children was 9.9.

Eleven respondents felt the definition for Potential for Enhanced Spiritual Well-being was adequate. The responses of the 12 chaplains who felt it was inadequate fell into three categories. First, the chaplains could not envision the definition without a reference to God or a 'Higher Power'. Second, they disagreed with the definition in that it sounded like spiritual well-being was a 'process'. Third, the definition was too vague. One chaplain admitted that he/she had a harder time assessing the frequencies of the characteristics under this label.

The weighted ratios of the defining characteristics for the diagnosis are listed in Table 1. No defining characteristics were identified as major for the diagnosis of Potential for Enhanced Spiritual Well-being. Twelve items met the criteria for a minor defining characteristic (weighted ratio of 0.50-0.79) when all age groups were averaged together. The likelihood that a defining characteristic would meet the minor criteria increased through the age groups. No defining characteristics met the criteria in the 3-5 year old age group, and 15 of the defining characteristics met the criteria in the 13-18 year olds. Table 2 lists additional defining characteristics identified by the chaplains.

Table 3 lists the responses by the chaplains

Table 3

Reasons Chaplains are Called to Work with Children (N=19**)			
Category Label	Number of Chaplains Who Identified	Number of Occurrences	Inter-rater Reliability
Death/Dying	11	17/17	100
Serious Illness	6	13/11	85
Referrals by Others	3	7/7	100
Behavioral Matters	5	7/6	86
Parental Issues	5	7/5	71
Emotional Matters	2	6/5	83
Multi-disciplinary team member	4	4/4	100
Trouble within the family	3	4/4	100
Child Asking Religious Questions	3	3/3	100
To Perform Religious Rituals	2	3/3	100
Made Routine visits	3	3/3	100
No requests to visit	1	3/1	33
Personal Clergy Issues	2	2/2	100
Eccentric Religious Practices	2	2/2	100
To Enhance Child's Spirituality	1	2/1	50
Birth of New Sibling	1	1/1	100
To Play Parental Role	1	1/1	100
Overall Percent Agreement		94	

*Total Number of themes found in that category/Number of common themes for both raters.

**N represents the actual number of chaplains who did respond to this question.

concerning when they are called upon to assess the spirituality of children (Pehler, 1997). The responses to the question dealing with the related factors of the nursing diagnosis provided rich data on how chaplains are used in the clinical setting, and some insight as to the related factors of the nursing diagnosis. Since this diagnosis is wellness focused, related factors were not listed in NANDA (1994). Chaplains did confirm that the enhancement of a child's spirituality can occur through routine visits and the performing of religious rituals.

Discussion

The chaplains were split as to the adequacy of the definition for Potential for Enhanced

Spiritual Well-being. Like the validation of the definition for Spiritual Distress (Pehler, 1997), the definition for Potential for Enhanced Spiritual Well-being also needs to be clarified.

None of the defining characteristics met the criteria as a major defining characteristic (> 0.80 weighted ratio). The issue of age-related characteristics is sharply realized when examining the defining characteristics that met the minor and major criteria under Fehring's (1987) methodology for the nursing diagnosis of Potential for Enhanced Spiritual Well-being. In the 3-5 year old group, no defining characteristic met the criteria. The 13-18 year old group had the highest number of defining characteristics that met the criteria for minor.

The chaplains' suggested lists of defining characteristics obtained in this study provides suggestions that might appear more in the 3-5 year olds, i.e. energy, playfulness, imagination, and trust (Table 2). Burkhardt (1989) proposed that indicators to spirituality include peace, hopefulness, creativity, joy, enthusiasm, courage, sharing with others, and flowing easy with change. The chaplains' support these additions as evidenced by Table 2, where optimism/hope, energy/resiliency and playfulness were their top three additions to the defining characteristics. Since no other validation studies could be found for the nursing diagnosis label of Potential for Enhanced Spiritual Well-being, there is no comparison of previously published results. Issues of clarity, population and age specific defining characteristics need to be addressed in future research studies.

Implications and Recommendations

Holistic care and health promotion are areas that nursing has claimed as essential to their domain of practice. When it is identified that children can have a spiritual response to a life changing event it can lead to interventions that enhance their spiritual well-being. Chaplains in this study have shown that this is possible. They have done this by seeing the defining characteristics in the patients they serve and identifying the related factors when they are called upon to work with children in their spiritual growth. Nursing should be instrumental in insuring that their patients receive the appropriate spiritual as well as physical and psychosocial care. This can only be done if the diagnoses that nurses work with are clear and truly describe the phenomena that nurses treat.

Ongoing research is needed to clarify the standardized languages that nurses use. Effectiveness studies of nursing interventions are also needed to achieve positive patient outcomes once nursing has defined the phenomena the patient is exhibiting. Future research should avoid the perception biases of others by having the children describe their own spiritual response(s) (Fehring's, 1987). Other research must look at the difference between spiritual care and psychological support (Spilka, Sprangler, & Nelson, 1983). Outcome data needs to show whether or not patient's quality of care and quality of life are increased when spiritual care is implemented. Spiritual research must also describe and validate the assessment strategies, interventions, and outcomes in spiritual care for children.

Underlying the research needs are the educational needs of nursing. Nursing's comfort in assessing spiritual issues with patients must be valued as equal to the physical or psychosocial assessments. For effective assessment, studies show a nurse must identify her or his own spirituality and receive additional education in spiritual assessment and interventions. These will be tools for the nurse to provide the spiritual care needed in holistic health care (Greshik, 1994; Kennison, 1987).

References

Burkhardt, M.A. (1989). Spirituality: An analysis of the concept. *Holistic Nursing Practice, 3*(3), 69-77.

Clark, C.C., Cross, J.R., Deane, D.M., & Loury, L.W. (1991). Spirituality: Integral to quality care. *Holistic Nursing Practice, 5*(3), 67-76.

Coles, R. (1990). *The spiritual life of children.* Boston: Houghton Mifflin Company.

Crosby, F.E., Ventura, M.R., & Feldman, M.J. (1989). Examination of a survey methodology: Dillman's total design method. *Nursing Research, 38*(1), 56-58.

Dillman, D.A. (1978). *Mail and telephone surveys: The total design method.* New York: John Wiley & Sons.

Ebmeier, C., Lough, M., Huth, M.M., & Autio, L. (1991). Hospitalized school-age children express ideas, feelings, and behaviors toward God. *Journal of Pediatric Nursing, 6*(5), 337-349.

Emblen, J.D. (1992). Religion and spirituality defined according to current use in nursing literature. *Journal of Professional Nursing, 8*(1), 4147.

Farran, C., Fitchert, G., Quiring-Emblen, J., & Burck, R. (1989). Development of a model for spiritual assessment and intervention. *Journal of Religion and Health, 28*(3), 185-194.

Fehring, R.J. (1987). Methods to validate nursing diagnoses. Heart & Lung: The *Journal of Critical Care, 16*(6), 625-629.

Fehring, R.J. (1994). The Fehring model. In R.M. Carroll-Johnson (Ed.). *Classification of nursing diagnoses,* Proceedings of the tenth conference, North America nursing diagnosis association. (pp. 55-62). Philadelphia: J.B. Lippincott Company.

Fowler, J. (1981). *Stages of faith.* San Francisco: Harper & Row.

Glaser, B.G., & Strauss, A.L. (1967). *The discovery of grounded theory: Strategies for qualitative research.* Chicago: Aldine publishing Company.

Greshik, J.G. (1994, November). *Care of the human spirit: Nurses' attitudes toward spiritual intervention. Spiritual Care: Does it Make a Difference?* Symposium sponsored by Saint Marys Hospital Sponsorship Board, Joint Chaplain Services, Saint Marys Hospital and Rochester Methodist Hospital, Rochester, Minnesota.

Harms, E. (1944). The development of religious experience in children. *The American Journal of Sociology, 50*(2), 112-122.

Heller, D. (1986). *The children's God.* Chicago: University of Chicago Press.

Kennison, M.M. (1987). Faith: An untapped health resource. *Journal of Psychosocial Nursing, 25*(10), 28-30.

Lane, J. (1987). The care of the human spirit. *Journal of Professional Nursing, 3,* 332-337.

Lincoln, Y.S., & Guba, E.G. (1985). *Naturalistic inquiry.* Beverly Hills, California: Sage.

Nagai-Jacobson, M.G., & Burkhardt, M.A. (1989). Spirituality: Cornerstone of holistic nursing practice. *Holistic Nursing Practice, 3*(3), 18-26.

Nagy, M.H. (1951). Children's ideas of the origin of illness. *Health Education Journal, 9,* 6-12.

NANDA. (1994). *Nursing diagnoses:*

Definitions and classification. Philadelphia: North American Nursing Diagnosis Association.

Neuman, B.M. (Ed.). (1989). *The Neuman systems model* (2nd ed.). Norwalk, Connecticut: Appleton & Lange.

Pehler, S.R. (1997). Children's spiritual response: Validation of the nursing diagnosis Spiritual Distress. *Nursing Diagnosis, 8*(2), 55-66.

Reed, P. (1992). An emerging paradigm for the investigation of spirituality in nursing. *Research in Nursing and Health, 15*(5), 349-357.

Sommer, D.R. (1989). The spiritual needs of dying children. *Issues in Comprehensive Pediatric Nursing, 12*(2/3), 225-233.

Spilka, B., Sprangler, J.D., & Nelson, C.B. (1983). Spiritual support in life threatening illness. *Journal of Religion and Health 22*(2), 98-104.

Webb-Mitchell, B. (1993). *God plays piano, too: The spiritual lives of disabled children*. New York: Crossroad.

Influence of Patients' Medical Status and Age on Content Validation of Anxiety, Pain, and Sleep Pattern Disturbance: A Study in Japan

Shigemi Sato, PhD, RN

This research was funded by a grant from 1994 & 1995 Fumiko Yamaji Memorial Trust for Nursing Research. An earlier draft of this paper was presented in Japanese at the annual conference of the Japanese Nursing Association, July 1997, Sapporo, Japan.

Are defining characteristics of nursing diagnoses general or population specific? This question was raised by Warren (1991) and Goyette-Vincent (1991) at the ninth conference of North American Nursing Diagnosis Association (NANDA). Nurses work with patients whose medical status and ages differ widely. It is likely that patients with different medical status or different age present different manifestations of a health problem. However, there is a single set of NANDA defining characteristics on which to base our clinical judgment. Thus, the validity of the current list of NANDA (1996) defining characteristics can be questioned.

Although there are many NANDA diagnoses which have never been tested clinically, various researchers have already examined content validity of Anxiety, Pain, and Sleep Pattern Disturbance. Nevertheless, only a few studies have addressed the influence of patient factors on these nursing diagnoses. The patient age factor has been studied by Wieseke et al. (1994) for Sleep Pattern Disturbance. These investigators have found that both the major and minor defining characteristics differed between adult patients and children. Another study by Whitley (1994) examined content validity of Anxiety and Fear between two nursing specialties, psychiatric-mental health and medical-surgical nursing. Whitley's study addressed how nurses perceived the influence of patient medical status on two diagnoses. Yet, no differences between the two nursing specialties were reported.

Purpose of the Study

The purpose of this study was to discover whether patients' medical status and age influence the major and minor defining characteristics of the selected NANDA diagnoses, namely Anxiety, Pain, and Sleep Pattern Disturbance. This study asked specifically the following research question:

Do major and minor defining characteristics of Anxiety, Pain, and Sleep Pattern Disturbance differ across patients' medical status and age?

Methods

This study, a part of a larger study of NANDA nursing diagnoses (Sato, 1996), utilized a modified Fehring's Diagnostic Content Validation (DCV) model (1987). Fehring (1994) emphasized that the use of master's prepared clinical nurse experts is desirable for content validation of nursing diagnoses. However, the paucity of master's prepared Japanese nurses, due to lack of educational opportunities in Japan, made their recruitment into the study impossible. Therefore, Japanese registered nurses (RNs) with various educational backgrounds were included.

This study assumed that (1) nurses in different practice areas take care of patients with different medical status, (2) nurses know diagnostic concepts and the relative frequency of their characteristics, (3) nurses are able to utilize this information to rate the degree to which defining characteristics represent a diagnostic concept. Therefore, it is assumed that nurses caring for each patient population can identify major and minor defining characteristics of the selected nursing diagnoses across different patient populations.

Sample and Setting

The convenience sample (n = 886) who used nursing diagnosis at least one year was drawn from 1,908 Japanese RNs who participated in another study (Sato, 1996). These subjects were attendees of a two-day nursing diagnosis seminar. The seminar participants were asked to give informed consent to complete the survey.

The subjects ranged in age from 22 to 70 years old with an average age of 36 (SD = 8.7) years. They had 13 (SD = 7.8) years of clinical experience. They used nursing diagnosis an average of 2.5 (SD = 1.5) years. The majority of subjects (91%) practiced as staff nurses (56%) in hospital medical or surgical related units (50%). Most of the subjects (78%) graduated from diploma nursing programs. Geographically, the subjects represented all but one of the 47 prefectures in Japan.

Instruments

The original study, from which these data were drawn, used a self-administered demographic form and the Diagnostic Concept Study Form (DCSF) based on Gordon's (1996) Nursing Diagnosis: Defining Characteristics Instrument. The development of the DCSF and its reliability and validity can be found elsewhere (Sato, 1996). The DCSF included 12 NANDA diagnoses and their 168 defining characteristics. Nurse subjects, requested to think of a representative sample of patients in their practice with the condition, rated how representative each defining characteristic was to the diagnosis. A five-point scale, ranging from (1) not at all characteristic (not present) to (5) very characteristic (nearly always present) was used for the rating.

Data Analysis

Based on Fehring's DCV model (1987), raw scores were converted into ratio scores, and means and standard deviations were calculated for each defining characteristic. In this paper, the mean ratio score for each defining characteristic is indicated as a DCV score. Fehring's DCV model uses a score .80 as the criterion for a major defining characteristic, but it was modified to .70 or above in this study. Accordingly, a defining characteristic with a DCV score of less than .70 or greater than .50 was considered as a minor defining characteristic.

To compare major and minor defining characteristics of the three diagnoses across

Table 1

Defining Characteristic	Medical-Surgical (n=102)	Medical (n=171)	Surgical (n=151)	Rehab (n=104)	Critical Care (n=63)	Maternal-Child (n=104)	Kruskal-Wallis H Chi-Square
DCV Scores of Anxiety by Area of Practice							
1. Insomnia	.76	.76	.79	.74	.82	.64	36.55****
2. Reports feeling anxious/apprehensive/tense/scared	.68	.72	.74	.65	.75	.71	10.56
3. Reports vague, uneasy feeling of concern/distress /fear of unspecified consequences	.63	.69	.70	.58	.69	.63	16.85**
4. Reports inability to relax, feeling of jittery	.59	.65	.64	.57	.66	.58	13.66*
5. Express concern/regret about changes in life	.57	.60	.62	.55	.58	.55	6.64
6. Facial tension	.55	.55	.56	.52	.68	.56	16.44**
7. Over excited, increased verbalization	.54	.57	.58	.49	.59	.46	19.89**
8. Irritable	.52	.56	.56	.50	.60	.49	14.83*
9. Tearful, voice quivering	.51	.52	.55	.46	.50	.56	10.06
10. Sympathetic response	.51	.54	.51	.46	.64	.45	25.33**
11. Increased muscle tension, restless, foot shuffling, hand/ arms movements, trembling	.51	.51	.51	.45	.56	.40	18.71**
12. Reports feeling of panic	.52	.53	.54	.45	.58	.51	10.34
13. Easy to get angry	.50	.54	.53	.47	.55	.41	23.04***
14. Lack of concentration	.50	.51	.48	.46	.53	.43	10.74
15. Glancing about, increased wariness	.49	.46	.46	.39	.54	.42	15.61**
16. Focus on self	.49	.58	.54	.58	.52	.48	10.39
17. Pallor or flushed	.49	.52	.46	.45	.59	.47	16.93**
18. Reports palpitation	.49	.52	.45	.41	.53	.38	29.68***
19. Poor eye contact	.45	.45	.44	.38	.43	.39	7.91
20. Reports feelings of helplessness/ inadequacy	.44	.46	.48	.41	.47	.40	7.17
21. Startles easily	.44	.41	.41	.36	.47	.39	11.49*
22. Urinary frequency or diarrhea	.44	.48	.47	.49	.42	.40	9.70
23. Diaphoretic, chills	.43	.48	.46	.39	.55	.42	18.50**
24. Distorted time sense	.42	.45	.43	.44	.63	.32	42.54****
25. Dry mouth	.37	.47	.43	.35	.50	.35	28.13****
Major/Minor Defining Characteristics	1/11	2/15	3/11	1/6	2/17	1/7	

Note. * $p < .05$, ** $p < .01$, *** $p < .001$, **** $p < .0001$

patient populations, descriptive and statistical analysis were used. In order to examine the differences across patient medical status, nurses were grouped according to their specialty or practice areas reflecting the patients' condition. A comparative number of the following six areas were identified: medical-surgical (n = 102), medical (n = 173), surgical (n = 155), rehabilitation (n = 103), critical care (n = 63) and maternal-child (n = 105). To compare across patients' age, nurses were divided into the following three age-range groups according to the clinical populations with whom the nurses worked: children (zero to 15 years, n = 70), adult (16 to 64 years, n = 339), and elderly (65 years or above, n = 362).

DCV scores of each practice area and age group were compared using the Kruskal-Wallis analysis of variance with a significance level of p < .05. A nonparametric test was chosen because the data were at the ordinal level of measurement and did not have normal distribution

Table 2

DCV Scores of Anxiety by Age Groups				
Defining Characteristic	Children 0-5 (n=71)	Adult 16-64 (n=346)	Elderly 65 or < (n=359)	Kruskal-Wallis H Chi-Square
1. Reports feeling anxious/apprehensive/tense/ scared	.70	.71	.71	.15
2. Insomnia	.66	.73	.78	15.29***
3. Reports vague, uneasy feeling of concern/ distress/ fear of unspecified consequences	.64	.65	.66	.29
4. Tearful, voice quivering	.59	.51	.53	4.82
5. Reports inability to relax, feeling jittery	.57	.61	.64	3.86
6. Facial tension	.57	.55	.56	.28
7. Express concern/regret about changes in life	.54	.57	.59	2.77
8. Focus on self	.51	.53	.55	1.76
9. Irritable	.50	.53	.56	3.98
10. Over excited, increased verbalization	.50	.51	.56	7.89*
11. Pallor or flushed	.50	.46	.52	6.30*
12. Reports feeling of panic	.49	.52	.53	.80
13. Sympathetic response	.45	.51	.56	11.51**
14. Lack of concentration	.47	.47	.51	4.61
15. Increased muscle tension, restless, foot shuffling, hand/arms movements, trembling	.44	.49	.52	5.62
16. Easy to get angry	.44	.48	.53	8.77*
17. Diaphoretic, chills	.44	.46	.46	.65
18. Reports feelings of helplessness/inadequacy	.42	.44	.46	2.41
19. Glancing about, increased wariness	.41	.44	.48	5.74
20. Poor eye contact	.41	.42	.44	.82
21. Startles easily	.41	.40	.41	.02
22. Urinary frequency or diarrhea	.40	.45	.49	7.01*
23. Dry mouth	.37	.42	.44	4.36
24. Reports palpitation	.34	.48	.50	19.89****
25. Distorted time sense	.34	.42	.48	16.34***
Major/Minor Defining Characteristics	1/7	2/10	2/14	

Note. * p < .05, ** p < .01, *** p < .001, **** p < .0001

(Munro & Page, 1993). The Mann-Whitney U test was used for the post-hoc comparison. To protect against a Type I error during multiple comparisons, the Bonferroni correction was used (Munro & Page); thus, a significance level was set at p < .0033.

Results

The results of analysis are shown in Tables 1 through 6, and the numbers of major and minor defining characteristics are indicated at the bottom of each table. Tables also include the actual number of subjects analyzed. Sixty-

Table 3

	DCV Scores of Pain by Area of Practice						
Defining Characteristic	Medical-Surgical (n=102)	Medical (n=173)	Surgical (n=155)	Rehab (n=103)	Critical Care (n=63)	Maternal-Child (n=105)	Kruskal-Wallis H Chi-Square
1. Report of severe discomfort/pain	.75	.74	.78	.77	.78	.74	2.56
2. Rubbing area	.70	.70	.73	.71	.65	.68	5.17
3. Facial mask of pain	.69	.74	.75	.69	.78	.69	8.51
4. Protecting area	.66	.68	.71	.67	.67	.64	4.89
5. Blood pressure changes	.64	.63	.64	.63	.76	.56	22.42***
6. Heart rate changes	.63	.64	.62	.60	.76	.59	19.22**
7. Diaphoretic	.62	.60	.59	.57	.66	.59	6.61
8. Crying/moaning	.59	.60	.61	.60	.61	.62	.66
9. Respiratory rate changes	.57	.59	.57	.52	.66	.54	16.84**
10. Unusual posture/fetal position	.57	.56	.55	.51	.52	.53	3.49
11. Clenched teeth	.54	.57	.55	.56	.58	.51	3.11
12. Irritable	.53	.63	.60	.60	.59	.48	28.04****
13. Guarding behavior	.52	.54	.54	.49	.60	.45	15.00*
14. Focus on self	.51	.57	.52	.61	.46	.50	18.29**
15. Muscle tension increased	.51	.54	.52	.56	.58	.50	6.03
16. Restless	.49	.56	.53	.51	.54	.47	10.42
17. Pale skin	.45	.49	.47	.44	.52	.47	6.62
18. Hostile	.43	.54	.51	.48	.49	.40	26.57***
19. Altered time perception	.40	.48	.45	.47	.52	.37	20.99***
20. Pacing	.36	.38	.37	.34	.24	.28	21.45***
21. Dilated pupils	.34	.34	.32	.29	.42	.27	12.18*
22. Quiet/withdrawn	.33	.41	.43	.35	.36	.36	13.57*
Major/Minor Defining Characteristics	2/13	3/14	4/13	2/13	4/13	1/10	

Note. * $p < .05$, ** $p < .01$, *** $p < .001$, **** $p < .0001$

nine defining characteristics of the three nursing diagnoses were compared descriptively as well as statistically across six practice areas and three age groups. This section reports the major findings.

Content Validity of Anxiety

Across practice areas: As seen in Table 1, the numbers of major and minor defining characteristics of Anxiety varied across practice areas. The Kruskal-Wallis analysis of variance showed that the DCV scores of the 16 defining characteristics were significantly different ($P < .05$) among six practice areas. "Insomnia" was a major defining characteristic in all areas except the maternal-child area, which had a significantly lower DCV score than other areas ($p = .0000-.0001$). "Reports feeling anxious/apprehensive/tense/scared" was a major defining characteristic in four areas, but the differences in DCV scores were not significant. "Reports vague, uneasy feeling of concern/distress/fear of unspecified consequences" was a major defining characteristic only in the surgical area, and its DCV score was significantly higher than the rehabilitation area ($p = .0015$). Statistical differences were also found in various minor defining characteristics. For instance, "distorted time sense" was a minor

Table 4

DCV Scores of Pain by Age Groups			
Defining Characteristic	Children 0-5 (n=71)	Adult 16-64 (n=349)	Elderly 65 or < (n=365)	Kruskal-Wallis H Chi-Square
1. Report of severe discomfort/pain	.76	.73	.77	2.45
2. Facial mask of pain	.70	.71	.73	.57
3. Rubbing area	.66	.68	.70	.97
4. Crying/moaning	.65	.58	.61	4.38
5. Protecting area	.64	.66	.68	1.78
6. Heart rate changes	.63	.61	.64	2.35
7. Diaphoretic	.61	.57	.61	6.04*
8. Blood pressure changes	.57	.62	.65	4.78
9. Unusual posture/fetal position	.56	.51	.56	5.49
10. Respiratory rate changes	.56	.55	.59	4.61
11. Focus on self	.52	.51	.56	6.12*
12. Clenched teeth	.51	.53	.58	5.26
13. Muscle tension increased	.51	.52	.54	.90
14. Pale skin	.49	.45	.49	5.82
15. Irritable	.48	.56	.60	11.15**
16. Restless	.48	.50	.55	7.90*
17. Guarding behavior	.45	.52	.55	5.80
18. Hostile	.43	.46	.51	10.02**
19. Altered time perception	.36	.42	.48	15.75***
20. Quiet/withdrawn	.34	.37	.40	5.31
21. Pacing	.27	.34	.36	7.53*
22. Dilated pupils	.25	.30	.36	10.28**
Major/Minor Defining Characteristics	2/11	2/13	3/14	

Note. * $p < .05$, ** $p < .01$, *** $p < .001$, **** $p < .0001$

defining characteristic in only the critical care area, and its score was significantly higher than those found in other practice areas ($p = .0000-.0001$).

Across patient age groups: As seen in Table 2, the numbers of major and minor defining characteristics in the children's group were half of those found in the elderly group. DCV scores of eight defining characteristics differed significantly ($P < .05$) among the three groups.

"Reports feeling anxious/apprehensive/tense/scared" was a major defining characteristic in all three groups, and its DCV scores did not differ statistically. "Insomnia" was a major defining characteristic in the adult and the elderly groups, and DCV scores differed significantly between the children and the elderly groups ($p = .0002$). Three age groups had seven common minor defining characteristics, and these DCV scores did not differ statistically. When statistical

Table 5

DCV Scores of Sleep Pattern Disturbance by Area of Practice							
Defining Characteristic	Medical-Surgical (n=102)	Medical (n=172)	Surgical (n=150)	Rehab (n=102)	Critical Care (n=63)	Maternal-Child (n=103)	Kruskal-Wallis H Chi-Square
1. Reports not feeling well rested	.74	.78	.77	.70	.79	.65	20.26**
2. Frequent interruptions during sleep	.74	.73	.72	.71	.80	.64	16.02**
3. Reports difficulty falling asleep	.74	.75	.75	.72	.71	.62	10.54
4. Sleep pattern reversal	.74	.69	.71	.71	.79	.53	35.91****
5. Reports interrupted sleep	.65	.63	.68	.63	.68	.52	17.78**
6. Reports awakening earlier than desired	.63	.68	.71	.63	.62	.50	31.91****
7. Increasing irritability	.57	.63	.58	.56	.65	.49	27.01***
8. Reports fatigue	.57	.61	.59	.56	.59	.52	7.63
9. Lethargic, falls asleep during activities	.56	.52	.52	.57	.60	.38	28.76****
10. Frequent yawning	.53	.53	.51	.47	.52	.47	4.45
11. Hallucinations/delirium/paranoia	.51	.44	.44	.47	.60	.25	65.98****
12. Change in behavior/performance	.50	.47	.44	.47	.56	.37	22.82***
13. Expressionless face	.48	.51	.48	.50	.54	.41	13.86*
14. Restless	.47	.53	.50	.46	.56	.44	18.57**
15. Disoriented	.45	.41	.38	.50	.53	.24	51.23****
16. Thick speech	.42	.39	.35	.41	.40	.26	27.67****
17. Dark circle under eyes	.41	.41	.41	.38	.39	.41	3.31
18. Incorrect word usage	.36	.35	.30	.35	.38	.24	19.92**
19. Hand tremor	.30	.30	.27	.30	.32	.25	6.71
20. Mispronunciation of words	.30	.29	.27	.33	.38	.18	32.79****
21. Mild, fleeting nystagmus	.29	.28	.28	.27	.32	.24	5.55
22. Ptosis of eyelids	.28	.26	.26	.28	.32	.20	16.00**
Major/Minor Defining Characteristics	4/7	3/9	5/5	4/5	4/11	0/6	

Note. * p < .05, ** p < .01, *** p < .001, **** p < .0001

differences were found in minor defining characteristics, they were usually between the children's group and the elderly group.

Content Validity of Pain

Across practice areas: The result of analysis is shown in Table 3. The numbers of major and minor defining characteristics of Pain differed slightly across practice areas. DCV scores of the 11 defining characteristics differed significantly (P < .05) among six practice areas. "Report of severe discomfort/pain" was a major defining characteristic in all areas, and its DCV scores did not differ statistically among six areas. Three additional characteristics, "rubbing area," "facial mask of pain," and "protecting area," were not always major defining characteristics in the six areas. Yet, differences of the DCV scores of these characteristics were not significant. "Blood pressure changes" and "heart rate changes" were major defining characteristics only in the critical care area. The critical care DCV score was significantly higher on "blood pressure changes" than all other areas (p = .0000 -.0010), except the medical-surgical area's score, and higher on "heart rate changes" than all other

Table 6

	Defining Characteristic	Children 0-5 (n=70)	Adult 16-64 (n=339)	Elderly 65 or < (n=362)	Kruskal-Wallis H Chi-Square
DCV Scores of Sleep Pattern Disturbance by Age Groups					
1.	Reports not feeling well rested	.61	.73	.77	16.57***
2.	Frequent interruptions during sleep	.59	.71	.74	12.67**
3.	Reports difficulty falling asleep	.56	.71	.74	14.03***
4.	Sleep pattern reversal	.53	.66	.73	28.42****
5.	Frequent yawning	.49	.51	.52	.96
6.	Increasing irritability	.49	.56	.60	10.54**
7.	Reports fatigue	.48	.58	.58	8.40*
8.	Reports interrupted sleep	.47	.64	.65	18.43***
9.	Reports awakening earlier than desired	.46	.64	.66	23.74****
10.	Lethargic, falls asleep during activities	.44	.49	.57	15.00***
11.	Restless	.44	.49	.51	3.92
12.	Expressionless face	.42	.47	.51	8.41*
13.	Change in behavior/ performance	.38	.45	.49	9.82**
14.	Disoriented	.38	.41	.41	.80
15.	Hallucinations/delirium/paranoia	.30	.43	.49	23.42****
16.	Thick speech	.29	.34	.41	21.18****
17.	Correct word usage	.26	.31	.35	10.21**
18.	Dark circle under eyes	.25	.38	.46	32.48****
19.	Hand tremor	.25	.29	.31	5.53
20.	Mild, fleeting nystagmus	.21	.29	.30	8.42*
21.	Mispronunciation of words	.21	.28	.32	14.69***
22.	Ptosis of eyelids	.19	.25	.29	12.09**
	Major/Minor Defining Characteristics	0/4	3/6	4/8	

Note. * $p < .05$, ** $p < .01$, *** $p < .001$, **** $p < .0001$

areas (p =.0010 - .0014). Statistical differences were also found in various minor defining characteristics.

Across patient age groups: Table 4 shows the result of analysis. The number of major defining characteristics across groups were similar, but the number of minor defining characteristics across groups differed slightly. DCV scores of the eight defining characteristics differed significantly (P < .05) among the three groups. "Report of severe discomfort/pain" and "facial mask of pain" were major defining characteristics in all three groups. "Rubbing area" was a major defining characteristic only in the elderly group, but the differences in DCV scores among the groups were not significant. Ten minor defining characteristics were common to all three age groups, and most of their DCV scores did not differ statistically. When statistical differences were found in minor defining characteristics, they were usually between the children's group and the elderly group.

Content Validity of Sleep Pattern Disturbance

Across practice areas: As seen in Table 5, the numbers of major and minor defining characteristics varied across practice areas. DCV scores of 16 out of 22 characteristics were significantly different ($P < .05$) among six areas. "Reports not feeling well rested," "frequent interruptions during sleep," "reports difficulty falling asleep," and "sleep pattern reversal," were major defining characteristics in five areas, but not in the maternal-child area. Post-hoc comparisons revealed that the DCV score differences on "reports not feeling well rested" and "frequent interruptions during sleep" were between the maternal-child and the other five areas. Although it was not a major defining characteristic in the maternal-child area, the DCV score of "reports difficulty falling asleep" in all six areas did not differ statistically. In various minor defining characteristics, statistical differences were also found between the critical care area and the maternal-child area.

Across patient age groups: As may seen in Table 6, the numbers of both major and minor defining characteristics varied across three age groups. DCV scores of 18 out of 22 defining characteristics differed significantly ($P <. 05$) among the three groups. While there were four major defining characteristics in the elderly group, none was found in the children's group. "Reports not feeling well rested," "frequent interruptions during sleep" and "reports difficulty falling asleep" were major defining characteristics in both the adult and the elderly groups. The adult and the elderly groups' DCV scores on these three characteristics were significantly higher than the score of children's group ($p = .0001 - .0044$). "Sleep pattern reversal" was also a major defining characteristic in the elderly group, and its DCV score was significantly higher than the other two groups' ($p = .0000 - .0030$). The adult and the elderly groups had five common defining characteristics, and the DCV scores of these characteristics were significantly higher than in the children's group. Differences were also found in several minor defining characteristics. For instance, "lethargic, falls asleep during activities" was a minor defining characteristic only in the elderly group, and its DCV score was significantly higher ($p = .0013 - .0032$) than other group scores.

Discussion

Although the Japanese nurses in this study used nursing diagnosis for only an average of 2.5 years, they were familiar with the three diagnoses which are commonly seen in patients. Therefore, it is unlikely that the nurses' insufficient experience with nursing diagnosis had a major effect on the results.

Content validation studies for nursing diagnoses have been conducted by obtaining a consensus from nurses working with various clinical populations. This consensus from nurses is usually based on a heterogeneous sample of nurses in that they work with patients whose medical status and age differ widely. This study used a large sample of nurses and divided them into groups reflecting patients' different medical status and age-range.

Patients' Medical Status and Major Defining Characteristics

The nurses' practice areas, which reflected patients' medical conditions and levels of acuity, influenced the number and content of major and minor defining characteristics for the three diagnoses. The clear influence of patients' medical status was found in the following two major defining characteristics: "blood pressure changes" and "heart rate changes" in the diagnosis of Pain. These were identified as major defining characteristics only in the critical care area, and statistical differences were also found between the critical care area and the other areas. The nurses in the critical care area take care of patients who are intubated or sedated from anesthesia and who may not be able to verbally communicate pain; therefore, autonomic responses, such as vital sign changes, may become important indicators.

Patients' Age and Major Defining Characteristics

Age of patients also influenced the number and content of major and minor defining characteristics of the diagnoses. The apparent influence of patients' age on major defining characteristics was "insomnia" in Anxiety. Although "insomnia" was identified as a major defining characteristic in both the adult and the elderly groups, it was not in the children's group. In contrast to the adult patients, pediatric patients are unlikely to exhibit "insomnia" as a manifestation of Anxiety. Statistical differences of DCV scores between children and the elderly age groups further support the population-specific nature of this characteristic. Another influence of patients' age on major defining characteristics is "sleep pattern reversal." This characteristic was identified only in the elderly group's Sleep Pattern Disturbance. Statistical differences of DCV scores support the uniqueness of this characteristic to this age group.

Minor Defining Characteristics

In this study, patients' medical status and age influenced minor defining characteristics as well. For instance, "distorted time sense" of Anxiety in the critical care area, and "lethargic, falls asleep during activities" of Sleep Pattern Disturbance in the elderly group were distinctive minor defining characteristics in each patient population. Statistical significance also supported the uniqueness of these minor defining characteristics. Since most of the content validation studies have focused on major defining characteristics to establish diagnostic criteria, minor defining characteristics have been somewhat disregarded. Fehring (1987) suggested discarding the characteristics with DCV scores of .50 or below. Sparks and Lien-Gieschen (1994) proposed raising the minimum score from .50 to .60 to further limit the number of characteristics associated with a diagnosis. However, the result of the present study suggested that discarding characteristics based on a consensus from nurses working with various clinical populations may conceal characteristics unique to a certain patient population.

Diagnoses for Children

Since 64% of the nurses in the children's group practiced in maternal-child areas, findings regarding this practice area and the children's group were similar. Fewer major defining characteristics were identified in the maternal-child practice area and in the children's age group than in other practice areas. This may be attributed to the underdevelopment of the current NANDA diagnoses with the pediatric population. Age group differences were more obvious in Sleep Pattern Disturbance than in other diagnoses. As Wieseke et al. (1994) demonstrated, defining characteristics of Sleep Pattern Disturbance in children are probably different from those in adults. However, this study did not include any age specific characteristics, such as "frequent awakening during night," "reluctance to retire," and "desire to sleep with parents." In future studies, when the diagnosis of Sleep Pattern Disturbance is validated in children, characteristics suggested by Wieseke et al. should be included.

Commonalities of Defining Characteristics
Warren (1991) made the following statement regarding the age factors on defining characteristics of a diagnosis: "There is probably a core of commonalities, but there also may be critical differences depending on age" (p.40). The findings of this study provided evidence of differences in major and minor defining characteristics of diagnoses not only across age groups, but also across patients' medical status. The results of this study can also provides support for Warren's statement.

"Report of severe discomfort/pain" was identified as a major defining characteristic in all practice areas and age groups; therefore, this defining characteristic can be considered as a core of commonalities of a diagnosis of Pain. When determining the commonalities of defining characteristics across patients' population, examination of the DCV score alone may not be sufficient. There were some defining characteristics found as a major characteristic in some, but not in all practice areas or age groups, but their DCV scores did not differ statistically. For example, "reports feeling anxious/apprehensive/tense/scared" in Anxiety was identified as a major defining characteristic in all age groups and in five practice areas except the medical-surgical area. Its DCV scores were not significantly different across practice areas and age groups. This statistical evidence may be also used to determine the commonalities of defin-

ing characteristics across patients' population. When the statistical measurement is used, three additional common defining characteristics across patients" population were found in the diagnosis of Pain: "facial mask of pain," "protecting area," and "rubbing area."

Conclusions
Although not a random sample from which generalization can be drawn, the large number of subjects in this study, their broad geographic representation, and their general familiarity with these three nursing diagnoses suggest the usefulness of the findings. Both the patients' medical status and age influenced the number and content of major and minor defining characteristics of Anxiety, Pain, and Sleep Pattern Disturbance. However, there were also major and minor defining characteristics found across patients' medical status and age. These findings suggest that not only common defining characteristics across patient populations exist, but also population specific defining characteristics exist.

References
Fehring, R. J. (1987). Methods to validate nursing diagnoses. *Heart & Lung, 16*(6), 625-629.

Fehring, R. (1994). The Fehring model. In R. M. Carroll-Johnson & M. Paquette (Eds.), *Classification of nursing diagnoses: Proceedings of the 10th conference.* (pp. 55-62). Philadelphia: J. B. Lippincott Company.

Gordon, M. (1996). Report of an RNF study: Diagnostic criteria for selected rehabilitation nursing diagnoses. *Rehabilitation Nursing Research, 5*(3), 80-91.

Goyette-Vincent, K. (1991). Defining characteristics: General or population specific. In R. M. Carroll-Johnson (Ed.),

Classification of nursing diagnoses: Proceedings of the ninth conference. (pp. 76-78). Philadelphia: J. B. Lippincott.

Munro, B. H., & Page, E. B. (1993). *Statistical methods for health care research.* (2nd ed.). Philadelphia: J. B. Lippincott.

North American Nursing Diagnosis Association (1996). *Nursing diagnoses: Definitions & classification 1997-1998.* Philadelphia: North American Nursing Diagnosis Association.

Sato, S. (1996). *Diagnostic concept development: Content validation of North American Nursing Diagnoses in Japan.* Unpublished doctoral dissertation, Boston College.

Sparks, S. M., & Lien-Gieshen, T. (1994). Modification of the diagnostic content validity. *Nursing Diagnosis, 5*(1), 31-35.

Warren, J. J. (1991). Implications of introducing axes into a classification system. In R. M. Carroll-Johnson (Ed.), *Classification of nursing diagnoses: Proceedings of the ninth conference.* (pp. 38-44). Philadelphia: J. B. Lippincott.

Wieseke, A., Twibell, R., Bennett, S., Marine, M., & Schoger, J. (1994). A content validation study of five nursing diagnoses by critical care nurses. *Heart & Lung, 23*(4), 345-351.

Whitley, G. G. (1994). Expert validation and differentiation of the nursing diagnoses anxiety and fear. *Nursing Diagnosis, 5*(4), 143-150.

Moving Beyond Content Validation of Nursing Diagnoses

Laurence Parker, PhD
Margaret Lunney, PhD, RN, CS

The 25th anniversary of the North American Nursing Diagnosis Association (NANDA) makes it appropriate to consider the work that was already done to develop and refine the NANDA taxonomy and the work that still needs to be done. The NANDA taxonomy was created and refined over the last 25 years through motivation, scholarly efforts, and commitment to name the phenomena of nursing's concern. The NANDA taxonomy is advancing in the direction of other, more sophisticated classifications, such as the International Classification of Diseases (ICD-9), albeit slowly. The purpose of this paper is to briefly review the state of the art of validation research for ongoing development of the NANDA taxonomy, to suggest that we may be "stuck" at the stage of nurse validation surveys, and to prompt nurses to move beyond this stage to other types of validation studies.

Background and Significance

The motivation and commitment to develop the NANDA taxonomy will continue into the 21st century because identification to human responses to health problems and life processes is the basis for nurses' decisions on how to help people. Nurses cannot know what interventions to select or which outcomes to project unless they have accurate representations of what patients are experiencing. Accuracy of interpreting the human responses of patients is facilitated by the naming of responses (Lunney, In press). In a theory of linguistics, Hayakawa and Hayakawa (1990) explained that naming improves thinking which improves actions. Thus the naming of responses to health problems and life processes helps nurses to think more clearly, cooperate more effectively with patients and others, and communicate patient experiences to self and others as the basis for selection of interventions and outcomes.

Development of the NANDA taxonomy through the naming of human responses spearheaded the development of two other important taxonomies, the Nursing Intervention Classification (NIC) (Iowa Intervention Project,

1996) and the Nursing Outcomes Classification (NOC) (Iowa Outcomes Project, 1997). The usefulness of these other two taxonomies in the provision of quality nursing care is dependent, however, on the accuracy of nurses' interpretations of the experiences of patients (Lunney, In press). Nurses interpret the experiences of patients whether or not these interpretations are named as nursing diagnoses. If these interpretations are not accurate, the most effective interventions and outcomes will not be selected. Accuracy of interpretations of human responses is supported by a research-based taxonomy of diagnostic labels with signs and symptoms.

Standardized languages such as NANDA, NIC and NOC are important for the Computer-Based Patient Record (CPR) which was projected to be in place by the year 2000 (American Nurses Association, 1995). Yet nursing care may not be represented in the CPR if the nursing classification systems are not valid and reliable. If nursing wants to be represented in the CPR in the future, studies must be done to establish the construct validity, criterion-related validity, and reliability of standardized nursing languages such as NANDA.

The need for research of NANDA labels and the taxonomy of labels was already explained in Gordon's book (1994), in many papers at previous conferences (e.g., Kerr, 1991; Kerr, 1994; Symposium..., 1994), in papers presented at an invitational conference on research methods (e.g., Alexander, 1989), in manuscripts by members of the Taxonomy Committee (Hoskins et al., 1992; Kerr et al., 1992, 1993), in a review of nursing diagnosis research (Dougherty, Jankins, Lunney, & Whitley, 1993), and in papers by Whitley (1995, 1998). The information from these papers can be used to plan a research program for refinement of spe-

cific diagnoses and the overall taxonomy. This paper is to remind nurses that much of this work still needs to be done and to give examples using the diagnoses of Ineffective Breathing Pattern (IBP), Ineffective Airway Clearance (IAC), and Impaired Gas Exchange (IGE).

State of the Art: Validation Research

The human responses on the NANDA list need to be validated for ongoing knowledge development of these concepts. Some of the concepts have been studied extensively in other fields, e.g., anxiety and fear. Other diagnostic concepts, e.g., IBP, IAC and IGE, were developed for the NANDA taxonomy based on knowledge of physiology. Regardless of the source of concepts, however, incorporation in a nursing taxonomy with signs and symptoms requires validation research.

In the early days of validation research, nurse researchers studied the content validity of diagnoses by doing retrospective chart reviews, i.e., studying which diagnoses were being used in clinical practice and what were the signs and symptoms that promoted use of the diagnoses. Examples of such studies are York (1985) and McDonald (1985). Later studies focused on nurse surveys. With the respiratory diagnoses, the studies of Boisvert (1995), Brukwitzki, Holmgren, and Maibusch (1996), Capuano, Hitchings, and Johnson (1990), Clark (1994), Matsuki and Otani (1995), and Wake, Fehring and Fadden (1991) were nurse validation studies. Some of the findings from these studies were similar and others were inconsistent, indicating a need for empirical data from patients rather than from nurses.

In respect to all diagnoses on the NANDA list, there have been few clinical validation studies as described by Hoskins (1989) and Carlson-

Catalano and Lunney (1995). A study by Carlson-Catalano et al. (1995; In press) was the first reported clinical validation of the three respiratory nursing diagnoses. Studies of the frequencies of diagnoses used in clinical settings (Gordon & Hiltunen, 1995; Hoskins et al., 1986; Lutjens, 1993), however, showed that one or more of these three diagnoses are frequently used by nurses. Many patients in many types of settings (critical care, acute medical and surgical care, long term care, home care) are at risk of these diagnoses; yet the research bases to guide use of these diagnoses is insufficient.

There have been few construct validation studies and criterion-related studies of any diagnoses and none are available for knowledge development of IBP, IAC, and IGE. Examples of construct validity are studies by Change (1989) and Whitley (Whitley & Tousman, 1996). The case control method used by Wooldridge et al. (1998) to distinguish the characteristics of Risk for Aspiration is an example of criterion-related validation.

Knowledge Development
Steps in the Process of Knowledge Development

Knowledge development of diagnoses in the NANDA taxonomy means that a series of studies need to be done for each individual diagnosis as well as groups of diagnoses. The steps in the process are: conduct concept analysis, develop hypotheses, obtain empirical data, use varied settings, examine reliability, incidence and outcome, aggregate and compare findings, reformulate hypotheses for further testing, and reformulate diagnostic categories.

In 1995, Whitley explained the importance of starting with concept analysis. Concept analysis explicates the conceptual base of a diag-

nosis to understand its meaning and helps to identify the defining characteristics (DCs). Concept analysis leads to the next step, that of developing operational definitions for each of the DCs. In preparation for the clinical study of the three respiratory diagnoses, paradiso (1992) did a concept analysis of IBP, IAC, and IGE which was reported at the 10th conference. This analysis provided the basis for conceptual and operational definitions of each of the 37 defining characteristics identified for the study. The definitions were used for the training of raters and the study protocols.

Three exploratory research questions/hypotheses were developed for testing (see Abstract, Appendix A). Both subjective and objective data were collected by expert raters from 76 patients on medical and surgical units in two hospitals who were identified as having one or more of the three diagnoses. In testing these hypotheses, it was determined that the 37 possible DCs identified from the literature were present in many patients with the diagnoses, but the large majority of possible DCs were not considered by the raters as important for making the diagnoses. Much fewer DCs met the criteria as important for making the diagnoses than studies using the nurse validation method. The subjective cues of "expresses fatigue" and "expresses anxiety" were considered important for making these diagnoses. These cues had not been identified in nurse validation studies but the concept analysis had indicated that they may be important. The study needs to be replicated in other settings to determine whether the findings are generalizable. Based on these data, more sophisticated hypothesis-testing studies can be conducted.

In order to achieve reliability, Carlson-Catalano et al. (1995, In press) did extensive training of eight clinical experts for achievement

Appendix A

Abstract

Purpose:
The three nursing diagnoses ineffective breathing pattern (IBP), ineffective airway clearance (IAC), and impaired gas exchange (IGE) are among the most frequently used, yet there has been no clinical research to validate the defining characteristics of these diagnoses. The purpose of this clinical study was to answer the research questions: (1) what are the defining characteristics of IBP, IAC and IGE?, (2) what are the etiologies of IBP, IAC, and IGE?, and (3) what are the most important interventions for IBP, IAC, and IGE?

Design:
The clinical validation method (Fehring, 1987) and standardized methods for quantitative studies (Carlson-Catalano & Lunney, 1995) were used. The population was 76 persons from two hospitals in two cities with medical and surgical diagnoses who were identified as having one or more of the diagnoses. Data were collected by eight master's-prepared nurses who were trained for accurate diagnosis of the responses and reliable completion of the study tool.
Methods: A literature-based concept analysis generated 37 possible defining characteristics (DCs) for the three diagnoses which were included in the instrument. Content validity ratings, using the method of item-objective congruence, by four nationally known experts, yielded as estimate of .92. For each patient, the clinical judgment of nurse experts was used to decide the presence or absence of the 37 possible DCs and the degree of importance of each for making each diagnosis. Clinical judgments of etiologies were described and 30 nursing interventions were judged for importance to each diagnosis and each patient.

Findings:
The findings were that the three diagnoses occurred in subjects with a variety of medical and surgical problems. A majority of the patients (55.2%) were experiencing either ineffective breathing pattern or ineffective airway clearance, while the remainder were experiencing two or more of the three responses. No patients were experiencing impaired gas exchange without IBP or IAC. Inter-rater reliability was estimated as .63, using Cohen's Kappa, for IBP and IAC with 11 randomly selected patients. Test-Retest reliability was estimated as 1.0 with a second assessment done within three hours. Of the 37 possible DCs identified through concept analysis, few met the criterion of a weighted mean of .50 or above when compared with nurse validation studies. In contrast to the defining characteristics approved by NANDA, the subjective cue of "expressive fatigue" was considered as important for making the three diagnoses; "expresses anxiety" was important for making the diagnosis of IAC.

Conclusions and Implications:
It was concluded that clinical validation methods are more discriminating than nurse validation methods. Implications are: (1) data that are present are not necessarily characteristic of diagnoses, and (2) subjective cues may be important for making these diagnoses.

of accuracy of the diagnoses. Six case studies were developed and validated; three were used in training procedures and three were used for evaluation of training. The study began when raters achieved at least 90% agreement with expert opinions related to the diagnoses and DCs represented in the case studies. In the study, both test-retest and inter-rater reliability were measured in two random samples of 10% of the total cases.

The occurrence and co-occurrence of the diagnoses were determined but outcomes were not measured (see Abstract, Appendix A). To this point, the data cannot be aggregated with data from other studies since no similar studies were reported. In respect to the last step of the process, reformulation of the diagnoses, small group work was conducted at the eleventh NANDA conference to incorporate the findings of previous validation studies with IBP, IAC, and IGE (Johnson et al., 1995).

Types of Validity Studies

Methodology texts distinguish between three types of validation studies — content, criterion-related, and construct validity. Content validity is the agreement of a construct or measuring instrument with expert judgment, or with common sense, so-called face validity. Most academic or personnel tests are constructed in this way. Criterion related validity lies in demonstrating that there is a predictive relationship with another variable. The relationship between the Scholastic Aptitude Test (SAT) and college Grade Point Average (GPA) is often cited as an example. Construct validity lies in developing a body of scientific theory related to the construct, and demonstrating that the theoretical relations hold. As with any scientific argument, it relies on the weight of empirical evidence. The

Authoritarian Personality (Adorno, 1950), one of the first great studies of modern social psychology, is a set of numerous types of empirical studies about this construct derived from psychoanalytic theory.

Since content validity requires only expert judgment, it is less elaborate and expensive to establish than criterion-related or construct validity, which require the study of an appropriate group of subjects and the measurement of other criteria or constructs. For a personnel test, appropriate use of expert opinion produces a content valid test. In contrast, establishing criterion-related validity involves developing an appropriate measure of job performance and following a group of tested subjects over time. Criterion-related and construct validity are more convincing than content validity, which is, after all, just a systematic process of exploring the assumptions that experts have. This is codified in federal regulations about personnel testing, which require criterion-related or construct validity studies if a personnel test differentially selects protected minorities.

An example from Foucalt (1970) illustrates why it is necessary to go beyond content validity in nursing diagnoses. He quoted a medieval taxonomy in which animals are divided into: (a) belonging to the Emperor, (b) embalmed, (c) tame, (d) sucking pigs, (e) sirens, (f) fabulous, (g) stray dogs, (h) included in the present classification, (i) frenzied, (j) innumerable, (k) drawn with a very fine camel hair brush, (l) et cetera, (m) having just broken the water pitcher, (n) that from a long way off look like flies. It may seem impossible that such a classification would be developed but this classification illustrates what can happen when classification depends only on content validity. Content validation only establishes that a group of experts think a certain way;

there is no assurance that their judgments match real world phenomena.

Construct validity, on the other hand, moves beyond assumptions. Cronbach (1990) stresses the similarity between construct validation and traditional scientific research. It involves developing plausible, rival hypotheses and testing them in empirical studies. Validation lies in the weight of evidence developed for a particular construct. A criterion-related validity study may be a piece of evidence in a construct validation argument, but generally criterion-related studies are concerned only with demonstrating predictive relationships and not with developing a body of scientific theory about the construct. From the perspective of criterion-related validity, it is sufficient to demonstrate the relationship of the SAT with college GPA; from the perspective on construct validity, a deeper understanding of the casual processes involved in this relationship is demonstrated. Construct validity studies explain that the SAT measures cognitive aptitude, as its developers have argued, or it measures the educational experiences or cultural backgrounds appropriate to college success.

Future Studies

Cronbach (1990) noted that construct validation is a fluid, creative process which cannot be reduced to rules. Construct validation develops in relation to specific problems. For nursing diagnoses, there are a variety of areas which should be explored. These areas include: reliability studies of the stability and coherence of the constructs; epidemiological studies of the occurrence and co-occurrence of diagnostic categories; outcome studies of the diagnostic categories and differential interventions; causal analysis in relation to other bodies of theory; and

generalizability studies over a variety of subjects and settings. Some of the directions that the fluid process of construct validation may take are described below.

Reliability Studies

In methodology texts, reliability is usually treated separately from validity, and the establishment of reliability is logically considered prior to validity studies. If a construct or measure is not repeatable or stable (test-retest reliability), or is not coherent (split-half reliability), than its validity or meaning is not worth exploring. However, reliability can also be considered a component of construct validation. While it may be desirable, in general, to have repeatable, internally consistent measures, the nature of the construct often influences which type of reliability is more important. Measurement of certain types of reliability may be important to demonstrate the correctness of a body of theory surrounding the construct. A scale which measures mood will not demonstrate test-retest reliability as will a scale which measures enduring characteristics of the person. A construct like authoritarianism, which involves many different types of behavior and underlying processes will not exhibit the same internal consistency as a factor analytic scale of introversion-extroversion. Finding the types of reliability one should find, and not finding the types one shouldn't find, is evidence for the correctness of the body of theory which defines the construct.

In respect to the respiratory diagnoses, internal consistency studies and long-term test retest studies were not conducted and they may have considerable theoretical importance. The former requires more subjects to permit factor analyses and the latter a design which allows following patients over long periods of time. Conducting these types of studies would address such theocratically important questions as whether these three diagnoses overlap, and whether one or more of the diagnoses are states or traits.

Epidemiological Studies

It is important to explore the empirical occurrence of the diagnostic categories in the fashion of traditional epidemiological research (Alesancer, 1989). These types of studies identify whether diagnostic categories are common or rare. They answer questions such as: What is the occurrence in different patients of different ages, sex and race? What is the occurrence in relation to other relevant demographics, such as educational level or SES? What are the interrelations of the NANDA categories? The respiratory studies that are cited found that IBP and IAC are common and that the three diagnoses co-occur. Much broader studies are required, however, to answer questions such as is IGE so rare that it is not very useful, or it is so intertwined with the other two categories that the three diagnoses should be redefined?

Outcome Studies

The value of a diagnostic system lies in its ability to organize a set of understandings about the phenomena it treats, to make differential predictions about the categories, and to choose appropriate interventions for them. The studies of respiratory diagnoses cited earlier have only touched on these issues by looking at expert opinion about interventions. Studies of prognosis and outcomes require longer time frames and a variety of data sources. Such studies might lead to descriptions of better nursing practices or might take the form of full clinical trails of differential interventions.

Causal Analyses

Ultimately, construct validation involves establishing the meaning of constructs. There are large bodies of theory about patient behaviors, such as self-care and locus of control; patient states, such as anxiety and fatigue, and underlying patient physiological states. The process of construct validation involves defining the relation of new categories to well-established categories. No such studies were done of IBP, IAC, and IGE. As research mounts, it becomes possible to move away from expert judgment of the categories to the development of diagnostic checklists and scales. The convergent-discriminant validity paradigm of Campbell and Fiske (1959) is a well known model for assessing convergences and divergences in constructs across measurement domains.

Generalizability

The ability to extend knowledge to other populations, generalizability, was termed external validity by Cook and Campbell (1979). In the past, respiratory diagnostic studies used convenience samples of patients, rather than sampling from the wide variety of patient domains, and, where they have been multi-institutional, sample size has not permitted comparison of institutions. The diagnostic categories need to be examined across institutions, for different ICD-9 categories, and for different clinical situations such as changes in body position (Robichaud, 1990). The question here is not just occurrence in different groups, but whether the same underlying causal and predictive relationship hold in different settings.

Controversies

One controversy to consider is the best type of research design, e.g., experimental/clinical trials, field studies, quasi-experiments. Cook and Campbell (1979) emphasized causal analysis and leaned toward the experimental model; Cronbach (1982) emphasized generalizability. There is always a tradeoff between precise causal analysis and the use of generalizable natural settings. To study a number of issues outlines above, more complex and larger designs are necessary. However, construct validation can be conducted by aggregation of a large number of small incremental studies using similar designs as described by Carlson-Catalano and Lunney (1995).

Another controversy is: should constructs be homogeneous or heterogenous? The opposing traditions in construct development are factor analysis, which emphasizes coherence of constructs, and the theory-based or rational approach, which emphasizes the scope of underlying theory. The variety of studies that are necessary for ongoing development of a classification system probably involves both sides of each of these controversies.

Implications

Nurses who are testing the validity of diagnostic concepts for the NANDA taxonomy need to move beyond content validation studies so the signs and symptoms of nursing diagnoses approved by NANDA are supported by a series of studies. Moving beyond nurse validation surveys to construct and criterion-related studies will increase the possibility, but does not guarantee, that nurses who use these concepts will make useful diagnoses as the basis for interventions and outcomes.

A systematic call for nursing diagnosis research by other organizations besides NANDA will help to advance this agenda. Nurses need to influence the reviewers of the National Institute of Nursing Research (NINR), National Institutes of Health, and private foundations who support nursing research to set nursing diagnosis research as a high priority for the next 25 years. The construct and criterion-related validity of diagnoses on the NANDA list, and other diagnoses not yet on the list, need to be studied to improve the overall validity of the taxonomy.

In order to accomplish these goals, research funds are needed. It is important that the importance of these issues are addressed in many forums so that funding sources will value the development of a valid and reliable taxonomy of human responses. Larger studies, involving more nurses, more patients, more settings, and more modalities of data collection need to be designed if a full program of construct validation is to be achieved.

One way that this can be done is to attend to the accuracy of nurses' diagnoses (Lunney, in press; Lunney, Karlik, Kill, & Murphy, 1997; Lunney & Paradios, 1995). Taking credit for high levels of accuracy that are occurring and taking responsibility for lower levels of accuracy may prompt funding agencies and agency administrators to focus on the NANDA taxonomy as a tool to facilitate continuous quality improvement. Even more important, perhaps, is a focus on outcomes. If nurses can demonstrate that the classification system leads to interventions which improve therapeutic outcomes, arguments for funding will be compelling.

References

Adorno, T.W. et al (1950). *The authoritarian personality*. New York: Harper.

Alexander, C. (1989). Epidemiological approaches to validation of nursing diagnoses. In *Monograph of the invitational* conference on research methods for validation nursing diagnoses* (pp. 121-136). Philadelphia: NANDA

American Nurses Association (1995). *Nursing data systems: The emerging framework.* Washington, DC: American Nurses Publishing.

Boisvert, C. (1995). Validation of four nursing diagnoses in France: A preliminaryreport. In M.J. Rantz & P. LeMone (Eds.), *Classification of nursing diagnoses: Proceedings of the eleventh conference* (pp. 182-188). Glendale, CA: CINAHL Information Systems.

Brukwitzki, G., Holmgren, C., & Maibusch, R. (1996). Validation of defining characteristics of the nursing diagnosis ineffective airway clearance. *Nursing Diagnosis, 7,* 63-69.

Campbell, D.T. & Fiske, D.W. (1959). Convergent and discriminant validation by the multitrait-multimethod matrix. *Psychological Bulletin, 56,* 81-105.

Capuano, T.A., Hitchings, K.S., & Johnson, S. (1990). Respiratory nursing diagnoses: Practicing nurses' selection of defining characteristics. *Nursing Diagnosis,1,* 169-174.

Carlson-Catalano, J., & Lunney, M. (1995). Quantitative methods for clinical validation of nursing diagnoses. Clinical Nurse Specialist: *Journal for Advanced Nursing Practice, 9,* 306-311.

Carlson-Catalano, J., Lunney, M., Paradiso, C., Bruno, J., Luise, B.K., Martin, T., Massoni, M., & Pachter, S. (1996). Abstract: Clinical validation of three respiratory nursing diagnoses. In M.J. Rantz & P. LeMone (Eds.), *Classification of nursing diagnoses: Proceedings of the eleventh conference,* North American Nursing Diagnoses

Association. Glendale, CA: CINAHL.

Carlson-Catalano, J., Lunney, M., Paradiso, C., Bruno, J., Luise, B.K., Martin, T., Massoni, M., & Pachter, S. (In press). Clinical validation of ineffective breathing pattern, ineffective airway clearance and impaired gas exchange. *IMAGE: Journal of Nursing Scholarship.*

Chang, B.L. (1989). Reliability and construct validity. In *Monograph of the invitational conference on research methods for validating nursing diagnoses* (pp. 217-234). Philadelphia: NANDA.

Clark, C.M. (1994). Validation of the defining characteristics of ineffective airway clearance. In R.M. Carroll-Johnson & M. Paquette (Eds.), *Classification of nursing diagnoses: Proceeding of the tenth conference* (p. 34). Philadelphia: J.B. Lippincott.

Cook, T.D. & Campbell, D.T. (1979). *Quasi-experimentation: Design and analysis issues for field settings.* Boston: Houghton Mifflin.

Cronbach, L.J. (1982). *Designing evaluations of educational and social programs.* New York: Jossey-Bass.

Cronback. L.J. (1990). *Essentials of psychological testing* (5th ed.). New York: Harper Collins.

Dougherty, C.M., Jankins, J.K., Lunney, M., & Whitley, G. (1991). Conceptual and research-based validation of nursing diagnoses: 1950-1993. *Nursing Diagnosis, 4,* 156-165.

Foucault, M. (1970). *The order of things.* London: Tavistock.

Gordon, M. (1970). *Nursing diagnosis: Process and application* (3rd ed.). St. Louis: Mosby-Year Book.

Gordon, M., & Hiltunen, E. (1995). High

frequency treatment priority nursing diagnoses in critical care. *Nursing Diagnoses, 6,* 143-154.

Hayakawa, S.I. & Hayakawa, A.R. (1990). *Language in thought and action* (5th ed.). San Diego: Harcourt Brace Company.

Hoskins, L.M. (1989). Clinical validation methodologies for nursing diagnosis research. In R.M. Carroll-Johnson (Ed.), *Classification of nursing diagnosis: Proceedings of the eighth conference* (pp. 126-131). Philadelphia: Lippincott.

Hoskins, L.M., McFarlane, E.A., Rubenfeld, M.G., Schreier, A.M., & Walsh, M.B. (1986). Nursing diagnosis in the chronically ill. In M.E. Hurley (Ed.), *Classification of nursing diagnoses: Proceedings of the sixth conference.* (Pp. 319-329). St. Louis: C.V. Mosby.

Iowa Intervention Project, J.C. McCloskey & G.M. Bulechek (Eds.) (1996).: *Nursing intervention classification (NIC)* (2nd ed). St. Louis: Mosby-Year Book.

Iowa Outcomes Project, M. Johnson & M. Maas (Eds.) (1997). *Nursing Outcomes Classification (NOC).* St. Louis: Mosby.

Johnson, S., Harkreader, H., Carlson-Catalano, J., Paradiso, C., Maibusch, R.M., Tyler, M.L., & Clark, C.M. (1995). Workgroup reports: Respiratory diagnosis. In M.J. Rantz & P. LeMone (Eds.), *Classification of nursing diagnoses. Proceedings of the eleventh conference, North American Nursing Diagnosis Association* (pp. 405-407. Glendale, CA: CINAHL.

Kerr, M. (1991). Validation of taxonomy. In R.M. Carroll-Johnson (Ed.), *Classification of nursing diagnoses: Proceedings of the ninth conference* (pp. 37-63. St. Louis: C.V. Mosby.

Kerr, M. (1994). How reliable are your reliability measures? In R.M. Carroll-Johnson & M. Paquette (Eds.), *Classification of nursing diagnosis: Proceedings of the tenth conference* (pp. 291-293). Philadelphia: Lippincott.

Kerr, M.E., Hoskins, L.M., Fitzpatrick, J.J., Warren, J.J., Avant, K.C., Hurley, M.E., Lunney, M., Mills, W.C., & Rottkamp, B.C. (1993). Taxonomic validation: An overview. *Nursing Diagnosis, 4,* 6-14.

Kerr, M.E., Hoskins, L.M., Fitzpatrick, J.J., Warren, J.J., Avant, K.C., Carpenito, L.J., Hurley, M.E., Jakob, D.F., Lunney, M., Mills, W., Rottcamp, B.C. (1992). Development of definitions for Taxonomy II. *Nursing Diagnosis, 3,* 65-71.

Lunney, M. (In press). Commentary: Accuracy of nurses' diagnoses: Foundation of NANDA, NIC, and NOC. Nursing Diagnosis: *The Journal of Nursing Language and Classification, 9(3).*

Lunney, M., & Paradiso, C. (1995). Accuracy of interpreting human responses. *Nursing Management, 6(1).* 48H-48K.

Lunney, M., Karlik, B., Kiss, M., and Murphy, P. (1997). Accuracy of nurses' diagnoses of psychosocial responses. *Nursing Diagnosis: The Journal of Nursing Language and Classification, 8(4),* 157-166.

Lutjens, L. (1993). The nature and use of nursing diagnosis in hospitals. *Nursing Diagnosis, 4,* 107-113.

Matsuki, M., & Otani, E. (1995). Diagnostic content validation for anxiety, hopelessness, and ineffective airway clearance. In M.J. Rantz & P. LeMone (Eds), *Classification of nursing diagnoses: Proceedings of the eleventh conference* (pp. 275-276). Glendale, CA: CINAHL.

McDonald, B.R. (1985). Validation of three

respiratory nursing diagnoses. *Nursing Clinics of North America, 20,* 697-710.

Paradiso, C. (1992, April). *Conceptual descriptions of respiratory diagnoses*. Paper presented at the tenth NANDA conference. Nashville, TN.

Robichaud, A.M. (1990). Alteration in gas exchange related to body position. *Critical Care Nursing, 10*(1), 56-59.

Schroeder, M.A. (1989). Tool development: Validity related to nursing diagnosis. In *Monograph of the invitational conference on research methods for validating Nursing diagnoses*. Philadelphia: NANDA.

Symposium on validation models (1994). In R.M. Carroll-Johnson & M. Paquette (Eds.), *Classification of nursing diangoses: Proceedings of the tenth conference*. (pp. 42-62). Philadelphia: Lippincott.

Wake, M.M., Fehring, F.J. & Fadden, T. (1991). Multinational validation of anxiety, hopelessness and ineffective airway clearance. *Nursing Diagnosis, 2,* 57-66.

York, K. (1985). Clinical validation of two respiratory nursing diagnoses and their defining characteristics. *Nursing Clinics of North America, 20,* 657-667.

Whitley, G.G. (1995). Concept analysis as foundation to nursing diagnosis. *Nursing Diagnosis, 6,* 91-92.

Whitley, G.G., & Tousman, S.A. (1996). A multivariate approach for the validation of anxiety and fear. *Nursing Diagnosis, 7,* 116-127.

Whitley, G.G. (1998, St. Louis). *Processes and methodologies for research validation of nursing diagnoses*. Paper presented at the thirteenth conference, North American Nursing Diagnosis Association.

Processes and Methodologies for Research Validation of Nursing Diagnoses

Georgia Griffith Whitley, EdD, RN

In her landmark texts on nursing diagnosis, Gordon (1982, 1987) spoke to issues of research. Initially, in her first edition, she addressed the need for reliability studies to produce clusters of highly reliable cues for accurate diagnoses. She went on to say that without these cues, diagnostic errors occur and lead to inadequate interventions. In this earlier edition, she cited four studies which address this issue (Burgess, 1974; Guzetta & Forsyth, 1979; Martin, 1979; Nicoletti, Reiz, & Gordon, 1981).

In the second edition, Gordon again addressed the need for research on the proposed diagnoses and provided an overview of the types of studies needed to develop an empirical base for diagnoses. The first type of research discussed was identification studies in which the clinician repeatedly observes a condition not labeled by an existing diagnosis. This identified pattern should then be studied through concept analysis. Gordon discussed the phenomena of clustering of diagnoses in patterns and the need to investigate these patterns and clusters. A sec-

ond type of research discussed was refinement studies, beginning with concept analyses of the diagnoses. In addressing issues of reliability, she emphasized the need for intra- and inter-rater reliability studies. She identified internal, external, and construct validity of defining characteristics as essential areas of research on nursing diagnoses. Fehring's models for content validity research were reviewed in her later edition, including nurse expert validation, clinical validation, and patient validation models. In addition, Gordon suggested epidemiological studies designed to document the base-rate occurrence of diagnoses in the population, diagnostic process studies designed to investigate how nurses collect, interpret, cluster, and name their diagnostic judgments, and diagnosis-based process and outcome studies. These suggestions regarding the diagnosis-based process and outcome studies can now be actualized in the study of NANDA, NIC, and NOC as we now know them. Lastly, she proposed the study of the ethics of diagnosis and treatment, specifically the ethical dimensions of practice in which nurses do not have time for assessment beyond that required for their collaborative role.

Historical Perspectives
Research Conference

An invitational conference on research methodologies for validating nursing diagnoses was held 1989 with two purposes: (a) to analyze existing research methodologies for the development and validation of nursing diagnosis, and (b) to generate new research methodologies for the development and validation of nursing diagnosis (Chang, Kim, Jones, & McFarlane, 1989). The categories of the methods presented included qualitative, quantitative, and integrated approaches. Presenters included researchers currently involved in nursing diagnosis research as well as researchers with expertise in an area of research methodology but no previous involvement in nursing diagnosis research. A great deal of enthusiasm was generated at this meeting and participants requested to have another conference to address other nursing diagnosis research issues.

The Journal

The birth of the NANDA journal, *Nursing Diagnosis*, in 1990 provided a vehicle for the publication of nursing diagnosis research, as well as for articles giving direction for the conduct of this research. In a survey of the literature, Dougherty, Jankin, Lunney, and Whitley (1993) identified 242 articles dealing with conceptual and research-based validation of nursing diagnoses. These articles consisted of 103 studies of existing diagnoses, 108 studies of potential diagnoses, and 31 studies of a general investigative nature on the overall topic of nursing diagnoses (Whitley, 1996). Since this survey of the literature, many more articles on diagnoses and investigational strategies have appeared in the NANDA journal and proceedings books alone.

In reviewing the *Nursing Diagnosis* since 1990, 15 articles are identified that specifically address issues of research methodologies and processes. In the first issue of the journal, Maas, Hardy, and Craft (1990) presented methodologic considerations in nursing diagnosis research and call for consistency among research questions, setting and sample, data collection methods, and data analysis and interpretation. In the second issue of the journal, another article on research methods appeared, this one on the use of magnitude estimation scaling (MES) to examine the validity of nursing diagnoses (Grant, Kinney, & Guzetta, 1990). A second article in this issue (Avant, 1990) explored the art and science of nursing diagnosis development and addresses concept formation and formalization, validation, refinement, and modification of diagnoses, and linking of related diagnoses through concurrent study of related diagnoses.

Chang and Hersch (1994) wrote about the development of a research tool for studies on nursing diagnosis by the Computer-Aided Research in Nursing (Carin) project. Patient information, nursing diagnoses, and a statistical interface are linked in a computer program for multiple types of analysis. This system offers the potential of providing large data sets for the study of nursing diagnoses. In the same issue of the journal, Sparks and Lien-Gieschen (1994) proposed modifications of the Fehring diagnostic content validity model for nursing diagnosis research. These modifications were to make the model more stringent in eliminating lower rated defining characteristics, thus producing a more concise and descriptive set of characteristics for a diagnosis. In 1996, Whitley also addressed the issue of reduction of the defining characteristics of two diagnoses into sets of smaller, more manageable and more meaningful variables for clinical use and further investigation. This was done with the use of a multivariate approach, specifically principal components analysis (PCA).

Four journal articles specifically addressed the theoretical/conceptual bases of diagnoses. Gordon (1990) stated that diagnostic categories are derived from concepts and represent theoretical formulations or models for giving meaning to observations, thus conceptual work is needed to develop diagnostic concepts and restructure diagnostic categories. In that same issue, Lunney (1990) approached the concept of accuracy of nursing diagnoses through concept development and emphasized the concept of accuracy of nursing diagnoses as a first step of nursing diagnosis theory development. Avant (1991) proposed three pathways to diagnostic concept development with principles and methods for each path. She stated that no concept or diagnosis should be submitted to NANDA until it has adequate concept validity. Whitley (1995) focused on the importance of concept analysis as a foundation for validation research on a specific diagnosis particularly as it can be used in identifying defining characteristics and developing their operational definitions. The critical need for operational definitions of defining characteristics was articulated by Grant and Kinney (1991) who stated that operational definitions provide the bridge between incidental observation and scientific validation of nursing diagnoses.

Another article in the journal with relevance for the research and development processes is one by the taxonomy committee (Hoskins et al., 1992). Axes to be considered for addition to the taxonomy describe the human condition and include unit of analysis (individual, family or community), age group (growth

and development), and wellness and illness (two axes). Acuity and chronicity were also discussed as axes. The question of whether to implement axes in the taxonomy has now progressed to the proposal and decision-making stage.

The Conference Proceedings

The NANDA Conference Proceedings provide an historical record of the progression of research on nursing diagnoses. Hundreds of papers on specific diagnoses are memorialized in the Proceedings. In addition, there are several papers contained in these Proceedings dealing with nursing diagnosis research processes and methodologies.

An early research project was completed between the First and Second National Conferences on Nursing Diagnoses, when the Clearinghouse in St. Louis coordinated a study aimed at receiving feedback from practicing nurses regarding the labels in common use for identifying nurse-treated problems and the signs and symptoms associated with these labels (Gebbie, 1976). Data were collected in 28 agencies from a wide geographic area on 588 patients. There were 2,338 diagnoses made with an average of 3.97 diagnoses per patient. Eighty-one percent of the diagnoses were directly related to the diagnoses identified at the First National Conference.

In the proceeding of the third and fourth NANDA conferences, Kim (1982) discussed the needs for research on the diagnostic process itself, and for research on the diagnostic nomenclature. She presented two methodological approaches to examine the cognitive processes in the identification of a nursing diagnosis, information processing and the mathematical approach to concept identification. She discussed the inductive and deductive approaches in relation to identifying, validating, and establishing the reliability of nursing diagnoses. Kim presented the models proposed by Gordon and Sweeny (1979) were presented, the retrospective identification model, the clinical model, and the nurse validation model. Also in the proceedings of the third and fourth conferences is a paper by Castles (1982) which discussed the need to establish inter-rater reliability in nursing diagnosis research.

The proceedings of the fifth conference contain some novel and helpful materials in the area of research on nursing diagnoses. A section is included on issues, research suggestions, and references for 44 "approved" diagnoses and 19 diagnoses to be developed (Kim, McFarland, & McLane, 1984). Following this section is one by McLane and Fehring (1984) on the state of the art of nursing diagnoses. They conclude that the paucity of nursing diagnosis research, especially diagnostic validation studies and inquiries into the diagnostic process, is a cause for great concern. It was also at the fifth conference that the use of the Delphi method appeared when Shoemaker (1984) presented her important work on the essential features of a nursing diagnosis. She sought group consensus through a series of mailed questionnaires to a panel of experts. Repeated questionnaires provided feedback from previous rounds regarding positions taken by respondents and reasons for these positions, and further opportunities to change their positions as more thought was given to the questions.

Clinton (1986) articulated nursing diagnosis research methodologies at the sixth conference to deal with issues of practical feasibility, reliability, including internal consistency, inter-rater reliability, and intra-rater reliability, validity, including construct validity testing, external criterion validity, and discriminate validity. In the arena of validity, she addressed the issues of stratifying variables (axes), a current issue in the development of the taxonomy, and identified stratifying variables that are germane to discriminate validity testing (developmental stages, gender, setting, social class, and ethnicity).

Also at the sixth conference, Fehring (1986) presented his paper on standardized methodology to validate diagnostic labels. This methodology basically further delineated and quantified the research methodology work of Gordon and Sweeney (1979) and provided a practical and useful set of models which spawned dozens of studies using two of the approaches. The approaches were diagnostic content validity (DCV) and clinical diagnostic validity (CDV). The DCV is retrospective evidence from experts on the characteristics of a given label; the CDV is prospective evidence on the characteristics from a clinical perspective.

Lackey (1986) discussed Q-sort methodology and its usefulness in validating defining characteristics of specific diagnoses. She gave an historical overview of the method, applied it to nursing diagnoses, and discussed various statistical analyses which may be applicable with Q-sort methodology, as well as advantages and disadvantages of the methodology.

Lo and Kim (1986), at the sixth conference, offered a study of sleep pattern disturbance as an example of a methodological approach using three phases, a comprehensive literature review, an expert validation phase, and a clinical validation phase. Data generated from all three phases were subjected to three analyses, Cronbach's alpha, inter-item correlations, and item-total correlations to test the homogeneity of the defining characteristics and their quality.

At the eighth conference, Kinney and Guzetta (1989) addressed the use of magnitude estimation scaling (MES) as a technique for estimating validity and reliability of defining characteristics and their operational definitions. Using MES, subjects numerically estimated the magnitude of defining characteristics on various dimensions (importance in identifying the diagnosis, frequency of occurrence when the diagnosis is present, and competency of the nurse in identifying each defining characteristic). The authors concluded that MIES is a useful technique for estimating validity and reliability of defining characteristics and their operational definitions and identified advantages of this technique over Likert-type scales.

Hoskins (1989) presented an invited paper on clinical validation methodologies at the eighth conference. In this paper she outlined the phases of concept analysis, expert validation, and clinical validation. She stated that design within the three phases can vary and emphasized the need for funding of nursing diagnosis research.

At the ninth conference, McFarlane (1991) delivered a synthesis of the three papers on the use of qualitative research methods in nursing diagnosis research presented at the invitational conference on methods for validating nursing diagnoses research (Dreher, 1990; Knafl, 1990; Strauss & Corbin, 1990). These qualitative methodologies included ethnographic methods, concept development, and grounded theory. In a review of the three papers, Kerr and Fitzpatrick (1990) identified four domains in which qualitative methods can be used to enhance the development of nursing knowledge. These were clinical judgment, contextual issues, clinical application, and philosophic inquiry. Factors influencing nurses' abilities to make diagnoses can be identified, thus identifying process and content of clinical judgments. The influence of context on nursing diagnoses can be thoroughly examined qualitatively, as can new and existing diagnoses. The level of abstraction of diagnoses, a still unanswered question, can be addressed qualitatively, and philosophic critiques of nursing knowledge can assist in examining the assumptions, methods, and contextual issues.

Also at the ninth conference, Schroeder (1991) recounted the papers on quantitative methods for nursing diagnosis research presented at the invitational conference. These papers addressed reliability and validity issues related to nursing diagnoses, the potential for using epidemiological research designs to validate nursing diagnoses, and the need for more sophisticated statistics for validation research. Schroeder created a trajectory of quantitative methods for clinical validation of nursing diagnoses with three stages of developmental research.

Stage I uses descriptive statistics and correlation coefficients associated with content validity and inter-rater reliability. Stage II uses multivariate quantitative statistical methods that further establish the predictive criterion and construct validity of actual nursing diagnoses. Stage III has added quantitative methods using prevalence rates to predict potential nursing diagnoses and Bayesian statistics to provide data for decision making for issues such as interventions. There is a developmental progression within the stages with inter-rater reliability and content validity preceding predictive and construct validity.

Kim (1991), in summarizing the presentations on qualitative and quantitative methods and their uses in nursing diagnosis research, states that an integrated approach using both qualitative and quantitative methods for validation of nursing diagnoses allows study of the holistic essence/nature of nursing. She recommends the use of a hybrid model consisting of a theoretical phase, a fieldwork phase, and an analytical phase, and also the use of methodologic triangulation. A symposium of three invited papers was presented at the tenth conference. The first of these papers, by Guzzetta, Kinney, and Grant (1994), addressed the use of magnitude estimation in nursing diagnosis research. The second paper, by Creason (1994), addressed the necessity for operational and conceptual definitions of nursing diagnoses and their defining characteristics, and presented an exemplar tool for use in the definition of nursing diagnosis terminology. The third paper was by Fehring (1994). He reviewed the models that he had presented at the sixth conference in 1984 and discussed some of the studies subsequently conducted using his models. He pointed out the strength of being able to compare several studies using the same model to study the same diagnosis. He also discussed problems and proposed refinements for the models. He emphasized the need to use true experts for the DCV method. This means at least a master's degree in nursing and expertise in the diagnosis as demonstrated by clinical experience, research, research presentations, publications, or education on the particular diagnosis. The strength of this model rests on the raters. In the CDV model, diagnostic accuracy and timeliness must be addressed. If the diagnosis is not accurate or is no longer present, the research is not valid. Both the DCV and CDV models require operational definitions in order for the expert raters or observers responses to be valid. Another issue for many diagnoses is redundancy of defining characteristics. By using both models and adhering to rigorous standards, redundancy of characteristics will be eliminated and critical characteristics will be identified. Lastly, Fehring addressed the

need to base all validation studies on an initial literature review and concept validation.

Magnan (1995) presented an application of Bayesian methods in a validation study at the eleventh conference. In Bayesian statistics the mechanics of increasing or decreasing one's confidence in the truth of a hypothesis are realized in the application of a precise mathematical formula used to calculate the degree of change that should take place in one's belief about the truth of the hypothesis. In nursing diagnosis research, that is the probability of a nursing diagnosis given information about the prior probability of the diagnosis and cue (defining characteristic)-diagnosis relationship.

Hoskins (11997) updated her presentation on how to do a validation study for the twelfth conference. She discussed concept analysis, nurse expert, and clinical validation as appropriate phases of diagnosis validation research. She reinforced the Fehring proposal regarding the qualifications of nurse experts and the use of the data from the concept analysis as the basis for the development of the research instrument. In addition, she emphasized the necessity of operationally defining all variables for proper measurement of these variables. Factor analysis was presented as an appropriate method of data analysis and this suggestion was accompanied by cautions about the necessary sample size to carry out factor analysis.

Where Are We Going?

A review of the relatively short history of nursing diagnosis research provides some clear and important direction for the future. A repeated theme is the need for conceptual clarity and development in the first stages of diagnosis development and research. The conclusion here is that nursing diagnosis research must start with a concept analysis before any other methodologies are attempted. The data generated by a concept analysis and subsequently used in instrument development provide a solid conceptual base appropriate for most research designs. The literature also clearly reveals that the majority of studies have been based upon the Fehring models, and most studies involve relatively small samples. For purposes of replication and comparison, further use of these models is appropriate. The need to use large standardized data bases is clear. The increasing availability of standardized data bases offers more opportunities to access large, good quality data sets more easily.

The literature review indicates that the majority of the studies have been based upon the DCV model. This model should involve the use of nurse experts. As previously mentioned, Fehring defined the term nurse experts and developed a rating system to determine who they are. It is critically important that the samples for initial studies use nurse experts. Non-expert nurses may be surveyed and analyzed separately or other identified groups of nurses may be surveyed later and these results compared with the results produced in the use of nurse experts. Instruments developed for use in the Fehring models should be based upon the results of careful literature review and concept analysis. Operational definitions must be based upon these data and these definitions should be reviewed and critiqued by the nurse respondents. Instruments must be pilot tested for reliability before being used for the study. Graduate students in nursing may provide an appropriate and willing sample for the pilot testing of instruments.

Because the CDV model is much more complicated to execute, there is an abundance of DCV studies and few clinical studies. It is appropriate that the concept analysis and the

nurse expert (DCV) research precede clinical validation. The concept has been analyzed, the instrument has been developed, the defining characteristics have been operationally defined, some may have been added, and some may have been subtracted. The instrument must be modified for use by trained nurse experts in the clinical setting and inter- and intra-rater reliability must be achieved. A system must be established for determining that the patients being observed do have the diagnosis being studied and that it is current. This may involve validation by both clinical staff and members of the research team.

Another clinical validation model which may be used is clinical validation by the patient. Obviously, only some diagnoses are appropriate for this approach and not all patients are able to participate in a study using this model. Again, the concept analysis, expert validation, and perhaps expert clinical validation will have been completed. The instrument must be modified so that instructions and operational definitions are changed from those appropriate for nurses to those appropriate for patients. The reading level of the instrument should be at the sixth or seventh grade level. A software program that assists in this conversion is invaluable in the process. The instrument should be available in large print for patients who need it. The instrument may need to be translated into more than one language, depending on the patient sample. If a patient cannot read or write his or her responses but wishes to participate, the nurse data collectors should have a procedure worked out so that they can read to the patient, mark the answers, and maintain the research protocols. A clinical study large enough to achieve a sample appropriate for higher level statistical analyses is very time intensive and should be planned with appropriate resources available to reach the desired $\underline{n}$.

The combination of concept analysis, nurse expert validation, and clinical validation, by both nurses and patients, when appropriate, yields several data sets and will, hopefully, identify patterns which direct the identification of a smaller, more manageable number of defining characteristics with some identified as critical characteristics. Through coordinated efforts and information sharing, these tasks are much less onerous. In addition to the use of the previously described methodologies, there is a need for researchers to design and test other strategies and methodologies for nursing diagnosis research. The Delphi method, Q-sort, and magnitude estimation scaling have all been used to a limited degree. These may merit further trials, other proven methodologies can be applied to nursing diagnosis research, and new approaches can be developed and pilot tested.

As previously mentioned, most studies have used only descriptive statistics. Schroeder (1989) called for the use of multivariate techniques to increase the construct validity of nursing diagnoses. This direction was echoed by Polit and Hungler (1995) who encouraged nurses to use and explain multivariate processes and results in comprehensible terms. Consideration must be given to the choice of statistical analyses during research design. Many current studies do not provide data sets that are appropriate for multivariate analysis. Whitley (1996) used principle components analysis (PCA) in a secondary analysis of data that had previously been analyzed using descriptive statistics. PCA proved to be effective in identifying patterns within defining characteristics and providing consolidation of characteristics into meaningful, usable sets. Researchers need to explore more powerful means of data analysis for nursing diagnosis research.

There is a need for large studies of nursing diagnoses and for replication and comparison of studies. A research team headed by Craft-Rosenberg and Delaney (1997) exemplifies this larger picture approach to nursing diagnosis research. The team who gave birth to the Nursing Diagnosis Extension and Classification project (NDEC) has entered into a collaborative agreement with NANDA to extend the work of NANDA. The goal is to improve the comprehensiveness, scope, specificity, clinical usefulness, and clinical testing of the NANDA taxonomy. All NANDA diagnoses and others will be subjected to concept analyses and expert validation using both clinical specialists and staff nurses. This is one example of a large scale approach to nursing diagnosis research. Others are needed. With the ease of electronic communication, researchers in various locations could team together to study diagnoses of common interest. Teams need not be restricted to common geography.

The study of related diagnoses or of clusters of diagnoses is a conceptually sound approach which can address when overlapping of definitions, defining characteristics, and related factors is appropriate and when is it the result of the underdevelopment of diagnoses. Gordon (1982, 1987) pointed out the usefulness of this approach but there is little evidence of it in the literature with the exception of the work on anxiety and fear. The study of both of these diagnoses by the same researchers and the consideration of both diagnoses by the small work groups has moved the knowledge bases forward for both anxiety and fear.

Two important issues which the NANDA Taxonomy Committee has dealt with throughout its history are the framework for the Taxonomy and the issue of axes within the framework. Axes which have been proposed at various times include acuity (acute to chronic), unit of care, (individual, family, community), developmental stage (fetus to elder), potentiality (actual, risk for, or potential for growthlenhancement), and a descriptor axis (altered, decreased, increased, deficit, depleted, excessive, disturbed, ineffective, effective). These are critical issues that need to be addressed and issues which call for solid research to validate or reject decisions on framework and axes.

Another very promising development has been the work of the small groups on specific diagnoses immediately preceding the NANDA conferences. Experts and interested persons come together to review and discuss the literature and research on particular diagnoses with the ultimate goal of submission of the results of their work to the NANDA Diagnosis Review Committee. Continuation and expansion of these small work groups offers a continuing forum for input and development of diagnoses for NANDA members and moves the work of the organization forward.

The involvement of nursing specialty groups in the development and research validation of diagnoses has been a very positive developmental link for NANDA. Further and more intense linkages with specialty groups will contribute to the development of better diagnoses and will move the process ahead. In the future, specific processes for this linkage would strengthen and hasten the achievement of the goals of both NANDA and the specialty groups.

The systematic development of a research agenda which addresses the related issues of nursing diagnosis research could help to move the research forward in a coordinated fashion. This agenda would provide direction for faculty in their mentorship and collaboration with graduate students in nursing who wish to pursue research in nursing diagnosis, and it could provide direction for those wishing to seek funding for nursing diagnosis research. With explicit information about the state of the art, both experienced and novice researchers are more likely to launch a study of nursing diagnoses. The development of a panel of expert advisors who are willing to consult and provide feedback regarding research proposals, on-going projects, and grant applications is another facilitative mechanism which can be implemented to promote nursing diagnosis research. At a time when interest and excitement about nursing diagnosis has spread in the international nursing community and the needs for common nursing languages is more apparent, we must facilitate and promote nursing diagnosis research to strengthen our bases for practice.

References

Avant, K. (1990). The art and science in nursing diagnosis development. *Nursing Diagnosis, 1*(2), 51-56.

Avant, K. (1991). Paths to concept development in nursing diagnosis. *Nursing Diagnosis, 2*(3), 105-110.

Burgess, A., & Homstrom. L. (1974). Rape trauma syndrome. *American Journal of Psychiatry, 131*, 981-986.

Chang, B. & Hirsch, M. (1994). Nursing diagnosis research: computer-aided research in nursing. *Nursing Diagnosis, 5*(1), 6-13.

Castles, M. (1982). Interrater agreement in the use of nursing diagnosis. In M. Kim, & D. Moritz (Eds.), *Classification of nursing diagnoses: Proceedings of the third and fourth national conferences* (pp.153-158). New York: McGraw-Hill.

Chang, B., Kim, M., Jones, P., & McFarlane, E. (1989). Proceedings of the conference. In

Monograph of the invitational conference on research methods for validating nursing diagnoses, (pp. 1-2). St. Louis: North American Nursing Diagnosis Association.

Clinton, J. (1986). Nursing diagnoses research methodologies. In M. Hurley (Ed.), *Classification of nursing diagnoses: Proceedings of the sixth conference* (pp. 159-167). St. Louis: Mosby.

Craft-Rosenberg, M., & Delaney, C. (1997). Nursing diagnosis extension and classification. In M. Rantz, M. & P. LeMone (Eds.), *Classification of nursing diagnoses: Proceedings of the twelfth conference* (pp.26-31). Glendale, CA: CINAHL.

Creason, N. (1994). Operational and conceptual definition tool development in nursing diagnosis validation research. In R. Carroll-Johnson, & M. Paquette (Eds.), *Classification of nursing diagnoses: Proceedings of the tenth conference* (pp. 47-54). Philadelphia: Lippincott.

Dougherty, C., Jankin, J., Lunney, M., & Whitley, G. (1993). Conceptual and researchbased validation of nursing diagnoses: 1950-1993. *Nursing Diagnosis, 4*(4), 156-165.

Dreher, M. (1990). Ethnographic methods as differentiated from phenomenology. In *Monograph of the invitational conference on research methods for validating nursing diagnoses* (pp. 78-97). St. Louis: North American Nursing Diagnosis Association.

Fehring, R. (1986). Validating diagnostic labels: standardizing methodology. In M. Hurley (Ed.), *Classification of nursing diagnoses: Proceedings of the sixth conference* (pp. 183-190). St. Louis: Mosby.

Fehring, R. (1994). The Fehring model. In R. Carroll-Johnson, & M. Paquette (Eds.),

Classification of nursing diagnoses: Proceedings of the tenth conference (pp. 55-62). Philadelphia: Lippincott.

Gebble, K. (Ed.), (1976). *Summary of the second conference: Classification of nursing diagnoses* (pp. 19-21). St. Louis: National Group for Classification of Nursing Diagnoses.

Gebbie, K. (1984). Approved nursing diagnoses and small group work on diagnostic labels. In M. Kim, G. McFarland, & A. McLane (Eds.), *Classification of nursing diagnoses: Proceedings of the fifth national conference* (pp.469-524). St. Louis: Mosby.

Gordon, M. (1982). *Nursing diagnosis: Process and application* (2nd ed.). New York: McGraw-Hill.

Gordon, M. (1987). *Nursing diagnosis: Process and application* (3rd ed.). New York: McGraw-Hill.

Gordon, M. (1990). Toward theory-based diagnostic categories. *Nursing Diagnosis, 1*(1), 5-11.

Gordon, M., & Sweeney, M. (1979). Methodological problems and issues in identifying and standardizing nursing diagnoses. *Advances in Nursing Science, 2*(1), 115.

Grant, J., Kinney, M., & Guzetta, C. E. (1990). Using magnitude estimation scaling to examine the validity of nursing diagnoses. *Nursing Diagnosis, 1*(2), 64-69.

Grant, J., & Kinney, M. (1991). The need for operational definitions for defining characteristics. *Nursing Diagnosis, 2*(1), 181-185.

Guzetta, C., & Forsythe, G. (1979). Nursing diagnostic pilot study: Psychophysiologic stress. *Advances in Nursing Science, 2*, 27-44.

Guzzetta, C., Kinney, M., & Grant, J., (1994). Validating nursing diagnoses using magnitude estimation. In R. Carroll-Johnson, & M. Paquette (Eds.), *Classification of nursing diagnoses: Proceedings of the tenth conference* (pp. 42-46). Philadelphia: Lippincott.

Hoskins, L. (1989). Clinical validation methodologies for nursing diagnosis Research. In R. Carroll-Johnson, (Ed.), *Classification of nursing diagnoses: Proceedings of the eighth conference* (pp. 126-131). Philadelphia: Lippincott.

Hoskins, L. (1997). How to do a validation study. In M. Rantz., & P. LeMone, (Eds.), *Classification of nursing diagnoses: Proceedings of the twelfth conference* (pp. 79-86). Glendale, CA: CINAHL.

Hoskins, L., Kerr, M., Fitzpatrick, J., Warren, J., Avant, K., Carpentino, L., Hurley, M., Jakob, D., Lunney, M., Mills, W., & Rottkamp, B. (1992). Axes: focus of taxonomy II. *Nursing Diagnosis, 3*(3), 117-123.

Kerr, M., & Fitzpatrick, J. (1990). Qualitative research methodologies: Synthesis and recommendations. In *Monograph of the invitational conference on research methods for validating nursing diagnoses* (pp. 114-120). St. Louis: North American Nursing Diagnosis Association.

Kim, M. (1982). Issues related to research on the classification of nursing diagnosis. In M. Kim, & D. Moritz, (Eds.), *Classification of nursing diagnoses: Proceedings of third and fourth national conferences* (pp. 124-137). New York: McGraw-Hill.

Kim, M. (1991). Integrated methods for nursing diagnosis research. In R. Carroll-Johnson, (Ed.), *Classification of nursing diagnoses: Proceedings of the ninth conference* (pp. 201-206). Philadelphia: Lippincott.

Kim, M., McFarland, G., & McLane (Eds.), (1984). *Classification of nursing diagnoses: Proceedings of the fifth national conference.* St. Louis: Mosby.

Kinney, M., & Guzetta, C. (1989). Testing a measuring technique to study nursing diagnosis. In R. Carroll-Johnson (Ed.), *Classification of nursing diagnoses: Proceedings of the eighth conference* (pp. 419-420). Philadelphia: Lippincott.

Knalf, K. (1990). Concept development. In *Monograph of the invitational conference on research methods for validating nursing diagnoses* (pp.37-63). St. Louis: North American Nursing Diagnosis Association.

Lackey, N. (1986). Use of the Q methodology in validating defining characteristics of specified nursing diagnoses. In M. Hurley (Ed.), *Classification of nursing diagnoses: Proceedings of the sixth conference* (pp. 191-196). St. Louis: Mosby.

Lo, C. & Kim, M. (1986). Construct validity of sleep pattern disturbance: a methodology approach. In M. Hurley (Ed.), *Classification of nursing diagnoses: Proceedings of the sixth conference* (pp. 197-206). St. Louis: Mosby.

Lunney, M. (1990). Accuracy of nursing diagnosis: Concept development. *Nursing Diagnosis, 1*(1), 12-17.

Magnan, M. (1995). A Bayesian methodological approach to validation of a nursing diagnosis: activity tolerance. In M. Rantz., & P. LeMone (Eds.), *Classification of nursing diagnoses: Proceedings of the eleventh conference* (pp. 97-111). Glendale, CA: CINAHL.

Martin, K. (1978). Nursing diagnosis of impaired parenting relative to the preschool child: A pilot exploration. In *Sigma Theta Tau, Monograph Series 79, Clinical Nursing Research: Its Strategies and Findings II. Proceedings of the Sixth Annual Nursing Research Conference* (208-220). Indianapolis, IA: Sigma Theta Tau.

Mass, M., Hardy, M., & Craft, M. (1990). Some methodologic considerations in nursing diagnosis research. *Nursing Diagnosis, 1*(1), 24-30.

McFarlane, E. (1991). Qualitative methods for nursing diagnosis research. In R. CarrollJohnson (Ed.), *Classification of nursing diagnoses: Proceedings of the ninth conference* (pp. 185-191). Philadelphia: Lippincott.

McLane, A., & Fehring, R. (1984). State of the art of nursing diagnosis. In M. Kim, G. McFarland, & A. McLane (Eds.), *Classification of nursing diagnoses: Proceedings of the fifth national conference* (pp. 525-540). St. Louis: Mosby.

Nicoletti, A., Reitz, S., & Gordon, M. (1982). A descriptive study of the parenting diagnosis. In M.. Kim, & D. Moritz (Ed.), *Classification of nursing diagnoses: Proceedings of the third and fourth national conferences* (176-183), New York: McGraw-Hill.

Polit, D., & Hungler, B. (1995). *Nursing research: Principles and methods* (5th ed.). Philadelphia: Saunders.

Schroeder, M. (1989). Tool development: validity related to nursing diagnosis. In *Monograph of the invitational conference on research methods for validating nursing diagnoses* (pp. 114-120). St. Louis, MO: North American Nursing Diagnosis Association.

Schroeder, M. (1991). Qualitative methods for nursing diagnosis research. In R. CarrollJohnson (Ed.), *Classification of nursing diagnoses: Proceedings of the ninth conference* (pp. 192-200). Philadelphia, PA: Lippincott.

Shoemaker, J. (1984). Essential features of a nursing diagnosis. In M. Kim, G. McFarland, & A. McLane (Eds.), *Classification of nursing diagnoses: Proceedings of the fifth national conference* (pp. 104-112). St. Louis, MO: Mosby.

Sparks, S., & Lien-Gieschen, T. (1994). Modification of the diagnostic content validity model. *Nursing Diagnosis, 5*(1), 31-35.

Straus, A., & Corbin, J. (1990). Grounded theory's applicability to nursing diagnostic research. In *Monograph of the invitational conference on research methods for validating nursing diagnoses* (pp.4-24). St. Louis: North American Nursing Diagnosis Association.

Whitley, G. (1995). Concept analysis as foundational to nursing diagnosis research. *Nursing Diagnosis, 6*(2), 91-92.

Whitley, G. (1996). A multivariate approach for the validation of anxiety and fear. *Nursing Diagnosis, 7*(3), 116-124.

Learnings From The Field: The Impact of Using Two New Nursing Diagnosis, Organized Infant Behavior and Disorganized Infant Behavior (abstract)

Kathy Wyngarden
Mary DeWys, RN, BSN
Margaret Padnos, RN, BA, BSN

Over the last four years, two new nursing diagnoses — Organized Infant Behavior and Disorganized Infant Behavior — have been used in a variety of health care settings, including a neonatal intensive care unit (NICU), a developmental assessment clinic (DAC) that follows NICU graduates and other high-risk infants, community health centers and pediatric practices.

From the use of these diagnoses, a guidelines for care has emerged for interventions and expected outcomes. Together, the diagnoses and the guideline for care have provided an excellent foundation to education parents, nurses and other health care professionals in various settings including the community.

In and of themselves, the two nursing diagnoses provide a window for observing a myriad of parent and infant/child behaviors and interactions. Thus, these diagnoses find a logical link with other diagnoses recognized by NANDA, namely Ineffective Infant Feeding and Altered Parent Infant/Child Attachment.

Outcomes for parents include greater confidence in caring for their infant and a higher degree of satisfaction in the parental role. Outcomes for infants include increased organization of the neurobehavioral subsystems resulting in calmer, less irritable infants who can then interact positively with their families and their environment.

Section 5

Poster Abstracts

Most Frequent Defining Characteristics for the Diagnosis *Decreased Cardiac Output*: A Study Developed in Brazil

Emilia Campos de Carvalho

Introduction: There are few studies about the nursing diagnosis *"decreased cardiac output"* in Brazil. The aim of this study was to identify the frequency of the possible defining characteristics in patients with cardiovascular diseases in a Brazilian hospital. Methods: We analyzed 50 cases of patients from a Cardiological Unit of the University Hospital – Faculty of Medicine at Ribeirao Preto (University of Sao Paulo/Brazil). Data were collected (using a tool developed by the teachers) by undergraduate students during the course "Medical Nursing," offered by the University of Sao Paulo at Ribeirao Preto College of Nursing, Brazil. These study cases used NANDA I Taxonomy (1990). Results: We have selected 22 study cases (44%) with the diagnosis of *decreased cardiac output* from the 50 cases. The sample consisted of 50% male and 50% female patients; age ranged from 20 to 80 years old. These patients presented the following medical diagnoses: valvular heart diseases (27.3%), heart failure (22.7%), coronary artery disease (22.7%), cardiomyopathies (18.2%), arrhythmias (13.6%), hypertension (9.1%), congenital heart disease (4.5%) and chronic obstructive pulmonary disease (4.5%). The study case of each patient was analyzed by only one observer, the teacher of the mentioned course, who was looking to identify clinical evidence that matched those presented in the data collection tool described by Jesus et al., which has the NANDA's proposed defining characteristics and other ones referring to this diagnosis. From the 49 defining characteristics for the nursing diagnosis of *decreased cardiac output* presented in the data collection tool, we did not identify 19 (38.9%); among those, 6 were proposed by NANDA's Taxonomy and 13 were described by Jesus et al. The most frequent defining characteristics observed were: dyspnea (50%), arrhythmias (45.5%), fatigue (40.9%), edema (27.2%), chest pain (27.2%), labile blood pressure (27.2%), weakness (18.9%), cough (18.2%), restlessness (13.6%), abnormal heart sounds (13.6%), vertigo (13.6%), abnormal chest radiography (13.6%). All defining characteristics with a frequency greater than 25%, except chest pain, were proposed by NANDA's Taxonomy. The other defining characteristics had a frequency below 10%: rales (4.5%), nocturnal paroxistic dyspnea (4.5%), use of accessory muscles to breathe (4.5%), elevated creatinine level (4.5%), elevated urea level (4.5%), change in mental status (4.5%), abnormal electrolytes (4.5%), elevated cardiac enzymes (9.5%) and EKG changes (9.1%).

Comments and conclusion: The data collection tool allowed identification of defining characteristics for the nursing diagnosis *decreased cardiac output* and it facilitated the diagnostic process. These results show the need to review the defining characteristics for this diagnosis with further validation clinical studies.

Validation in Spain of *Dysfunctional Ventilatory Weaning Response* (DVWR)

Ana Gimenez

Objective: To validate the nursing diagnosis content of *Dysfunctional Ventilatory Weaning Response* in Spain.

Design: An observational descriptive study through a survey of opinion.

Setting: Nine hospitals from six autonomies communities in Spain.

Instrumentalization: Elaboration of two questionnaires based on the defining characteristics and related factors published by NANDA plus an appendix containing operational definitions. Fehring's Content Validity Model was reproduced and consensus among subjects was reached through Delphi technique. Mean calculation for each defining characteristic was analyzed. Factor analysis to decrease the number of moderate DVWR was performed. The percentage of agreement upon factors proposed as related or associated with these diagnosis was calculated.

Results: The grades mild and moderate of DVWR did not have "major" defining character-istics, but mild grade had 4 and grade moderate had 33 "minor" characteristics. The factor analysis developed 7 factors that explained 70.8% of the total variance. There was 0.6 to 0.9 percentage agreement regarding 16 associated factors which could influence this diagnosis and the independent nursing treatments which could be used to modify them.

Conclusions: The general content of DVWR is also valid in Spain, although defining characteristics of each grade could not be determined by Fehring's model. The factor analysis has been useful to reduce the number of defining characteristics and also to describe the levels of severity of this dysfunctional response. The results of this study will be used to construct a questionnaire to determine the incidence of DVWR among our population and to identify which characteristics are critical for each grade of dysfunctional response.

A Grounded Theory Study of Hardiness in Women with Breast Cancer

Carol A. Craft

The purpose of this study was to expand the theoretical development of hardiness. Social psychologists defined hardiness as a stress-resistance resource comprised of commitment, control, and challenge. They developed the concept solely through the study of male executives. Nurses and other social scientists have used the concept extensively, but many concerns remain about the concept, including its definition. The qualitative method of grounded theory was used to investigate the nature of hardiness as manifested by women with breast cancer. Thirteen women, identified by nurses as having handled their experience of cancer particularly well, were recruited from a university medical center. Semi-structured interviews were audiotaped, transcribed, and analyzed through the method of constant comparison. Recorded field notes, theoretic and analytic memos, and personal reflections were compiled to create an audit trail. Two major characteristics of hardiness were identified: a strong sense of purpose, and the ability to endure. These characteristics were described in terms of their internal dimensions, manifestations, and outcomes. A strong sense of purpose had as its internal dimension the needs of others. It was manifested in the women's caring for themselves, engaging in meaningful activities, and striving for normalcy, and its outcomes included the determination to go on and a growth in inner strength. The ability to endure had as its internal dimension the acceptance of breast cancer. It was manifested through a variety of strategies: physically making it through, self-talk, creating appropriate expectations, personal control through choosing, optimism, and hope. The outcomes of the ability to endure included positive and negative alterations in relationships, positive outcomes through a change in life perspective, and personal growth. Comparisons of the findings were made with the original conceptualization of hardiness. For women demonstrating feminine hardiness in a life-threatening illness, commitment and control were evident, but not as major characteristics. Commitment was seen as one of the manifestations of the broader characteristics of a strong sense of purpose, and control was reflected as one of the manifestations of the ability to endure. Challenge was not evident in the women's presentation of hardiness, although it is conceivable that the stressor of breast cancer posed a challenge which evoked their hardiness. The ability to endure had not been included in the original conceptualization. The findings of this study offer a conceptual portrait of feminine hardiness. The key elements of this hardiness are not reflected in current measures of the concept, but clearly need to be. Future theory and research are needed on the relationships within the characteristics, for example, the place and significance of inner strength and the priority of personal control through choosing. The concept of hardiness is an important one for nurses because of its potential for explaining why some individuals handle well the major stress which illness can create. But to serve as that explanations, a fully developed and articulated concept is needed. A description of feminine hardiness has been offered which expands, extends, and modifies the original concept of hardiness.

Diagnosis Incidence in Surgical Patients Care of the HCUFMG/Brazil

Tania Couto Machado Chianca
C.B. Solange Godoy
Miguir T.V. Donoso

This abstract refers to a descriptive study conducted by three professors of nursing specializing in the medical surgical area and interested in studying the taxonomy of nursing diagnosis proposed by the North American Nursing Diagnosis Association (NANDA) and the International Classification of the Nursing Practice (ICNP). A retrospective research of 33 case studies done by 77 graduate students of the Nursing School of the Federal University of Minas Gerias (UFMG/Brazil), in the March 1995 to June 1997 period. The objectives were to identify the affected basic human necessities and to establish the nursing diagnosis presented by the patients operated in the "Hospital das Clinicas" of the same Brazilian university (HCUFMG). The patients were submitted to gynecological (33.3%), digestive system (27.3%), plastic (15.2%), urological (15.2%), cardiovascular (6.1%) and orthopedical (3%) surgical procedures. Therefore, 57 diagnosis were identified, 9 from NANDA and 48 from ICNP. The patients in the perioperative period were affected by 15 human necessities. This fact is supported by Horta (1979) who describes the Surgical Syndrome, categorized by physical and emotional security necessities (81%); tissue-mucous membrane integrity (60%); thermal and vascular regulation (46%); painful and sensorial perception (44%) and health education (42%). Among the most significant nursing diagnoses were *surgical wound* (44%); *anxiety* (35%); *lack of knowledge* (28%); *risk for fluid volume deficit* (16%); *risk for infection* (14%); *partial immobility* (12%); *high blood pressure* (12%); *fear* (11%) and *health seeking action* (11%) were found in this study. The identification of the basic human necessities and the nursing diagnosis of patients in perioperative period enables the nurses to plan interventions that will contribute to the better quality of the care and the unifying of the nursing language.

Implementation of Strategies to Enhance Clinical Reasoning and Decision Making in Nursing Practice

E.P.L. Albersnagel-Thijssen

M. den Boer

M. C. Kastermans

C.A.M. Mulder

J.E. Schoemaker

H.A. Stallinga

Aim of the project: A project, funded by the Ministry of Education and Science, has been carried out to implement clinical reasoning and decision making in nursing practice. The aim of this project was twofold:

— to develop implementation strategies

— to test educational material concerning clinical decision making and the use of unified nursing language (diagnoses, outcomes and interventions) and management skills (decisions making on patient-allocation and delegating care).

Method: The project has been carried out in 13 different health care institutions: four general hospitals, four home health care agencies, three mental health hospitals and two different nursing homes. At the start of the project an analysis of every practice situation was made. This analysis was directed at nurses' attitudes towards the nursing process and towards the use of nursing diagnoses on the one hand and at the use of nursing care plans on the other. Based on this analysis different implementation plans for each specific situation were developed (top-down versus bottom-up). These implementation plans were focused on:

— the way nurses had to be supported in the practice field;

— education in the use of nursing diagnoses, outcomes and interventions, based on a Dutch classification of diagnostic terms (derived from the ICIDH), a Dutch translation of the NIC and the NOC);

— teaching management skills.

To be able to evaluate the effects of this strategy the same analysis was repeated at the end of the project.

Results: Nurses appeared to have a very positive attitude towards nursing diagnoses and the nursing process. The decision making model can be considered to give a firm grip on diagnosing patient problems. The PES-structure and a unified nursing language are frequently used. Nursing care plans are increasingly applied in every practice situation. The motivation of nurses appeared to depend on the chosen implementation strategy. If only a top-down strategy was used, nurses were less motivated and results were less encouraging, while nurses were very motivated when a bottom-up implementation strategy was chosen. When a combination of a top-down and a bottom-up strategy was used results appeared to be more embedded in both policy and practice.

The Frequency and Importance for NANDA's Nursing Diagnoses in Japan

Eiko Otani

Mitsuko Matsuki

Yuko Yamamoto

Chie Ogasawara

Takako Egawa

Yuko Ohno

The purpose of this study was to examine the actual situation of the utilization of nursing diagnoses in Japan, and to obtain basic information for a validation study.

Methods: Sample: 497 nurses who have experience in using nursing diagnosis. 109 NANDA nursing diagnoses were evaluated in terms of frequency and importance. Both of these variables were rated on a five-point scale; (5: very often used - 1: never used) (5: very important - 1: not important).

Results and Discussion: 1. High and low frequency diagnoses: There are 14 high frequency nursing diagnoses (frequency score > 3.0); *Pain, Anxiety, High Risk for Infection, Impaired Skin Integrity, Constipation, Knowledge Deficit, Bathing/Hygiene Self Care Deficit, Toileting Self Care Deficit, Sleep Pattern Disturbance, Dressing/Grooming Self Care Deficit, Activity Intolerance*. The reason is that their definitions and interventions are thought o be clear and concrete. Low frequency diagnoses (frequency score < 2.0) were *Rape-Trauma Syndrome, Post-Trauma Syndrome, Altered Sexuality Pattern*. 2. High and low importance diagnoses: There were 22 high importance nursing diagnoses (important score > 3.5). There was no diagnosis which was rated less than 2.0. The lowest was rape-trauma syndrome (mean score 2.3).

Conclusion: There were 31 nursing diagnoses which showed high frequency and importance (combined score > 6.0). This suggests that it is necessary to conduct validation studies of these nursing diagnoses in Japan.

The Relevancy for NANDA's Nursing Diagnoses in Japan

Yuko Yamamoto
Mitsuko Matsuki
Eiko Otani

Takako Egawa
Chie Ogasawara
Yuko Ohno

The purpose of this study was to investigate the relevancy for NANDA's nursing diagnoses, and the problems of using them in Japan. The sample consisted of 380 nurses who had experience using nursing diagnosis. The relevancy of 109 NANDA's nursing diagnoses (1992-1993, translated to Japanese by Mitsuko Matsuki) were evaluated. The problems in using them were collected by open-ended question. The findings were as follows:

1. Nursing diagnoses with highest relevancy: nursing diagnoses that over 95% of subjects reported "relevant" were *diarrhea, sleep-pattern disturbance, constipation, anxiety, impaired swallowing, impaired verbal communication, self-toileting deficit, self-bathing-hygiene deficit.*

2. Nursing diagnoses with lowest relevancy: nursing diagnoses that below 50% of subjects reported "relevant" were *unilateral neglect, spiritual distress, rape-trauma syndrom: compound reaction, rape-trauma syndrome: silent reaction.*

3. Problems of using NANDA's nursing diagnoses: 1639 open-ended comments were classified into 8 categories. (1) The translation to Japanese was unsuitable. (2) The diagnoses could be covered by another one. (3) Nurses could not understand the definition of the diagnoses. (4) Nurses felt difficulties in diagnosing. (5) Nurses regarded the diagnoses as collaborative problems. (6) The diagnoses were rarely used in nursing practice. (7) There was a cultural gap between North American and Japan. (8) Nurses could not find nursing interventions for the diagnoses.

These findings suggest that development of nursing diagnoses reflecting Japanese cultural perspective is needed.

To Examine Content Validity of the Defining Characteristics of *Activity Intolerance*

Takako Egawa

Mitsuko Matsuki

Yuko Yamamoto

Eiko Otani

Chie Ogasawara

Yuko Ohno

Diagnostic labels which were developed by the North American Nursing Diagnosis Association (NANDA) have become more familiar to most Japanese nurses and are being used in nursing practice at many facilities. The diagnostic labels and defining characteristics provide not only the language, but also a basis, for nurses' clinical judgement. However, in order to disseminate in Japan, the defining characteristics must be examined for validity and relevancy in our culture. Our previous research showed that *"Activity Intolerance"* was the most frequently used in our country. The purpose of this study is to examine the diagnosis content and validity on *"Activity Intolerance."* Fehring's Diagnostic Content Validity Model (DCV) was used to identify major or minor defining characteristics for *Activity Intolerance.* Each listed defining characteristic ranked the relevancy on a five point scale with the end points being "not at all relevant (1)" to "very relevant (5)," and used weighted ratios for each listed characteristic provides for ratings between 0 and 1. Then, the responses of all of answers were weighted and the weight for each item were summed.

We found that listed characteristics receiving weighted ratios of above 0.75 were dyspnea, verbal report of fatigue and weakness, and abnormal increase of respiration rate, while weighted ratios between 0.60 to 0.75 were found for 10 defining characteristics such as complaint of tiredness, exterional, pallor, cyanosis and dizziness. These results were quite similar to preceding studies for defining characteristics of *"Activity Intolerance"* in USA. These findings suggested that the defining characteristics could be used in Japan; however, in order to use them effectively in clinical areas, each defining characteristic must continuously be studied for further clinical validation and develop more objective defining characteristics.

Integrating Nursing Diagnoses and Interventions in Public Health Nursing Practice

Kathleen M. Parris

The Public Health Field Nursing Program of Orange County, California changed a 20-year-old mode of documenting public health nursing activities to a standardized data collection system which is family/client centered with the capacity to accommodate regulatory compliance of multiple health mandates including those needed to measure outcomes and obtain reimbursement for services provided by the public health nurses. A group of ten public health nurses, using a Total Quality Management approach, researched the available body of knowledge published in the nursing literature and decided to integrate the Taxonomy II of Nursing Diagnoses developed by NANDA and the Nursing Interventions Classification (NIC) published by the Iowa Intervention Project. The decision to use the two classification systems was based on the strength that they are supported by research or a review and consensus process.

A set of forms designed and adapted from NANDA diagnoses and NIC systems documents the nursing process in a public health nursing setting. The forms are based on the NANDA nursing model, using the nine Human Response Patterns, and clusters of activities from the NIC list of interventions. The comprehensive minimum data collection recorded in family and client profiles reflects subjective and objective information necessary to identify nursing diagnoses leading to nursing care plans for intervention and to attain expected outcomes. The documents are designed to be used for single and multiple visits and to assist the public health nurses in documenting their assessments, diagnoses, interventions, and evaluations of the family/client status using a common framework of reference and a universal nursing language.

'Natural Decline' as a Potential Nursing Diagnosis: The Conceptual Analysis of Dying as it Relates to the Phenomenon of 'Natural Decline' in the Elderly

(Name of presenter not available on abstract)

Research has identified that most of the people in the United States die at a relatively old age after a prolonged period of physical decline and chronic disabilities. This conflicts with much of the research surrounding dying that is focused on those who die of either cancer or HIV. Dying is a complex process involving complex nursing interventions, especially for the geriatric client. The purpose of this analysis of dying is to identify a phenomenon of 'natural decline' which may be used as a potential nursing diagnosis. This can be a useful label to guide nursing toward interventions for the chronically declining elderly in order to assist with a peaceful death. Review of the literature related to dying is conducted to reach a clearer definition. Critical attributes of the concept are discussed as well as the antecedents and consequences. Finally, interventions for dying as it relates to 'natural decline' are suggested.

Clinical Validity of the Nursing Diagnoses *Impaired Mobility and Impaired Ambulation* in Post Hospital Experience

Jean A. O'Neil

This study compared the defining characteristics of *impaired mobility* and *impaired ambulation* with the cues presented by same day surgery patients undergoing arthroscopy. It was an inductive study via secondary data analysis of how patients describe their experience.

Purpose: The purpose of this investigation was to validate the cues used by nurse experts to identify dysfunctional responses to the experience of same day surgery (SDS). The nurses used a symptom rating scale and open ended interview at 72 hours post surgery to formulate nursing diagnoses. This study analyzed the data for correlation of cues with the defining characteristics published by NANDA for *impaired mobility* and *impaired ambulation*.

Methodology: 100 patients in an ambulatory day surgery setting in a large urban medical center participated. Doctoral students and faculty expert in the use of diagnostic reasoning conducted home telephone calls 24 and 72 hours following surgery, using a semi-structured interview and a symptom rating scale to collect data. Data were completed for 77 subjects. Secondary analysis of generated cues and formulated nursing diagnoses addressed clinical validation through descriptive statistical techniques.

Results: *Impaired mobility* is a long accepted nursing diagnosis. Recently, rehabilitation nurses proposed differentiation of this diagnosis including *impaired ambulation*. Results from the current study support the differentiation of ambulation as a specific form of *impaired mobility*.

Toward Measurement of Diagnostic Reasoning

Marjory Gordon

Diagnostic reasoning became an important and visible part of nursing practice with the publication of the American Nurses Association Standards of Practice and a social policy statement to consumers. These documents were validated by developments in practice, such as the classification and use of diagnostic nomenclature, as well as the development of the nurse practitioner and advanced practice role. When responsibility for nursing diagnosis is assumed, there is an accountability for continuous improvement in diagnostic skills and the need to assure the public that nurses have the competencies required. Accountability for these skills is important to both educators and practitioners.

The purpose of this paper is to review current efforts to measure the cognitive abilities used in diagnostic reasoning and judgment. The literature review will cite some important methods used in nursing and other health-related disciplines. The authors' current work on developing an instrument to measure diagnostic reasoning and judgment will be discussed. Their model for item construction, sample items and methods for measuring reliability and validity of items will be included. The measurement of cognitive skills may provide an understanding of how these abilities develop and could lead to important studies on the relationship between nurses' clinical judgments and health-related patient outcomes.

Chronic Pain: Related Nursing Diagnoses

Cibele de Mattos Pimenta
Dina de Almeida Lopes Monteiro da Cruz

The aim of this study was to analyze the differences in nursing diagnosis for patients with oncologic and non-oncologic pain. The convenience sample was 114 patients with chronic pain in treatment in the ambulatory care setting. The mean age was 53.1 years and 45.6% of the patients were male. The patients were interviewed and examined to collect the defining characteristics of the nursing diagnoses. Five hundred forty four nursing diagnoses (mean 4.8/patients) were accepted. There were 36 different nursing diagnoses categories. The frequencies of nursing diagnoses were compared between the two groups by chi-square test. The frequency of seven nursing diagnoses were statistically (p>0.05) different between patients with oncologic and non-oncologic pain. Risk for *obstipation* and *altered sexuality patterns* had higher frequency in patients with non-oncologic pain. The patients with oncologic pain had higher frequency of *sensory/perceptual alteration (gustatory)*, *risk for aspiration, impaired swallowing* and *altered thought processes*. The etiology of chronic pain may determine specific clusters of nursing diagnoses.

Coping with Chronic Pain: An Exploratory Study

Cibele de Mattos Pimenta
Dina de Almeida Lopes Monteiro da Cruz
Geana P. Kurita
Ana Claudia Oiveira
Kathia C. Leite

The aim of this study was to identify the pain coping strategies used by patients to cope with chronic pain, to analyze associations between coping strategies categories and sex, age, educational level, pain etiology, and the intensity and duration of pain complaint. Eighty-nine patients in treatment in a pain ambulatory care setting were evaluated. The patients were women in 55.2 of the cases with an average of 51.6 years of age for all subjects. The etiologies of pain were oncologic (35.9%), myofascial (24.7%), neurophatic (13.5%), and undetermined (25.9%). The chronic pain patients coping strategies were evaluated by the questions: What do you do to cope with pain? Are there important spiritual practices to you? Do they help you in pain control? The strategies expressed by patients were classified as proposed by Rosenstiel & Keefe (CSQ, 1983). The coping strategies most utilized were increasing pain behavior (92.4%), praying or hoping (4.7%), and increasing activity levels (2.9%). Descriptive statistical data suggest there are no differences in general coping strategies and the variables of sex and age. There seems to be differences between the average coping strategies and the variables of education, etiology, intensity, and duration of pain. The number of coping strategies were lower in patients with less schooling, neurophatic or oncologic pain, pain of longer duration, and mild or severe pain. A lower number of coping strategies was observed per patient (average 1.47) and a small diversity of strategies and maintenance of pain, which can be characterized as ineffective coping.

Pain: Clinical Validation with *Post-Operatory* Cardiac Surgery Patients

Dina A.L. Monteiro Da Cruz
Consuelo Garcia Correa

The objective of this study was to estimate the content validity of pain defining characteristics. The sample consisted of two groups of 40 post-operatory cardiac surgery patients, of which one was composed of patients with no pain during the assessment period, and the other was composed of patients with pain. Thirty-three possible defining characteristics were identified in the literature. Operational definitions and measurement criteria were developed for each defining characteristic, and these were validated by a panel of experts. Every patient was observed and interviewed with regard to the presence of each defining characteristic, and non-parametric tests were performed in order to identify the differences between groups according to the defining characteristics. The group with pain had statistically different results than the group without pain because there was a higher occurrence frequency of higher scores in the following 14 defining characteristics: elevated cardiac frequency, decreased respiratory expansion, anxiety, depression, altered body mobility, protective posture, self-focusing behavior, altered concentration, feeling of frustration, change in feeding, grimace, altered muscle tonus, diaphoresis and altered comfort. These results contribute to validate the content of the diagnosis of pain in the context of an acute situation. The principal limitation of this study is the possibility of confounding factors related to the sample studies. Studies of the same defining characteristics in other sample groups of acute and chronic pain patients might be useful in the development of knowledge in this field.

Critically Ill Patients: Nursing Diagnoses of Patients of Critical Care Units

Dina A.L. Montiero da Cruz

Dolores Pasini

Iracema Alvim

Luiza Kanda

Rita do Socorro Pereira Mendes

Nursing diagnoses express nursing care needs. The knowledge of the nursing care requirements of a specific group is useful for the development of nursing knowledge concerning these groups. The aim of this study was to identify the nursing diagnoses of critically ill patients as there are few studies carried out directly with patients of critical care units. The sample group consisted of 32 conscious patients admitted to intensive care units (66.5% male; mean age 52.5 years; the most frequent principal medical diagnoses were related to the cardiovascular system). The data were collected by means of interview and physical examination and Functional Health Patterns formed the framework nursing diagnoses for each patient and only diagnoses where at least the authors were in agreement were accepted. Two hundred and six diagnoses were accepted counting for more than 40% of the sample were: *high risk for infection* (96.85%); *altered skin integrity* (96.8%); *altered physical mobility* (81.2%); *sleep pattern disturbance* (75%); *pain* (62.5%); *activity intolerance* (43.5%); *self-care deficit* (43.5%); and *knowledge deficit* (40.6%). Twenty-three diagnoses are present in less than 40% of the sample. These results show that critical care patients have specific nursing care needs. The composition of the nursing diagnoses for each patient is specific although there were some categories that seem to constitute the core of care needs for critically ill patients. It is necessary to replicate this study with samples composed of a wider variety of critically ill patients. The control of variables as well as the utilization of multivariate analysis would be interesting in the identification of the principal nursing diagnoses of these patients.

Nursing Diagnoses in Neonatal ICU

Iane Nogueira Do Vale
Sandra Regina Souza
Sonia Mara dos Santos Cardoso
Maria Helena Baena de Moraes Lopes

INTRODUCTION: In accordance with North American Nursing Diagnosis Association (NANDA) taxonomy, nursing diagnosis is used in the Neonatal ICU to the entire support center of women's heath (CAISM/UNICAMP) since 1993.

OBJECTIVES: The purpose of this study was to verify which and the frequency of nursing diagnosis, used by the nursery staff, compared with those that weren't identified, although there were defining characteristics in the nursing appointments. SUBJECTS AND METHODS: The data was retrospectively collected, looking into the documents of infant that were discharged from the hospital in April, May, and June of 1996 in the CAISM Neonatal ICU.

RESULTS: A total of 67 infant documents were analyzed. Thirteen diagnosis were identified, and related to the patterns: CHANGE, MOVE and PERCEIVE. It was verified that some related factors as: umbilical stump not scarred, prematurely and the use of protector glasses as well as the diagnoses of ineffective breast-feeding risk, altered perception sense risk (visual) and changed oral mucous risk weren't related in the taxonomy, but were identified in children in the Neonatal ICU. Several known and already identified diagnoses were not identified by nurses, although there were defining characteristics.

CONCLUSIONS: It is necessary to evaluate the nursing diagnosis and the nursing intervention more often, once it is Intensive Critical Unit. The use of nursing diagnosis must be done by reflective form and not by the routine. The mother and the family have to be provided with assistance.

Examining the Wounded Healer Archetype: A Case Study in Expert Addictions Nursing Practice

Marion Cont D'Hare

The theme of the wounded healer was elicited from a phenomenological study of the lived experience of therapeutic use of self in expert addictions nurses caring for addicted clients in early recovery. A case study methodology was subsequently used to examine the research question "How is the wounded healer archetype manifested in expert addictions nursing practice?" The conceptual frameworks used to support the analysis were Brenner's Novice to Expert Model, Martha Rogers' Science of Unitary Human Beings and Carl Jung's archetypal theory. The purpose of the study was to illustrate how the process of healing is facilitated or inhibited through the nurse's own wounding, especially from early childhood trauma in the alcoholic family. The in-depth case study examined one of five expert addictions, nurses using practice case scenarios, interview data and nurse's biographical data. It was suggested that the wounded healer archetype is facilitated when nurses accept their own wounds, are open to the client's wounding and experience openness from the client within the therapeutic relationship. The wounded healer is inhibited when the nurse has not recovered from personal trauma that mirrors the client's trauma within the clinical situation and when the client is not open to healing in the moment. Healing takes place when the nurse is aware of her own health patterns and participates in deliberative mutual health patterning with the client. The case study provides a qualitative analysis of therapeutic and less therapeutic nurse-client relationships using the wounded healer archetype as a framework. Nurses at all levels of proficiency can benefit by applying these concepts to their work with addicted clients.

Managing the Impact of Health Problems on Daily Living

Marijke C. Kastermans
Roel H. Bakker

A central focus of nursing practice is assisting clients to manage the impact of health problems on their daily lives. The North American Nursing Diagnoses Association (NANDA) has accepted several diagnoses concerning this area.

In April 1992 the nursing diagnosis *ineffective management of therapeutic regimen* was accepted. The development of the nursing diagnosis *ineffective management of therapeutic regimen* can be seen as an attempt to overcome part of the ethical and professional drawbacks that are associated with the related nursing diagnosis *noncompliance*. There are indications that the idea behind the diagnosis *ineffective management of therapeutic regimen* is widely recognized (Bakker & Kastermans, 1996). One validation study of this diagnosis has been conducted on the level of signs and symptoms, using Fehring's DDV-method (van der Werff et al, 1997). According to this study nurses make no difference between *ineffective management of therapeutic regimen* and *noncompliance*. Another related diagnosis is *impaired adjust-*

ment. Impaired adjustment has to do with a refusal to accept a change in health status and can lead to a denial of health problems. When this refusal thereby leads to neglecting lifestyle advices of the health expert, the person involved could be diagnosed as noncompliant. But is there also a link between *ineffective management of therapeutic regimen* and *impaired adjustment*?

By analyzing the concept of management of therapeutic regimen an answer will be given to this question. Even so attention will be paid to the concept of self-management. Self-management is used in different ways: sometimes it is synonymous to management of therapeutic regimen; sometimes it is used in the context of the desired outcomes of an intervention program. The term self implies that there is also a management of someone else: the health professional. But how far should the health expert's involvement go without interfering with the focus of nursing: helping the patient to direct his/her own life and health!

Performing Nursing Diagnoses in the Coronary Critical Care Patient

V.L.R. Maria

E.A.M. Arcuri

The present investigation was intended to characterize either the patient's assessment, evaluation phase or their related diagnoses, to analyze the diagnostic adequacy, to identify the most frequent diagnostic categories found out in that unit's patients, and to discuss the Human Response Patterns and their diagnoses. Based on 100 records of hospitalized patients in the Coronary Care Unit of "Instituto Dante Pazzanese de Cardiologia" - Brazil, 100 selected assessments and 487 nursing evaluations were studied. Data were analyzed in accordance with the proposed objectives using specific criteria able to classify the adequacy of those nursing diagnoses. Research findings showed that all (100.0%) of the assessments were carried out by the permanent nurses in the unit, most assessments (74.5%) were filled out up to 48 hours following the patient's hospitalization and predominantly during the morning shift (55.0%), and that nurses could achieve a mean of 8.0 diagnoses per assessment. Most (94.2%) of the evaluations were carried out by permanent nurses while the proxy ones identified new diagnoses in all (100.0%) of the evaluations which they performed.

Thus, 868 diagnoses (47 categories) were identified within the assessments and 3.686 diagnoses (38 categories) in the evaluations. According to the criteria established by the present investigator most (71.8%) diagnoses were classified as Adequate while 56.1% were related to NANDA and 15.7% were not included within this taxonomy; 21.5% were Incomplete and 6.7% Inadequate. A predominance (64.7%) of the real nominal categories was observed in relation to the potential (35.3%) ones. Those categories identified as Adequate but not included within the NANDA classification were: Altered cardiac tissue perfusion (40.5%), Risk for decreased cardiac output (27.2%), and Risk for constipation (27.2%). Coronary patients presented the following most frequent diagnoses: Risk for infection (90.0%), Impaired tissue and skin integrity (83.0%), Altered protection in the coagulation mechanism (68.0%), Altered cardiac tissue perfusion (55.0%) and a Hygiene self care deficit (50.0%). The Exchanging Pattern included the higher frequency of diagnoses (71.0%) with the 34 described categories either in the assessments and evaluations.

The Development of a Regional Information Resource Using the Intranet Services of the NHS Net to Support Parents and Clinicians in the Care of Premature Babies

(Name of presenter not available on abstract)

This abstract outlines a research development using the Intranet services of the newly established NHS Network in the UK to provide information for clinicians and carers involved in providing treatment and care for neonates. This application would be used to deliver information to support clinical practice and decision-making for nursing staff across the northwestern region of the UK coordinated from the regional unit neonate unit at St. Mary's Hospital, Manchester. This would incorporate diagnostic and clinical, transport and referral protocols, information used for the updating of professional practice, parental support and telemedicine developments such as telemetry transfer. This is a national project supported by NHS Executive - Information Management Group.

Advances in nursing and medical diagnostics, interventions together with technology improvements in the area of monitoring and life-support, have dramatically improved the positive outcomes for premature babies. However, the benefits from these advances are essentially dependent upon two areas. These are:

— The quality of the updating and information processes made available to clinicians involved in the care of these infants.

— The degree of support and information given to parents and careers of this group.

In both areas, information is the key process whereby these benefits can be achieved. This paper outlines a proposal to use information and communications technology as a means to offer tangible benefits to both parents and the clinicians within the area of neonatal care.

Within the North West & Mersey Regional Health Authority in the UK it had been recognized by clinicians that there needed to be a means of communicating and disseminating areas of good practice emerging in one centre to the rest. As a result, a North West Neonatal Outreach program was formed with the aim of providing forums where practice developments could be discussed and shared.

The project had achieved its aims in initially linking the neonate units together through establishment of a human network. However, at the end of this program there currently exist problems in maintaining a dynamic and sustained dialogue and information exchange between clinicians over a large geographical area. This creates problems in taking the work of the outreach program further due to a lack of coherent communications infrastructure.

The aim of the research project is to formalize the work of the outreach program for clinicians and parents by establishing a targeted Intranet application within the UK North West segment of the NSH Network. The information server will be run from the St. Mary's Hospital Regional Neonatal Unit, Manchester with access at each neonatal unit in the North West region.

Identification and Validation of the Defining Characteristics of the Nursing Diagnosis *Ineffective Airway Clearance*

Ivete Martins

Maria Gaby R. de Gutierrez

Alba Lucia B. L. de Barros

The utilization of nursing diagnoses as proposed by NANDA for systemized care delivery and provided by Dante Pazzanese Institute of Cardiology, originated discussions and the need for validation of clinical studies. This study purpose was to approach the diagnosis *Ineffective Airway Clearance* to verify which of the defining characteristics proposed by NANDA were more frequently identified by that health care setting nurses in order to establish the above diagnosis. The sample included 30 patients with or without diagnosis who were separated into two groups by two expert nurses. Data were collected by the expert nurses and five practitioner nurses. The conclusion attained by the statistical analysis showed that the more frequently identified defining characteristics in the with-diagnosis group were rales, changes in rate of respiration, dyspnea, changes in depth respiration, *tachypnea*, and ineffective coughing; no significant statistical difference was seen between one of the expert's groups of patients. However, when analyzing the occurrence of each of the defining characteristics, there was a significant difference between both groups' characteristics. Regarding the consonance of opinions between the practitioner and the expert nurses as to the establishing or not of the diagnosis, it was observed that in the with-diagnosis group, the mean percentage was 78% of the agreement and, in the without-diagnosis group, only 44%.

Nursing Diagnosis: Minimum Standard Nursing Diagnosis in the Emergency Department of a Cardiology Hospital

M.S. Peixoto

G.I.D.C.E. Urrutia

M.P.G. Costa

V.L.R. Maria

The purpose of this study was to identify the most frequent nursing diagnosis of hospitalized patients in the emergency department of a cardiology hospital. Based on data obtained from 100 nursing reports of hospitalized patients during May 1994, the authors established the minimum standard nursing diagnosis. The most frequent nursing diagnoses were: hygiene self care deficit (90%), potential for infection (82%), impaired skin integrity (81%), impaired physical mobility (74%), and knowledge deficit (71%). The nursing diagnosis consensus were: potential for trauma, potential for altered nutrition, potential for constipation, potential for altered sleep, impaired familiar interaction, potential for altered vital signs. The authors also established the nursing interventions for each diagnosis, as well as a new presentation for the nursing evolution and prescription.

Nursing Process: How Nurses Perceive the Assessment and Nursing Diagnosis

F.A.C. Farias

E.A.M. Arcuri

The present study was carried out within the "Instituto Dante Pazzanese de Cardiologia" Sao Paulo, Brazil, and was intended to: verify the way nurses perceive the significance of the Nursing Process and the factors likely to interfere in the nursing assessment and diagnosis implementation according to the model developed by this institution. A semi-structured interview was used to learn nurses' perception (29 nurses) on the subject. Regarding nurses' perception on the Nursing Process, it was evidenced that: it regulates the tasks (55.2%), enables a more careful observation of the patient's evaluation (37.9), is an essential care tool (17.2%), and as well the process improves care (17.2%). Based in the model, the nursing assessment at patients' admission was carried out by 41.1% of the nurses; however, all the nurses (100%) working in the Emergency Department performed the assessment in the records. Reasons for not carrying out those assessments at admission were: lacking time (82.4%); inadequate nurse/patient interac-

tion (17.6%); organizational deficiency (11.8%). Causes for the failure in carrying out hospitalized patient's assessment were: lacking time (72.4%); organizational deficiency (20.7%) and nurses' non-involvement (13.8%). In relation to the nursing assessment advantages, nurses reported that: them it is a mean to know the patient better (51.7%); assessment is an essential step for prescription (31.0%); assessment promotes individualized care (27.6%); assessment generates higher patient/nurse reliability (17.2%); it is essential to the nursing diagnosis performing (17.2%). Regarding the physical examination, 51.7% reported no difficulty in performing it, while 69% of the nurses carry out interviews without any difficulty. Regarding nurses' perception on nursing diagnosis, it is considered as important for 62.1% and very important for 37.9% since this stage promotes: professional advancement (41.4%), knowledge deepening (34.5%); professional appreciation (20.7%) and reasoning power (20.%).

Use of Nursing Diagnosis in an Interdisciplinary Plan of Care Across the Continuum

Diane Hanson
Kathy Wyngarden

Health care is changing rapidly, with a multitude of external forces. In the noise of this chaos it is critical to not only respond to these changes but to proactively design a system that will support quality health care across the continuum. A systems-thinking framework can provide the foundation for practice clarity and coordination of individualized care. Short- and long-term outcomes will be impacted by diagnosing and treating the human response in partnership with the client and family.

This presentation will provide an overview of an integrated systems thinking framework. This framework includes an interdisciplinary plan of care using interdependent and independent (nursing diagnosis) guidelines and education records for a select patient population across care settings. A high risk pregnant woman and her journey beginning with community based care in the home, through the health care system during her perinatal experience and back home with the newborn infant, will be featured as an example.

This presentation will explore and uncover the actual and potential outcomes for women, infants, family units, health care providers and the community. Actual documentation, practice guidelines and education tools will be shared. This systems-thinking framework can be applied to any patient population.

Integrated Interdisciplinary Care and Outcomes Management for Patients with Chronic Pain

Diane Hanson
Kathy Wyngarden

Outcomes management, care management, clinical pathways, nursing diagnosis, practice guidelines, interdisciplinary plan of care and patient teaching... how do all of these fit together? The heart of this starts with knowing the story of the individual person and mutually identifying the human response(s) of the person. To facilitate planning care and outcomes management for individuals with chronic pain, a practice guideline and education record was developed. This guideline delineates the related risk factors, defining characteristics, expected outcomes (health/activity and teaching) and interventions. A consensual validation process of the guidelines was done by health care providers in 20 settings across the USA and Canada. The practice guideline was foundational in the development of a clinical pathway for chronic pain. The interdisciplinary team uses a report card to follow progress toward outcomes related to patient satisfaction and outcomes, process, utilization of resources, cost and length of stay. Diagnosing and treating the human response is a vital foundation for quality care process across the continuum of care.

Importance in Nursing Care Methodology Concepts and Practice of Nursing Diagnoses

Glaucia Borges Seraphim
Valdirene Polonio

This study attempts to unveil the nursing practice as it refers to nursing diagnoses (ND) in hospitals of Curitiba/Parana/Brazil. The purpose was to identify the resources that serve as basis for the development of nursing interventions utilized by nurses in those institutions as well as their conceptions and expectations in regards to ND. Previous studies developed by Seraphim, Holts, Mendonca & Polonio (1996) searched for answers for such questions among faculty in the same city, leading the authors to pursue studying the same questions in the hospitals, attempting to identify convergent and divergent view points between teaching and practice of ND. This is an exploratory field research that used the method of systematic observation to look at the way nurses act, followed by subjects' answers to a questionnaire containing identification and four open-ended questions. It is concluded that the majority of hospitals studied do not offer working conditions for nurses in order to make it possible to apply a systematic process of nursing care, therefore, they do not offer possibilities for the implementation of ND. The reasons for such results are attributed to the reduced number of nursing staff, the overload of activities, and the lack of professional recognition. Nurses defined ND as the core of nursing actions, but they consider that actual reality of Brazilian hospitals makes this task hard to be performed. However, they consider this an important subject that needs further discussion along with the nursing process.

Nursing Diagnoses in the Nursing Diplomature

Alorda Carmen

M. Crespf

P. Ferrer de Sant Jordi

D. Forteza

G. Gallego

J. Garcia

P. Jaramillo

A. Maya

M. Marrugat

E. Ponsell

C. Vidal

Introduction: Since 1992, the Nursing School of the University of the Balearic Islands has followed the NANDA taxonomy for course curricula within the nursing Diplomature. A descriptive study was planned with the aim of unifying criteria among professors, in order to provide an improved teaching quality, and to allow the initiation of works designed to validate the nursing diagnoses most frequently found during the clinical practices performed in hospitals by students attending Medical-Surgical Nursing and Maternal and Children's Nursing. The second poster shows the nursing diagnoses most often encountered during practical course work in Community Nursing and Geriatric Nursing, carried out in the community and at geriatric residences, respectively.

Objectives: To identify the nursing diagnoses most frequently encountered by students during clinical practices in the Intensive Care Units, Urgency Unity, and adult and maternal and children's Hospitalization Units.

Material and Method: Location: Intensive Care Units, adult Urgencies, and adult and maternal and children's Hospitalization, Adult and maternal and children's buildings, Son Dureta Hospital, National Institute of Health, Palma de Mallorca. Study population: 246 clinical cases (164 from Medical-Surgical Nursing, 82 from Maternal and Children's Nursing). Data were collected randomly by students in a nursing format structured by Marjory Gordon's 11 health functional patterns. Each student gave a presentation of a clinical case to be corrected by the teacher.

Results: The most frequent nursing diagnoses in the Intensive Care Units were: High risk for infection, Disuse syndrome, High risk for aspiration, High risk for impaired skin integrity, Impaired skin integrity. In the Urgency units: High risk for infection, Bathing/hygiene self care deficit, Toileting self care deficit, Anxiety, Ineffective family coping, Risk for injury. In the adult Hospitalization units: High risk for infection, Bathing/hygiene self care deficit, High risk for altered health maintenance, Feeling alteration (pain), Sleep pattern disturbance. Maternal and Children's Units: High risk for impaired for impaired skin integrity, High risk for infection, Ineffective breast-feeding, Sexual dysfunction, High risk for altered health maintenance. Further results and discussion will be reported in the presentation.

The Utilization of Social Representation Theory in Teaching Psychiatric Nurses How to Intervene with the Client with a Nursing Diagnosis of *Risk for Violence*

Marga S. Coler
Antonia S. Paredes

Maria de Oliveira Ferreira Filha

Social Representation Theory has been under-utilized in nursing. However, it is one of the key educational strategies that will be used to teach practicing psychiatric nurses in the Northeastern Brazilian State of Paraiba how to identify clients who are at *Risk for Violence* (*Self-Directed* or *Directed at Others*). In the postgraduate course, NANDA risk factors will be used as landmarks to help the nurses identify body language, attitudes, and verbalizations used both by the caregiver and care recipient during the data collection stage in order to help the nurse arrive at an objective nursing diagnosis. The phenomenon, violence, has recently been identified as a universal problem by 10 psychiatric nurse leaders, representing nine countries at a Rockefeller Foundation funded team residency in Bellagio, Italy. The purpose of their meeting was to identify common mental health problems within all of the represented cultures and to plan post-graduate educational models for nurses practicing in the specialty in these countries. The educator representing Brazil has adapted the generic framework for the module on violence to the culture in Paraiba. The methodology for teaching the nurses about their social representations related to the diagnosis will begin with analyses of their thematic perceptions through pictures, drawings and case studies. Content analysis of the descriptions will serve to validate the risk factors proposed in the NANDA diagnosis and in the identification of culture-specific risk factors. From the content analysis and subsequent identification of the social representations, the nurses will become equipped with a skill of identifying and therapeutically intervening in the risk reduction of a client's violence.

Aggregate Nursing Diagnoses of a Population of Practicing Psychiatric/Mental Health Nurses in a Northeastern State in Brazil as a Basis for Interventions and Outcomes in Graduate Nursing Education

Marga S. Coler

Maria de Oliveira Ferreira Filha

Maria Miriam Lima da Nobrega

The proposed presentation will justify the use of aggregate nursing diagnoses based on the NANDA taxonomy to succinctly identify problems within nursing. A justification is that nursing interventions (in this case, nursing education) will be used by nurses. The diagnoses serve as a focal point for the planning of post-graduate nursing education. In Brazil, content and skill educational standards in psychiatric nursing education are ill-defined at the undergraduate level. At this juncture, there are no standards for basic, nor advanced practice in the specialty. Inadequate nursing care and limited contribution of nursing personnel are two factors that have been targeted to be addressed through permanent programs of post-basic education in the Countries of the Southern Cone by the Pan American Health Organization (Pan American Health Organization [PAHO], 1995). The publication, Analysis of the PAHO Mental Health Program, begins with a statement citing an urgent need for commitment to intervention programs that are creative and scientifically sound (1995). This can only be accomplished with an informed group of caregivers, in this case, practicing psychiatric nurses in the state of Paraiba, Brazil. A preliminary step in the identification of the status of nursing practice psychiatric/mental health nursing in the "developing" Northeastern State, Paraiba, Brazil, was the development of a questionnaire. Because of the lack of standards of practice in any specialty in Brazil, the Standards of Psychiatric-Mental Health Clinical Nursing, published by the American Nurses' Association, were used in the capitol of the state were NANDA diagnoses of:

- Knowledge Deficit due to a lack of focused education in the specialty... especially in the area of deinstitutionalization and the identification and utilization of community resources.

- Risk for care-giver role strain (modified for the aggregate) due to lack of development for the care-giver role.

- Self esteem disturbance due to dependency on the physician, marginal salary, lack of power.

Having identified these nursing diagnoses as typifying the practicing psychiatric nurses in Joao Pessoa has given the educators a point of embarkation in the planning of sound educational intervention at the post-graduate level. The presentation will identify the development of the three nursing diagnoses at the aggregate level and how diagnostic formulation aided in the planning of data-based modules.

Nursing Diagnosis and its Utilization in the Development of a Community

Marga S. Coler
Neuza Maria Correra Paula
Cizone Maria Carneiro Acioly

The exploratory study utilizing structured interviews of a randomly selected sample in a perimeter community of the Capital city of the State of Paraiba, Brazil, identified problems which impaired the natural development of the community. Nursing diagnoses were formulated from the identified risk factors (i.e., a high presence of parasitic and infectious disease, degenerative diseases; subhuman living conditions such as dirty water tossed indiscriminately into the street, garbage thrown into fields, untreated drinking water, proliferation of flies, mosquitoes), and lack of community infrastructure. These were validated as such through a review of the literature since there is no NANDA protocol. Interventions were identified for one of the diagnoses. From the data is was concluded that pathology of social nature can negatively affect the health of a community. Some of the identified nursing diagnoses were: 1) Risk for infectious/contagious diseases related to lack of sanitation, standing waste water in front of houses, lack of pavement, consumption of untreated water and garbage deposition under the open sky in a nearby field; 2) Risk for Violence, Directed at others; Knowledge Deficit; Recreational deficit and Risk for social marginalization. Interventions are proposed as generic, covering all nursing diagnoses (i.e., education in the prevention of illness; assertiveness training/ consciousness raising) and diagnosis-specific (i.e., proper methods of garbage disposal when there is a lack of public transportation and public garbage pick-up services). To help resolve these are needed action of the health authorities; good will of the politicians who determine budget priorities and consciousness of the population about their rights for optimal health. The authors conclude that, aside from consciousness-raising efforts and the support of the community leaders, only a multidisciplinary team can help resolve the problems which are those of social order and not solely within the practice of community health nursing. Although the nurse can act as a team leader and/or participant it is egotistical to think the profession of nursing can resolve all the problems by itself.

Dysfunctional Health Patterns and Nursing Diagnoses in Young Adults

Elizabeth Archambault

Gina Ankner

Diane Berry

Michelle Lyden

Lila Raamot

Dorothy Jones

The health status of the young adult populations is poorly understood. Clinical assessment and information based on this population suggest potential disruptions in health patterns.

Purpose: The purpose of this study was to describe functional health patterns in college age young adults and to identify potential nursing diagnoses.

Sample and Method: One hundred eighty-four male and female participants at a college health fair in the Northeast, age 18 to 25, completed the 58-item Functional Health Pattern Assessment Screening Tool (Foster & Jones, 1996). Responses were reviewed by advanced practice nursing students to determine areas of pattern dysfunction, isolate cues, and identify potential nursing diagnoses.

Data Analysis and Results: Frequency distributions were generated to describe responses to each pattern. Significant cues were identified to suggest dysfunction in three health pattern areas. They were the nutritional-metabolic pattern, the health perception-health management pattern, and the coping-stress tolerance pattern. Other areas of potential dysfunction suggested by the data were sleep-rest, activity-exercise, and self perception. Analysis of the cues generated tentative hypotheses resulting in the following nursing diagnoses: *Altered nutrition: less than body requirements, altered health maintenance,* and *ineffective individual coping.*

Implications: This study identified three major areas of concern for nurses working with the young adult population. These issues involved nutrition, stress and coping, and health promotion. Further research should include replication of the study with larger sample, and formulating strategies for intervention.

Emphasis Breastfeeding: Nurturing, Nourishing, Protecting

Kathleen L. Powers

The purpose of this multidisciplinary project implemented at San Bernardino County Medical Center (SBCMC) is to increase the incidence and duration of breastfeeding mothers and their infants as recommended by the Healthy Children 2000 Project. In addition, use of *Effective Breastfeeding* and *Ineffective Breastfeeding* nursing diagnoses were implemented in the inpatient setting.

The national incidence of breastfeeding during a 24-48 hour inpatient stay averages 52% to 56%. The incidence of breastfeeding at SBCMC in 1996 was 30% to 40% using the same parameters. Studies that describe methods to increase the number of breastfeeding mothers are scant. One method concerns an initiative by the WHO and UNC called the Baby-Friendly Hospital Initiative (BFHI). It describes ten ways in which to support, promote and protect breastfeeding in the hospital setting and improve breastfeeding practices. SBCMC utilized the BFHI as a framework for establishing key project components: 1) development of a 5-part assessment tool that describes and tracks breastfeeding behaviors on 6 different occasions, 2) implementation of breastfeeding nursing diagnoses, 3) implementation of an education plan to address both staff and mothers' learning needs, 4) establishment of telephone follow-up within 48 hours by nursing staff, 5) access to a lactation consultant and 6) use of incentives in the outpatient arena. In addition to these key elements, a mechanism for reporting results was established through the development of quality indicators through SBCMC's Performance Improvement program

The need for a multidisciplinary standardized approach to the development of breastfeeding policies and practices was realized through assessment of the current process throughout the continuum of care. Assessment findings included 1) duplication of efforts across care areas, 2) identification of barriers supported by the literature, 3) fragmentation of education to staff and mothers due to the lack of individualized teaching plans based on the needs of staff and mothers, 4) lack of prenatal care in as much as 50% of mothers, thereby making pre-delivery education and decision making difficult, and 5) breastfeeding mothers or mothers having problems with breastfeeding were not identified using the appropriate nursing diagnoses.

Data collection is on-going and the statistical impact on outcomes will be summarized. Preliminary data, however, has shown that there has been an increase in breastfeeding women who are discharged from the hospital. Mothers gave positive feedback during phone follow-up conversations as well as when they received their incentives for continuing to breastfeed.

Increasing breastfeeding is a realistic goal for the year 2000 and necessitates a multidisciplinary approach. Breastfed infants have a superior start in life and, in general, maintain a better state of health. Breastfeeding is a simple and cost-effective health practice that improves infant and child health. The use of nursing diagnosis in short stays is an effective strategy to focus the nurse on one of the most important components of discharge planning and documentation of the nursing process.

Descriptions of Sleep Pattern Disturbance and Related Factors in Intensive Care

Stephanie J. Richardson

With increasing recognition that sleep patterns of the critically ill adult are disturbed, it becomes important to document sleep descriptors and related factors from the patient's point of view. A secondary qualitative analysis of data from an exploratory study provided information about the patient's perception of sleep.

Thirty-six adults with differing diagnoses and lengths of stay in intensive care were purposively recruited into the study for three days, and were randomly assigned to two groups. The experimental group received a relaxation and imagery intervention on two successive nights. On three mornings, all subjects were asked, "In your own words, what was the last night like for you?" Answers were immediately confirmed for accuracy with each subject. Data were analyzed using an iterative approach, collapsing groups for the purpose of describing sleep pattern disturbance and related factors. Multiple perspectives were used to protect against bias.

This study provided more evidence that the sleep patterns of adults in critical care are very disrupted. Descriptors for the night were vividly negative in most cases, though sleep disturbance improved somewhat for most subjects as time passed. Interruptions were consistently described over time as the most important factor in sleep disturbance. Many subjects described emotional factors, uncertainty, and worry as contributing to insomnia. Factors of pain, urinary urgency, cold, dyspnea, thirst, and discomfort from devices were described by some subjects. A small number experienced temporal distortion at night, which worsened over three nights.

There are gender differences in the experience of insomnia in intensive care. Males described dozing or light sleep, while females described difficulty in getting to sleep. For males, sleep improved more quickly. Initially, males tended to describe being bothered by pain and difficulty finding a comfortable position, while some females initially were bothered by urinary urgency. Later, many females related being keep awake by the presence of devices, emotions and worry.

Identification of Factors and Values Which Interfere in the Conditions of Daily Living of a Community Through Community Nursing Diagnoses

Marga S. Coler
Maria do Carmo Andrade Duarte
Maria do Socorro M. Lins Silva

For the nurse to develop any program or purpose an intervention in a community, it is necessary to know and label those factors which interfere with the achievement and promotion of optimal health in that community and interact with the individuals within it. For this reason this qualitative exploratory study was initiated in three villas located in Joao Pessoa, Paraiba, Brazil. The objectives of the study were to identify those factors and values which interfere in the life of the community, identify community nursing diagnoses based on those factors, and propose nursing interventions based on the diagnoses. Data collection was realized in 1996, utilizing structured interviews and systematic observation. The data were analyzed quantitatively from which two community nursing diagnoses were formulated according to NANDA protocol. *Diversional Activity Deficit* and *Knowledge Deficit* of the populace regarding how to obtain resources. Proposed intervention strategies were shared with community leaders. It must be emphasized that student projects in a community must go beyond diagnostics. The nurse must be attentive to the importance of implementing the interventions by sharing the responsibility with community inhabitants. In this case, communication with community leaders through conscious-raising meetings which would focus on methodology of 1) initiating, preventive and therapeutic educational programs and 2) obtaining space and resources for leisure activities were proposed.

Nursing Diagnosis and Social Representation: A Methodology of Diagnostic Formulation

Antonia S. Paredes
Antonia Regina Furegato
Marga S. Coler

Social representations are modalities of internalized knowledge which determine behavior and communication among individuals. The multidisciplinary nature of these representations mandates that, in the process of formulating nursing diagnoses, the diagnostician must consider not only observed behavior but also the verbal and nonverbal communication of and between the nurse and the client. In this study the authors analyzed the process of diagnostic formulation based on the Theory of Social Representations as was forwarded by Moscovici in 1978. The conventional and prescriptive strength of social representations as related to the reality in which the diagnostic process occurs will be presented. In such a context, thought processes are the environment in which daily life develops. Presented also will be a proposition on how interventions can be planned. Examples will be presented from the NANDA taxa of Communicating, Knowing and Relating.

NANDA Nursing Diagnosis *Impaired Physical Mobility* in Hospitalized Clients in Brazil and a Proposal for Nursing Interventions

Marga S. Coler
Maria Auxiliadora Pereira

As the taxonomy of NANDA gains worldwide acceptance as a diagnostic vehicle, validation studies are increasingly creative in order to conform with the culture in which the taxonomy is being used. In the case of this study, the NANDA nursing diagnosis *Impaired Physical Mobility*, was validated in Brazil according to the Basic Human Needs theory of Wanda Horta, a Brazilian nursing theorist of the late sixties and early seventies. The sample was comprised of hospitalized patients. Defining charac- teristics, related factors and functional levels were evaluated according to those described in the NANDA nursing diagnosis. The findings of the study indicated that, aside from physiological (i.e., preoccupation with physical appearance, especially in arthritic clients) and social (anger at the dependence on family members or friends) components. These are considered in the proposed interventions from the intervention system of the Iowa Interventions Project, NIC (Nursing Interventions Classification).

High Incidence Nursing Diagnoses in Women with Surgical Breast Biopsy & Monitored Anesthesia

Mary J. Costa
Dorothy A. Jones

An individual's responses to surgical interventions are unique. Stress associated with surgery is an integral component of the experience potentially compounded by the uncertainty associated with the biopsy reports and dysfunction.

The purpose of this investigation was to describe function and postoperative responses of women (24-72 hours) following surgical breast biopsy. The sample consisted of approximately 100 adult females, 18 years of age or older receiving monitored anesthesia at a large medical center in the Northeast.

Data collection followed informed consent and IRB approval. Information was collected on the surgical day, intra-operatively and 24 hours post surgery. For women having a positive biopsy report, a 72-hour follow-up phone interview was obtained.

Instrumentation included the use of "Functional Health Pattern Assessment Screening Tool" and a 24-hour Post-Operative Interview Schedule. Data analysis included frequency, distributions, tests of significance and content analysis.

Preliminary results are currently being evaluated and early nursing diagnoses include *anxiety, fear* and *ineffective individual coping.* Implications for nursing intervention across the perioperative experience indicate the importance of preoperative preparation and continued contact with the nurse following surgery and until final diagnosis.

The Discussion about Nursing Diagnosis Opens

J.L. Van Der Heyden

A necessary condition for the development of nursing diagnosis and the measurement of its value to the profession of nursing is the possibility of exchanging thoughts and point of views and to discuss them. On balance, there aren't many opportunities, especially when you look at the international character of the subject. The chances are limited to writing or reading in professional journals, visiting congresses which handle (or not) specifically about nursing diagnoses. Further the discussion is held in direct contact with colleagues who are interested and experts. The identified possibilities have their own disadvantages which impede the transfer of knowledge.

To contribute to the development of nursing diagnosis, the working-group World Wide Nursing Diagnosis Forum (WWNDF) wants to use the medium of Internet for exchange in knowledge, experience and point of view. Qualities of Internet are speed, accessibility and that it is world wide. Because of these qualities, the Internet has great value in relation to the communication on nursing diagnostics, next to the already existing mediums. World wide, one can easily address an interested audience, by which a greater accessibility to the discussion is warranted. Added to that, information from the discussion can be fast found, measured in seconds, and accurately be found on the right spot and it is possible to respond to that directly and prompt.

The WWNDF was founded on completion of the 12th NANDA Conference on the Classification of Nursing Diagnoses, which was held in April 1996, in Pittsburgh (PA), USA. During this conference, a working group under the supervision of Marjory Gordon about how the discussion about nursing diagnostics could be held in the broadest way, how it could be internationally formed, faster and more accessible than it is at the time. The members of the working group WWNDF, who were at this meeting, made the suggestion to start and guide such a thing on their own initiative in Holland, to give form to the discussion about nursing diagnosis by means of the medium Internet. In the first instance the attention will be focused on the Netherlands itself, but in a later phase the discussion will be internationalized. This initiative was received in Pittsburgh with much enthusiasm. In cooperation with the foundation Care Net Holland (CNH, http://www.cnh.nl) the WWNDF has created a special site for the communication about nursing diagnostics on Internet, on the home-page of CNH, to be reached at the Internet e-mail address: http://www.cnh.nl/wwndf.

Beginning July 1997 the conference area is officially declared open on a national base. At this moment the conclusion can be made that it is possible to set up a discussion about nursing diagnosis by means of the medium Internet. The impact at a national level is somewhat below expectations, but can be explained. Beginning January 1998 the conference area will be internationalized. Results will be available at the 13th NANDA conference at St. Louis, MO. Besides the results also the development of the conference area shall be discussed.

Developments on Language and Classification, the European Perspective: ACENDIO

June Clarke

Nico Oud

When ICN surveyed its members' national nurses associations in 1991 to find out what was happening around the world in the development of nursing classifications and computerized informations systems concerning diagnosis interventions and outcomes, there appeared to be very little happening in Europe. By 1997 this situation has changed dramatically, and it is about this change that we like to inform our colleagues during NANDA's anniversary celebration. In this way Europe likes to participate in the celebration of our colleagues in North America and present the European Perspective: ACENDIO, being the Association for Common European Nursing Diagnoses, Interventions, and Outcomes.

After a brief overview of the development of a common language in several European countries, information will be given about the first European Conference on Nursing Diagnoses in 1993 and the second European Conference on Nursing Diagnoses and Interventions in 1995, which led to the First European Conference of the Association for Common European Nursing Diagnoses, Interventions and Outcomes in May 1997 which had the following theme: "From Diagnoses to Outcome: Nurses Network Across Europe." This May 1997 conference appeared to put ACENDIO on a firmer footing within Europe, both as a professional network and as an organization which can achieve realistic goals.

ACENDIO's stated mission became: "To develop and promote a common European terminology and taxonomy for the description and classification of nursing, expressed as nursing diagnoses, interventions and outcomes." Links to European National Nurses Associations and to the Standing Committee of Nurses of the European Union were discussed and positively welcomed, as well as the active collaboration in the development and use of the International Classification for Nursing Practice (ICNP).

After a brief summary of the May 1997 conference a description will be given of the mission, purposes and the objectives of the association. Next a synopsis of its membership, board of directors, committees, organization and activities.

To finish it all the future role and activities of ACENDIO within the European nursing framework and perspective will be discussed, and also its relation to the other nursing organizations across Europe and within countries. At the end ACENDIO will announce the date and place of the second European Conference of ACENDIO in the spring of 1999 in Italy.

Workgroup Reports

Diagnosis Work Group Reports: 1998 NANDA Conference

Elizabeth Hiltunen, MS, RN, CS

Marjory Gordon, PhD, RN

Susan Chase, EdD, RN, CS

At the thirteenth North American Nursing Diagnosis Association conference the tradition of pre-conference diagnosis work groups was continued. The overall purpose of the work-groups has been refinement of nursing diagnoses in the NANDA taxonomy. For this conference, work group participants had an opportunity to pre-select from six diagnoses which were chosen for revision based on research base in the literature, lack of specificity in diagnosis, previous recommendations of work groups, and potential for improving the clinical usefulness of the diagnoses. Based on the interest of the participants, four work groups were convened at this pre-conference session.

Participants who indicated an interest in participating in the work groups were mailed instructions and were asked to select a diagnostic area in which they had a high interest and one or both of the following: significant clinical experience with the diagnostic area and/or have done extensive literature review or clinical research. The purpose of the work groups was to analyze the components of selected diagnoses, compare and contrast similar diagnoses, prepare a bibliography, and make recommendations. Guidelines for preparation for the work groups were included in the mailing to participants. This included the Chart for Summarizing Research Literature and the Criteria for Staging Nursing Diagnoses (NANDA, 1996). In preparation for the work groups, participants were asked to: 1) review research literature in the selected diagnostic area, 2) utilize NANDA's Criteria for Staging Nursing Diagnoses in critique of the components of the selected diagnoses, 3) bring critical articles, summary chart, and critique to the work group for discussion, and 4) bring a typed reference list of critical articles to the group.

Experts who had published research or significant clinical experience in one of the selected diagnostic areas were contacted and invited to participate in the diagnosis work-group. Experts were also offered the opportunity to submit contributions to the work group,

Table 1

NANDA Work Group Discussion Guide

Goals of Work Groups
Critically analyze label, definition, defining characteristics, related factors utilizing discussion guide.
Make recommendations for changes.
Make recommendations for staging.
Make recommendations for future research.
Prepare and submit reference list.
Present report.

Discussion Guide
1. Conceptual Basis of Diagnostic Category
   a. What is current state of knowledge/research in area?
   b. Is there consistency between:
      1.) the current concept description in the literature and
      2.) the diagnosis label, definition, characteristics and related factors?
2. Structure of Diagnostic Category
   a. Label
      1.) Is the label clear and concise? Is the conceptual meaning reflected in the label?
      2.) Is the category stated at a level useful for planning treatment? Is it too inclusive of multiple conditions/diagnoses? Is it too abstract?
      3.) Does the label represent a condition district from other categories within the taxonomy?
      4.) Does the label represent a condition that nurses are able to obtain data needed for diagnosis and treatment and can assume responsibility for outcomes? (Consistent with the current NANDA definition.)
   b. Definition
      1.) Is the definition clear; concise; clinically useful?
      2.) Is there consistency between the meaning of the label and the definition?
      3.) Does the definition represent a condition distinct from all other diagnoses in the taxonomy?
   c. Defining Characteristics
      1.) Is each defining characteristic concrete, distinct and measurable?
      2.) Is there internal consistency among the defining characteristics, label and definition?
      3.) Do the (major/critical) characteristics permit discrimination between the presence and absence of the phenomena?
      4.) Does at least one (major/critical) characteristic distinguish the category from all others?
      5.) Is the list of defining characteristics concise? Does it conserve memory resources?
   d. Related Factors
      1.) Is there support for the related factors in the literature?
      2.) Are the factors defined?
      3.) Are they clear, distinct, observable?

References

Dougherty, C.M., & Kerr, M.E. (1997). Diagnosis workgroup reports: 1996 NANDA conference. In M.J. Rantz and P. LeMone (Eds.). *Classification of nursing diagnoses: Proceedings of the twelfth conference* (pp. 413-414). Glendale, CA: CINAHL Information Systems.

Gordon, M. (1994). Nursing diagnosis. Process and application (3rd ed.) (pp. 291-297). St. Louis: Mosby.

Kerr, M., & Dougherty, C. (1995). Diagnosis workgroup reports. In M.J. Rantz and P. LeMone (Eds.). *Classification of nursing diagnoses: Proceedings of the eleventh conference* (pp. 393-437). Glendale, CA: CINAHL Information Systems.

North American Nursing Diagnosis Association. (1996). *NANDA Nursing diagnoses. Definitions and classification 1997-1998* (pp. 92-93). Philadelphia: Author.

which was done by three individuals through submissions of extensive bibliographies, research articles, and commentary.

The work group sessions were held from 9:00 a.m. to 3:30 p.m. on April 22, 1998 in St. Louis, MO. An orientation session was held and the following goals of the work groups were reviewed: utilizing the discussion guide critically analyze label, definition, defining characteristics, and related factors; make recommendations for changes; make recommendations for staging; make recommendations for future research; prepare and submit reference list; and present report. The groups were given a guideline, the Work Group Discussion Guide (see Table 1), to facilitate discussion. Groups were encouraged to consider the strength of the evidence when reviewing literature and making recommendations. One format, utilized by the U.S. Department of Health and Human Services, AHCPR Clinical Practice Guidelines (1994), was reviewed. Although this guideline has been used as a rating for interventions, the model for describing the type of evidence (types of studies or reports) and rating the strength and consistency of the evidence was suggested as a key component of the process. Each work group had a recorder, who was a doctoral student, to document discussion and to facilitate the group work. A summary of the reports prepared by each group was presented in a general session on April 24, 1998.

During the sessions the groups also made recommendations to facilitate the processes of future work group preparation and sessions. These recommendations included:

- maintain standing groups to continue work on diagnoses of their interest
- develop mechanism for diagnostic interest groups to maintain communication, e.g., utilize e-mail. (One group at the session established an e-mail list).
- identify future work group diagnostic areas at the end of the conference to allow at least 6 months to 1 year for preparation and literature review for the next conference.
- continue to invite experts to participate and develop mechanisms (e.g., e-mail or mail) for their participation if unable to attend conference.
- encourage and facilitate work groups who want to work locally on a diagnostic area and then submit their work to the work group convening at the conference.
- include international participants in the work groups. (Three of the four groups had international members and their contributions were very helpful in identifying translation problems and clarifying meaning).

The following reports are a summary of the work and recommendations of the four work groups convened at the 1998 NANDA conference. We would like to thank all the participants for their interest and enthusiasm, the volunteer recorders (listed by work group), Anne Perry, the coordinator of the volunteers, and Eileen Gebbie for her assistance.

References

North American Nursing Diagnosis Association. (1996). *NANDA Nursing diagnoses: Definitions and classification 1997-1998* (pp. 92-93). Philadelphia: Author.

U.S. Department of Health and Human Services, Public Health Service, Agency for Health Care Policy and Research. (1994, March). *Management of cancer pain: Clinical practice guideline*, Number 9 (p225). Rockville, MD: Author

Altered Thought Process

Rose Harvey, DNSc, RN

Peggy McComb

Dorcas McLaughlin, MSN, RN, CS, CID

Mary Moorhouse, RN, CRRN

Lina Rahal, MEd, BSCN

Nancy Semenza, MSN, RN

Asta Thoroddsen

Catherine Hancock, MS, RN, CS

Recommendations for Altered Thought Process

1. Continue to consider and develop four subcategories recommended by NANDA Work Group, 1994, (see 11th Conference Proceedings): distorted thought process, cognitive impairment, altered level of consciousness, acute confusion.
2. Support recommendations and research by Hancock (1998, 1994) for development of more specific nursing diagnoses to replace altered thought processes, which was critiqued as being too general.

Distorted Thought

Taxonomy:

°Recommend Change: 5.2 Cognition

                      5.2.4 Distorted Thought

   (°per proposed Taxonomy 2)

Recommended Definition:

A state in which a person expresses or reports fixed false individually held beliefs or experiences inconsistent with reality.

Defining Characteristics (As evidenced by):

The following recommendations of the NANDA Work Group, 1994, were supported:°

    Delusions

    Hallucinations

    Ideas of reference

    Magical thinking

    Obsession

    Thought insertion

    Distorted memory

    Egocentricity

    Loosening of association

    Thought broadcasting

Other characteristics for consideration:

    Illusions

    Bizarre behaviors

    °Not yet able to divide into major versus minor without research base.

Related factors:

Not yet identified until research based literature is reviewed.

Cognitive Impairment, Altered Levels of Consciousness, Acute Confusion

Not reviewed.

Comments/Concerns:

1. Current knowledge based on research in the area of psychoneurobiology supports distorted thought as a cognitive domain.
2. A group should be convened to directly address research based articles concerning distorted thought with the objective of identifying major and minor defining characteristics as well as related factors.
3. Additional diagnostic categories need to be formulated to address a) level of consciousness and b) attention. This would assist in addressing a more holistic perspective.
4. Another option is to have Impaired Cognition as an overriding diagnosis (such as elimination) with more specific diagnoses beneath this.
5. Build on work of the NANDA Taxonomy Committee, Taxonomy 2, proposed for discussion/vote at this conference. If the proposed Taxonomy 2 does not become an accepted framework, we recommend retaining Altered Thought Processes, but raising it to a second order category header at _________, with Distorted Thought to follow at the next level as a nursing diagnosis.

For example: 8. _________Altered Thought Process

8. _________ _________Distorted Thought

6. Need to identify research resources outside the psychiatric nursing area.

References

Berry, K. (1987). Let's create diagnoses psych nurses can use. *American Journal of Nursing, 87,* 707-708.

Bondy, K., Maas, M., & McCourt, A. (1995). Altered thought process. In M.J. Rantz and P. LeMone (Eds.). *Classification of nursing diagnoses: Proceeding of eleventh conference* (pp.401-404). Glendale, CA: CINAHL Information Systems.

Hancock, C.K., Munjas, B., Berry, K., & Jones, J. (1994). Altered thought processes and sensory perceptual alterations: A critique. *Nursing Diagnosis, 5,* 26-30.

Other References:

Hancock, C.K. (1998) Personal communication. Letter to discussion group of recommendations and comments.

North American Nursing Diagnosis Association. (1998). Taxonomy 2 (proposed), Taxonomy Committee. Unpublished manuscript.

Caregiver Role Strain

Marga Simon Coler, EdD, RN, CS, CTN, FAAN
Martha Craft-Rosenberg, PhD, RN, FAAN
Susan Hinck, MSN, RN
Cibele Pimenta, RN, PhD
Patricia Potter, MSN, RN
Danielle Schmouth, MED, BScN

Recommendations for Caregiver Role Strain

1. Revise the definition of caregiver role strain in order to resolve translation difficulties and to eliminate the construct label from the definition.
2. Conceptualize caregiver role strain to include both informal as well as professional caregivers. As a result the utilization of family caregiver terminology should be excluded.

Caregiver Role Strain

Recommended Definition:

A subjective experience or exhibited difficulty in providing care and/or services to a care receiver.

Recommended Defining Characteristics:

The following defining characteristics are based upon the work groups' literature review and discussion:

fatigue (18)°
conflicting expectations regarding
role performance (6)
frustration (9) (G,CV)#
feeling stress (1)
guilt (McFarland)
difficulty in meeting role
obligations (9) (G, CV)
tension (9) (G, CV)
anxiety (9) (G, CV))
competing role commitments (4)
decrease in self esteem (10)
emotional liability (18)
anger (feeling of being manipulated
interpreted as anger) (2)
apprehension about the future of care
receivers health (18)
apprehension about care receivers care
when caregiver is ill or deceased (18)
apprehension about possible
institutionalization of care receiver
(18)
unrealistic expectations of caregiver by
care receiver (18)
depression (15)

Recommended Related Factors:

willingness of caregiver/care receiver to accept help from an outside caregiver (McFarland,17)

perception of crisis situation by caregiver (17)

role conflict (2)

lack of resources (2)

mismatched expectations (2)

lack of knowledge about caregiving tasks (11)

amount of direct care required (4)

deviance from role expectations (6)

lack of mutuality (reciprocity?) between caregiver and care receiver (2,4)

economic burden (2) lack of preparedness of caregiver (2,4)

(*See References)

(#G=Other Research Methods; CV=Construct Validity)

A revised list of defining characteristics and related factors was drawn from a review of literature. A cross comparison with the previous NANDA list of defining characteristics and related factors was not made.

Relevant issues to consider in further development:

1. Does role strain differ across the different populations who provide care, i.e. spouse, adult children, parents of children, and nurses?

2. Is the experience of caregiver role strain the same for caregivers of elderly and caregivers of ill children?

3. Defining characteristics of role strain may vary by the acuity of burden/stress. For example, acute role strain may exhibit more psychological stress and chronic role strain may exhibit more physical stress.

4. Proposed defining characteristics need further review research and cross comparison with current characteristics.

References

Aneshensel, C., Pearlin, L., & Schuler, R. (1993). Stress, role captivity, and the cessation of caregiving. *J Health Soc Behav, 34*, 54-70.

Archbold, P., Stewart, B., Greenlick, M., & Harvath, T. (1990). Mutuality and preparedness as predictors of caregiver role strain. *Res Nurse Health, 13*, 375-84.

Burack-Weiss, A., (1995). The caregiver's memoir: A new look at family support. *Social Work, 40*, 391-396.

Bums, C., Archbold, P., Stewart, B., Shelton, K. (1993). New diagnosis: Caregiver role strain. *Nursing Diagnosis, 4*, 70-76.

Chen, M. (1977). Hypothesis on nurse role strain: Are knowledgeable patients necessarily pests in hospitals? *Med Care, 15*, 350-353.

Egeland, J., & Brown, J. (1988). Sex role stereotyping and role strain of male registered nurses. *Res Nurse Health, 1*, 2-16.

Goode, W. (1960). A theory of role strain. *American Sociological Review, 25*, 483-496.

Gates, M., & Lackey, N. (1998). Youngsters caring for adults with cancer. *Image: Journal of Nursing Scholarship, 30*, 11

Lengacher, C.A. (1993). Development and study of an instrument to measure role strain. *Journal of Nursing Education, 32*, 71-77.

Lengacher, C. (1993). Comparative analysis of role strain and self-esteem across academic programs. *Nursing Connections, 6*, 33-46.

Miller, G. (1976) Patient knowledge and nurse role strain in three hospital settings. *Med

Care, 14, 662-673.

Piscopo, B. (1994). Organizational climate, communication, and role strain in clinical nursing faculty. *J Prof Nurse. 10*, 113-119.

Russell, J., Hezel, L. (1994). Role analysis of the advanced practice nurse using the Neuman Health Care Systems Model as a framework. *Clinical Nurse Specialist. 8*, 215-220.

Schumacher, K, Stewart, B., & Archbold, P., (1998). Conceptualization and measurement of doing family caregiving well. *Image: Journal of Nursing Scholarship. 30*, 63-69.

Smith, J. (1979). Role stain of US nurse tutors. *Nurse Times. 75*, 521.

Vrabec, N. (1997). Literature review of social support and caregiver burden, 1980 to 1995. Image: *Journal of Nursing Scholarship. 29*, 383-388..

Other References:

Richard, N., Fortin, F., & Bonin, J-P. (1995). *Fardeau subjective et etat de sante des aidants naturels de personnes afteintes de troubles mentaux en situation de crise et de remission.* Universite de Montreal, Faculte des sciences infirmieres.

NDEC. *Nursing diagnosis extension and classification.* University of Iowa. Unpublished manuscript.

Altered Sexuality Patterns/Sexual Dysfunction

Marilynn Doegnes, RN, MA, CS, APN

Paul Wibbenmeyer, RN, BSN

Janice DeMasters, PhD (c),RN,CS

Kay Gaehle, PhD (c), RN

Recommendations for Altered Sexuality Patterns/Sexual Dysfunction

1. Further research review is needed to recommend other changes.
2. Clinical research needed to further refine and validate defining characteristics of the category and subcategories.
3. Further develop taxonomy under Pattern 3: Relating. Examine differentiation of sexual dysfunction and altered sexuality patterns. Examine placement of sexual dysfunction under altered role performance. Need development of subcategories for altered sexuality patterns.

Altered sexuality patterns

Taxonomy:

Taxonomy 1 R -Relating: Altered sexuality patterns 3.3*

(Diagnostic Division: Sexuality)

*Note: Differentiation between Sexual Dysfunction vs. Altered Sexuality Patterns. Group expressed concerns regarding the taxonomy and suggests that development is needed in assignment of the altered sexuality patterns to the Relating 3.3 category. Not all altered sexuality patterns can be placed into one diagnostic label at that level of abstraction in the taxonomy. Need further development of subcategories. A greater degree of specificity of diagnosis in necessary to be clinically useful.

Label:

No change recommended. Patterns suggests a dynamic on-going process which "altered sexuality" does not.

Definition:

No change recommended. Current definition supported: The state in which an individual expresses concern regarding her/his sexuality.

Defining Characteristics:

Major

Subjective Criteria:

Reported difficulties, limitations, or

"

changes in sexual behaviors or activity

Recommended Defining Characteristics:

Self-expression of alienation, loneliness, loss, powerlessness and/or anger

Difficulty in verbalizing sexual concerns

Change in interest in sexual activities

Self-expressed lack of knowledge of sexual information

(*See References, #1 (LeMone, 1993) for all four characteristics)

Objective criteria

None (diagnosis has a subjective focus).

(*See References for support in the literature).

Related factors:

No change:

Knowledge/skill deficit about alternative responses to health-related transitions, altered body function or structure, illness or medical treatment

Lack of privacy*

Impaired relationship with a significant other; lack of significant other*

(Difficult to observe; comes more from self-report than observation.)

Ineffective or absent role models

(Support in the literature, particularly in parenting literature — Dr. Tom Gordon).

Conflicts with sexual orientation or variant preferences*

(Social, cultural and religious context needs to be considered in this related factor.)

Recommend change in Related Factors:

Fear of unintended pregnancy or of acquiring a sexually transmitted disease*

(Unclear differentiation of intensity of the fear and focus on "unintended" pregnancy. Not clear, distinct, observable).

(*Literature support for the related factors, see References. Related factors were defined, clear, distinct, and observable, except as noted above).

Comments or concerns:

1. Current state of knowledge/research: The level of knowledge in nursing at this point is underdeveloped. There exists great potential for growth in understanding in this area. Nurses seldom assess actual or potential alterations of sexual patterns in their clients.

2. The concern is clarification, further development and differentiation in the taxonomy for Relating Pattern... Sexual dysfunction is subcategory of altered role performance. Altered sexuality patterns is at the same level as altered role performance and has no subcategories.

3. This diagnosis label should not include gender specificity. Gender specificity should occur at a low, clinically useful level of abstraction.

4. Recommendations for work group process: Convene work group at least 6 months prior to conference to allow lead time to review relevant research. Have access to health sciences libraries at meeting site. Encourage individuals who are unable to attend to participate through research review, bibliographies, and other means of communication.

References:

LeMone, P. (1993) Validation of the defining

characteristics of altered sexuality patterns, *Nursing Diagnosis 4*, 56-62.

LeMone, P., & Jones, D., (1997, July-September) Nursing assessment of altered sexuality: A review of salient factors and objective measures. *Nursing Diagnosis, 8,* 120-128.

LeMone, P., & Weber, J. (1995, April-June) Validating gender-specific defining characteristics of altered sexuality. *Nursing Diagnosis 6,* 64-69.

Medlar, R. (1998, Spring). *Sexuality and disability, 16*(1), Appendix A, 43-66.

Spiritual Distress

Heather Herdman, PhD, RN
Joanne M. Johnson, RNC, MSN
Audrey M. McLane, PhD, RN
Geralyn Meyer, PhD(c), RN, CS
Vivianne Saba, M. Sci. Info. (NM)
Rita Wunderlich, MSN, RN
Carol Smucker

Recommendations for Spiritual Distress

1. Recommendations for future research: Further studies across the lifespan. Need more studies on diverse populations (not only on cancer patients). Focus research on patient centered data (not just data collected from nurse survey).
2. Recommendations for Related Factors: Further studies needed to validate related factors. Consider inclusion of definition of related factors.

Spiritual Distress
Recommended Definition:

Disrupted sense of harmonious connectedness with all of life and the universe in which dimensions that transcend and empower the self have been disrupted.

(° See References: 6, 7, 13, 14)

Defining Characteristics:

All NANDA defining characteristics supported by two or three research studies with DCV scores of 0.5 or greater; except for Gallows Humor, supported by only one study.

(° See References: 5, 9, 12, 18)

There are 17 additional defining characteristics that were reported in at least one research study with DCV score of 0.5 or above.

(°See References: 9, 12, 18)

Recommendations for Changes in Defining Characteristics:

Use of humor that indicates spiritual need (gallows humor).

(Alternative: use of term "morbid humor,") (Change from: gallows humor.)

Anger toward guiding spirit/deity. (Change from: anger toward God.)

Verbalizes concerns about relationship with guiding spirit/deity. (Change from: verbalizes concerns about relationship with deity.)

Recommendations for Changes in Related Factors:

Related factors were edited and refined for clarity:
Challenged belief and value system; separation from support and/or cultural/religious ties; intense suffering; ethical/moral implication of therapy.

Recommendations for Staging:

Stage at 2.2, with possibility of 2.3 with access to other research studies.

References:

Dossey, B. et al. (1994). American Holistic Nurses Association. In R.M. Carroll-Johnson & M. Paquette. *Classification of nursing diagnoses: Proceedings of the tenth conference*, (pp. 160-167). Philadelphia: J.B. Lippincott.

Engebretson, J. (1996). Considerations in diagnosing in the spiritual domain. *Nursing Diagnosis, 7*, 100-107.

Fehring, R., & McLane, A. (1997). Functional health pattern: Value-Belief. In J.M. Thompson, et al., *Clinical nursing*, 4th ed., (pp. 1762-1766).

Hall, B.A. (1998). Patterns of spirituality in persons with advanced HIV disease. *Research in Nursing and Health, 21*, 143-153.

Hensley, L.D. (1994). Spiritual distress: A validation study. In R.M. Carroll-Johnson & M. Paquette. *Classification of nursing diagnoses: Proceedings of the tenth conference* (pp. 200-202). Philadelphia: J.B. Lippincott

Hungelman, J., et al. (1989). Development of the JAREL spiritual well-being scale. In R.M. Carroll-Johnson (Ed.). *Classification of nursing diagnoses: Proceedings of the eighth conference* (pp.393-398), Philadelphia: J.B. Lippincott Company.

Labun, E. (1988). Spiritual care: An element in nursing care planning. *Journal of Advanced Nursing, 13*, 314-320.

Mansen, T.J. (1993). The spiritual dimension of individuals: Concept development. *Nursing Diagnosis, 4*, 140-147.

McHolm, F. A. (1991). A nursing diagnosis validation study: Defining characteristics of spiritual distress. In R. M. Carroll-Johnson (Ed.). *Classification of nursing diagnosis: Proceedings of the ninth conference* (pp. 112-119). Philadelphia: J.B. Lippincott.

NANDA. (undated) *Category: Matters of spirituality. Original submission of "Spiritual Concerns" for consideration as a nursing diagnosis.*

NANDA Research Committee: C.M. Dougherty et al. (1993). Conceptual and Research-based validation of nursing diagnoses: 1950-1993. *Nursing Diagnosis,4*, 156-165.

Pehler, S. (1997). Children's spiritual response: Validation of the nursing diagnosis spiritual distress. *Nursing Diagnosis, 8*, 55-66.

Reed, P.G. (1992). An emerging paradigm for the investigation of spirituality in nursing. *Research in Nursing & Health, 15*, 349-357.

Smucker, C. (1995). A phenomenological description of the experience of spiritual distress. In M.J. Rantz & P. LeMone (Eds.). *Classification of nursing diagnoses: Proceedings of the eleventh conference* (pp. 136-149). Glendale, CA: CINAHL Information Systems.

Smucker, C. (1996, April-June). A phenomenological description of the experience of spiritual distress. *Nursing*

Diagnosis, 8, 81-91.

Stolte, K. (1994). Health-oriented nursing diagnoses: Development and use. In R.M. Carrol- Johnson & M. Paquette (Eds.). *Classification of nursing diagnoses. Proceedings of the tenth conference* (pp. 143-148). Philadelphia: J.B. Lippincott.

Sumner, C.H. (1998). Recognizing and responding to spiritual distress. *American Journal of Nursing, 98,* 26-3 1.

Weatherall, J., & Creason, N.S. (1987). Validation of the nursing diagnosis, spiritual distress. In A.M. McLane (Ed.). *Classification of nursing diagnoses: Proceedings of the seventh conference* (pp. 182-185). St. Louis: C.V. Mosby Company.

Wesorick, B. (1995). Consensual validation of interventions categorized by nursing diagnoses. In M. J. Rantz & P. LeMone (Eds.). *Classification of nursing diagnoses: Proceedings of the eleventh conference* (pp. 115-124). Glendale, CA: CINAHL Information Systems.

Younger, J.B.(1995). The alienation of the sufferer. *Advances in Nursing Science, 17* (4), 53-72.

Business of the Organization

Agenda of the NANDA General Assembly

Saturday, April 25, 1998, 2:30-4:00 PM
Marriott Pavilion Hotel, St. Louis, MO

I. Welcome
II. Establishment of a Quorum
III. Adoption of Agenda
IV. Adoption of Rules, Catherine Murphy
V. Approval of Business Meeting Minutes:
Saturday, April 13, 1996, Pittsburgh, PA
Meridean Maas, Secretary
VI. Report of the President, Judith Warren
VII. Report of the Treasurer, Sheila Sparks
VIII. Management Services Report,
Joseph Braden
IX. Standing Committee Reports
   A. Publications Committee,
Janet Weber
   B. International Affairs Committee,
Cecile Boisvert
   C. Membership Committee,
Gloria Antall
   D. Bylaws Committee, Susan Suchy
   E. Taxonomy Committee, Kay Avant
   F. DRC Committee, Marjory Gordon
   G. Nominating Committee,
Gail Davis
X. Old Business
   A. Report of the NANDA
Foundation, Dorothy Jones
   B. Other
XI. New Business
   A. The Hidden Pearl: The
Keystone, Judith Warren
   B. Other items from the membership
XII. Adjournment

NORTH AMERICAN NURSING DIAGNOSIS ASSOCIATION, 13th Biennial Conference, St. Louis, MO

Biennial Business Meeting Minutes, April 25, 1998

TOPIC	DISCUSSION	Action
President Warren called the meeting to order at 2:40 PM.		
Quorum		The president declared a quorum present.
		K. Avant moved the adoption of the agenda as printed. Seconded by Derry Ann Moritz. Motion Carried.
Minutes of 1996 Biennial Business Meeting		Audrey McLane moved that the minutes of the 1996 biennial business meeting be approved as printed and circulated with Jane Kelley's name corrected. Seconded by Helen Cox. Motion Carried.
President's Report	J. Warren moved the approval of the President's Report as written in the Book of Reports.	Motion adopted.
Report of the Treasurer	M. Briody requested more detailed information about the financial status of NANDA & asked that in the future a more detailed budget be provided in the book of reports. J. Braden provided information verbally about changes in accounting structure.	S. Sparks moved approval of the Treasurer's report presented in the book of reports with the appended remarks & material presented by the Treasurer during session. Seconded by K. Avant. Motion Carried.
	S. Sparks supplied more detail regarding NANDA's finances.	
Report of the NANDA Management Service	M. Briody requested that the detailed report from the Treasurer be provided to members. S. Sparks agreed to add the detailed report to the Treasurer's Report.	J. Braden to explore possibility. H. Cox moved approval of the Management Service Report as printed. Seconded by K. Avant. Motion Carried.
	Dorothea Jacob requested a 1-800 number be implemented.	

NORTH AMERICAN NURSING DIAGNOSIS ASSOCIATION, 13th Biennial Conference, St. Louis, MO

Biennial Business Meeting Minutes, April 25, 1998

TOPIC	DISCUSSION	Action
	The impending Web Page for NANDA was discussed. NDEC, research team at Iowa, discussed their Web Page. E-mail & FAX numbers are included in the membership list database if the information comes in.	Web page to be developed during the coming months and will be reviewed by the incoming Board of Directors. J. Braden to revise needed forms to include request for e-mail & Fax numbers.
Report of the Publication Committee	Correction noted in the report, "21 manuscripts received." According to contract with CINAHL for Proceedings, papers published in the Proceedings can also be submitted to a journal for publication.	Report approved with corrections.
Report of the International Committee	Funding received from Rockefeller Committee to convene nurse leaders in Bilagio, Italy to study cross-cultural violence.	Report approved.
Membership Committee Report	Report read from the podium. Investigating dual membership between NANDA and specialty nursing organizations. Will seek to publicize NANDA in specialty organization journals. Members encouraged to advertise for NANDA at ANA convention, e.g., wearing special 25th Anniversary pins.	Report approved.
By-Laws Committee Report	No activity during last 2 years.	As printed, By-Laws, p 26, Sec 3, "Treasurer is omitted and should be added"; p 28 "insert April 1996" at end of paragraph.
Report of the Diagnostic Review	C. Dougherty questioned the DRC process and the disposition of small group work and comments of discussion groups at the Conference.	Revision by small groups at previous Conference should have been reviewed and incorporated if appropriate.

NORTH AMERICAN NURSING DIAGNOSIS ASSOCIATION, 13th Biennial Conference, St. Louis, MO

Biennial Business Meeting Minutes, April 25, 1998

TOPIC	DISCUSSION	Action
	M. Gordon & J. Warren indicated that '94 small group work was included.	Lois Hoskins moved the Reports of Committees as printed & amended be accepted. Seconded by Sheila Sparks. Motion Carried.
	Concern was expressed by the Chair regarding impending time constraints and the need to adjust times of meeting to complete the business of the organization.	Lois Hoskins moved that the time of adjournment be changed to 4:45 PM. Seconded by Derry Moritz. Motion Carried. Meeting recessed at 4:45 pm.
Meeting reconvened 4/? at ??		Lois Hoskins moved to reorder the agenda and move to New Business. Seconded. Motion Carried with 1 abstention. (2/3 majority???)
New Business	Need for dialogue among members and for communication between committees discussed.	In the spirit of increasing dialogue among nurses internationally, Lynda Carpenito moved that the developers of the World Wide Web Nursing Diagnoses Forum be advised that: NANDA strongly endorses this Web site as a forum for discussion. Seconded by A. McLane. Motion Carried.
Process of review and approval of diagnoses and taxonomy	Discussion of members supported the need for Taxonomy II. J. Warren indicated that the Board will continue to discuss this. Taxonomy II in its current format has not been formally approved.	M. Lunney moved that this year's publication be held up until Taxonomy II can be included. Seconded. Motion Withdrawn by M. Lunney.
	J. Warren discussed the process in detail with the assembly, noting Board and membership authority as defined in the NANDA By-Laws.	Tina Kurkowski moved to amend the motion to include Domains and Classes in this year's publication. Motion to amend withdrawn by T. Kurkowski.

NORTH AMERICAN NURSING DIAGNOSIS ASSOCIATION, 13th Biennial Conference, St. Louis, MO

Biennial Business Meeting Minutes, April 25, 1998

TOPIC	DISCUSSION	Action
	It was noted that legal consul is available and is advising regarding copyright law. The question of the availability of legal advice regarding international publishing and copyright was raised.	Cecile Boesvert and the international affairs committee move to convey NANDA's concerns to ICN that the ownership of nursing language belongs to the worldwide nursing profession (not to computer vendors, publishing companies). Seconded by Ann Kelley. The motion passed by a vote of 37 to 32, with 12 abstentions.
		Marguerite Eleufors moved to amend the main motion by changing "ICN-P" to "nursing language" unless there is some licensing agreement that would preclude that. Seconded by Eleanor Borkowski. Amendment withdrawn.
Report of Taxonomy Committee	Membership discussed the need for Taxonomy II. Recognized that it was not perfect but "good enough" to help us move forward.	A. McLane moved the formal adoption of the proposed Taxonomy II, the multiaxial health pattern taxonomy, as proposed by the Taxonomy Committee. Seconded. Motion Carried.
		The question was called and passed 84 to 28 with one abstention. Motion Carried. 1 abstention.
		Meeting recessed by J. Warren at 4:30 PM.
J. Warren reconvened the 1998 biennial business meeting, 8:20 a.m. Election results	Those elected were announced by Eleanor Borkowski as follows: *President-Elect*: Kay Avant *Secretary*: Meridean Maas *Board Directors*: Marjorie Gordon, Mary Ann Lavin, Judith Warren	S. Sparks moved to accept the election results as stated. Seconded by G. Whitley. Motion Carried. S. Sparks moved to destroy the ballot. Second by H. Cox. Motion Carried.

NORTH AMERICAN NURSING DIAGNOSIS ASSOCIATION, 13th Biennial Conference, St. Louis, MO

Biennial Business Meeting Minutes, April 25, 1998

TOPIC	DISCUSSION	Action
	By-Laws Committee: Sylvia Weber *Diagnosis Review Committee*: Susan Chase, T. Heather Herdman *International*: Dickon Weir-Hughes *Membership*: Michael Bleich, Roberta Cavendish *Nominating*: Roberta Cavendish Victoria Cole Schonlau *Publication*: Jane Timm, Helen Harkreader *Taxonomy*: Lois Hoskins, M. Anne Woodtli	
Foundation Report	D. Jones discussed the success of the Foundation Gala on Friday, 4/24/98. Indicated approval of tax status and that the Board will formalize structure in coming year.	D. Jones moved to accept the report of the Foundation. Kay Avant Seconded. Motion Carried.
	It was encouraged that a forum on Web page for discussion of diagnosis review submissions.	
	Winnie Mills urged NANDA for the next Conference to consider ways to include members or persons from specialty organizations to be included in the program and work of NANDA and to give this a high priority. She also suggested that a memorial book be developed to recognize the contributions of persons who have contributed to NANDA and are no longer living.	

NORTH AMERICAN NURSING DIAGNOSIS ASSOCIATION, 13th Biennial Conference, St. Louis, MO

Biennial Business Meeting Minutes, April 25, 1998

TOPIC	DISCUSSION	Action
	Judy asked that an abstract of each Dx label be included in the Conference packet, including rationale, need. Also asked that Community Health nurses be included among specialty organizations that are asked to participate.	
	Dorothea Jacob suggested that in future conferences more time be allotted for the business meeting.	
	Cindy Dougherty asked the DRC to publish the entire and complete list of diagnoses submitted with the name of the submitter and all action taken to date. She asked that the process of decision and action by the DRC be explicated and disseminated.	Board to review all of the Membership recommendations in subsequent meetings.
	Stephanie Richardson recommended that NANDA take full advantage of the WWW to communicate information between NANDA Conferences, holding a forum on the Web page for discussion.	
Adjournment		Meeting adjourned at 9:30 am. Submitted by Meridean Maas, Secretary

Report of the President

Submitted by Judith J. Warren, President

I assumed the Presidency at the end of the Twelfth NANDA Conference for a two-year term. During this current conference we are celebrating the 25th Anniversary of NANDA and the accomplishments we have achieved together. At the end of this conference I will conclude my term and Dorothy Jones will become the new President and take NANDA into the new millennium, 2000 AD, another joyous celebration.

We have had several changes on the Board. Three members' terms expired in 1994: Margaret Briody, Mary Kerr, and Cindy Dougherty. Sheila Sparks was elected Treasurer and Helen Cox and Georgia Whitley were elected as Members of the Board for the term of 1996-2000. Joan Fitzmaurice resigned from the Board and the DRC Committee in August 1996. Per operating guidelines, Peggy Wetsch was appointed by the Board to finish her Board term. Ms. Wetsch, a member of the DRC Committee, was then appointed as the new DRC chairperson. In October, 1997, Ms. Wetsch also resigned. Since her term was to be completed this April, the Board chose not to appoint a replacement and appointed Marjory Gordon as chair of the DRC for the remaining portion of the term. The final composition of the Board, with new and continuing members, included Dorothy Jones, President-Elect; Sheila Sparks, Treasurer; Meridean Maas, Secretary; and as Directors: Kay Avant, Marjory Gordon, Helen Cox, and Georgia Whitley. I extend my heartfelt thanks to these members who have served on the Board during my Presidency.

Organizational Affairs

The Board met once during the 1996 conference in Pittsburgh. It has met five times since: August 1996, November 1996, July 1997, November 1997 (in conjunction with the NANDA, NIC, NOC Conference), and February 1998. During the August meeting the Board began developing a new strategic plan that will take the organization into the new millennium.

The Board continues to be satisfied with the services provided by Resource Management Plus (RMP), a subsidiary of Nursecom. The services of

(a) associations affairs and management plus (b) publishing support has provided us with the daily support and confidence for running our business and organization. They have sought sources of income through licenses and sales of the Taxonomy; provided guidance in publishing for the taxonomy book, the journal, and our proceedings; facilitated legal counsel to finalize the IRS approval of our Foundation; negotiated contracts for foreign language translations; and sought financial support for the conference and Foundation. NANDA, through RMP, has contracted to develop an Internet web site. The development of this web site will be a priority for the coming year. We do have an address, though nothing exists at the moment. Watch the Journal for the announcement of the implementation of "www.nanda.org". Finally, RMP sponsored a conference that brought together for the first time NANDA, NIC, and NOC. This very successful conference was held last November, 1997 and may be the beginning of a wonderful new venture. The Board expresses gratitude to Joseph Braden and his staff for their support and belief in us.

Two years ago, President Lois Hoskins reported that she had spent much of her Presidency ensuring the financial viability of NANDA. I am pleased to report that I received NANDA with a small positive balance and, through the efforts of the Board and RMP, have been able to increase the financial reserves of NANDA. The income has primarily come from the sales of the Taxonomy book, copyright fees, licensing agreements with software vendors, and translation rights. The income from membership dues is still low and needs to be improved. The Board continued to conserve expenses by sharing costs for their meetings. However, finances were sufficient to suppport one face-to-face meeting in November 1997 for the Board, the Taxonomy Committee, and the DRC. This face-to-face meeting greatly accelerated the work of the DRC and Taxonomy Committees. All other committees have worked by e-mail, telephone conferences, and regular mail. The commitment of these people to the success and work of NANDA is phenomenal and I want to acknowledge them all for their contributions that went far beyond what is reasonable to expect.

The DRC spent 1996 refining the processes of reviewing and recommending new and revised nursing diagoses. In 1997, they have been working closely with numerous submitters of new diagnoses. They also have reviewed the work submitted to them by NDEC (Nursing Diagnosis Extension and Classification research team who NANDA has contracted with for this work). The Taxonomy Committee has completed their work on evaluation of the current classification structure and is proposing an alternative structure at this conference.

The Publications Committee has been very busy. First, they have taken on the production of a special edition of the Journal to commemorate NANDA's 25th Anniversary. Second, they searched for and hired a new Editor for the Journal and changed the name of the journal to "Nursing Diagnosis: The Journal of Nursing Language and Classification." This new name emphasizes the new leadership role NANDA is taking in promoting the use and research of standardized languages. Finally, they continue to provide guidance to all publication efforts of NANDA.

Interorganizational Affairs

NANDA continues to be a member of NOLF (Nursing Organization Liaison Forum) in order to network with other specialty nursing organizations and to promote the development and use of nursing languages and classifications. NANDA collaborates closely with ANA and its Steering Committee on Databases Supporting Clinical Nursing Practice. The Steering Committee has included NANDA in several major lobbying efforts. First, as NANDA President, I received an invitation to testify before the National Committee on Vital and Health Statistics about the need for and use of nursing nomenclatures in patient data sets used by HCFA. A copy of my report is appended. Second, NANDA was asked to submit a report to the ANSI-HISB (American National Standards Institute-Healthcare Informatics Standards Board) to be included in their compilation of standards to submit to the Department of Health and Human Services. This compilation will be used to set policy and regulations for the implementation of the Health Insurance Portability and Accountability Act of 1996 which requires that HCFA use standards. A copy of my report is appended. I have also been asked to present information about NANDA at the American Academy of Nursing in 1997, the American Medical Informatics Association in 1996 and 1997, and the ANA 1997 Convention. With the advent of computer-based patient records the need for standardized language has been a necessity in healthcare.

International Affairs

At the last NANDA conference it was stated that interest in nursing diagnosis on an international basis was burgeoning. At this conference I can report that interest is now exploding. In 1996, NANDA presented a panel at the International Council of Nursing. The room was packed and the dialogue was fabulous. We found an empty room and hosted "A Conversation about Nursing Diagnosis and International Collaboration." Again the room was packed and the discussion lasted a couple of hours. As a result, ACENDIO and NANDA will exchange institutional memberships and we are exploring a similar relationship with ATENDE (the Spanish nursing diagnosis association). NANDA continues to dialogue with the International Classification for Nursing Practice team from ICN. This has been a very fruitful experience.

Conclusion

During the past two years I have been privileged to serve as your President and to work with the NANDA Board and a group of nurses dedicated to nursing diagnosis and willing to commit extensively of their time and other personal resources. I am deeply grateful for the opportunity and their support. I also thank the committee members who have worked productively under fiscal restraint.

I thank all of those who have offered sponsorships, auction gifts, and monetary donations to this conference, and those who have committed funds to the Foundation. I thank RMP for their unfailing support during good times and times of challenge for both them and the Board.

Finally, I thank you, the membership, the heart of NANDA, for trusting me with the resources and future of NANDA for the last two years. It has been an experience I will never forget!

President's Report Appendix

NORTH AMERICAN NURSING
DIAGNOSIS ASSOCIATION TESTIMONY
by Judith J. Warren, PhD, RN, FAAN, President
NCVHS Hearing on Clinical Coding and
Classification Issues

Thank you for inviting NANDA to give testimony at this hearing from the perspective of a classification developer. NANDA began its work

24 years ago when a group of nurses met to develop a vocabulary that captured nursing's contribution to patient care and was coded to enable computerization. A nursing diagnosis is a clinical judgment about individual, family, or community responses to actual and potential health problems and/or life processes. Nursing diagnoses provide the basis for selection of nursing interventions to achieve outcomes for which the nurse is accountable (NANDA, 1990). There have been twelve biannual conferences where the membership has approved additions to the NANDA Nursing Diagnosis Taxonomy (1996). Though a consensus process is used and the membership provides major input to the development and acceptance of a new nursing diagnosis, the criteria for inclusion are stringent. The new diagnosis must be research and/or evidenced based. NANDA developed a staging system, based on the DSM 4 system, to facilitate the development and maintenance of the Taxonomy. NANDA was the first nursing classification to be recognized by the American Nurses Association.

The following are the questions I was asked to address:

1. What clinical codes and classifications do you use in administrative transactions now? What do you perceive as the main strengths and weaknesses? Of current methods for coding and classification of encounter and/or enrollment data?

Nursing has never had clinical codes used in administrative transactions. This has been a major problem in nursing. The charges for nursing care have always been embedded in room charges or some other charge, i.e., physician service. Therefore, a major resource in our health care system has never been captured so that impact to the system can be projected. Many policy analysts believe this contributes to the various rounds of nurse shortages and overages (the pendulum must swing widely since there is no statistical way to predict need). Recently, advanced practice nurses who have a master's degree (nurse practitioner, clinical nurse specialist, nurse midwife, and nurse anesthetist) have achieved the ability to charge for service. They use CPT 4 codes. ANA has lobbied the AMA for many years and now has advanced practice nurses sitting on CPT panels. However, 80-90% of the nurses in this country have no administrative codes that cover their practice. The impact of nursing care on patient care is enormous, yet our administrative codes fail to capture this contribution to patient outcomes. Several major studies have demonstrated that they can predict allocation of resources and patient outcomes when nursing care is factored in (Halloran; Knaus [APACHE]).

2. What clinical codes and classifications do you recommend as initial standards for administrative transactions, given the time frames in the HIPAA? What specific suggestions would you like to see implemented regarding coding and classification?

NANDA is a "niche" classification, designed to capture the conditions for which nursing is accountable to treat. As such, we have been collaborating with other classifications to produce more comprehensive codes for health care. We have been working with the editors of SNOMED International and have placed nursing diagnoses in the Functional Axis. In two recent coding studies conducted by the CPRI (in which I participated) the addition of NANDA to SNOMED significantly strengthened its performance in capturing data from patient records. Those classifications which did not have nursing content — ICD-9-CM and CPT 4 — performed at a significantly less capability.

Since nursing does not participate in coding, we have no recommendations for

implementation. However, NANDA is in every nursing textbook, taught in our schools, and is throughout our licensing exams, nurses know the terms and can select them rapidly from a code list.

3. Prior to the passage of HIPAA, the National Center for Health Statistics initiated development of a clinical modification of ICD-10 (ICD-10-CM), and the HCFA undertook development of a new procedure coding system for inpatient procedures (called lCD-10-PCS), with a plan to implement them simultaneously in the year 2000. On the pre-HIPAA schedule, they will be released to the field for evaluation and testing by 1998. If some version of ICD is to be used for administrative transactions, do you think it should be ICD-9-CM or ICD-10-CM and ICD-10-PCS, assuming that field evaluations are generally positive?

NANDA has looked at ICD-10 (proposals for both ICD-10-CM and ICD-10-PCS) and is in favor of using it since it codes more human-level conditions, not just disease or organ-level content. Nursing diagnoses treat human responses to health conditions, not the disease conditions. ICD-10 supports this view. When ICD-10 was being developed, NANDA submitted its work for inclusion and even developed a translation of our work into ICD-10 code format. This work was not accepted as only the International Council of Nursing could submit work to the WHO. Only the

ANA could submit work to the ICN, and this work was done prior to ANA recognition of NANDA's work. Since then the ANA and NANDA have developed close working relationships. However, the ICN has decided to create its own classification, the International Classification of Nursing Practice. The team producing this work is European, and while Americans participate, they are not leaders. NANDA has offered assistance to this group. As a result of our willingness to collaborate, we have become, along with the ANA, reviewers of this work. I will be meeting with this team in a few weeks to discuss issues of coding approaches.

While many are in favor of initially keeping ICD-9-CM and CPT 4 due to implementation readiness and the short-time frame, that reluctance to change will always be there. If practicality forces that decision and it is known that the ICD-10 will replace the ICD-9-CM and the CPT 4, that announcement with a tentative time line for implementation must be released as soon as possible. The health care industry must know that the change is coming or it will always be put off and fought against. Worse yet, resources will be used to develop new classifications instead of being used to collaboratively develop the ICD-10-CM and ICD-10-PCS.

4. Recognizing that the goal of HIPAA is administrative simplification, how, from your perspective, would you deal with the current coding environment to improve simplification, reduce administrative burden, but also obtain clinically meaningful information?

NANDA supports the migration to the CPR as rapidly as possible. In my own institution, I am co-chair of a team to develop and implement a computerized, multidisciplinary problem list. The clinician will select from a list of problems the appropriate problem to add to the patient's record. This list is already mapped to the ICD-9-CM, SNOMED, NANDA, and UMLS. Our billing office is also involved in this project to insure that administrative transactions are assured. In this way, clinical need for data are met as well as administrative needs.

5. How should ongoing maintenance of code sets and the responsibility, intellectual input and funding of maintenance be addressed for the classification systems included in the standards? What are the arguments for having these systems in the public domain versus the private sector, with or without copyright?

NANDA supports a modification of the public domain system. Our system is copyrighted. Royalties are collected from publishers and other vendors who use our work to develop products that are sold for profit. This income is used to find the ongoing development and maintenance of NANDA since there is no other current source of money for this work. Clinicians may use the work by requesting permission for use, but there is no fee. We want the work used. The copyright allows us quality and version control. We and other groups publish textbooks and manuals for using the NANDA Taxonomy as other sources of income to support the work.

We have problems with proprietary systems that are a major source of income for an organization and that are required for use by the federal government and other payers. The classification should be copyrighted but be free to users. Money to support development should result from sales of tools and educational products concerning the use of the classification or the funding should come from a government/private sector collaboration.

6. What would be the resource implications of changing from the coding and classification systems that you currently are using in administrative transactions to other systems? How do you weigh the costs and benefits of making such changes?

As a developer, NANDA would need to re-evaluate its strategic plan and budget. We have several collaborative projects underway with the ICN, SNOMED, the ANA, the UMLS, and three research teams at the University of Iowa (Nursing Diagnosis Extension Project, the Nursing Intervention Classification, and the Nursing Outcome Classification) that would need to be reconsidered. However, we are deeply committed to serving the data and information needs of the nursing profession and will work collaboratively to achieve that goal. We believe that as these systems capture more clinical variance to facilitate control over the process and outcomes of care, health care costs will decrease and this will offset any start-up costs or costs of changing systems. We are also collaborating with the American Medical Informatics Associationís Nursing Specialty Group to hold an invitational conference at the end of May 1997 to assess the state of the art of nursing classification devopment and to make recommendations for future work. I will send a conference summary to you the first of June.

7. A Coding and Classification Implementation Team has been established within the DHHS to address the requirements of HIPPA. Does your organization have any concerns about the process being undertaken by DHHS to carry the law in regard to coding and classification issues? If so, what are those concerns and what suggestions do you have for improvements? We have no concerns about

the process. At this time, the Department seems to be listening to all the stakeholders for which we are very pleased. We plan on monitoring the process and are willing to provide whatever assistance we can to this process. We see this activity as a major way to standardize health care data, both administrative and clinical, which will improve the quality of care and hopefully reduce its costs.

We do caution the Committee to be aware of the implications of word use. Please be concerned about the health care community, not just the medical community, and about health care in this country, not just medical care. We have become a country that is concerned about wellness and health promotion, not just disease and disease prevention. Let us strive to develop codes and classifications that reflect the needs of the country.

Additional questions for NCVHS Hearing on Coding and Classification Systems:

1. Can one system serve most if not all purposes e.g, clinical care, surveillance, quality assessment/improvement, clinical research, billing/management? If not, which systems can serve most of these functions?

No one current system can serve all needs. NANDA supports mapping efforts between systems if the owners of the systems allow that to occur. We are currently working with UMLS, SNOMED, and the ICN to develop mappings between our systems. These organizations are willing to collaborate. We do not have access to work with WHO on any ICD project but would if it were possible.

2. Is it administratively simpler to use same disease classification for administrative and statistical reporting?

Not for nursing data, since we do not treat disease but the human response to it. Statistical reporting, if I understand what that means, must include clinical data; administrative data is skewed to the billing process and does not accurately reflect clinical data. Nursing is not represented in any administrative system. We have worked with Werley as she developed the Nursing Minimum Data Set (NMDS), of which nursing diagnosis is one data element and NANDA is a set of appropriate values, and we have worked with the American Organization of Nurse Executives to create the Nursing Management Minimum Data Set which captures workload and work force data to be used with the NMDS. Again, whatever classification system(s) is used must include nursing diagnoses and nursing interventions.

3. To what extent do you feel that your discipline and practice setting are well represented by the current systems for coding health conditions, diagnoses, services and procedures in administrative and financial transactions?

Nursing is invisible in the current systems, yet significantly influences patient care and outcomes. The only way to capture this influence is through research which is very expensive to conduct. The National Institute of Nursing Research in NIH no longer funds this type of research, nor do they fund classification development research.

4. What issues do you encounter linking data coded with different classification systems and trying to crosswalk between (or among) classification systems?

NANDA has participated in several projects. A previous president assisted the NLM in adding and cross walking NANDA into the UMLS which required mapping to the Home Health Care Classification and the Omaha System (two other ANA recognized nursing diagnosis classifications) and I have been working with one of the editors of SNOMED to do the same thing (including mapping the fourth ANA recognized classification, Nursing Intervention Classification). In the first project a set of filters was developed that facilitated an accurate mapping. These were used to facilitate mapping in SNOMED but using their rules of classification, not UML's rules. We are still working on developing the filter or other approach to cross walking the interventions.

The major issue in cross walking between a medical and a nursing classification is the issue of disease versus human response. The nursing diagnosis of Pain is classified as a symptom in SNOMED; however, the scope of treatments between the medical and nursing clinicians is different. Mapping between different scopes of practice is like mapping behaviors between different cultures — it can lead to great misunderstandings. You need experts from each discipline that are open to understanding and learning about the classifications in the other disciplines.

5. What are the impact on and implications for current (and emerging) medical/clinical classifications as we migrate towards computer-based patient records (CPR)? To what extent can the major classification systems currently in use serve, in part, as vocabulary for the CPR, and if another system is recommended as the vocabulary for the CPR, how can we assure that it crosswalks relatively easily to the classification systems currently used in

administrative and financial transactions?

It is very difficult to change codes and the database structure for the codes. We must design structures that facilitate ease of changing codes (because that will be a fact of life as health care science and knowledge evolves). However, as migration occurs to a CPR, the computer can provide the code (unseen to the user) when the clinician directly enters the patient's diagnosis and interventions/orders. As a result of the two CPRI studies, a recommendation was made that SNOMED was an excellent clinical classification and could be used to provide decision support to the clinician. UMLS can also be mapped to the clinical data and thus provide bibliographic retrieval support for the clinician by organizing literature and information searches around the actual patient data in question. These and other advantages have all been noted in the Institute of Medicine's report on the computer-based patient record. NANDA fully endorses this report and vision of the CPR. The CPR can support nursing classifications and make visible nursing's contribution to patient care and outcomes. One note of caution that NANDA would give to other developers, since we have committed the error ourselves, concerns the development of code structures for the classification systems. There are two issues about coding: 1) ease of the human user and 2) ease of the machine user. Coding is the abstract representation of a concept. Classification is commonly used to reveal the relationships between concepts. When a human user is considered, classification trees reveal these relationships in a pictorial way that can be readily grasped and understood. A code can be developed that represents the location of each concept within the classification. The problem begins when the basic understanding of the classification system changes or evolves to include new relationships or the creation of different relationships. The classification trees must change to help the human understand the new relationships. Therefore, the code structure must also change as it encodes information about the concepts. For humans we can provide new understandings and map the changes from the old to the new even though the mapping is not a precise translation of the new location/relationship of the concept. A machine user cannot "understand" this new relationship unless it is a one-for-one change (which rarely occurs in the world). Changes are usually "kaleidoscopic" in nature — same elements, very different patterns and relationships. Therefore, codes for the machine user need to be without meaning or random. Only the concept is coded not the relationships or locations in the classification systems. The humans may change the classification system (relationships with other concepts) without changing the identification of the concept. Classification trees assist human understanding and confound machine handling of the concept. As developers of classification systems, we should code concepts for the ease of the user. Today the user is a machine. The quantity of information has grown too large for a human to remember and/or manipulate. A machine does this very well. Humans manipulate large quantities of information with metaphors or models — machines cannot. Therefore codes should have no information about the classification model encoded in them. NANDA after consultation with the NLM, recommends a multi-digit (alphanumeric) code (for machine use only) as the true code for the concept and a conceptual model to communicate the concept relationships to the human user. To rephrase, as long as a concept keeps the same code and codes are not reused when concepts are deleted, how we display NANDA to nurses/humans may

change over time without having to completely recode and handle mapping of same concepts from one version to another. Secondarily codes without meaning will facilitate different cultural views or relationships of the same concepts so that all nurses can use NANDA and share data about the concepts (which are language neutral, much like the GALEN project) while exploring how relationships are the same and/or different.

A final note of concern as more of health care migrates to the home and families become the major caregivers, they will need a language to document the observations and care they deliver. As our health care system evolves, we must make sure that all care providers, whether professional or family, contribute to the documentation of clinical care and the resources given to support that care. Without a doubt, a traditional clinical classification filled with professional jargon will not serve this group of care givers. The CPR has a goal of becoming a life long record across many sites. Let us not forget to consider these sites that are not hospital or clinic based.

6. For presenters recommending a particular coding or classification system what is the market acceptance for the system and current scope of use? What are mechanisms for low cost distribution?

NANDA is widely used in schools of nursing, by all major textbook publishers, and numerous hospitals and other sites of practice. We actively encourage all nurses to submit candidate nursing diagnoses for the ongoing development of the NANDA Taxonomy. The ANA has recognized NANDA as the nursing organization responsible for developing and maintaining a nursing diagnosis classification. We are a member of the Nursing Organizations Liaison Forum which brings together all the nursing speciality organizations to address common concerns. A major concern is the classification of nursing phenomena and the creation of clinical guidelines. As a result, the specificity of some of our diagnoses is developing and the flow of new diagnostic submissions is growing.

NANDA does not charge a fee for using the Taxonomy in schools of nursing or facilities that provide nursing care. We require permission for use so that we can ensure quality and version control. Only organizations that use the Taxonomy in the development of a product that generates income/profit for that organization must pay royalty fees.

7. How might NCVMS work with DHHS to assure that the USA coordinates development of an international medical dictionary, classification/coding system, etc., including the terms, a process to keep continuously such terminology updated, and a server to deliver the content to whoever needs access?

Any international effort should be coordinated through WHO. It is arrogant to think that the United States should coordinate an international medical system. This approach did not work for nursing. NANDA strongly supports that all discussion concerning coding and classification be focused on clinical systems not just medical. There is discussion of the formation of a new International Standards Organization (ISO) committee. NCVHS and the DHHS might join the ANSI-HISB (American National Standards Institute-Health Information Standards Board) effort to become sponsors of this ISO committee and that way provide leadership in this effort — this will require money and resources.

8. Is it practical to move to a single procedure classification system on the timetable required for initial implementation of administrative standards or should the standards continue the current practice of requiring different procedure coding systems for the ambulatory and inpatient sectors?

It is practical only if the procedures of all disciplines are included, not just the ones that currently receive reimbursement. Also, one discipline must not be in control of the entire system and make a profit on the sales of that classification system. Development and maintenance must be multidisciplinary.

9. If a clinical code set or classification system is selected as a standard, should providers be able to use all the available codes within the set or system or should those requiring the information (e.g., payers) be allowed to restrict reporting of certain codes?

NANDA supports the clinician being able to accurately describe and code the care given. They should not be forced to use Procrustean measures that distort the work in order to be reimbursed for their work. The implications of this question are enormous. The ANA published a monograph (Zielstorff, R.D., Hudgings, C.I., & Grobe, S.J. (1993). Next-generation nursing information systems: Essential characteristics for professional practice.) that described a data pyramid. At the bottom was accurate clinical data. At the top the data had been abstracted, coded, and summarized for policy makers to use. This data no longer represents the actual clinical conditions but only those that administrative transactions allow. Yet the United States determines public policy and laws based on that flawed data as if it is accurately represented the health of our country.

NANDA Nursing Diagnosis Taxonomy (submission to ANSI-HISB Compilation of Healthcare Standards)

I.   **Name of the code set including the associated vocabulary. Include the version, if available.**
NANDA Nursing Diagnosis Taxonomy, revised

II.   **Name of the Development organization**
North American Nursing Diagnosis Association
1211 Locust St.
Philadelphia, PA 19107

III.   **Status of ANSI accreditation. Indicate one of the following: ANSI accredited, ANSI accreditation applied for, or not ANSI accredited.**
This taxonomy is not ANSI accredited

IV.   **Description of the code set/vocabulary. Include separate statements for:**
Though not ANSI accredited, NANDA has been officially recognized by the American Nurses Association as an appropriate nursing terminology to use in documentation of care. The taxonomy is a registered trademark owned and copyrighted by the North American Nursing Diagnosis Association. The organization is involved in developing a standardized nursing diagnosis vocabulary and taxonomy but is not involved in standards development.

Purpose or objective (for example, patient care, decision support, integration of data across systems, research, and so forth).
NANDA Taxonomy is recognized throughout the world as a classification of the conditions that nurses diagnose and treat. A nursing diagnosis is defined as "clinical judgment about individual, family, or community responses to actual or problems/life processes. Nursing diagnoses provide the basis for selection of nursing interventions to achieve outcomes for which the nurse is accountable" (NANDA, 1990).

Type of code set (for example, vocabulary, classification system, knowledge representation, and so forth).
This is a taxonomy (classification) of nursing diagnoses. Each diagnosis has a definition, defining characteristics (similar to signs and symptoms), risk factors if appropriate, and etiologies.

Clinical topics addressed (for example, anatomy, diseases, procedures, results, and so forth).
The classification framework is comprised of nine patterns of human responses to health and illness. The diagnosis and treatment of human responses to health and illness have been defined by the American Nurses Association to be the scope of practice for nursing in the USA (ANA, 1991, 1997). Under these nine patterns there is a structure in which to classify each diagnosis and give it a unique code number.

Domain focus (for example, general medicine, surgery, emergency care, home health, and so forth).
The domain focus is for nursing practice only across all specialties and practice sites and across the continuum of care.

How often is this code set updated or

enhanced?

The Taxonomy is updated every two years.

How are these updates or enhancements distributed?

The revision announcement is sent to NANDA members and all major health care publishers, published in NANDA's journal, and published by NANDA as a monograph.

What is the source of funding for these updates or enhancements?

The NANDA membership dues and other income (conference fees and publications) support the majority of this work. Individual members donate their work on specific diagnoses and their time.

Are there regular user group meetings? If so, how frequently do they meet?

NANDA has a conference every two years. This conference is open to members and nonmembers.

Is the code set/vocabulary copyrighted?

Yes, by the organization.

Does the License allow derivative works, such as the creation of a database?

Yes, each license is negotiated to provide flexibility in this area.

Other relevant characteristics such as are terms coded in a fixed structure, does it support synonyms, is it concept-oriented (that is, do codes correspond to meanings), does it include multiple hierarchies, and so forth).

It is a hierarchal classification; it does not support synonyms; it is concept-oriented; there is a defined code structure. Under the nine patterns of the taxono-

my there is a structure in which to classify each diagnosis and give it a unique code number.

How is this code set different from or superior to others that it may compete with.

This code set is specific to nursing and to nursing diagnoses. It was the first nursing classification to be developed and most others have based their work on this early development. The only other ANA recognized classifications to have nursing diagnoses in them have been developed for specific sites of care: home health (Home Health Care Classification) and community health (Omaha System). NANDA can be used in all settings.

V.   Readiness of the code set/vocabulary. Include the following:

What portions of the code set are complete and implementable now?

The entire set is ready for implementation when it is published.

What portions or versions are under development?

There are always new diagnosis submissions under review, but these are not released until they are ready for implementation.

When will these new portions or versions be published or available?

The new portions/versions are published every two years.

How do users obtain the code set?

They contact the NANDA office for a copy or they may find a copy in the numerous nursing textbooks that publish NANDA's work. NANDA publishes the Taxonomy in: Nursing Diagnoses: Definitions & Classification (NANDA), 1997-1998.

What tools are available (for example, encoders, browsers, translators, modeling tools, maintenance tools, and so forth)?

At present, none are available. An electronic database and browser are under development by NANDA.

What organizations develop and maintain each of these tools?

An electronic database and browser are under development by NANDA.

Which of these tools is provided with the code set?

It is anticipated that these tools will be sold separately in order to support the development of the Taxonomy.

What tools are required that are not provided with the code set?

None.

If the tool is not provided, how is it acquired?

N/A

Is a user guide available?

N/A

Is the user guide approved by the development organization?

N/A

Are there any other indicators of readiness that may be appropriate?

NANDA is the oldest nursing taxonomy in the profession. The first versionwas published in 1973.

VI.   Indicators of market acceptance of the code set/vocabulary. Include the following:

What number or percentage of relevant vendors have adopted it?

Since nursing care is not reimbursable, vendors have been very slow to incorporate nursing vocabularies. With the implementation of HIPAA this is beginning to change. However, Ergo Inc., Cerner Corporation, HealthMaster, CINAHL, and Health Sciences Consortium have licenses to incorportate NANDA into their electronic systems. Most of the other major vendors have fields available for each institution to insert a nursing diagnosis or they have starters sets that are small enough not to require a copyright fee.

What number or percentage of healthcare institutions use it?

This is difficult to determine. NANDA does not charge a copyright fee for institutional use (we charge only for derivative work). JCAHO does recommend in their accreditation criteria that using NANDA is one way to meet documentation and care planning criteria in nursing. Kaiser-Permanente has permission to use the Taxonomy internally throughout their system without a fee. University of Nebraska and University of Iowa Medical Centers use NANDA in their computer-based patient records (others may also use it, but these two institutions regularly publish their experiences).

What number or percentage of health professional societies refer to it?

ANA recognizes it as one of five recognized nursing classifications. NANDA is also a member of the Nursing Organization Liaison Forum (NOLF) which has over 75 nursing organizations as members. We have received diagnoses submissions from several of these organizations.

What number or percentage of government agencies use it or refer to it?

The DOD and VA use NANDA in their care planning tools. NCVHS has asked NANDA to testify as to its usability as code sets are being considered under the HIPAA legislation.

Is the code set being used in other countries? If so, which ones?

NANDA has been translated into French, Dutch, Chinese, Taiwanese, Portuguese, Spanish, Japanese, Italian, and German. It is also being used in the United Kingdom, Korea, Sweden, Norway, Iceland, Australia, New Zealand, Mexico, Brazil, Belgium, and Canada (NANDA is composed of USA and Canadian membership).

Approximately one third of the attendees to the NANDA conferences are from other countries.

Are there any other relevant indicators of market acceptance?

NANDA is one of five nursing classifications recognized by the American Nurses Association. This recognition lead to its incorporation in the National Library of of Medicine's Metathesaurus for a Unified Medical Language. Both the Cumulative Index to Nursing and Allied Health Literature (CINAHL) and Index Medicus have added NANDA diagnostic terms to their indexes. NANDA is included in the Joint Commission on Accreditation for Healthcare Organization's (JCAHO). As one nursing classification system that can be used to meet the requirements of the the Information Management criteria. Many health care agencies are using NANDA in standards, care plans, and nursing information systems. All major nursing textbooks use NANDA to discuss the conditions that nurses diagnose and treat (Mosby, Lippincott, Sage Publishers, PDR, Addison-Wesley, Springhouse, Franklin Electronic Books, Appleton-Century-Crofts, Saunders). The textbook exceptions are in community health which primarily uses the Omaha System (since it is specifically for this practice area) and home health which uses the Home Health Care Classification (since it is specifically for this practice area). As a result nursing education programs teach the NANDA Taxonomy. There is enough interest to support a conference every two years. NANDA publishes their own journal: *Nursing Diagnosis: The Journal of Nursing Language and Classification*.

VII. Level of specificity of the code set/vocabulary. Include the following:

Describe its clinical specificity and/or granularity.

All diagnoses have undergone clinical validation and so have established specificity. The level of the diagnoses is still at a conceptual or abstract level. We are beginning to see submissions of diagnoses that are at a more granular level.

Does it reference or assume other code sets?

No.

C. If so, what are they? Why are they being referenced?

N/A

VIII. Relationships with other code sets/vocabularies. Include the following:

Describe the relationships, such as inclusion, dependency, interface, overlap, conflict, or coordination.

Preliminary conversations are beginning with the Nursing Intervention Classification (NIC) and the Nursing Outcome Classification (NOC) to develop linkages between the three systems so that they may be used together to provide a more comprehensive set of codes to capture nursing data. Each NANDA diagnosis has been linked with NIC interventions and mapped to the other nursing classifications with nursing diagnoses (Omaha System and the Home Health Care Classification) in the Unified Medical Language System.

Describe any coordination or reconciliation activities.

NANDA has established a collaborative relationship with SNOMED International. This nomenclature incorporated NANDA before it was copyrighted. We are now working to model the NANDA updates into SNOMED International. NANDA is also included in the UMLS. NANDA also collaborates with nursing organizations in other countries: Japanese Nursing Diagnosis Association; Association of Common European Diagnoses, Interventions, and Outcomes; and the International Council of Nursing (a component of the World Health Organization). NANDA has been a contributor and reviewer of the International Classification of Nursing Practice (ICNP).

What portion of the code set is affected by this coordination?

NANDA continues to be an independent code set.

D. What conditions are assumed in order for this coordination to be effective?

What gaps exist among related code sets that should be addressed?

The patient's signs and symptoms are not captured in any of the nursing classifications. SNOMED International appears to have a relevant terminology for this purpose.

F. Describe what is being done to address these gaps.

There is no formal work, just informal discussions among nursing developers.

IX. Relationship to message format standards. Are your codes or terms used within specific message formats standards? If so, which ones?

NO

If your code sets or terms are used, are they specified as required, preferred, or optional by the message format standard?

N/A

Has this code set been adopted for use within a vendor or end-user system? If so, which ones?

Ergo Inc., Cerner Corporation, HealthMaster, CINAHL, and Health Sciences Consortium

How are the links between your code set and specific message formats maintained?

N/A

In which message format standards organizations do you regularly participate?

ANA represents NANDA's interest in these organizations — ANSI-HISB, ASTM, and HL7.

X. Identifiable costs. Indicate your best estimate for the following: Cost of Licensure.

This is negotiable depending on scope and derivative products. The range is $650.00 and up for two years.

Cost of acquisition (if different from licensure).

N/A

Cost of tools.

N/A

Cost/time frames for education and training.

Nurses are taught the Taxonomy in their basic educational programs. Minimal inservicing is required after that. The only intensive training that seems to be required is if a computerized form is being introduced but the bulk of training is for the application not the taxonomy.

Cost/time frames for implementation.

No estimate is available as nurses have been mandated to do care planning for the last 25 years (the same time that NANDA has been in existence). Professional coders are not used as in ICD-9CM. The current electronic applications automatically code as the nurse selects the nursing diagnosis.

Any other cost considerations, such as annual or usage fees, updates, maintenance, and so forth.

No estimate is available as nursing has always integrated this type of maintenance into their workflow and staffing patterns. This may change with the advent of more CPRs.

XI. Who to contact for more information. Include name, E-mail address, phone and fax number. Position in developing organization.

Judith J. Warren, PhD, RN, FAAN
President 1996-1998, NANDA
E-mail: ejwarren@navix.net

Dorothy Jones, EdD, RN, FAAN
President, 1998-2000, NANDA
E-mail: dorothy.jones@bc.edu

Joe Braden, Nursecom, Inc.
Account Manager for the North American Nursing Diagnosis Association
1211 Locust St.
Philadelphia, PA 19107
FAX: 215-545-8107
E-mail: joe.braden@nursecominc.com

Report of the President-Elect

Dorothy A. Jones, EdD, RN, C, FAAN

During the past two years there have been many opportunities to share in the work of NANDA as President-Elect. In addition to becoming familiar with current organizational activities, there were several projects that became the focus of my activities. Over the past two years I served as Board liaison to the Membership Committee. Although there were no committee meetings due to limited funds, discussions with the committee chairperson impacted on strategic planning for the coming two years.

Much time was also spent exploring opportunities to preserve NANDA's history and related documents, now and in the future. To this end, an archive site was eventually selected by the NANDA Board. Marjory Gordon, Helen Cox and myself spent time in Philadelphia going through boxes of NANDA materials sent from the St. Louis office. These documents were then forwarded to the Burns Archive Library on the Boston College Campus.

Preparation for NANDA's 25th Anniversary Celebration at the 13th Conference was the major Board focus during the past year. Many activities surrounded preparations including the development of a videotape highlighting NANDA's History; selection of outstanding contribution and leadership award recipients; preparation of historical materials for sale and viewing at the conference; preparation of materials such as a "NANDA Historical Timeline" for inclusion in a special conference issue of the Journal; and facilitating projects such as the convening of the specialty groups at the conference.

In addition, the NANDA Foundation Gala was organized and will be held during the conference (Friday, April 24th) at the Adams Mark Hotel in St. Louis. This event will be co-hosted by Dr. Lucille Joel, former ANA President and current First Vice President of ICN. During this event special recognition will be given to outstanding nurse leaders who have advance the work of NANDA over the past 25 years.

The Board worked to generate a Strategic Plan that will guide the organization through 2000 and beyond. A preliminary plan will be presented to the membership during the President's address at the conference, on Sunday, April 26th, 1998. Over the past year I had many opportunities to participate in the work of NANDA as President-Elect. Many thanks to Judy Warren and the Board for support during these past two years.

Management Support Services Report

Resource Management Plus, Inc. (RMP) provides association management services to the North American Nursing Diagnosis Association (NANDA) under direction of the President of NANDA or a designated liaison. RMP has provided administrative, financial, membership and conference management services to NANDA since 1993. Implicit in all action undertaken by RMP is the understanding that all policy matters and major business decisions remain under the control of NANDA.

The administrative services provided by RMP focus on the implementation of the policies and procedures of the Association. This support is provided with direction from the President of NANDA, its Board of Directors, and its elected officers and committee chairs. Some of the functions undertaken during the past year have included:

- preparing and distributing written communications
- disseminating information on membership criteria, costs, benefits

- coordinating, publishing and printing books and other products
- arranging and supporting meetings of the Board of Directors
- acting as liaison among NANDA Board, CPA and legal advisors, including coordinating the process of having the NANDA Foundation designated as a charitable organization
- marketing and negotiating licensing agreements with domestic publishers
- marketing and negotiating the sale of foreign language rights

The membership services performed by RMP are structured to give each member an accessible contact point with their Association. Both members and nonmembers can reach the NANDA office from 8:00 AM to 6:00 PM (EST) Monday through Friday by calling the toll free 800 telephone number, 800-647-9002. Calls received after hours and on weekends are handled by voice mail and the call is returned promptly on the next business day. During the past year an average of 185 calls per month have been handled by RMP.

In addition, RMP provides the following services to maintain contact with NANDA members:

- preparing and mailing annual dues (RMP can accept dues payments by either VISA or Mastercard)
- maintaining up-to-date memberships listing
- preparing labels for mailings to the members
- replacing undelivered copies of *Nursing Diagnosis*
- handling address changes and inquiries about membership status
- responding to new member inquiries and mailing of membership information
- preparing newsletter section for *Nursing Diagnosis*
- processing orders for Taxonomy and other NANDA publications

The financial services provided by RMP are essentially the implementation of the fiscal policies and procedures of the Association. These services are provided with direction from the NANDA board and its elected officers. Some of the functions performed during the past year have included:

- handling accounts receivable, accounts payable, maintaining Association checking account and processing funds from dues payments
- preparing monthly and quarterly financial statements
- preparing the annual budget in collaboration with the Treasurer
- preparing all information for annual tax returns

The conference management services provided by RMP include coordinating all conference activity and providing support to the program chairperson. "Coordinating" includes handling the details of site selection; negotiating accommodations, meeting rooms, air and ground transportation; soliciting exhibitors; preparing and sending out conference brochures and general management of the conference. Some of the functions performed for the 1998 conferences include:

- developing a conference budget and monitoring all expenses
- designing and coordinating printing and mailing of brochures promoting the conference
- handling all speaker arrangements (honorariums, audiovisuals and handouts)
- working with the Marriott to arrange all meeting rooms and food functions and visiting the hotel staff to assure a well managed conference
- accepting program abstracts, duplicating and distributing to the Committee
- maintaining records and coordinating abstract review cycle
- contracting with a CE provider to provide ANCC accepted CEs
- selling and coordinating exhibit space
- preparing all conference registration materials (badges and packet information)
- contracting with suppliers (audio-visual and computer rental)
- handling site selection for future conferences based on cities recommended by the membership and Board

NANDA Foundation. RMP coordinated the process of applying to Internal Revenue Service to have the NANDA Foundation designated as a charitable organization. This acceptance of the NANDA Foundation as a 501 c 3 by the Internal Revenue Service permits all donations to the NANDA Foundation to be tax deductible. The process was completed in November, 1997.

RMP is pleased to be furnishing management support to NANDA. We understand the reality of the limited time that leaders of the Association can volunteer to make the organization successful. Our function is to provide administrative support to NANDA's leadership so that the time they do dedicate to the organization can be effectively utilized.

RMP supports NANDA's goal to maximize member retention by delivering superior membership services. By providing the toll-free 800 telephone number members can access those services by calling the office at their convenience. Knowledgeable staff can answer their questions or will refer them to the proper resource should the question be better handled by another NANDA member.

RMP is here to serve you. As a member or officer of NANDA we are available to assist you.

Thank you for your confidence and support.
Joe Braden, Executive Director
Margo Neal, Publisher
Joe Mason, Association Services Coordinator
Lanie Meriwether, 1998 Conference Coordinator
Scott Andress, Business Manager
Tim Bower, Marketing Manager

Treasurer's Report

July 1, 1995 to June 30, 1996
Actual vs. Budget

REVENUE

		($) Actual	($) Budget	$ Diff	% Diff
Dues	Dues-Member	21,787	20,748	1,039	5%
	Dues-Associate	0	0	0	NA
	Dues-Student	151	0	151	NA
	Dues-Institution	648	0	648	NA
	Dues-Affiliate	945	0	945	NA
	TOTAL DUES	**23,531**	**20,748**	**2,783**	**13%**
Publishing	Subscription Fee	14,686	13,832	854	6%
	Taxonomy	27,555	15,500	12,055	78%
	Returns	0	-3,500	3,500	-100%
	Bad Debt	0	0	0	NA
	Proceedings	3,465	1,500	1,965	131%
	Royalty & Rights	7,000	7,000	0	0%
	License Agreements	8,002	0	8,002	NA
	Translations	3,500	0	3,500	NA
	Translation Royalties	6,382	0	6,382	NA
	TOTAL PUBLISHING	**70,590**	**34,332**	**36,258**	**106%**
Conference	Fees	21,787	20,748	1,039	5%
	Allowance for Returns	0	-1,500	1,500	-100%
	Donation	5,501	6,000	-499	-8%
	Advertising	900	1,500	-600	-40%
	Exhibits	5,900	7,500	-1,600	-21%
	TOTAL CONFERENCE	**89,492**	**85,525**	**3,967**	**5%**
Donations	Donation-Individual	0	0	0	NA
	Donation-Corporate	0	0	0	NA
	NANDA Foundation Donation	15,421	0	15,421	NA
	TOTAL DONATION	**15,421**	**0**	**15,421**	**NA**
Other Income	Interest Received	628	600	28	5%
	Miscellaneous	1,465	1,000	465	47
	TOTAL OTHER INCOME	**2,093**	**1,600**	**493**	**31%**
	TOTAL REVENUE	**201,127**	**142,205**	**58,922**	**41%**

Continued…

NANDA Revenue and Expenses   *(continued)*

EXPENSES

		($) Actual	($) Budget	$ Diff	% Diff
Administration	Marketing & Promotion	2,921	2,550	371	15%
	Postage & Shipping	1,772	3,000	-1,228	-41%
	NANDA Foundation	8,322	0	8,322	NA
	Professional Fees	985	1,000	-15	-2%
	Management Fees	37,122	37,080	42	0%
	Telephone	1,507	1,000	507	51%
	Stationery	1,377	1,000	3,77	38%
	Admin. Other	4,115	2,000	2,115	106%
	TOTAL ADMINISTRATION	**58,121**	**47,630**	**10,491**	**22%**
Comm./Board	Board Expenses	763	2,500	-1,737	-69%
	Committee Expenses	2,642	4,000	-1,358	-34%
	President's Office	162	400	-238	-60%
	TOTAL COMM./BOARD	**3,567**	**6,900**	**-3,333**	**-48%**
Publications	Member Subscription	16,694	15,379	1,315	9%
	Editor's Stipend & Expenses	7,402	7,000	402	6%
	Taxonomy Mfg. & Dist.	8,937	4,938	3,999	81%
	Proceedings	2,000	0	2,000	NA
	Publications Other	830	400	430	108%
	TOTAL PUBLICATIONS	**45,798**	**33,297**	**12,501**	**38%**
Conference-1996	Conference Promotion	10,497	10,000	497	5%
	Registration & Program	4,803	10,000	-5,197	-52%
	Meeting Room Charge	0	0	0	NA
	Conf. Equip. Rental	4,542	3,500	1,042	30%
	Speaker Fees	315	2,500	-2,185	-87%
	Food & Beverage	17,287	20,100	-2,813	-14%
	Conference Postage	1,492	2,500	-1,008	-40%
	Exhibitor Cost	811	1,000	-189	-19%
	Conference Mgt. Fee	5,865	6,450	-585	-9%
	Travel	1,030	4,500	-3,470	-77
	Conf. Other	802	2,000	-1,198	-60%
	TOTAL CONFERENCE	**47,444**	**62,550**	**-15,106**	**-24%**
	TOTAL EXPENSES	**154,930**	**150,377**	**4,553**	**3%**
	NET INCOME	**46,197**	**-8,172**	**54,369**	**665%**

NANDA Revenue and Expenses

July 1, 1996 to June 30, 1997
Actual vs. Budget

REVENUE

		($) Actual	($) Budget	$ Diff	% Diff
Dues	Dues-Affiliate	212	925	-713	-77%
	Dues-Member	20,494	21,998	-1,504	-7%
	Dues-Retired/Student	151	920	-769	-84%
	Dues-Institution	882	1,000	-118	-12%
	TOTAL DUES	**21,739**	**24,843**	**-3,104**	**-12%**
Publishing	Subscription Fee (Members)	10,317	10,687	-370	-3%
	ND Royalty & Rights	7,000	7,000	0	0%
	Proceedings	2,045	500	1,545	NA
	Definitions and Classifications	36,336	36,750	-414	-1%
	D&C Returns	0	-4,500	4,500	-100%
	D&C License Agreements	13,230	15,000	-1,770	-12%
	D&C Translations	1,000	11,000	-10,000	-91%
	D&C Translation Royalties	12,362	0	12,362	NA
	TOTAL PUBLISHING	**82,290**	**76,437**	**5,853**	**8%**
Conference	Fees	45	0	45	NA
	Allowance for Returns	0	0	0	NA
	Advertising	0	0	0	NA
	Donation	0	0	0	NA
	Exhibits	0	0	0	NA
	TOTAL CONFERENCE	**45**	**0**	**45**	**NA**
Donations	Donation-Individual	0	0	0	NA
	Donation-Corporate	0	0	0	NA
	NANDA Foundation Donation	0	0	0	NA
	TOTAL DONATION	**0**	**0**	**0**	**NA**
Other Income	Interest Received	3,203	1,000	2,203	220%
	Miscellaneous	1,904	1,600	304	19
	TOTAL OTHER INCOME	**5,107**	**2,600**	**2,507**	**96%**
	TOTAL REVENUE	**109,181**	**103,880**	**5,301**	**5%**

Continued...

NANDA Revenue and Expenses *(continued)*

EXPENSES

		(\$) Actual	(\$) Budget	\$ Diff	% Diff
Administration	Marketing & Promotion	860	2,000	-1,140	-57%
	Postage & Shipping	1,727	3,000	-1,273	-42%
	Professional Fees	465	815	-350	-43%
	Management Fees	39,147	40,000	-853	-2%
	Telephone	987	1,600	-613	-38%
	Stationery	683	1,600	-917	-57%
	Admin. Other	166	1,000	-834	-83%
	Returns/Allowances	7,011	0	7,011	NA%
	TOTAL ADMINISTRATION	**51,046**	**50,015**	**1,031**	**2%**
Comm./Board	Board Expenses	2,501	2,000	501	25%
	Committee Expenses	686	4,000	-3,314	-83%
	President's Office	0	400	-400	-100%
	TOTAL COMM./BOARD	**3,187**	**6,400**	**-3,213**	**-50%**
Publications	Member Subscription	11,703	15,400	-3,697	-24%
	Editor's Stipend & Expenses	7,543	7,200	343	5%
	D&C Mfg. & Dist.	8,992	9,300	-308	-3%
	D&C Pre-Press	383	750	-367	-49%
	D&C Publishing Fee	10,022	10,910	-888	-8
	Publications Other	3,803	1,000	2,803	280%
	TOTAL PUBLICATIONS	**42,446**	**44,560**	**-2,114**	**-5%**
Conference	Conference Promotion	0	0	0	NA
	Registration & Program	0	0	0	NA
	Meeting Room Charge	0	0	0	NA
	Conf. Equip. Rental	0	0	0	NA
	Speaker Fees	0	0	0	NA
	Food & Beverage	0	0	0	NA
	Conference Postage	0	0	0	NA
	Exhibitor Cost	0	0	0	NA
	Conference Mgt. Fee	0	0	0	NA
	Travel	0	0	0	NA
	Conf. Other	0	0	0	NA
	TOTAL CONFERENCE	**0**	**0**	**0**	**NA**
	TOTAL EXPENSES	**96,679**	**100,975**	**-4,296**	**-4%**
	NET INCOME	**12,502**	**2,905**	**9,597**	**330%**

NANDA Foundation
Treasurer's Report

Purpose: The primary purpose of the NANDA Foundation is to promote the development, refinement, and use of standardized nursing diagnoses in the patient care.

Tax Status: The NANDA Foundation was incorporated on April 23, 1996 in the Commonwealth of Pennsylvania for educational purposes within the meaning of section 501 (c) (3) of the IRS code. Donations to the NANDA Foundation are tax deductible.

Revenue Sources: The main source of revenue for the NANDA Foundation has been the gala event held at the biennial conference.

Fund Balance: As of March 31, 1998 there was $5,655.88 in the Foundation's treasury.

Employer Identification Number: 23-2845901

Committee Reports: Bylaws Committee

There have been no requests for changes in bylaws.

DRC COMMITTEE

The DRC has had one meeting, November, 1997. Committee process and policies were reviewed and a list of activities were generated to be completed by May, 1998. Some of the activities were the proposal to change the format for diagnosis labels (NDEC proposal) and the development of 3.0 in the staging criteria. Ten diagnoses were reviewed out of a total of 21 currently in process. One did not meet the NANDA definition. In addition there is a set of 21 wellness diagnoses from one submitter. The committee plans to try an e-mail review process.

In November, 1997, 21 new diagnoses were received (NDEC), 39 revisions of diagnosis (NDEC), and one deletion (NDEC). Diagnoses already received were assigned to Committee members for e-mail review.

Ten of the new NDEC diagnoses raised the question/controversy of medical diagnoses that some nurses believe they diagnose and treat (i.e., protocols). Should these be called nursing diagnoses? Consideration has to be given to the conceptual focus of human responses, the larger care delivery system beyond nursing, the impact it will have on information systems, and the legal ramifications.

Submitted by Dr. Marjory Gordon

INTERNATIONAL COMMITTEE

Members:	Term expires
Cecile Boisvert, chair	2000 (elected).
Marga Coler	1998 (appointed).
Nancy Creason	1998 (elected).
Beverley O'Connell	2000 (elected)
Cecile Lambert	2000 (appointed).

Meetings

The Committee will have a meeting of the entire committee during the St. Louis Conference 98. One face-to-face meeting occurred during the Spring 1997 at the ICN

Conference in Vancouver (Bev. O' Connell, Cecile Lambert, and past member Josc. Matthewman). All business was conducted by e-mail or by telephone.

Activities 1996
Presentations workshops at international conferences by committee members: C. Boisvert was guest speaker at the foundation Conference of the Spanish Association on Nursing Diagnoses, AENTDE, May 1996, Barcelona.

With Marjory Gordon's collaboration, we were able to gather a group of experts from the NANDA Board of Directors and offer an "Ask the Expert" type of session at the ICN Conference on June 18th, 1997. The small groups discussions were very lively and contributed to NANDA's International image.

The networking with nurses from several cultures and countries in Vancouver provided the groundwork for an International Panel presentation during the St. Louis Conference. The issues of meaning, linguistic structure, cultural diversity and methodology for translation and validation will be discussed with the reference to the translation of NANDA's Taxonomy into Dutch, French, Japanese, Portuguese and Spanish. We feel that the feedback from the International community given to NANDA could be used to refine the language of nursing that relates to diagnoses.

Collaboration was established with the NDEC principal investigators during the Chicago Premiere Conference on Nursing Diagnoses, Interventions and Outcomes. Nurses from Spain and England were suggested to give feedback about the refinement and development of diagnoses. The languages spoken in various countries may be different but many of the concerns are often similar.

In 1996, the International Committee established an award to commemorate the work of Elisabeth A. Mottet, DNSc. (C.) M.S., R.N., former chair of the committee. I had the great pleasure of being awarded this distinction and this year we have proposed the name of an outstanding individual who has contributed to the international advancement of nursing diagnosis use, research and/or development. Her name will be disclosed at the Award Banquet.

In February 1998, the Board has accepted a motion proposed by our Committee and seconded by Marjory Gordon. In the future, the International Committee will be formally consulted in the diagnostic review process.

The main objectives are the following:
- To involve the international NANDA members in the refinement and development of the nursing diagnoses.
- To encourage feedback and input of nurses from different cultures and clinical fields.
- To facilitate the dissemination, translation and use of NANDA's Taxonomy around the world.

Cecile Boisvert
Chair Person

MEMBERSHIP COMMITTEE
Total number of members: 450. The committee met via telephone conferences. One recruitment exhibit was staffed at the International Council of Nursing Conference in June, 1996.

NOMINATING COMMITTEE
The ballot being used at this conference for voting reflects the work of the Nominating Committee with good support from Mr. Joe Mason, NANDA Services Coordinator. In addition to myself, the members of this year's

Committee were as follows:

    Judy Carlson-Catalano, EdD, RN
    Regina Maibusch, MS, RN, CS
    Eleanor Borkowski, RN

Gail Davis
Chair, Nominating Committee

TAXONOMY COMMITTEE

April, 1998

The Taxonomy Committee met in November 1997, after the first NANDA, NIC, NOC Conference in Pheasant Run, Illinois. Members in attendance were Kay Avant, chair, Martha Craft-Rosenberg, Rona Levin, and Rose Harvey. Joan Norris was not in attendance.

Our purpose was to do three Q-sorts that we had not completed at our previous meeting at the last NANDA conference, to make a decision about the new taxonomic structure to be recommended, and to meet with the DRC to discuss some issues of joint concern.

Three Q-sorts were completed. As a result of this work, two recommendations were sent to the Board for action.

Recommendation #1. The Taxonomy Committee joins the DRC in recommending that "diagnoses submitted which conceptually already appear on other classifications (ICD, DSM, etc.) will be included in the NANDA Taxonomy and be double coded to the referent classification." The Board approved the recommendation.

Recommendation #2. The Taxonomy Committee recommends that the proposed multi-axial Health Patterns framework be adopted as Taxonomy 2. This recommendation was not supported but the Board did vote to have the Taxonomy Committee present this new taxonomic framework at the Conference so that the membership would have an opportunity for discussion and input.

The Taxonomy Committee will present the new framework at the 13th Conference and provide multiple opportunities for member input.

Respectfully submitted,

Kay Avant, Chair

HISTORICAL ARCHIVES REPORT

Dorothy A. Jones, EdD, RN, C, FAAN — President-Elect

Over the years, the NANDA Board of Directors along with NANDA members have been concerned about the preservation of NANDA's history. During the past year, the Board of Directors investigated several available sites interested in archiving NANDA documents. At the Summer Board meeting (1997), the Board unanimously agreed to accept Boston College's offer to archive NANDA historical documents into an historical Nursing Collection at the Burns Library, on the Boston College Campus.

In January 1998 NANDA documents were brought to Boston College and are currently being cataloged. Nurses around the world will have access to a description of these holdings through the WWW. Dr. Barbara Munro, Dean of the Boston College School of Nursing, will formally present information about the library to NANDA members at the Thirteenth National Conference in St. Louis. In the future, all nurses will have access to the history of NANDA's contribution to nursing language development and classification.

It is also anticipated that the Library will be offering small stipends to scholars who wish to come to the Burns Archival Library and study available historical docments. As time progresses, additional papers and association materials will be added to the collection. This is an exciting opportunity for NANDA members to share in the contributions and continued developments of the many nurses who have advanced the work of NANDA and nursing diagnosis around the world. http://www.bc.edu/bc-org/avp/ulib/Burns/msslist.htm/ttnursmedethics

NANDA Foundation TREASURER'S REPORT

Purpose:	The primary purpose of the NANDA Foundation is to promote the development, refinement, and use of standardized nursing diagnoses in the patient care.
Tax Status:	The NANDA Foundation was incorporated on April 23, 1996 in the Commonwealth of Pennsylvania for educational purposes within the meaning of section 501 (c) (3) of the IRS code. Donations to the NANDA Foundation are tax deductible.
Revenue Sources:	The main source of revenue for the NANDA Foundation has been the gala event held at the biennial conference.
Fund Balance:	There is currently $5,655.88 in the Foundation's treasury.

Employer Identification Number: 23-2845901

PROGRAM COMMITTEE REPORT

Program Committee

Mary Ann Lavin, ScD, RN, CS, FAAN, Chair
Georgia Griffith Whitley,
   EdD, RN, Board Liaison
Vici Cole Schonlau, RN, DNSc
Ros Alfaro-Lefevre, MSN, RN
Carol Matz, MSN, RN
Anne G. Perry, EdD, RN

Report

To prepare for the 1998 NANDA Conference, the Program Committtee met by means of phone and e-mail over the course of the past two years. One new contribution has been to build into this conference time for great escapes, i.e., the "Art Walk" sponsored by Saint Louis University and coordinated by Dottie James, PhD, RN and "Revisit St. Louis" sponsored by the University of Missouri - St. Louis and coordinated by Mary Ellen McSweeney, PhD, time for individually planned excursions, and post-conference tours.

Other program functions accomplished were: development of a two-year program plan, coordination of activities with NANDA Board and with Nursecom, publication of pertinent material as needed or requested, preparation of program committee reports, and distribution of conference tasks. The latter included:

- coordinating with Board members specific conference tasks, e.g., establishing communication with specialty groups and identifying specialists to serve as conference panelists, Awards Committee work, and Voting Committee work
- meeting with hotel management and facilitating coordination of layout with Nursecom and hotel
- selecting conference menus
- assigning concurrent sessions to rooms
- selecting a Gala site and its music

- recruiting and preparing volunteers for assisting the program chair and serving as room monitors, registration helpers, and vote counters. These volunteers include students and faculty from universities in the conference area as well as volunteers solicited through *Nursing Diagnosis*
- assigning a program committee person for each conference day (duties include making any necessary daily announcements, serving as a conference resource person/troubleshooter, and finding back-up volunteers, when needed)
- assuring effective communication among Program Committee members and volunteers at the conference

In brief, it has been a full but most rewarding two-year period in which the Program Committee plus people from universities and organizations across the United States have pulled together to present a 25th Anniversary program. A most sincere thanks to the entire Program Committee, to the NANDA Board and its liaison, Georgia Griffith Whitley, EdD, RN, and to Lanie Meriwether and Joe Braden of Nursecom.

PUBLICATION COMMITTEE REPORT - April 23, 1998

MEMBERS:

Janet Weber, Chair (2000)

Lois Hoskins (1998)

Winnifred Mills (1998)

Marilyn Rantz (1998)

Jolene Simon (2000)

Meetings

All correspondence with committee members has been by mail and phone. The only formal meeting held was April 23, 1998 at the 13th conference in St. Louis. (Present: J. Weber, L. Hoskins, M. Rantz, J. Simon, M. Neal, H. Cox, J. Warren, D. Jones; Absent: W. Mills)

Journal

Jolene Simon reported that for 1997, 21 manuscripts were accepted and 17 accepted (See attached publishers' report).

The committee recommended that a call be make for potential guest editors for future issues.

A memorial column was recommended for the journal. This idea was well received and will be directed to the NANDA NEWS.

Jolene Simon has had difficulty getting NANDA NEWS. A process was established to resolve this problem. Joe Mason will be asked to send new diagnoses and committee reports to the editor. The president will send the editor a president's report and information from the board minutes to be included in future news prior to the publication of each issue.

Steps have been taken to streamline and shorten the editorial process for the journal editor. The publisher will now send author queries directly to the author with a FYI copy to the editor. Author will send responses directly to the publisher. Jolene Simon has a new FAX number: 630/462-4521. She should have e-mail set up within a month.

Jolene Simon agreed to work with Noreen Frisch, former journal editor, to complete the application process for the journal to be accepted to the Index Medicus. One of the requirements to do this is that the newsletter and information be moved to the back of the journal, which has been done.

The board requested that the committee develop an editor evaluation tool. A sample was reviewed by the committee. Margo Neal, journal publisher, agreed to revise the sample tool from her perspective and forward it back to the committee for review and approval. There will be a call for a yearly written editor evaluation by the publisher, editorial board and chair of the Publications Committee. The journal editor will also do a yearly self-evaluation. Jolene will inquire of other editors at the upcoming INANA meeting regarding processes used for evaluations of editors.

The lettering design of the journal title and mission statement has been revised by the publisher as recommended by the committee and approved by the Board and Publications Committee. The editorial board recommends that by the next conference that the journal title eliminate the words nursing diagnoses. We are requesting the boards approval to make the words "nursing diagnosis" smaller in the next issues as a transition to this change.

Anniversary Issue

The anniversary issue of the journal is in press and will be mailed to the members with the April/June regular issue. It was intended to be available at the conference but many delays were encountered, including delayed communication of acceptance of the proposal by the board and delayed submission of manuscripts by authors.

Proceedings

The Board approved that the 13th proceedings be edited by Marilyn Rantz and Priscilla LeMone and published by CINAHL. Thank you Marilyn, Priscilla, and CINAHL for doing an outstanding job and for once again taking on this task!

Sales to date for the 11th proceedings are 475; for the 12th proceedings, 156.

June Levy from CINAHL will send the standard publication and license agreement for this edition, which allows authors to publish their work in both the NANDA Proceedings and the journal, to the President for signature.

Taxonomy

The Board requested a proposal from the chair of the Publications Committee for editing the new edition of the taxonomy (NANDA Nursing Diagnosis: Definitions & Classifications 1999-2000). This proposal was rejected. The Board of Directors agreed to serve as editor of the next edition. They will also determine what small group work will be incorporated into it.

Monographs

The Board recommended that monographs (e.g., How to submit a diagnoses, What is a diagnosis?, History of nursing diagnoses, Invitational 1989 Research Conference) be developed to sell in the future. Proposals for future monographs will be submitted to the publications committee for review and approval. This recommendation will be forwarded to the Board.

Margaret Lunney submitted a proposal to the Publications Committee to publish a monograph consisting of reprints of case studies, submitter's analysis and commentaries that have been published in the column: "You make the Diagnosis" in the journal. The publications committee approved and strongly recommends that the Board review and accept her proposal.

Historical Preservation

An update of the Archives will be submitted to the journal for inclusion in the NANDA NEWS.

Dotty Jones has collected a copy of past NANDA NEWSLETTERS, which has been bound and sells for $35.00. A few copies are still missing. If you have a copy you would be willing to donate to the collection, please contact Dotty.

Thank you to Dotty Jones and Marjory Gordon for preparing the NANDA Historical Video to be shown at the NANDA Dinner Meeting on Saturday Night at the 13th Conference. Another thank you goes to Dotty Jones for developing the historical preservation proposal, which was approved and supported by Boston College. This is a major accomplishment!

Respectfully submitted,
Janet Weber, Chair, Publications Committee

Diagnostic Review Committee Report

Submitted by Dr. Marjory Gordon

Business Meeting 1998

I assumed the Chair of the Diagosis Review Commitee (DRC) in November 1997 to serve until April 1998. Because of the extent of activities since this time and the time restraints this morning, I will confine my comments to the period of the last seven months.

Your DRC Members, 1996-1998, were:

Susan Chase

Leann Scroggins

Barbara Kranovitch Miller

Connie Delaney (appointed 1997)

Kathy Sheppard

Kay McCash

Marlene Lindeman

Joan Fitzmaurice (resigned)

Peggy Wetch (resigned)

The DRC were funded for one meeting in November. At this meeting the committee became a working group and this facilitated the diagnosis review work for the next seven months that was done by e-mail. The e-mail discussion was satisfactory but can be improved.

Review takes time and in NANDA we are not creating labels or just words, we are creating concepts that are used in thinking. These are the building blocks of nursing science. Both DRC and submitters must keep in mind that concept development takes time and is an onging process.

The following was the work in priority rank:

1. The first priority was to review the 96 diagnoses or diagnosis revisions in the cycle. This was completed and will go to Forums at this conference. After reviewing conference participants suggestions (Forums)the diagnoses will go to the NANDA Board.

2. Priority 2 was to prepare the materials for the Pre Conference Work Groups. It was decided that broad, abstract categories would be selected: Sleep Pattern Disturbance, Altered Family Process, Altered Parenting, and Altered Role Performance. Participants in these work groups were asked to identify the more

specific, clinically useful diagoses in each of these categories. Elizabeth Hiltunen, Marjory Gordon, and Susan Chase prepared the material for the small groups.

3. The following activities were begun but not completed by March 1998. They will be forwarded to the next DRC Committee.

a. Diagnostic Staging. Susan Chase presented a proposal for staging the diagnoses at Stage 3. The criteria she proposed are based on those used by the Agency for Health Care Policy and Research in their clinical practice guidelines. This agency classifies their individual guidelines into 1) supported by research categories and 2) expert opinion. This looks promising and may allow us to stage the diagoses as well as the defining characteristics. Criteria are needed in the expert opion area until we have enough research. It is premature to delete characteristics until they have been studied across relevant age, sex, cultural, and illness groups.

b. The DRC Process of Review and the need to involve a broader number of nurse-experts in diagnosis review. We would like to establish expert panels from the United States, Canada, and other countries. The DRC and International Committee brought a motion to the NANDA Board to have diagnoses reviewed by representatives from language groups before acceptance. The rationale was that translation problems may be avoided during diagnostic review. This was passed by the Board and will commence with the next review cycle.

c. The DRC in a 5-2 vote accepted and sent to the Board the following motion: "When disease-focused diagnoses are submitted, and the DRC judges that the diagnosis is conceptually already in another taxonomy such as ICD, that it can be included in the NANDA Taxonomy using the already accepted term with a cross-reference to the other classsification." Passed by the NANDA Board.

d. The DRC-Submitter Working Process. During this review I have created the category, "Working with Submitter." Diagnoses submitted that are in an early state of diagnostic concept development may require more work until the elements are clearly defined. Similarly, diagnoses that are very similar or interrelated are sometimes submitted. DRC needs to put submitters in contact with each other.

Taxonomy Committee Report

REPORT OF THE TAXONOMY COMMITTEE TO THE NANDA MEMBERSHIP

APRIL, 1998

Over the last four years, the Taxonomy Committee forwarded to the Board four Q-sorts of the diagnoses using different frameworks (naturalistic; Jenny's proposed framework from the tenth conference; the Nursing Outcomes Classification framework; and the Functional Health Patterns framework used by Gordon). None of the four frameworks was entirely satisfactory. However, Gordon's functional health patterns worked better than the other three since it is an assessment based in framework. With Gordon's permission, we modified her framework and it is this modified Health Patterns framework that we are recommending become the new Taxonomy 2. The Board has approved the new taxonomy to be brought for discussion to the membership. The Board has NOT approved the taxonomy for general use at this time. As you will see from our report, it is

still a work in progress. There are several issues that need to be considered before final approval can be sought. Nevertheless, we felt it was sufficiently developed to be brought to the membership for discussion and feedback.

The new taxonomy is composed of a synthesis of several things we liked in the different frameworks we evaluated. It is currently composed of 12 Domains, each divided into two or more Classes. The new taxonomy is designed to be multi-axial in its form. Using multiple axes will substantially improve the flexibility of the nomenclature and allow for easy additions and modifications. The five axes proposed are:

Axis 1 Acuity – acute to chronic

Axis 2 Unit of care – individual, family, community

Axis 3 Developmental stage – fetus to elder

Axis 4 Potentiality – actual, risk for, opportunity or potential for growth/enhancement

Axis 5 Descriptors – altered, decreased,

increased, deficit, depleted, excessive, defective, disturbed, impaired, ineffective, effective, ability, inability, intermittent, continuous, dysfunctional, functional (more descriptors can be added as needed)

A multiaxial model was chosen because it is easily incorporated into computer databases and because it is much more flexible and "user friendly" than the current system. However, there are several issues that arise when considering a multiaxial model.

The first is that by placing all the descriptors into an axis two things happen. Many of the current labels become nouns that may require the addition of another work to make the diagnosis understandable, and several of the current labels will be collapsed into a single noun or noun phrase (management of therapeutic regimen is a case in point). Using nouns or noun phrases is recommended by all taxonomy experts as the only logical means to classify anything. Using nouns and noun phrases for the actual diagnoses of human responses is also more efficient in explaining what the human response of the patient/client actually is. On the other hand, removing the descriptor from the current diagnosis does potentially alter the original label chosen by the developer of that diagnosis.

The second issue is related to the first. Placing the descriptors into an axis potentially allows the nurse to choose any of the available descriptors for any of the nouns (diagnoses) in the list. The "good news" is that it increases the usefulness and flexibility of the diagnoses considerably. The "bad news" is that it also increases the actual number of potential diagnoses in the taxonomy, many of which will not have defining characteristics, related factors, etc.,

available. Our diagnostic list would have many more "empty cells" than it currently does. For instance, the current diagnosis of "altered parenting" becomes simply "parenting" in the new taxonomy, with the potential for any one of several modifiers available for the nurse to use. Potential descriptors of "impaired," "disturbed," or "ineffective" might be chosen by the nurse rather than the current descriptor "altered." However, there are currently no defining characteristics, risk factors, etc., developed for "impaired, disturbed, or ineffective parenting," a situation that leaves much to be desired in terms of making sound clinical judgments. One way to handle this problem might be to block the use of certain descriptors with certain of the diagnoses by programming the computer to offer only those descriptors with each diagnosis for which there are defining characteristics available. On the other hand, leaving the options open (but indicating that no defining characteristics are available for some options) would allow nurses to see where additional work needs to be done and might stimulate some of them to contribute to the diagnostic list.

The third issue is that the use of a multiaxial system requires a means for numbering all potential descriptor choices for each diagnostic label and for numbering any additions/subtractions to the list. This may get complex. All the numbers in the current taxonomy will have to change to accommodate the new structure and to make the diagnoses independent of taxonomic placement. The structure that we are recommending at this time does not have a numbering system in place. The taxonomy committee may need to consult a specialist in computer-based taxonomy design to develop a numbering system that will be flexible and still provide meaningful data. The new numbering system must then be "mapped" to the old numbering system so that any diagnosis in Taxonomy One-Revised can be traced to its new placement in Taxonomy 2. This is not an issue that will be of concern to the practicing nurse, as a rule. It is a pure taxonomic issue. But it will need to be addressed prior to final adoption of the new taxonomy.

As you can see there is still a lot of work to do. The proposed Taxonomy 2 is definitely a work in progress. We welcome any and all feedback from the membership as we continue to refine it and try to deal with the issues we delineated for you. For those members who were interested in working with the new taxonomy, we provided several sessions during the conference when members of the taxonomy committee were available and when individual NANDA members could come by to actually sort the diagnoses into the proposed taxonomic structure. The results of the membership sorts will be published later in the Journal. A further study is proposed using a Delphi method to assist us in coming to better agreement about placement of the diagnoses into the best domains and classes.

Below is the proposed multiaxial Health Patterns framework for Taxonomy 2 including the initial sorting of the diagnoses that was done by the taxonomy committee. Again, we welcome any and all feedback from members to help us in this work.

Proposed Taxonomy 2

Domain 1 Health perception – Health management

    Class 1 Health awareness – (diagnoses needed)

    Class 2 Health management behaviors – management of therapeutic regimen, health seeking behaviors (specify), noncompliance (specify), health maintenance, home maintenance management, growth and development status

    Class 3 Health promotion behaviors – (diagnoses needed)

Domain 2 Nutrition – metabolism

    Class 1 Indigestion – infant feeding pattern, breastfeeding, swallowing, nutrition – less than body requirements, nutrition – more than body requirement

    Class 2 Digestion – nutrition – less than body requirements

    Class 3 Absorption – nutrition – less than body requirements

    Class 4 Metabolism – nutrition – more than body requirements, tissue perfusion (specify renal, cerebral, cardiopulmonary, GI, peripheral), body temperature, thermoregulation, hypothermia, hyperthermia

    Class 5 Hydration – fluid volume status

    Class 6 Integumentary system – tissue integrity, skin integrity, oral mucous membrane status

Domain 3 Elimination

    Class 1 Urinary – urinary elimination status, urinary retention, total incontinence, functional incontinence, stress, incontinence, urge incontinence, reflex incontinence

    Class 2 Bowel – bowel incontinence, diarrhea, constipation, colonic constipation, perceived constipation

    Class 3 Skin – (diagnosis needed)

    Class 4 Lung – (diagnosis needed)

Domain 4 Energy Maintenance

    Class 1 Sleep-rest – sleep pattern, fatigue

    Class 2 Activity-exercise – activity intolerance, disuse syndrome, physical mobility status

Class 3 Cardio-respiratory – peripheral vascular function, cardiac output, gas exchange, breathing pattern, airway clearance, ventilatory weaning response, maintenance of spontaneous ventilation

Class 4 Activities of daily living – self care dressing/grooming, self care – feeding, self-care – bathing/hygiene, self care – toileting, diversional activity status

Class 5 Energy field – energy field status

Domain 5 Cognitive – Perceptual

Class 1 Sensation – perception – unilateral neglect, impaired environmental interpretation syndrome, sensory/perceptual status (specify visual, auditory, kinesthetic, gustatory, tactile, olfactory)

Class 2 Cognition – confusion, memory, thought processes, knowledge status (specify)

Class 3 Communication – verbal communication

Domain 6 Self-perception – Self-concept

Class 1 Self-concept – personal identity, powerlessness, hopelessness

Class 2 Self-esteem – self-esteem status, low self-esteem, situation low self-esteem

Class 3 Body-image – body image status

Domain 7 Role relationships

Class 1 Caregiving roles – caregiver role strain, parenting

Class 2 Family relationships – family processes, family processes – alcoholism, parent/infant/child attachment, parental role conflict

Class 3 Role performance – role performance status

Class 4 Social relationships – social interaction, social isolation, loneliness

Domain 8 Sexuality – Reproduction

Class 1 Sexuality patterns – sexuality pattern, sexual dysfunction

Class 2 Reproductive function – (diagnosis needed)

Domain 9 Coping – Stress tolerance

Class 1 Post-trauma responses – relocation stress syndrome, rape trauma syndrome, rape-trauma syndrome – silent reaction, rape-trauma syndrome – compound reaction, post-trauma response

Class 2 Coping processes – fear, anxiety, denial, grieving, anticipatory grieving, adjustment, coping status, compromised coping, defensive coping, disabling coping

Class 3 Neuro-behavioral stress responses – dysreflexia, infant behavior status, intracranial adaptive capacity

Domain 10 Values – Beliefs

Class 1 Spiritual values/beliefs – decisional conflict, spiritual well being, spiritual distress

Class 2 Health values/beliefs – decisional conflict

Class 3 Personal values/beliefs – decisional conflict

Domain 11 Safety – Protection

Class 1 Infection – infection (specify)

Class 2 Physical injury – protection status, trauma (specify), injury (specify), perioperative positioning injury, suffocation, aspiration

Class 3 Violence – self mutilation, violence-directed to others

Class 4 Environmental hazards – poisoning

Domain 12 Comfort

Class 1 Pain – pain (specify)
Class 2 Nausea/vomiting – diagnoses
    needed
Class 3 Itching – diagnoses needed

Respectfully submitted,
The Taxonomy Committee
Kay C. Avant, Chair
Rose Mary Harvey
Rona Levin
Joan Norris
Martha Craft-Rosenberg

Board Meeting Minutes

Members present: J. Warren, D. Jones, H. Cox, M. Gordon, S. Sparks, K. Avant, M. Maas, and G. Whitley

North American Nursing Diagnosis Association, April 25, 1998 Board Meeting Minutes		
TOPIC	**DISCUSSION**	**Action**
President Warren called the meeting to order at 7:15 a.m.		
DRC report	Marjorie Gordon, chair of the Diagnostic Review Committee, presented the results of the small group discussions and actions of the DRC.	
	The Board discussed the "Potential for Enhanced" diagnoses as presented and felt that as written reflected manifestation of a conceptual focus yet to be described.	H. Cox moved that the "Potential for Enhanced" diagnoses be returned to M. Lunney and the NDEC group for further clarification. Second. Motion carried. It was recommended that M. Gordon & D. Jones talk with M. Lunney about these recommendations.
		H. Cox moved that M. Lunney be asked to head up a Task Force to study and make recommendations

North American Nursing Diagnosis Association, April 25, 1998 Board Meeting Minutes

TOPIC	DISCUSSION	Action
		to the next Conference regarding the "Potential for Enhanced" diagnoses, otherwise known as the "Enhanced Wellness" diagnoses. Second. Motion carried.
	M. Gordon presented a list of proposed rejected diagnoses from DRC.	Overflow Urinary Incontinence was rejected as a diagnosis on the basis that it is a defining characteristic for Urinary Retention. Members of the Board voted 3 members "aye" and 1 member "nay" for rejected the diagnosis. 3 members abstained.
	J. Warren cautioned Board members that some members of foreign delegations may be seeking NANDA representatives to give endorsements of products. She advised that if this occurs, the individual be asked to submit something after the conference in writing.	H. Cox moved that the DRC recommendations of rejected diagnoses be accepted. Second. Carried.
	J. Warren asked the Board if NANDA should publish the new Taxonomy as "a work in progress" in the NANDA Taxonomy book, ask for comments from members, and be sure it is clear that it has not been accepted by the Board and Conference.	J. Warren & M. Gordon will have the DRC diagnoses that are recommended for approval reproduced and circulated to members of the Board. Members will return comments and indicate approval or disapproval. J. Warren will review the feedback, collate the voting, and call an additional Board meeting to resolve remaining issues if required. J. Warren will prepare a draft for inclusion in the Taxonomy book and circulate it to the Board for approval prior to publication.
		Meeting adjourned at 8:30 a.m.
		Submitted by Meridean Maas, Secretary.

Members present: J. Warren, D. Jones, M. Gordon, K. Avant, G. Whitley, H. Cox, S. Sparks, and M. Maas

North American Nursing Diagnosis Association, Post Convention Board Meeting Minutes, April 26, 1998		
TOPIC	**DISCUSSION**	**Action**
Newly elected President Dorothy Jones called the meeting to order at 2:15 p.m.		Members requested more time for the biennial business meeting and 1/2 blocks of free time for sightseeing/fun.
Evaluation of Conference	The Board discussed the evaluations and concluded that overall the conference went very well. The Program Committee is to be congratulated for a job well done. The Board also agreed to convey to Joe Braden and his staff (Lanie & Joe Mason) appreciation for doing such a good job. (More detailed evaluation comments appended).	
		D. Jones to write letter to J. Braden acknowledging contributions of Lanie & Joe M. to conference.
		Recommendations will be given to Program Committee.
	It was agreed that a registered parliamentarian should be oriented prior to the business meeting and sit for consultation and support of the presiding officer during the meeting.	These recommendations were supported by the Board and will be included in planning for the 2000 conference.
	Suggestions for the next conference included more content on Informatics, research methods, review of the definition of nursing diagnosis, a phenomenon describing person experience, discussion of how the NANDA, NIC & NOC taxonomies relate and how they might be pulled together into one taxonomy.	

North American Nursing Diagnosis Association, Post Convention Board Meeting Minutes, April 26, 1998		
TOPIC	**DISCUSSION**	**Action**
	The Board also discussed developing stronger collaborative relationships with specialty organization and ways that joint endeavors to support nursing diagnosis research might be developed.	D. Jones will pursue this with J. Mason.
Dates for Board Meetings		The Board agreed to hold the next meeting August 7,8,9, 1998 in Boston.
	The Program Committee suggested that Ann McCourt be placed on the Program Committee for the 14th Conference since she lives in middle Florida.	Program Committee to contact Ann in the near future.
	Meeting dates for meetings subsequent to the August 1998 Board meeting will be determined at that meeting.	Meeting dates for Board meetings to be held between the 1998 and 2000 Conferences were discussed.
Publications Committee	The Publication Committee again recommendeds that the Journal title include the word "nursing diagnosis" in a smaller font. The number and quality of manuscripts is a concern and lack of recognition as a premier research journal.	Helen Cox moved that the Board approve the Publication Committee request to make the words "nursing diagnosis" smaller on the cover than the other words in the journal's title. Second. Motion withdrawn.
		The Board asked the Publication Committee to send 2 mock-ups of the journal cover for the Board to consider at August meeting.
Margaret Lunney publication of community health case studies.		Helen Cox moved Board approval of Margarent Lunney proposal to publish a monography of Community Health case studies. Second. Motion carried.
Taxonomy Committee	Kay Avant requested that the Board consider approval of funding of a Taxonomy validation Delphi study.	K. Avant to present a proposal including a budget at the August Board meeting.

North American Nursing Diagnosis Association, Post Convention Board Meeting Minutes, April 26, 1998		
TOPIC	**DISCUSSION**	**Action**
Diagnosis Review Committee	Marge Gordon requested in behalf of the DRC that all small group preconference group work be published in a journal article.	The Board agreed with the proposal.
	DRC also requested to see the galleys of the NANDA taxonomy book.	J. Warren to prepare Taxonomy Book. Sent disk with galleys to M. Gordon & D. Jones.
	A report from DRC should be published immediately in the Proceedings of the 13th Conference.	Marge Gordon will prepare a proposal for what needs to be done with DRC activities, an action plan, and a budget to support the actions to be considered at the next Board meeting.
		The Board directed Sheila Sparks, Treasurer, to include interest from the CD as operating funds.

Approval of new diagnoses	New Dx/proposed Dx from DRC for approval by Board presented by M. Gordon.
	    Autonomic Dysreflexia Risk
	    Sleep Deprivation
	    Spiritual Integrity
	        Enhancement Potential
	    Decreased Myocardial
	        Tissue Perfusion
	    Nausea
	    Impaired Walking
	    Impaired Wheelchair
	        Mobility
	    Impaired Wheelchair
	        Transfer Ability
	    Impaired Bed Mobility
	    Chronic Sorrow
	    Adult Failure to Thrive
	    Death Anxiety
	    Developmental	

NANDA Board of Directors

1999 – 2000

President:
Dorothy Jones, EdD, RN, FAAN
Braintree, MA   exp. 2000

President Elect:
Kay Avant, PhD, RN, FAAN
Waco, TX   exp. 2002

Secretary:
Meridean Maas, PhD, RN, FAAN
Iowa City, IA   exp. 2002

Treasurer:
Sheila Sparks, DNSc, RN, CS
Sterling, VA   exp. 2000

Directors:
Helen Cox, EdD, RN, C
Lubbock, TX   exp. 2000

Marjory Gordon, PhD, RN
Brighton, MA   exp. 2002

Mary Ann Lavin, ScD, RN, CS, ANP, FAAN
St. Louis, MO   exp. 2002

Judith Warren, PhD, RN, FAAN
Plattsmouth, NE   exp. 2002

Georgia Griffith Whitley, EdD, RN
Plainfield, IL   exp. 2000

1998 Unique Contribution Awards

Priscilla Boykin

Priscilla Boykin's nomination for NANDA's Unique Contribution Award was supported by the Washington Area Nursing Diagnosis Association. "Mike" Boykin has contributed to the advancement of nursing diagnosis through her leadership on the Board of Directors in the local nursing diagnosis group, WANDA, and through her tireless efforts to promote and facilitate the use of nursing diagnosis at the Clinical Center of the National Institutes of Health. Certified in Informatics by the American Nurses Association, Priscilla has continued to promoted a better understanding of nursing diagnosis, taxonomy development, and integration of nursing diagnoses in clinical information systems.

Since 1978, Priscilla has been actively involved in the education of local and international visiting nurses. In particular she has focused on content related to nursing process, nursing diagnosis, and quality assurance. At the NIH Clinical Center, she was awarded the Magnuson Clinical Center Director's Award for Outstanding Contributions.

Mike Boykin has been an active member of the Washington Area Nursing Diagnosis Association since 1984, serving as Secretary from 1990-1996. It was primarily through her efforts that WANDA was able to continue publishing a newsletter, the WANDA News. During time of decreased member participation, the newsletter has maintained its reputation for high quality throughout Priscilla's tenure as editor. For over 20 years Priscilla Boykin has enhanced the image of NANDA and promoted its chief goal, facilitating the use of nursing diagnosis in clinical practice. For all of her efforts, I am pleased to present Priscilla "Mike" Boykin for the NANDA Unique Contributors Award.

Cindy Dougherty

Cindy Dougherty is a voice for nurses at any NANDA Conference. Over the years she has contributed to the development, validation, and use of nursing diagnoses in a number of ways.

First, she has been a long time member of NANDA and has served on NANDA committees as well as the Board of Directors. Throughout her master's, doctoral, and post-doctoral education, Cindy has continued to work on the development, validation, and refinement of physiological diagnoses, particularly Decreased Cardiac Output.

Cindy has published journal articles and authored book chapters describing the development, validation, and use of nursing diagnoses. While a member of the NANDA Board of Directors, Cindy, along with fellow Board member Mary Kerr, initiated the Small Work Groups. These groups have become a part of the Pre-Conference activities and have focused on review and refinement of the NANDA diagnoses. This work has been published in the NANDA Proceedings along with an annotated bibliography of nursing diagnosis research.

For her many contributions to the advancement of nursing diagnosis, NANDA is pleased to present the Unique Contribution Award to Cindy Dougherty.

Janet Weber

Janet Weber currently is an Associate Professor at Southeast Missouri State University where she received the "Outstanding Researcher Award" in 1993. She has been a member of NANDA since 1981 and a member and Chairperson of the NANDA Publications Committee since 1993. She has focused much of her research on clinical reasoning, particularly around specific nursing phenomena like spiritual well being and hardiness. In addition, she has conducted research related to the diagnostic reasoning skills in students and developed and tested gaming simulation tool for teaching nursing diagnoses.

Dr. Weber has published extensively in scholarly journals nationally and internationally including our own, *Nursing Diagnosis*. In addition, Janet has published in textbooks including Nurses' Handbook of Health Assessment, for which she received the AJN "Book of the Year" Award. Dr. Weber is a strong advocate for nursing diagnosis and has presented on the subject nationally and internationally including Brussels, China and Japan.

As Chairperson of the Publications Committee, Janet has coordinated the work of this committee, facilitating the publication of the Proceedings and the journal, particularly the 25th Anniversary issue. She is continually available to the Board for consultation and is a role model for conducting committee work.

Dr. Weber has participated in numerous activities that have advanced the image of NANDA and nursing diagnosis. For endless hours of dedicated work and commitment on behalf of NANDA and for her leadership in disseminating the work of NANDA, we would like to present the Unique Contribution Award to Dr. Janet Weber. She is a most worthy recipient.

Marilyn Rantz

Marilyn Rantz was well supported to receive the NANDA's Unique Contribution Award at the 25th Anniversary Conference. Marilyn has contributed uniquely to the development, validation, and use of nursing diagnoses in a variety of ways. She has been a long time member of NANDA. While she served as an Administrator of a long term care facility, she implemented nursing diagnoses in that facility, developed a computerized nursing clinical planning and documentation system including nursing diagnoses, and published a substantial number of articles describing the implementation and the prevalence of specific nursing diagnoses that characterized residents in long term care facilities.

As an academic, Marilyn has continued her work with diagnoses development and refinement, by integrating this work with research using the Long Term Care Minimum Data Set in Missouri. This has been an important contribution to quality care for the chronically ill. Finally, Marilyn has made significant contributions as co-editor of NANDA's Eleventh, Twelfth, and soon to be Thirteenth Conference proceedings. It is therefore with pleasure that NANDA presents Marilyn Rantz with the Unique Contribution Award.

Priscilla LeMone

Priscilla LeMone has been active in the development, validation, and dissemination of nursing diagnoses for many years. In her faculty role, she uses nursing diagnoses in her teaching and program of research. Priscilla has an active program of research in the area of Altered Sexuality among women with chronic disorders. She has reported seminal studies of concept development and validation of altered sexuality. Priscilla integrates nursing diagnoses in her teaching of undergraduate and graduate nursing students, focusing on developing skills in diagnostic reasoning.

Most recently, Priscilla has co-edited with Marilyn Rantz several editions of NANDA's conference proceedings. Her service and contributions to NANDA have indeed been unique and deserve to be recognized with the award. We are grateful for the contributions of Priscilla LeMone to nursing diagnosis and are pleased to her NANDA's Unique Contribution Award.

Mary Kerr

Mary Kerr has contributed uniquely to the development of nursing diagnoses in a number of ways. She has been a long time member of NANDA and has served on NANDA committees and as a member of the Board of Directors. Throughout her master's and doctoral programs, Mary has continued to work on the development, validation, and refinement of physiological diagnoses. She has published journal articles describing the development, validation, and use of these diagnoses in practice and research. Her service on the Taxonomy Committee resulted in the publication of seminal articles, that analyzed the issues and conceptualization of the NANDA Taxonomy.

While serving as a member of the Board of Directors, Mary and colleague Cindy Dougherty initiated the Preconference Small Group Work to review and further refine selected nursing diagnoses and published a review and annotated bibliography of related research. Mary adds scholarship to NANDA's work in the use in clinical research and practice to advance nursing diagnosis. For her many efforts in behalf of NANDA, we are pleased to present to recognize Mary Kerr's work with the Unique Contribution Award.

Mitsuko Matsuki

Dr. Matsuki's many contributions to NANDA and language development have led to the implementation of nursing diagnosis in a country many thousand miles away from North America. Through her efforts, the Society for Nursing Diagnosis (JSND) was established in 1995. This Society has established a research journal and holds well attended biennial conferences to discuss the issues of nursing diagnoses. Matsuki (sen sie, Professor Matsuki) has also contributed to development of nursing diagnosis through her research on the crosscultural validation of nursing diagnosis. This was the first study of nursing diagnosis in Japan, in fact, the first in

Eastern culture.

Over the years many Japanese nurses have participated in NANDA conferences. This is due to the work of Dr. Matsuki and her colleagues. For her many contributions to NANDA and the advancement of nursing diagnosis, we are pleased to recognize Dr. Mitsuko Matsuki with the Unique Contribution Award.

Mercedes Ugalde

Mercedes Ugalde has contributed to the development and implementation of nursing diagnosis in Spain. She has been an active member of NANDA and has presented papers at multiple NANDA conferences. Mercedes organized the first "Nursing Diagnosis Symposium" in Spain. Over 800 participants attended that meeting to discuss the issues associated with nursing diagnosis and language development.

Concerned with the need to disseminate nursing diagnosis information throughout Spain, Mercedes and her colleagues established the AENTDE. This association serves to coordinate the development and dissemination of nursing diagnosis. In addition they produce and distribute a newsletter that is circulated nationwide as well as internationally. For her leadership and vision, NANDA proudly presents the Unique Contribution Award to Mercedes Ugalde.

Nico Oud

Since 1991, Nico Oud has been involved in the development of nursing diagnoses, interventions and outcomes. In 1992, he and his colleague Leo Regeer attended the Tenth (10th) NANDA conference in San Diego. Following this meeting he organized the first Dutch Conference on the Classification of Nursing Diagnoses and Interventions, called "NANDA: Line of Action for the Netherlands."

Nico presented an article about the measurement methods used to validate nursing diagnoses. From here he went on to the organize (in collaboration with the Danish Institute of Health and Nursing Research) the First European Conference on Nursing Diagnoses: "Creating a European Platform" in November 1993 at Copenhagen. Later he helped organize the Second European Conference on Nursing Diagnoses and Interventions in Brussels, 1995. In 1997 he was elected Board Member (treasurer) of ACENDIO. This group held its First European Conference of the Association for Common European Nursing Diagnoses, Interventions and Outcomes: From Diagnosis to Outcome: Nurses Network Across Europe.

Nico addressed the 1994 NANDA conference on behalf of the Dutch NNA and focused on the developments of nursing diagnoses in the Netherlands during an international panel presentation. In 1995 he co-authored a handbook on nursing diagnoses, interventions and outcomes. As a result of this effort, he is now responsible for the translation of the NANDA diagnoses into the Dutch language. He is also publishing a newsletter in connection with this handbook on a quarterly basis.

Within the Netherlands Nico is an active member of a Network Nursing Diagnosis and an Association for Common Nursing Language in the field of the mentally handicapped. He continues to be an active NANDA member and is chairperson of the Publications Committee at ACENDIO. It is with great pleasure that NANDA presents the Unique Contribution Award to Nico Oud for his outstanding work in behalf of nursing diagnosis and language development.

Editor's Award

Rosemary Carroll Johnson has been a long and loyal friend to and member of NANDA. As the first editor of the *Nursing Diagnosis*, Rosemary was the perfect leader to launch this publication. Her editorial competence and talent enabled her to present a journal that received international visibility and recognition.

Rosemary had a unique ability to develop and shape young authors. Her comfort in sharing personal "know how" with compassion was a valued commodity for young as well as seasoned journal contributors. Rosemary also lent her talent to editing the NANDA Conference Proceedings for the Eighth, Ninth and Tenth conferences. She gave these proceedings a new look while maintaining readability and comprehensibility. For her leadership in helping to develop and influence the direction of nursing scholarship and nursing diagnosis, NANDA is very pleased to present Rosemary Carroll Johnson with NANDA's first Editor's Award. She is most deserving of this recognition.

Dr. Noreen Frisch is currently a fellow in the American Academy of Nursing and Professor and Chairperson of the Department of Nursing at Humboldt State University. She became the second editor of *Nursing Diagnosis: Journal of the North American Nursing Diagnosis Association* in 1993. She served in this role until 1997. During that time, Noreen brought vision and direction to the Journal. Her talent as an editor and her life-long commitment to Nursing Diagnosis made her most ready to assume the challenges of journal editor.

Like Rosemary Carroll-Johnson, Noreen was able to generate manuscripts and develop authors. She showcased their talents and conceptual abilities and helped nurses advance the work of NANDA through scholarly publications. For her years of service and for outstanding leadership in promoting the visibility of nursing diagnoses through scholarship, NANDA is proud to present the Editor's Award to Dr. Noreen Frisch.

International Award

This year the Better Mote International Award was presented to Dr. Mitsuko Matsuki by Cecile Boisvert for her outstanding contribution to the international community and her commitment to the advancement of nursing diagnosis globally.

25th Anniversary Outstanding Leadership Awards

North American Nursing Diagnosis Foundation Gala

The North American Nursing Diagnosis Foundation Gala was held on April 24, 1998 at the Adams Mark Hotel in St. Louis, MO. The event was co-hosted by Dr. Lucille Joel, First Vice President of ICN and Dr. Dorothy Jones, NANDA President-elect. During the Gala, 12 nurse leaders were recognized with the NANDA 25th Anniversary Outstanding Leadership Award for the Advancement of Nursing Diagnosis. The following are the names of the Award recipients and the citation as read for each recipient.

Linda Carpenito

Perhaps one name associated with the promotion and advancement of nursing diagnoses throughout North American and around the world is Linda Juall Carpenito. Linda found a way, both as a speaker and writer, to help nurses, particularly those within the practice settings, understand and use nursing diagnoses.

Professional developments around the nursing diagnosis movement provded Linda with a vehicle to share her personal talents with the work of language development. Linda's ability to connect with clinicians and students in particular is fueled by her own clinical expertise. This expertise, recently complemented by her completion of a Family Nurse Practitioner program, has broadened her ability to address the implications of nursing diagnosis across clinical settings.

Over time, Linda has become a sought after speaker around the world and a leader associated with advancement of nursing diagnosis. Currently, Linda continues to serve as President of LJC Consultant, Inc. in New Jersey and is the editor of *Nursing Forum*.

Her text *Handbook of Nursing Diagnosis* is currently in its sixth edition and has been translated Japanese and Italian. The text *Nursing Diagnosis Application to Clinical Practice* also in its sixth edition, has been translated into Spanish and Japanese. These publications continue to be used by nurses around the world.

Linda brought her commitment and talents to NANDA serving on the Board of Directors from 1986 to 1990. Linda served as Chair of the Diagnostic Review Committee, helping to establish policies and procedures that increased the credibility of those nursing diagnoses and improving the processes used to submit, approve and classify a nursing diagnoses.

Linda served as Chairperson of the Program Committee in 1993. She has been an integral part of the Awards Dinner every year. Those of you who will be at the dinner tomorrow night can judge for yourself. For those of us who have "been there before," you can expect to enjoy that special spark Linda brings to the evening's events. Her energy is contagious and it is equal to the enthusiasm she has used to promote the goals of NANDA and nursing diagnosis.

Linda has been an active participant in the work of NANDA Foundation and hosted the "grand opening" 1996 Gala in Pittsburgh, PA. For her dedication and commitment to nursing diagnosis and the international recognition brought to this Association by her work, NANDA proudly presents the 25th Anniversary Award for the Advancement of Nursing Diagnosis to Linda Jual Carpenito.

Dr. Marjory Gordon

What can one say about Marjory Gordon that does not immediately affiliate her with NANDA and the advancement of nursing diagnosis? Marge Gordon and nursing diagnosis have become inextricably linked, a fact known by our nursing colleagues worldwide. From the time she completed her dissertation on concept attainment and nursing diagnosis at Boston College, Marge has worked to describe the concept and content of nursing diagnosis as clinical judgments made by the professional nurse.

Marge was invited to attend and participate in the first conference facilitated by Gebbie and Lavin in St. Louis in 1973. Later she became the Chairperson of the Task Force of the National Conference Group on the Classification of Nursing Diagnosis. At each subsequent conference, Marge has presented compelling papers that challenged the current state of nursing diagnosis development, always remaining true to the philosophical and theoretical belief that it is through the use of nursing diagnosis that the uniqueness and independence of the nurse can be best articulated.

Marge has presented her ideas through multiple forums. Her numerous publications include *The Manual of Nursing Diagnoses*, translated in multiple languages, and the seminal work *Nursing Diagnosis: Process and Application* are, both known in the nursing community worldwide.

Marge is an internationally sought after world speaker. She is a unique traveler and all of you who have traveled with Marge have your own "Marge" stories... like that last minute purchase she needed to make at a gift shop about a half a quarter of a mile away from the plane's departure area. This of course as the plane has begun boarding. Of course, true to Marge's nature she successfully gets the gift and reaches the plane on time. While I share this humorous side of things, I must add that if you spend time with Marge on these trips you quickly realize how the world honors and respects Marge Gordon and the visability she has given nursing through her work with nursing diagnosis.

Marge has received numerous honors for all of her efforts. She was an early admittant to the American Academy of Nursing and has been recognized by national and state organizations as well as academic institutions and organizations for her achievemts. Boston College is proud to claim her as one of their own. Students at BC and clinicians, particularly in the Boston area, have been influenced by Marge's teaching and scholarship. Through Marge's leadership in the development of the doctoral program in nursing at BC, there is a strong emphasis on clinical judgment. Student dissertations guided by Marge have contributed significantly to research in the areas of diagnostic and ethical reasoning. For others, their nursing career expanded when they took a course or attended a workshop that Marge led. Through her presentation and unique style, Marge inspired the novice to think great thoughts and the expert to actually carry them out.

Marge Gordon is an international leader in the truest sense of the word. Her role as mentor, teacher and researcher is well known.

Personally, my journey to NANDA has been influenced by Marge's enthusiasm and commitment to advancing professional nursing and I thank her for that opportunity. It is therefore with a sense of great personal pride and great privilege that NANDA presents the 25th Anniversary Leadership Award for Outstanding Contribution to the Advancement of Nursing Diagnosis to Dr. Marjory Gordon. For nurses worldwide she remains nursing diagnosis's greatest ambassador.

Lucille Joel

When I first called Dr. Lucille Joel and asked her to serve as chairperson of this year's NANDA Foundation Gala, Lucille responded without hesitation, "Whatever you want, I'll do it." I have known Dr. Joel for any years and have had the privilege of serving on the Congress for Nursing Practice while she was President of the American Nurses Association. Over time I have witnessed dimensions of Lucille's distinguished careerr. Her efforts can be characterized as visionary, tempered by logic and reason.

Lucille has been a long-time supporter of NANDA's efforts. She was a participant in the 1973 inaugural conference in St. Louis and and continues in her role as First Vice-President of the International Council of Nursing (ICN) to address issues related to language development internationally. Just as an aside, when I reviewed early historical NANDA materials in preparation for this conference, I found several communications from Lucille, including a completed order form for conference proceedings.

Lucille has been an activist for nursing for many years. She continues to serve as Professor at Rutgers, The State University of New Jersey, College of Nursing. Early in career she wrote extensively on the once front-page news item DRG'S (Diagnostic Related Groups). She was a leader in receiving funding from the Robert Wood Johnson Nursing Home Demonstration Project and through her efforts this work helped make elder care more visable in the undergraduate nursing curriculum and across the state.

As many of you know Lucille, served two terms as President of the American Nurses Association. Besides being an incredible facilitator of the business meeting, Lucille sheparded many critical issues through the Association. She worked to promote the quality of nursing practice and improved patient care. She facilitated implementation of a new organizational structure at ANA including work on nursing standards and nursing diagnoses.

Lucille has received many honors. She is a Fellow in the American Academy of Nursing and currently as mentioned earlier, First Vice-President of the International Council of Nursing. One of the areas Lucille has addressed in many forums is the effort put forth by the international community on language development and ICNP (International Classification of Nursing Phenomena). Lucille has authored numerous articles, chapters and books. She is the editor of *Dimensions in Professional Nursing* and the current Editor-at- Large of the new and improved *American Journal of Nursing*.

Lucille has been an advocate for nursing over the years. She continues to give voice to the contributions of the practicing nurse and quality patient care. For her dedication and commitment to nursing and nursing diagnosis internationally and the global recognition brought to American Nursing by her presence, NANDA proudly presents the 25th Anniversary Award for the Advancement of Nursing Diagnoses to a most worthy recipient, Dr. Lucille Joel.

Dr. Norma Lang

Dr. Lang has held many influential positions in nursing throughout her long and successful career. Currently, she is the Margaret Bond Simon Dean and Professor at the University of the Pennsylvania School of Nursing. Previously, she was Dean and Professor at the University of Wisconsin Milwaukee School of Nursing.

In the late 1970's Dr. Lang chaired the American Nurses Association's (ANA) practice committee, which issued and implemented "Nursing: A Social Policy Statement." This document formed the definition of nursing and defined the scope of professional and practice. It was this document that guided ANA policy decisions through the 1980's and heavily influenced policy in England's Royal College of Nursing. Dr. Lang has served as a consultant to the International Council of Nurses (ICN) in Geneva, Switzerland and helped to foster the development of the International Classification of Nursing Practice (ICNP).

Over the years Dr. Lang has been a visible participant at many NANDA conferences. She has presented papers at NANDA and has spoken at international forums in behalf of nursing diagnosis.

Dr. Lang holds many national and international appointments on committees where the issues around the development and use of nursing diagnoses are discussed. These appointments include, but are not limited to, serving as ANA Chairperson of the National Data Base Steering Comittee (1989 to 1997), member of the National Center for Nursing Priority Expert Panel on Information Systems and her most recent leadership work with ICN and ICNP (Alpha Version) project.

Dr. Lang's research has addressed issues including quality assurance, nursing standards and outcome measures, peer review, the nursing minimum data set and development and evaluation of the ICNP. Her pioneering work in identifying standards to evaluate the quality of nursing care has served as the basis for nursing policy throughout the world. The seminal model for measuring and evaluating the quality of nursing care which bears her name has been adopted in the U.S., Canada, Australia, and the United Kingdom.

Dr. Lang is a prolific writer and has recently authored several articles with June Clark on the ICNP project in Europe. An article published in 1997 in *International Nursing Review* focused on the "International Classification for Nursing Practice: Classification for Outcomes."

It is with the recognition of the many contributions made by Dr. Norma Lang to the discipline of nursing and nursing diagnosis globally that NANDA enthusiastically presents the 25th

Anniversary Leadership Award for Outstanding Contribution to the Advancement of Nursing Diagnosis. Due to travel outside the country, Dr. Lang has asked that Dr. Judy Warren, our current NANDA President and close colleague, to accept this award on her behalf.

Ann McCourt

Ann McCourt is a native of Massachusetts and a graduate of Simmons College and Boston University. She has been a long-standing and loyal member of NANDA serving on many committees and task forces. From 1989-1993, Ann was a member of NANDA's Diagnostic Review Committee bringing her talent and leadership to this group's agenda. Ann is now become a resident of Florida... but remains in close contact with friends and family "up north." Since her move, Ann has served as Vice-President of the Southern Area Nursing Diagnosis Association, SANDA, and was the editor of their newsletter, the SANDA News.

Ann has brought two significant perspectives to promoting nursing diagnosis nationally and internationally. First, was her pioneering work with the American Nurses Association as well as NANDA on quality assurance and outcomes. These contributions were published in several NANDA proceedings and other journals including the *Nursing Clinics of North America*. As a result, Ann became a sought after speaker on this topic participating in over forty-five workshops related to the implementation of nursing diagnosis and quality assurance.

The second major career effort for Ann has been the advancement of nursing diagnoses with specialty organizations, in particular the Rehabilitation Nurses Association. As a long-standing member of this Association, Ann helped make visible the work of rehabilitation nurses. Over the years she has assisted in the development of five nursing diagnoses including "Total Self Care Deficit; Self Feeding Deficit" and "High Risk for Disuse Syndrome."

In addition to honors including the American Nurses Association's Honorary Membership Award, Ann received NANDA's Unique Contribution Award in 1996. For this recognition one of her nominator's wrote, "Through her commitment to nursing practice Ann has become a role model... tirelessly demonstrating the usefulness of nursing diagnosis in directing and describing practice."

Even though she is now retired, Ann remains a consultant to the Rehabilitation Nurses and continues to move the work of nursing diagnosis ahead within this forum. For a lifetime of service to nursing and nursing diagnoses, it is a pleasure to award Ann McCourt NANDA's 25th Anniversary Leadership Award for Outstanding Contributions to the Advancement of Nursing Diagnosis. She is most deserving of this recognition.

Hildegard Peplau

Dr. Hildegard Peplau has remained a steadfast and loyal supporter of the nursing diagnosis movement. Throughout her career, Dr. Peplau has been a public advocate for this effort in forums at the national and international levels. Recently, in her acceptance speech following the presentation of the Christian Reimann Award at the 1997 International Council of Nursing, Dr. Peplau expressed a commitment to the use of nursing diagnosis as a vehicle for disciplinary clarity and recognition for nursing contributions to patient care.

Dr. Peplau has had a long and distinguished career in nursing. She is a "Living Legend" in the full sense of the word. As a diploma graduate from Pottstown Hospital in Pennsylvania to her reciept of a master's in Psychiatric Nursing as well as a doctorate from Teachers College Columbia University, Dr. Peplau acquired both knowledge and perspective. But it is the faculty at Rutgers, The State University of New Jersey, College of Nursing who claim Dr. Peplau as their Professor Emerita.

Dr. Peplau's her impact on nursing has been global. Nurses worldwide, and I am sure even many at this conference, have been touched by Dr. Peplau's wisdom, compassion, friendship and above all, dedication to psychiatric mental health nursing. In a time when many wonder about nursing's future, Dr. Peplau will quickly remind us of the mission nursing plays in the improvement and direction of world health. As with the clinical nurse specialists she educated, her words continue to direct us and give clarity to an evolving discipline.

Dr. Peplau's honors are numerous and include honorary degrees from Boston College, Rutgers University, Alfred University, and Duke University. In 1974 she was inducted into the American Academy of Nursing and was recognized by the American Nurses Association for her many contributions to nursing with the establishment of the Hildegard Peplau Award. Dr. Peplau has held numerous positions and has spoken worldwide. Her publications capture a lifetime of changes in nursing. One article written during her tenure as Executive Director of the American Nurses Association (1980) focused on the impact of the social policy statement on the scope of nursing practice and diagnosis. This work is still very relevant today.

Dr. Peplau's efforts in behalf of nursing have been nothing short of remarkable. Unfortunately, Dr. Peplau now an active 88 year old living in California and unable to be with us tonight. But true to her nature, she assumed full responsibility for making sure that NANDA knew how much she appreciates tonight's honor. To this end, she prepared her remarks and sent them to her friend (and mine) and former Dean of Rutgers College of Nursing, Dr. Dorothy DeMaio. Dorothy is currently serving in the role as University Professor at Rutgers University. We would like to welcome her here tonight to accept NANDA's 25th Anniversary Award for Outstanding Contributions to the Advancement of Nursing Diagnosis in behalf of Dr. Peplau.

Audrey McLane

Dr. Audrey McLane is a lifetime member of NANDA, a scholar and major contributor to the shaping and development of nursing diagnosis. Over the years she has been recognized as an outstanding leader in nursing. She was honored by NANDA with the Unique Contribution Award to Nursing Diagnosis in 1996. She also received the St. Louis University Alumnae Merit Award and is Professor Emeritus of College of Nursing at Marquette University, Milwaukee, WI.

Audrey's publications are numerous and noteworthy. In 1984 she received the *American Journal of Nursing* "Book of the Year Award" for "A Pocket Guide to Nursing Diagnoses and Classification of Nursing Diagnoses." She completed an early definitive work on the nursing diagnoses related to elimination and spirituality. Audrey has authored many publications for textbooks and journals. She was an editor for the Proceedings from the 7th NANDA Conference.

Dr. Audrey McLane has been a member of NANDA since its inception and a member of national task force (1980-83). She served on the NANDA Board of Directors from 1983-1987, and again from 1992-1994. She was Vice-

President of NANDA from 1987-1991, Chairperson Regional Affairs Committee (1986-1989), member and Chairperson of the Program Committee (1983-1986) and Chairperson of the Diagnostic Review Committee (1990-1993). Audrey was also a member of the regional group SANDA from 1989-1990.

Audrey is a voice of reason on issues sensitive to NANDA. She has been a committed leader and has given years of dedicated service to advance the goals of the Association. For these efforts along with a lifetime of nursing accomplishments NANDA presents to Dr. Audrey McLane the 25th Anniversary Leadership Award for Outstanding Contribution to the Advancement of Nursing Diagnosis. She has brought NANDA vision in the past and remains a loyal member as we move to the next century

Winnifred Mills

Winnifred Mills has been a lifetime supporter of the North American Nursing Diagnosis Association. Through her efforts, the Canadian Nurses were brought into the early developments of the Association. Since that time she has remained a voice for NANDA in the United States and across Canada. This contribution was most evident in the leadership she provided to initiate the first International Conference on Nursing Diagnosis in Alberta, Canada in the mid-1980s. This effort helped to introduce the work of NANDA to the international community.

Winn was educated at Holy Cross Hospital in Alberta, Canada and received her Masters in Educational Administration at the University of Alberta in Edmonton, Alberta. Throughout her career Winn worked as both a clinician and educator in Canada. In addition she served as consultant for quality assurance across internationally. She is currently Principal Associate at the Western Counseling Associates and an educator. In 1989 Winn was project coordinator, assigned to plan and implement a research review of the Alberta nursing practice standards. This report was approved and accepted by the Association of Alberta Registered Nurses.

As one reviews NANDA's history, the impact of Winnifred Mills is clearly evdent. Many articles in the Proceedings of the 5th, 9th,10th and 12th conferences provide significant cotributions to the advancemant of nursing diagnosis development. Winn's scholarship has focused on issues related to Taxonomy development, classification of selected nursing diagnoses, diagnostic reasoning and quality assurance. Many of her co-authors have often been NANDA members. Winn will have a special article in the upcoming Anniversary issue of the NANDA journal. In addition, she has presented on many of these topics globally.

Winn Mills served on the first NANDA Board of Directors (1982) and served on many Association committees, including the first Taxonomy Committee. For her many contributions to she recieved NANDA's Unique Contribution Award in 1994.

Winn has been a kind and generous friend to NANDA and nursing diagnosis internationally. In her quiet but firm way she has provided this organization leadership, reason, direction and open communication. Tonight it is with admiration of friends and colleagues and recognition of a lifetime committment to nursing we of leadership that NANDA presents to Winifred Mills the 25th Anniversary Leadership Award for Outstanding Contribution to the Advancement of Nursing Diagnosis.

Harriet Werley

Rarely was there a NANDA conference where we did not see Harriet Werley at the microphone. Her words were always clear and profound. As one listened to Harriet you were always impressed by her knowledge and ability to "zero in" on the heart of the matter. She continued to help us refine our thinking about language and data management, through many a long deliberation at business meetings. What is most profound about Harriet's efforts has been the realization that her efforts have stood the test of time. As we move toward the next millennium, the direction of our future is clearly infused with the development of data sets and informatics.

Besides her watchful attendance at NANDA conferences, Harriet always made NANDA visible at national and international meetings. As chairperson of the committee to establish the Nursing Minimum Data Set, Harriet saw an immediate link to the work of nursing diagnosis and helped to bring visibility to the nursing diagnosis movement globally. In one of her many articles presented as an invited paper during the 5th NANDA Conference, Harriet addressed the issues around nursing diagnoses development and the Nursing Minimum Data Set.

It is very important for nurses to support and help put into effect nursing care that is based on sound clinical judgment and results in making a nursing diagnosis, thus leading to the nursing actions, or interventions, to be taken on the patient's behalf. It will be important for nurses to show a united front in promoting and using nursing diagnoses, if nurses are to convince federal officials who make health information policy that they should review the NMDS favorably support is being field tested nationally, and then implement it in a variety of their health care programs, such as Medicare and Medicaid.

Harriet has been retired from her academic position at the University of Wisconsin for several years. Until very recently, she continued to attend NANDA conferences. Her words of wisdom brought us clarity and offered vision to a growing Association. For those who were mentored by Harriet, her vision lives on. Throughout her life, Harriet has been a well-respected scholar, international leader and academician. Along with Fellowship in the American Academy of Nursing, Harriet has received many honors. We at NANDA would like to add one more recognition to her lifetime of achievements by presenting Dr. Harriet Werley with NANDA's 25th Anniversary Leadership Award for Outstanding Contributions to the Advancement of Nursing Diagnosis. Her faithful vigilance has helped to bring NANDA to this celebration.

Harriet is not able to be with us at this conference, but accepting this award for her friend and colleague is Dr. Marjory Gordon.

Dr. Kenneth Cianfrani

Dr. Kenneth Cianfrani brought excitement and enthusiasm to his work with the nursing diagnosis movement. This was most evident in the leadership he provided to nurses in the Midwest and in particular in his home state of Illinois. Ken was a leader and friend to many nurses, particularly to those within the NANDA network. He was always ready to lend a helping hand and had a smile that demonstrated a love for life and his commitment to knowledge development.

Ken was a member of the NANDA Board of Directors from 1988-1992 and was a former recipient of the Association's Unique Contribution Award. As a teacher, researcher and clinician Ken advanced the work of NANDA until his untimely death. The editors of NANDA's 10th Conference Proceedings seem to capture Ken's essence in a dedication they wrote in the introduction to the text. I would like to read what they wrote to you now:

> This book is dedicated to Kenneth L. Cianfrani, Ph.D., RN, for his belief in, commitment to, and support and value of nurses, nursing, and nursing diagnosis. His dedication to the continued growth and development of the discipline of nursing was imbedded in his leadership in NANDA at local, regional, national, and international levels. Through his enduring efforts to share knowledge about the development, implementation, use, and research of nursing diagnosis with all nurses, he founded and chaired the Midwest Nursing Diagnosis Task Force (1982-1991).

> May his zest for life, his effervescent spirit of inquiry, and his pursuit of personal and professional development live on in us and guide NANDA as we move toward the 21st century and the goal of a standardized language for nursing.

It is with gratitude that we award posthumously NANDA's 25th Anniversary Leadership Award for Outstanding Contributions to the Advancement of Nursing Diagnosis to Dr. Kenneth Cianfrani. His dedication to NANDA will live on in the nurses he taught, the scholarship he wrote and the spirit in which he demonstrated leadership and commitment. Accepting this award in Ken's memory will be Dr. Georgia Whitley, a personal friend of Ken and his family and current member of the NANDA Board.

Peggy Mehmert

We would like to also recognize the unique contributions of another NANDA member, Peggy Mehmert. Peg was a nurse administrator at Mercy Hospital in Davenport, Iowa (Genesis Medical Center). Peg was influential force in facilitating the implementation of nursing diagnosis at her hospital. Through her efforts, nursing diagnoses were put into a hospital-wide, computerized information system long before it was a mainstream effort. Peg worked with Ken Cianfrani at the University of Illinois and with the faculty at University of Iowa. These impressive connections gave her an opportunity to connect with leaders in the work of language development and to use this knowledge in her teaching and practice.

Peg was the President and Secretary of the Midwest Task Force on Nursing Diagnosis. She was also a member of the NANDA Board of Directors and contributed to many of the Association's committees. In all of her professional work Peg was a promoter of NANDA. She served as a mentor to other nurses, always bringing a cohort of nurses with her to conferences. She enjoyed her role as a NANDA ambassador and was able to get people excited about nursing diagnoses. Until her death, Peg Mehmert was a nursing administrator and colleague dedicated to the promotion of nursing diagnosis. For a lifetime of dedication and commitment to the work of NANDA, we are proud to present NANDA's 25th Leadership Award for Outstanding

Contribution to the Advancement of Nursing Diagnosis posthumously to Peggy Mehmert. In honor of this special award we are pleased to have two women who were mentored by Peg with us tonight. Mary Clark and Marilyn Wilerty will accept this award in honor of their colleague and friend, Peg Mehmert.

Jean Jenny

Jean Jenny has been a lifetime friend of NANDA. Over the years she has been recognized for the scholarship and her wisdom. Jean, like Winn, brought to NANDA the perspective of the Canadian nurses and was a voice for testing and validation of nursing diagnoses as well as Taxonomy development. Jean worked tirelessly in behalf of NANDA and was a member of many committees. She served on the first Editorial Advisory Board of *Nursing Diagnosis Journal* and contributed many articles throughout the tenure of the journal. Her articles always brought both clarity and vision to the reader.

Jean was a scholar who had the capacity to link nursing research and practice with ease. Even better, she could stand up at a national conference and in the midst of great confusion, make sense of complex issues. As one reviews issues of past Proceedings the name of Jean Jenny is a prominent one. Over the years Jean has given much to NANDA. She has done so with a sense of grace and charm, always respectful of another's point of view... and for this we are grateful.

Jean is unable to be with us tonight. She has retired to Florida since the death of her husband. I had a long letter from her in response to her receipt of our letter announcing tonight's award. She asked me to accept this honor in her behalf and to express to the membership her profound gratitude. In retrospect, she said, NANDA provided her with new friendships, memories to last a lifetime and created new opportunities for personal growth. She indicated that she was glad to be part of such a movement and wished us well in the future.

For her years of service to NANDA and the scholarship and knowledge she provided through her association with NANDA we are most appreciative. We are pleased to present to Jean Jenny our 25th Anniversary Leadership Award for Outstanding Contribution to the Advancement of Nursing Diagnosis.

Appendix

North American Nursing Diagnosis Association Bylaws

Article I
Title, Purpose and Function

Section 1. Title. The name of this Association shall be the North American Nursing Diagnosis Association, Inc.

Section 2. Purpose. This Association is organized to develop, refine, disseminate and promote nursing diagnostic terminology as well as taxonomic structure for use by professional nurses including, but not limited to:

- Conducting conferences
- Publishing a journal and other documents
- Facilitating research
- Serving as an information resource

Section 3. Restrictions. The Association qualifies as a tax exempt organization within the meaning of section 501(c) (6) of the U.S. Internal Revenue Code. The affairs of the Association shall be conducted in such a manner as to qualify for tax exemption under that provision.

Section 4. Equal Rights. The purposes of this Association shall be unrestricted by consideration of nationality, race, creed, lifestyle, color, sex, or age.

Article II
Membership

Section 1. Composition: The membership of NANDA will consist of Regular, Associate, Regional Affiliate, Student and Institutional Members.

Section 2. The membership shall be organized into seven (7) districts.

These districts will consist of:

District #1 — Northeastern

District #2 — Central Atlantic

District #3 — Southeastern

District #4 — North Central

District #5 — South Central

District #6 — North Pacific

District #7 — South Pacific

Section 3. Regular Member. A Regular Member is one who holds unrestricted licensure or a comparable credential to practice as a professional nurse and whose dues are current.

Nurses with inactive or retired status licensure may also be Regular Members. Regular Members are entitled to vote, hold office, serve on Committees, and otherwise actively participate in all other activities of the Association.

Section 4. Associate Member. An Associate Member is one who does not qualify as a Regular Member, who shares an interest in the purposes of the Association and whose dues are current. Unlicensed undergraduate students may also be Associate Members. Associate Members do not have a vote, may not hold office, and may not serve on Committees. They may participate in all other activities of the Association.

Section 5. Affiliate Members. A Regional Affiliate Member is a regional organization whose purpose, structure, and Bylaws are consistent with and meet the criteria of the Association. Affiliate Membership is established by application to and approval of the Board of Directors. Benefits of Affiliate Membership do not include the right to vote, hold office or serve on Committees.

Section 6. Student Member. A Student Member is a licensed professional nurse who is matriculating in an undergraduate, master's or doctoral program. Student Members are entitled to voting privileges.

Section 7. Institutional Member. An Institutional Member is an organization having a major purpose of providing nursing care to clients, such as a hospital; one engaged in the education of nurses, such as a nursing school, and/or engaged in nursing research. They shall have one vote.

Section 8. Membership Year. The membership year shall be a period of 12 consecutive months, beginning the first month of each quarter (July, October, January, April).

Article III
Financial Administration

Section 1. Fiscal Year. The fiscal year will be a period of 12 consecutive months beginning July 1 and ending June 30 of the following year.

Section 2. Dues. The dues of this Association shall be set by the Board of Directors with the approval of a simple majority of the General Assembly or by a majority of a mail ballot of the membership. Any member who fails to pay the dues within four (4) months after they become payable shall be dropped from the membership role.

Section 3. The Board of Directors delegates through a payment arrangement the directing and maintaining of the operations of the organization. This person(s) insures that all funds, physical assets and other property of the organization are safeguarded and administered as directed by the Board of Directors.

Article IV
Officers and Duties of Officers

Section 1. Composition. The Executive Committee of the Association will be the President, President-Elect, Secretary, and Treasurer. These officers are authorized to transact the business of the Association between meetings of the Board, and assist the President as needed. They shall also perform the duties usually performed by such officers as specified in these Bylaws or as designated by the Board.

Section 2. Vacancy. A vacancy in the office of President will be filled by the President-Elect. The offices of Secretary or Treasurer will be filled by appointment by the Board of Directors until the next regularly scheduled election for that office. A vacancy in the office of President-Elect will be filled only through the election process.

Section 3. Duties. The Executive Committee is authorized to assist the President with the business of the Association and to transact the business of the Association between meetings as may be required.

a) The President. The President is the Chairperson of the Board of Directors and ex-officio member of all Committees and task forces except the Nominating Committee. The President presides at all meetings of the Association, appoints ad-hoc Committees or task forces, serves as the Association's representative and performs other duties as assigned by the Board.

b) President-Elect. The President-Elect assumes the duties of the President in case of the President's absence and performs other duties as assigned by the Board.

c) Secretary. The Secretary is responsible for the minutes of all proceedings of the Association and the Board. The Secretary performs other duties as may be assigned by the Board.

Section 8. Compensation. Elected officers will not receive any compensation for their services but may be reimbursed for their expenses.

Article V
Board of Directors

Section 1. Composition. The Board of Directors of the Association shall be the officers (President, President-Elect, Secretary, and Treasurer) and five (5) directors.

Section 2. The term of office. The term of office of the Board of Directors of the Association will be four years. A member, who has served more than a half of a term, will be deemed to have served a term. The term of office will commence at the end of the Association's biennial conference and will continue until the expiration of their term of office or until their successor is elected. A member of the Board of Directors of the Association may be reelected one time with no more than eight consecutive years of service on the Board of Directors of the Association.

Section 3. Election of the Board. The President-Elect would be elected every two years. This individual would advance to the office of President at the end of the two years to complete the four year term in office. The offices of Secretary and three (3) Directors will be in opposite years from the Treasurer and two (2) Directors.

Section 4. Meetings. The Board of Directors shall meet at least annually during the fiscal year of the Association. Special meetings may be called with a ten-day notice to each of the Board members. Special meetings may be called by the President or by written request by four (4) or more Board members.

Section 5. Board Vacancy. Vacancy occurs in the case of resignation or absence of a member of the Board from one day or more of the two regularly scheduled meetings in succession unless excused by the President. Such vacancy except for the office of President and President-Elect will be filled by appointment of the Board.

Section 6. Duties of the Board. The Board of Directors shall have authority over the business of the Association between regular Association meetings, except that of modifying any action taken by the members. The Board will perform the following duties and others as delegated to it by the Association:

a) Delegate operations of the organization and fix compensation.

b) Establish administrative policies governing the affairs of the Association.

c) Develop/implement a strategic plan toward the accomplishment of the Association's purposes.

d) Transact the general business of the Association.

e) Provide a biennial report to the membership at a regular meeting of the Association.

f) Act as the custodian of the property, securities and records of the Association; select a place for the deposit of funds of the Association; provide for the annual audit of the books of the Association; provide for bonding of Board officials as it may deem necessary and provide for payment of authorized expenses.

g) Establish and dissolve task forces and appointments to accomplish the purposes of this Association.

h) Fill vacancies except the office of President.

i) Set date and place of General Assembly.

j) Adopt a biennial budget and review/revise said budget at least annually.

k) Perform other duties as assigned elsewhere in the Bylaws of the Association.

Section 7. Retiring Members. All retiring members of the Board shall deliver to the Association within one month all Association properties in their possession.

Article VI
Committees

Section 1. Composition. The Association will have the following standing Committees: Diagnosis Review, Membership, Nominating, International Affairs, Taxonomy, Publications, and Bylaws Committees. Ad-Hoc Committees and task forces will be formed by the Board as necessary to fulfill the functions of the organization.

Section 2. Terms of Memberships. The terms of memberships is for four (4) years. All members of the Membership Committee are elected. For other Committees, half of the Committee members are elected and one-half are appointed by the President in consultation with the Executive Committee. Appointments and elections are staggered so that one-half of the membership is elected every two years. A member may be elected/reappointed one time with no more than eight successive years of service on a Committee.

Section 3. Committee Selection. Each Committee will be composed of NANDA members. The President in consultation with the Executive Committee appoints a Chairperson to each Committee with attention to previous Committee involvement, geographic location and clinical expertise. The Committee Chairperson reports to the Board and to meetings of the Association.

Section 4. Duties.

a) Diagnosis Review. The Diagnosis Review Committee will review proposed diagnoses and make recommendations to the Board. The Committee will designate the format for submission and review of the proposed diagnoses or revision to previously accepted diagnoses. The

Committee will identify research priorities related to nursing diagnoses.

b) Membership. The Membership Committee will establish and promote strategies related to:

- Increasing membership
- Providing a mechanism for bringing communication of membership with Board and General Assembly
- Awarding recognition of NANDA awards for outstanding contributions to the advancement of Nursing Diagnosis.

c) Nominating. The Nominating Committee will solicit nominations and prepare the ballot biennially.

d) Taxonomy. The Taxonomy Committee will develop, review, revise and promote a taxonomic system for the diagnoses. The Committee will make recommendations to the Board for review. The Committee will collaborate with groups supporting other established health-related taxonomies and will identify research priorities.

e) Bylaws. The Bylaws Committee will solicit suggestions from the membership prior to biennial General Assembly. The Committee will review the Bylaws every two years and recommend changes to the Board and General Assembly.

f) Publications. The Publications Committee shall oversee the publications of the Association including but not limited to the journal of Nursing Diagnosis and the taxonomy publication.

g) International Affairs. The International Affairs Committee will promote networking with international nurses interested in nursing diagnosis, and promote information exchange between NANDA and other organizations with international scope related to NANDA interests.

Article VII
Elections

Section 1. Nominating Committee Membership. The President shall appoint one (1) member to the Committee. No member of the Committee may be a member of the Board of Directors. In addition, four (4) members shall be elected by the membership. The Chair will be the elected member with the most votes.

Section 2. Election Procedure. Regular elections will be held every two years in accordance with Association policies and Bylaws. An election is constituted by a plurality of voting members or by lot in case of a tie vote.

Section 3. Tellers. The tellers will be appointed by the President. Tellers will count ballots and cast lots for tie votes.

Article VIII
General Assembly

Section 1. Composition. The composition of the General Assembly shall be the voting members and associate members who are in attendance at the meetings of the Association.

Section 2. Purpose. The General Assembly will approve Bylaws and review and comment on proposed diagnoses from the Diagnosis Review Committee.

Article IX
Meetings

Section 1. General Assembly. The General

Assembly will meet at least once every thirty (30) months. The receipt of a written notice of the time and place of each regular meeting will be sufficient notice of the meeting.

Section 2. Waiver of Notice. Whenever any notice is required to be given under the provision of these Bylaws or under the provisions of the Articles of Incorporation or under the provisions of the laws of the State of Missouri, a waiver in writing signed by the person or persons entitled to such notice, whether before or after the time stated therein, shall be deemed equivalent to the giving of such notice. Further, the notice will be mailed to all members.

Section 3. Special meetings. Special meetings of the General Assembly may be called by the President upon majority vote of the Board or upon the written request of 100 members representing at least four districts. Each member will be sent a written notice of at least ten (10) days prior to the date of the meeting.

Article X
Quorum

Section 1. General Assembly. A simple majority of those registered for the day of the meeting will constitute a quorum at any regular meeting.

Section 2. Special meetings. A 2/3 majority of the one-hundred (100) members requesting the special meeting will constitute a quorum.

Section 3. Board of Directors. A majority of the members of the Board shall constitute a quorum at any meeting of the Board.

Article XI
Parliamentary Authority

The rules contained in Robert's Rules of Order, Newly Revised shall govern meetings of this Association in all cases to which they are applicable and in which they are not inconsistent with these Bylaws.

Article XII
Amendments

Section 1. Amendments. Proposal of Amendments. Proposed amendments from the Bylaws Committee will be submitted to the Board prior to submission to the membership. Proposed amendments will be sent to all members at least two-months prior to the General Assembly meeting. Amendments to the Bylaws may be proposed at the General Assembly by a majority vote of the voting membership present.

Section 2. No notice. These Bylaws may be amended without previous notice at any regular or special meeting of the General Assembly by a ninety nine percent vote of those members present and voting.

Article XIII
Dissolution

The Association may be dissolved by a two-thirds vote of the members upon recommendation of the General Assembly. Upon dissolution after payment of all liabilities, the remaining assets shall be distributed to any nursing organization provided that no distribution shall be made to any organization not then covered by Section 501(c)(3) of the Internal Revenue Service Code of 1954 or the corresponding provisions of any future federal or applicable tax law.

The North American Nursing Diagnosis Association adopted its Bylaws in March 1994. The Association replaced the National Group for the Classification of Nursing Diagnosis which was established in 1973. The Association incorporated in February 1985 and the Bylaws were amended in March 1986, March 1988; March 1990, April 1992, and March 1994.

Guidelines for Nursing Diagnosis Submission

The North American Nursing Diagnosis Association (NANDA) solicits nursing diagnoses for review by the Association. Proposed diagnoses or revisions of diagnoses undergo a systematic review for determination of consistency with criteria for a nursing diagnosis. All submissions are subsequently staged according to evidence supporting either the level of development or validation (see attached CRITERIA FOR STAGING NURSING DIAGNOSES and GLOSSARY OF TERMS).

You may submit at various levels depending on the level of completeness, e.g., label and definition, label, definition, and defining characteristics, or all of the above with clinical research. Submit your work on the ABSTRACT OF NURSING DIAGNOSIS form.

Upon receipt of your diagnosis, the Diagnostic Review Committee (DRC) will review and stage it. Diagnoses will be entered into the taxonomy at level 1.4. Prior to the development at level 1.4 you may seek consultation from the DRC and/or experts in the area of concern to assist you with further development and placement in the taxonomy.

MAIL TO: NANDA, 1211 Locust Street; Philadelphia, PA 19107 FAX TO: 215-545-8107

Definition of Terms: Nursing Diagnosis

Nursing diagnosis: a clinical judgment about individual, family, or community responses to actual or potential health problems/life processes. Nursing diagnoses provide the basis for selection of nursing interventions to achieve outcomes for which the nurse is accountable (approved at the 9th conference, 1990).

Actual nursing diagnosis: describe human responses to health conditions/life processes that exist in an individual, family or community. It is supported by defining characteristics (manifestations/signs and symptoms) that cluster in patterns of related cues or inferences.

Risk nursing diagnosis: describe human responses to health conditions/life processes which may develop in a vulnerable individual, family or community. It is supported by risk factors that contribute to increased vulnerability.

Wellness nursing diagnosis: describe human responses to levels of wellness in an individual, family, or community that have a potential for enhancement to a higher state.

Components of a Diagnosis

Label: provides a name for a diagnosis. It is a concise term or phrase that represents a pattern of related cues. It may include qualifiers (see below).

Definition: provides a clear, precise description, delineates its meaning, and helps differentiate it from similar diagnoses.

Defining Characteristics: observable cues/inferences that cluster as manifestations of a nursing diagnosis. These are listed for actual and wellness diagnoses. A defining characteristic is described as critical if it must be present to make the diagnosis, and is described as major if it is usually present when the diagnosis exists. It is described as minor if it provides supporting evidence for the diagnosis but may not be present. Critical and major defining characteristics need to be substantiated by research.

Related factors: conditions/circumstances that contribute to the development/maintenance of a nursing diagnosis.

Risk factors: environmental factors and physiological, psychological, genetic, or chemical elements that increase the vulnerability of an individual, family, or community to an unhealthful event.

Qualifiers for Diagnoses

(Suggested/not limited to the following)

Acute	severe but of short duration
Altered	a change from baseline
Chronic	lasting a long time, recurring, habitual, constant
Decreased	lessened, lesser in size, amount or degree
Deficient	inadequate in amount, quality or degree, defective, not sufficient, incomplete
Depleted	emptied wholly or in part, exhausted of
Disturbed	agitated, interrupted, interfered with
Dysfunctional	abnormal, incomplete functioning
Excessive	characterized by an amount or quantity that is greater than necessary, desirable, or useful
Increased	greater in size, amount or degree
Impaired	made worse, weakened, damaged, reduced, deteriorated
Ineffective	not producing the desired effect
Intermittent	stopping or starting again at intervals, periodic, cyclic
Potential for	(for use with wellness diagnoses)
Enhanced	made greater, to increase in quality or more desired

NANDA: Developmental Stages for Nursing Diagnoses

1.0		Received for Development (DRC Consultation)
	1.1	Label Only
	1.2	Label and Definition
	1.3	Label and Defining Characteristics or Risk Factors
	1.4	Label, Definition, and Defining Characteristics or

                       Risk Factors, References

2.0   Accepted for Clinical Development
         (Authentication/Substantiation)

      2.1   Label, Definition, Defining
               Characteristics and Literature
               Review

      2.2   Case Study

      2.3   Clinical Series

3.0   Clinically Supported
         (Validation and Testing)

      3.1   ° °

      3.2   ° °

      3.3   ° °

4.0   Revision
         (Refinement)

      4.1   ° °

      4.2   ° °

° °Criteria Under Development

NANDA: Criteria for Staging Nursing Diagnoses

1.0   Received for Development
         (DRC Consultation)

      1.1   Label Only

This stage is primarily intended for submission by organized groups rather than individuals. The DRC will consult with and educate potential developers through distribution of printed guidelines for diagnostic development, telephone consultation and referral to diagnostic development experts. At this stage the label would be categorized as received for development.

1.2 Label and Definition

The label is clear and stated at a basic level. The definition is consistent with the label. The label and definition should be distinct and contrast from other diagnoses. The definition differs from the defining characteristics and label, and these components should not be included in the definition. At this stage the diagnosis must be consistent with the current NANDA definition of nursing diagnosis and is screened for meeting this criteria. (Refer to Glossary of Terms.)

1.3 Label and Defining Characteristics or Risk Factors

The defining characteristics or risk factors (for risk diagnoses) should be consistent with the label. The defining characteristics should be distinct, observable and measurable. The list of defining characteristics may include both major and minor characteristics. The number of major characteristics should be limited to 5-7. (Refer to Glossary of Terms.)

1.4 Label, Definition, and Defining Characteristics or Risk Factors, References

The label, definition, and defining characteristics or risk factors are consistent. References are included. Criteria in 1.2 and 1.3 must be met. At this stage the label will be forwarded to the Taxonomy Committee for classification.

At stage 1.2, 1.3, 1.4 the content will be examined for consistency with the current nursing knowledge base. The content should be consistent with the Glossary of Terms. Collaboration with experts may be utilized. Consultation with the DRC is encouraged.

2.0   Accepted for Clinical Development
         (Authentication/Substantiation)

      2.1   Label, Definition, Defining
               Characteristics and Literature
               Review

A narrative review of relevant literature is required to demonstrate the existence of a substantive body of knowledge underlying the diagnosis. The literature review is consistent with the label and definition. Literature should include discussion and support of the defining characteristics or risk factors (for high risk diagnoses), and related factors (for actual diagnoses).

2.2 Case Study

The criteria in 2.1 are met. The narrative includes the description of an actual case that exhibits the nursing diagnosis and includes defining characteristics or risk factors. Related factors, interventions and outcomes are optional.

2.3 Clinical Studies

The criteria for 2.1 are met. The narrative includes the description of a series of at least 10 cases which exhibit the diagnosis and includes defining characteristics or risk factors, related factors, interventions and outcomes.

3.0 Clinically Supported
(Validation and Testing)

3.1 **

3.2 **

3.3 **

4.0 Revision
(Refinement)

4.1 **

4.2 **

**Criteria Under Development

NANDA Labels

NANDA Definitions & Classification 1997-1998 – Labels
This list represents the NANDA-approved nursing diagnoses for clinical use and testing (1994).

PATTERN 1: EXCHANGING

1.1.2.1	Altered Nutrition: More Than Body Requirements
1.1.2.2	Altered Nutrition: Less Than Body Requirements
1.1.2.3	Altered Nutrition: Risk for More Than Body Requirements
1.2.1.1	Risk for Infection
1.2.2.1	Risk for Altered Body Temperature
1.2.2.2	Hypothermia
1.2.2.3	Hyperthermia
1.2.2.4	Ineffective Thermoregulation
1.2.3.1	Dysreflexia
1.3.1.1	Constipation
1.3.1.1.1	Perceived Constipation
1.3.1.1.2	Colonic Constipation
1.3.1.2	Diarrhea
1.3.1.3	Bowel Incontinence
1.3.2	Altered Urinary Elimination
1.3.2.1.1	Stress Incontinence
1.3.2.1.2	Reflex Incontinence
1.3.2.1.3	Urge Incontinence
1.3.2.1.4	Functional Incontinence
1.3.2.1.5	Total Incontinence
1.3.2.2	Urinary Retention
1.4.1.1	Altered (Specify Type) Tissue Perfusion (renal, cerebral, cardiopulmonary, gastrointestinal, peripheral)
# 1.4.1.2.1	Fluid Volume Excess
# 1.4.1.2.2.1	Fluid Volume Deficit
1.4.1.2.2.2	Risk for Fluid Volume Deficit
# 1.4.2.1	Decreased Cardiac Output
1.5.1.1	Impaired Gas Exchange
1.5.1.2	Ineffective Airway Clearance
# 1.5.1.3	Ineffective Breathing Pattern
1.5.1.3.1	Inability to Sustain Spontaneous Ventilation
1.5.1.3.2	Dysfunctional Ventilatory

	Weaning Response (DVWR)
1.6.1	Risk for Injury
1.6.1.1	Risk for Suffocation
1.6.1.2	Risk for Poisoning
1.6.1.3	Risk for Trauma
1.6.1.4	Risk for Aspiration
1.6.1.5	Risk for Disuse Syndrome
1.6.2	Altered Protection
1.6.2.1	Impaired Tissue Integrity
1.6.2.1.1	Altered Oral Mucous Membrane
1.6.2.1.1.2	Risk for Impaired Skin Integrity
1.7.1	Decreased Adaptive Capacity: Intracranial
1.8	Energy Field Disturbance

PATTERN 2: COMMUNICATING

2.1.1.1	Impaired Verbal Communication

PATTERN 3: RELATING

3.1.1	Impaired Social Interaction
3.1.2	Social Isolation
3.1.3	Risk for Loneliness
3.2.1	Altered Role Performance
3.2.1.1.1	Altered Parenting
3.2.1.1.2	Risk for Altered Parenting
3.2.1.1.2.1	Risk for Altered Parent/Infant/Child Attachment
3.2.1.2.1	Sexual Dysfunction
3.2.2	Altered Family Process
3.2.2.1	Caregiver Role Strain
3.2.2.2	Risk for Caregiver Role Strain
3.2.2.3.1	Altered Family Process: Alcoholism
3.2.3.1	Parental Role Conflict
3.3	Altered Sexuality Patterns

PATTERN 4: VALUING

4.1.1	Spiritual Distress (Distress for the Human Spirit)
4.2	Potential for Enhanced Spiritual Well-Being

PATTERN 5: CHOOSING

# 5.1.1.1	Ineffective Individual Coping
5.1.1.1.1	Impaired Adjustment
5.1.1.1.2	Defensive Coping
5.1.1.1.3	Ineffective Denial
# 5.1.2.1.1	Ineffective Family Coping: Disabling
# 5.1.2.1.2	Ineffective Family Coping: Compromised
5.1.2.2	Family Coping: Potential for Growth
5.1.3.1	Potential for Enhanced Community Coping
5.1.3.2	Ineffective Community Coping
5.2.1	Ineffective Management of Therapeutic Regimen (Individuals)
5.2.1.1	Noncompliance (Specify)
5.2.2	Ineffective Management of Therapeutic Regimen: Families
5.2.3	Ineffective Management of Therapeutic Regimen: Community
5.2.4	Effective Management of Therapeutic Regimen: Individual
5.3.1.1	Decisional Conflict (Specify)
5.4	Health Seeking Behaviors (Specify)

PATTERN 6: MOVING

6.1.1.1	Impaired Physical Mobility
6.1.1.1.1	Risk for Peripheral Neurovascular Dysfunction
6.1.1.1.2	Risk for Perioperative Positioning Injury
6.1.1.2	Activity Intolerance
6.1.1.2.1	Fatigue
6.1.1.3	Risk for Activity Intolerance
6.2.1	Sleep Pattern Disturbance
6.3.1.1	Diversional Activity Deficit
6.4.1.1	Impaired Home Maintenance Management
6.4.2	Altered Health Maintenance
6.5.1	Feeding Self Care Deficit
6.5.1.1	Impaired Swallowing
6.5.1.2	Ineffective Breastfeeding
6.5.1.2.1	Interrupted Breastfeeding
6.5.1.3	Effective Breastfeeding
6.5.1.4	Ineffective Infant Feeding Pattern
6.5.2	Bathing/Hygiene Self Care Deficit
6.5.3	Dressing/Grooming Self Care Deficit
6.5.4	Toileting Self Care Deficit
6.6	Altered Growth and Development
6.7	Relocation Stress Syndrome
6.8.1	Risk for Disorganized Infant Behavior
6.8.2	Disorganized Infant Behavior
6.8.3	Potential for Enhanced Organized Infant Behavior

PATTERN 7: PERCEIVING

7.1.1	Body Image Disturbance
# 7.1.2	Self Esteem Disturbance
# 7.1.2.1	Chronic Low Self Esteem
# 7.1.2.2	Situational Low Self Esteem
7.1.3	Personal Identity Disturbance
7.2	Sensory/Perceptual Alterations (Specify) (Visual, Auditory, Kinesthetic, Gustatory, Tactile, Olfactory)
7.2.1.1	Unilateral Neglect
7.3.1	Hopelessness
7.3.2	Powerlessness

PATTERN 8: KNOWING

# 8.1.1	Knowledge Deficit (Specify)
8.2.1	Impaired Environmental Interpretation Syndrome
8.2.2	Acute Confusion
8.2.3	Chronic Confusion
# 8.3	Altered Thought Processes
8.3.1	Impaired Memory

PATTERN 9: FEELING

# 9.1.1	Pain
# 9.1.1.1	Chronic Pain
# 9.2.1.1	Dysfunctional Grieving
# 9.2.1.2	Anticipatory Grieving
# 9.2.2	Risk for Violence: Self-Directed or Directed at Others
9.2.2.1	Risk for Self-Mutilation
9.2.3	Post-Trauma Response
9.2.3.1	Rape-Trauma Syndrome
9.2.3.1.1	Rape-Trauma Syndrome: Compound Reaction
9.2.3.1.2	Rape-Trauma Syndrome: Silent Reaction
9.3.1	Anxiety
9.3.2	Fear

Diagnoses revised by small work groups at the 1994 Biennial Conference on the Classification of Nursing Diagnoses; changes approved and added in 1996.

Participants

13th NANDA Conference

Ackley, Betty...Jackson, MI
Adams, Priscilla..Lincoln, NE
Agretelis, Joan..Somerville, MA
Alfaro-LeFevre, Rosalinda ....Stuart, FL,
Alorda, Carmen..Baleares, Spain
Ander, Janice ....Hanover Park, IL
Antall, Gloria...Shaker Heights, OH
Arito, Yuri, Kanagawa ....Japan
Arnold, Jean...Towaco, NJ
Avant, Kay...Waco, TX
Baena De Maers Lopes,
    Maria Helena...Campinas, SP, Brazil
Baker, Laurie ....New York, NY
Bartlett, Beverly...Erie, PA
Becker, Ann..St Louis, MO
Berry, Pam...Clinton, IA
Beyea, Suzanne ....Tilton, NH
Biermann, Joan...Lakewood, NJ
Blanner, Janet...St Louis, MO
Bleich, Michael ....Lincoln, NE
Boisvert, Cecile...St Aubin, France
Borkowski, Eleanor.......................................San Benardino, CA
Boykin, Priscilla..Bethesda, MD
Braden, Joseph ....Philadelphia, PA
Briody, Margaret ....Rochester, NY
Brottmiller, William.......................................Albany, NY
Bulechek, Gloria ....Iowa City, IA
Bulette Coakley, Amanda ....Somerville, MA
Callista, Roy...Chestnut Hill, MA
Cameron, Karen..Portland, OR
Carlson Catalano, Judy ....Radford, VA
Carpenito, Lynda J. ....Clarksboro, NJ
Carroll-Johnson, Rose Mary ....Valencia, CA
Casteel, Britt..Tokyo, Japan
Cavendish, Roberta ....Brooklyn, NY
Chase, Susan..Chestnut Hill, MA
Chianca, Tania ....Belo Horizonte City, MG, Brazil
Cibele, Pimenta..Sao Paulo, SP, Brazil
Clark, June..Reading, United Kingdom
Clarke, Mary ....Davenport, IA
Clifton, Margaret..Exeter, RI
Clingerman, Evelyn ....Rochester, MI
Coakley, Edward...Boston, MA
Coenen, Chel..Nymegen, Netherlands
Cole-Schonlau, Victoria ......Rancho Palos Verdes, CA
Collins, Jim..Burlington, NJ

Collopy, Katherine ....Durham, NC
Conley, Virginia ....Palm Harbor, FL
Coomes, Jill.......................................Parsons, KS
Costa, Mildred Patricia...............Sao Paulo, SP, Brazil
Cox, Ruth ....Clinton, IA
Cox, Helen ....Lubbock, TX
Cox, Karen ....Beek, Netherlands
Craft-Rosenburg, Martha..........................Iowa City, IA
Creason, Nancy...........................Johnson City, TN
Cullen, Barbara ....St Louis, MO
D'Meza Leuner, Jean ....Charleston, SC
Daniels, Jessie............................Minneapolis, MN
Davis, Darlene ....Clearwater, FL
Davis, Gail.......................................Denton, TX
DeMaio, Dorothy................................Far Hills, NJ
DeWys, Mary.............................Grand Rapids, MI
Delaney, Connie................................Iowa City, IA
Deleeuw, Linda............................Grand Rapids, MI
Denehy, Janice................................Iowa City, IA
Dillon, Ann.....................................New Lenox, IL
Doenges, Marilynn....................Colorado Springs, CO
Dougherty, Cynthia.................................Seattle, WA
Dungan, Joyce.................................Evansville, IN
Egawa, Takako ...."Suita-City, Osaka", Japan
Ehnfors, Margareta...............................Orebro, Sweden
Ehrenberg, Anna.................................Falum, Sweden
Emick-Herring, Brenda ....Mechanicsville, IA
Emoto, Aiko.............................Mabara, Chiba, Japan
Esperti, Cathy ....Albany, NY
Fairchild, Nancy....................................Watertown, MA
Feit, Teri..Lincoln, NE
Fendrich, LuAnne..................................Peoria, IL
Ferrer de Sant Jordi, Pilar...............Baleares, Spain
Fitzpatrick, Sandra ....Winchester, VA
Flanagan, Jane ....Brookline, MA
Flint, Joan ....Warwick, RI
Ford, Susan ....Belvidere, IL
Foster, Frances.................................Weston, MA
Fox Jakob, Dorothea..............Toronto, ON, Canada
Frisch, Noreen.....................................Arcata, CA

Fujii, Naoko ....Tokyo, Japan
Fujimura, Ryuko..........................Karagawa, Japan
Fujisaki, Kaoru.............................Kobe, Hyogo, Japan
Gardner, Donna...............................Chesapeake, VA
Garriga, Xavier...........................Barcelona, Spain
Gebbie, Kristine..............................New York, NY
Gec, Tatjana....................2000 Maribor, Slovenia
Geissler, Alice ....Colorado Springs, CO
Gimenez, Ana...............................Ann Arbor, MI
Goas Diaz, Luisa..Spain
Gordon, Marjory..................................Brighton, MA
Grafft, Cyd....................................Cedar Falls, IA
Green, Pauline ....Edmonston, MD
Greiner, Joe......................................Coralville, IA
Griebenow, Linda ....Rochester, MN
Griffith Whitley, Georgia ....Plainfield, IL
Hanson, Diane ....Grand Rapids, MI
Harkreader, Helen ....Austin, TX
Harold, Stefan....................................Vienna, Austria
Harris, Marcelline.............................Wortham, MN
Harvey, Rose....................................Lexington, MA
Head, Barbara ....Iowa City, IA
Herdman, T. Heather ....Stevens Point, WI
Herpers, Theo.....................The Hague, Netherlands
Hesselink, Klein........................Nymegen, Netherlands
Hibben, Lynn.....................................Duluth, GA
Hidalgo, Gayle..................................Clinton, IA
Hiltunen, Elizabeth ....Ipswich, MA
Hinz, Mittie..Modesto, CA
Holleman, Gerda....................Blaricum, Netherlands
Hoops, Lynn.................................Philadelphia, PA
Hoskins, Lois ....Ashton, MD
Jennewein, Cel ....Minneapolis, MN
Johnson, Genie...........................Winchester, VA
Johnson, JoAnne..........................Cincinnati, OH
Johnson, Marion..............................Iowa City, IA
Jones, Dorothy...........................Chestnut Hill, MA
Judge, M. Kay.....................................Seattle, WA
Kataoka, Toshiyuki.............................Tokyo, Japan
Keihsler, Renate...............................Vienna, Austria

Kelley, Jane.....................................Cape Girardeau, MO
Keneally, Susan.................................Philadelphia, PA
Kennedy, Donna.......................................Peoria, IL
Kerr, Mary............................Cranberry Township, PA
Killen, Aileen ....Hanover, NH
Kimura, Tadashi.....................................Tokyo, Japan
Kume, Yasuko....................."Suita-City, Osaka", Japan
Kurkowski, Tina..Plover, WI
L'Ecuyer, Kris ....St Louis, MO
Ladwig, Gail..Jackson, MI
Lambert, Cecile ....Outremont, ON, Canada
Lavin, Mary Ann.....................................St Louis, MO
LeMone, Priscilla ....Columbia, MO
Lesh, Kathy ....Baltimore, MD
Levin, Rona.......................................Westberry, NY
Levine, Lois......................................Little Ferry, NJ
Lindeman, Marlene..................................Omaha, NE
Lippens, Beth ....Clinton, IA
Lubro, Mary Ann ....Minford, OH
Lukkarila, Mary Helen.........................Apple Valley, CA
Lunney, Margaret ....Staten Island, NY
Lutz, Carroll..Jackson, MI
Lyte, Victor ....Manchester, England
Maas, Meridean....................................Iowa City, IA
Madden, Gay ....Mission, KS
Martijn, LFJ....................Vlaardingen, Netherlands
Martins, Ivete ....Sao Paulo, SP, Brazil
Martone, Robert ....Philadelphia, PA
Mason, Joe...Philadelphia, PA
Matsuki, Mitsuko.................................Fukui, Japan
Matz, Carol...Boyertown, PA
McAllister, Connie......................................Liberty, MO
McCash, Kay ....Tijeras, NM
McCloskey, Joanne ....Iowa City, IA
McComb, Peggy........................Vancouver, WA
McCourt, Ann..............................Ormond Beach, FL
McFarlane, Elizabeth.....................Fairfax Station, VA
McLane, Audrey ....Hendersonville, NC
Meriwether, Lanie ....Philadelphia, PA
Meyer, Gerrie...St Louis, MO

Michel, Jeanne Liliang Marlene........Sao Paulo, SP, Brazil
Michel-Gaines, Olivia...............................Glendale, CA
Mills, Winnifred ....Vancouver, BC, Canada
Mittelstredt, M.E.....................................Rochester, MI
Miyamoto, Chizuko ....Kanagawa, Japan
Monteiro Da Cruz, Dina..............Sao Paulo, SP, Brazil
Moorhead, Sue......................................Iowa City, IA
Moorhouse, Mary ....Colorado Springs, CO
Moritz, Derry Ann.....................................Placitas, NM
Moudry, Sharon ....Minneapolis, MN
Munro, Barbara..................................Chestnut Hill, MA
Munten, Guus ....Venlo, Netherlands
Murphy, Catherine ....Chestnut Hill, MA
Murray, Ruth ....St Louis, MO
Nagamine, Atsushi..................................Tokyo, Japan
Nagueira Do Vale, Iane ....Campinas, SP, Brazil
Nakamura, Hideho....................................Tokyo, Japan
Neal, Margo ....Philadelphia, PA
Nemoto, Takiko...................................Tokyo, Japan
Nordorft, Jeanette....................................Cuba City, WI
O'Gara, Joanne..Clinton, IA
O'Neil, Jean...Watertown, MA
Oertel, Thomas......................................San Diego, CA
Ogasawara, Chie................."Suita-City, Osaka", Japan
Oliver, Catalina..Aloy, Spain
Osowski, Ron ....Madison, WI
Oud, N.E. ....Amsterdam, Netherlands
Paleotti-Fawcett, Margaret ....Nice, France
Palutke, Janet.....................................Winchester, VA
Parker, Laurence....................................Philadelphia, PA
Parris, Kathleen ....Santa Ana, CA
Pascal, Annie....................................Sint Etienne, France
Passos Guimaraes, Heloisa ....Sao Paulo, SP, Brazil
Pattison, Ivor..Groton, MA
Pehler, Shelley-Rae ....Davenport, IA
Perry, Amy ....Ann Arbor, MI
Perry, Anne..St Louis, MO
Powers, Kathlyn...........................San Benardino, CA
Pritchett-Gustafson, Nancy ....Mission, KS
Rahal, Lina ....Blainville, QC, Canada

Rantz, Marilyn ....Columbia, MO

Rausch, Michele...............................Norman, OK

Richardson, Stephanie....................Salt Lake City, UT

Ridgeway, Sharon...........................Minneapolis, MN

Rigol, Assumpta.............................Barcelona, Spain

Roberson, Nancy................................Albany, NY

Roche, Pam....................................Cape Giradeau, MO

Rours, Maria....................................Nynegen, Holland

Rowley, Frances ....Greenfield, WI

Saba, Vivianne...........................Montreal, QC, Canada

Saitoh, Akira ....Tokyo, Japan

Sakata, Naomi...............................Gifu City, Japan

Sato, Shigemi................................Nagano, Japan

Schmouth, Danielle..............Bellefeuille, QC, Canada

Schutte, Sheryl..................................Clinton, IA

Schwartz, Cathy ....Pleasant Plains, IL

Scroggins, Leann ....Rochester, MN

Seraphim, Glaucia......................Curitiba Arana, Brazil

Shaw, Michael...............................Springhouse, PA

Sheppard, Kathleen.......................Houston, TX

Simon, Jolene ....Warrenville, IL

Simon Coler, Marga.......................Paraiba, Brazil

Smith, Janet................................Philadelphia, PA

Smith, Louise................................Atlanta, GA

Smochek, Mary Rose...........Bryn Mawr, PA

Sparks, Sheila ....Sterling, VA

Sprengel, Ann.........................Cape Girardeau, MO

Strauman-Raymond, Karen............Coon Rapids, MN

Suchy, Susanne ....Southgate, MI

Swisher, Gena ....Winchester, VA

Takahasi, Shuichi ....Tokyo, Japan

Talley, Candace.........................Coal Valley, IL

Tanabe, Michiko..............................Fukui, Japan

Thoroddsen, Asta ....Reykjavik, Iceland

Tillman, Harry.............................Portsmouth, VA

Timm, Jane...................................Rochester, MN

Ugalde, Mercedes...........................Barcelona, Spain

Van Dyke Hayes, Kathryn ....Philadelphia, PA

Van Kuyh, Elle ....Nymeyen, Holland

Van der Heijden, J.L.....................Breda, Netherlands

Vassallo, Barbara ....Willingboro, NJ

Vilhena Abrao, Ana Cristina ....Sao Paulo, SP, Brazil

Wake, Madeline..............................Milwaukee, WI

Warren, Judy..................................Plattsmouth, NE

Watson, Donna ....Gig Harbor, WA

Weber, Janet...................................Jackson, MO

Weir-Hughes, Dickon.........................London, England

Wesorick, Bonnie.............................Grand Rapids, MI

Westbrook, Alex ....London, England

Wetsch, Peggy..................................Corona, CA

Wibbenmeyer, Paul........................Chicago, IL

Wilhelm, Tom................................St Louis, MO

Wilkinson, Judith............................Overland Park, KS

Willits, Marilyn.................................Davenport, IA

Wortham, Toni ....Madisonville, KY

Wyngarden, Kathy ....Grand Rapids, MI

Yamaguchi, Keiji ....Bryn Mawr, PA

Yocent, Christy.................................Cape Giradeau, MO

Yoshida, Seiji....................................Tokyo, Japan

Author Index

Subject Index